To Clarence Suellke,

With much gratitude for
giving that guy who walked into
your lab off the street wearing
overalls a chance. You took a
gamble. I hope this book shows
in a small way that it was a
good bet. Thanks for all that
you gave me... my balla and my career.

Warmly, your friend,

Comprehensive Cardiovascular Medicine in the Primary Care Setting

CONTEMPORARY CARDIOLOGY

CHRISTOPHER P. CANNON, MD
SERIES EDITOR

ANNEMARIE M. ARMANI, MD
EXECUTIVE EDITOR

For other titles published in this series, go to
http://www.springer.com/series/7677

COMPREHENSIVE CARDIOVASCULAR MEDICINE IN THE PRIMARY CARE SETTING

Edited by

PETER P. TOTH

*Preventive Cardiology, Sterling Rock Falls
Clinic, Sterling, IL, and
University of Illinois College of Medicine,
Peoria, IL USA*

CHRISTOPHER P. CANNON

*Harvard Medical School, Brigham and Women's
Hospital, Boston, MA, USA*

Foreword by Peter Libby

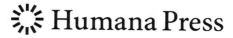 Humana Press

Editors
Peter P. Toth, MD, PhD
Preventive Cardiology
Sterling Rock Falls Clinic
101 East Miller Road
Sterling, IL 61081
Clinical Professor
University of Illinois College
    of Medicine
Peoria, Illinois
USA
peter.toth@srfc.com

Christopher P. Cannon, MD
Associate Professor
Harvard Medical School
Brigham & Women's Hospital
Cardiovascular Division
TIMI Trials
350 Longwood Avenue
Boston, MA 02115
USA
cpcannon@partners.org

ISBN 978-1-60327-962-8   e-ISBN 978-1-60327-963-5
DOI 10.1007/978-1-60327-963-5
Springer New York Dordrecht Heidelberg London

Library of Congress Control Number: 2010929621

Printed on acid-free paper

Humana Press is part of Springer Science+Business Media (www.springer.com)

Foreword

In *Comprehensive Cardiovascular Medicine in the Primary Care Setting*, Drs. Toth and Cannon provide a practical compendium to guide the primary practitioner through the rapidly evolving thicket of the management of patients with, or at risk for, cardiovascular disease. We practice in an environment of information overload: A relentless stream of print and electronic mail and ever-present Internet resources furnish us with a dizzying and sometimes distracting array of stimuli and overwhelming sources of medical information. Amid this cacophony, this focused volume provides a single well-organized source of authoritative information, in a highly accessible and practical form, to help practicing physicians in their care of cardiovascular patients.

The case-based approach provides a proven learning platform to help the practitioner link the complex maze of results of clinical studies and pathophysiologic discoveries with the kind of specific clinical situations they encounter on a regular basis. This pedagogical tool will certainly help physicians organize the content in their own minds and will aid their application of that information as they approach their patients in daily practice. The boxed "take-home messages" that populate this volume provide "bite-sized" summaries in a way that permits ready reference and promotes retention of information by the busy clinician. In addition to the liberal use of case studies that puts the learning into a clinical context, the practical key points at the beginnings of chapters provide an extremely useful framework for learning.

The comprehensive coverage of topics ranges from prevention through invasive management strategies. The section that features non-coronary vascular disease provides particular value and utility. This series of seven chapters will serve to bring clinicians up to date on this important aspect of cardiovascular practice, which has traditionally received less attention than coronary artery disease. The imaging section provides readily approachable summaries of some newer technologies, including cardiac computed tomographic angiography and magnetic resonance imaging. The section on risk factor management goes beyond the "usual suspects" by including chronic kidney disease and a particularly practical and useful chapter on obesity and therapeutic approaches to weight loss—which, in addition to the chapter on metabolic syndrome, reflects the changing face of cardiovascular risk in contemporary society.

While this book does not aim to provide a fundamental scientific background, Chapter 6 will no doubt prove useful for the busy clinician who strives to integrate the rapidly accumulating results of genomic studies into a broader context of cardiovascular care.

Drs. Toth and Cannon have assembled an authoritative team of experts from around the United States to provide a balanced and up-to-date compendium of the essential information that the interested internist or primary cardiologist on the front lines of clinical practice needs to bring his or her patients the fruits of the recent advances made in this fast-moving field. Their book fills an important gap in the universe of available learning tools and will no doubt elevate the practical platform from which practitioners can build the best cardiovascular care.

Peter Libby, MD

Preface

Cardiovascular disease is highly prevalent throughout the world. The American Heart Association estimates that in the year 2009, the direct and indirect costs of cardiovascular disease in the United States will approximate one-half trillion dollars. Despite a staggering series of discoveries and innovations over the last five decades, cardiovascular disease remains the leading cause of morbidity, disability, and mortality among men and women. The pace of progress in the field of cardiology is rapid and keeping up with medical, surgical, and diagnostic breakthroughs is quite challenging. Our ability to beneficially impact cardiovascular disease has grown exponentially. Clinical trials and novel insights from basic scientific and clinical investigation continually transform what, when, and how we have come to do things in cardiovascular medicine. The frequency with which national guidelines and recommendations of best practice are promulgated for a variety of cardiovascular disease states is accelerating and their complexity is growing. Unfortunately, adherence to national guidelines and levels of patient goal attainment nationwide tend to be relatively low. Many proven, highly efficacious therapies and interventions remain underutilized.

Primary care clinicians must play a larger role in the prevention, diagnosis, and management of cardiovascular diseases. A high clinical priority in contemporary medicine is the prevention of disease. It has now become routine to screen patients for such disorders as dyslipidemia, hypertension, metabolic syndrome, diabetes mellitus, heightened systemic inflammation, and albuminuria, all of which impact risk for atherosclerosis. Early identification of established disease is also critical so as to prevent progression and long-term adverse clinical sequelae, such as myocardial infarction, stroke, heart and renal failure, claudication and lower extremity amputation, and thromboembolic phenomena. In addition to laboratory measures of genetic and metabolic background, it is important to cultivate clinical skills and proficiency in using imaging modalities to characterize such anatomical abnormalities such as coronary artery and peripheral arterial disease, aortic aneurysms, and cardiac valvular disease. A critical feature of long-term care is ensuring that specific disease states remain optimally treated through lifestyle modification and pharmacologic intervention and that patients remain compliant with these therapies lifelong. Primary care clinicians play critical roles in all of these areas.

Comprehensive Cardiovascular Medicine in the Primary Care Setting was written for the busy, practicing clinician. There are numerous exceptional texts in cardiovascular medicine of encyclopedic scope, which are for the most part targeted toward specialist audiences. Given the high prevalence of cardiovascular diseases, we have developed a text in cardiovascular medicine that addresses the needs and gaps in knowledge of primary care clinicians. More and more cardiovascular diseases are being identified and managed by primary care clinicians in its subclinical, acute, and chronic stages. Our principal aim in this book is to provide comprehensive coverage of cardiovascular disease in an authoritative and easy to apply manner. Concept is intricately balanced with practical utility. The pathophysiology of specific cardiovascular diseases is explained. Algorithms, case studies, and recommendations on evidence-based best practice are presented in every chapter. There is appropriate emphasis on optimal approaches to pharmacologic management. Each chapter begins with a bulleted list of the 10–12 most important points for each disease state addressed. This volume is not intended to be encyclopedic; rather, it is designed to help the busy practitioner perform assessments, initiate and guide efficacious therapy, and know when referral to a cardiologist or cardiovascular surgeon is indicated. The book is divided into five main sections: cardiovascular disease risk factors, coronary artery disease, peripheral forms of venous and arterial disease, cardiac disease, and cardiac imaging. Improving the quality of patient care and expanding scope of practice are our ultimate goals. We sincerely hope this book also helps foster greater cooperation and synergy between primary care clinicians, cardiologists, and cardiovascular surgeons.

Peter P. Toth, MD, PhD
Christopher P. Cannon, MD

Contents

Contributors

RASHID M. AHMAD, MD, *Vanderbilt Heart and Vascular Institute, Nashville, TN, USA*

NIKOLAOS ALEXOPOULOS, MD, *Division of Cardiology, Department of Internal Medicine, Emory University Hospital, Atlanta, GA, USA*

ERIC R. BATES, MD, *Division of Cardiovascular Medicine, University of Michigan Medical Center, Ann Arbor, MI, USA*

JOHN G. BYRNE, MD, *Vanderbilt Heart and Vascular Institute, Nashville, TN, USA*

DAVID A. CARBALLO, *Department of Medicine, Cardiovascular Division, Brigham and Women's Hospital, Boston, MA, USA*

OTAVIO R. COELHO-FILHO, MD, *Department of Medicine, Cardiovascular Division, Brigham and Women's Hospital, Boston, MA, USA*

GEORGE D. DANGAS, MD, *Cardiovascular Innovation, Mount Sinai Medical Center, New York, USA*

PATRICK DONNELLY, MD, *Cardiac MR PET CT Program, Department of Radiology, Harvard Medical School, Massachusetts General Hospital, Boston, MA, USA*

DANIEL A. DUPREZ, MD, PhD, *Cardiovascular Division, University of Minnesota, Minneapolis, MN, USA*

KIM A. EAGLE, MD, *Division of Cardiovascular Medicine, Cardiovascular Center, University of Michigan Medical School, Ann Arbor, MI, USA*

BLAIR FOREMAN, MD, *Cardiovascular Medicine, Midwest Cardiovascular Research Foundation, Davenport, IA, USA*

ELI V. GELFAND, MD, *Division of Cardiovascular Medicine, Beth Israel Deaconess Medical Center, Boston, MA, USA*

JAY GIRI, MD, *Cardiovascular Division, University of Pennsylvania School of Medicine, Philadelphia, PA, USA*

IRFAN HAMEED, MD, *Division of Cardiovascular Medicine and Michigan Cardiovascular Research and Reporting Program, University of Michigan Medical School, Ann Arbor, MI, USA*

ERIC A. HELLER, MD, *Columbia University Medical Center, New York, USA*

UDO HOFFMANN, MD, *Cardiac MR PET CT Program, Department of Radiology, Harvard Medical School, Massachusetts General Hospital, Boston, MA, USA*

CALVIN HUANG, MD, *Department of Emergency Medicine, Brigham and Women's Hospital, Boston, MA, USA*

ERIC M. ISSELBACHER, MD, *Cardiac Unit Associates and Department of Medicine, Massachusetts General Hospital, Boston, MA, USA*

ANDREAS KASTRUP, MD, *Departments of Neurology, Klinikum Bremen-Ost and Klinikum Bremen-Mitte, Bremen, Germany*

ASLAM M. KHAJA, MD, *Department of Neurology and Rehabilitation, University of Illinois at Chicago, Chicago, IL, USA*

ROBERT A. KLONER, MD, *Department of Cardiovascular Medicine, Keck School of Medicine, Good Samaritan Hospital, University of Southern California, Los Angeles, CA, USA*

JOSHUA M. KOSOWSKY, MD, *Department of Emergency Medicine, Brigham and Women's Hospital, Boston, MA, USA*

WILLIAM E. KRAUS, MD, *Division of Cardiovascular Medicine, Department of Internal Medicine, Duke University Medical Center, Durham, NC, USA*

ROBERT F. KUSHNER, MD, *Department of Medicine, Northwestern University Feinberg School of Medicine, Chicago, IL, USA*

RAYMOND Y. KWONG, MD, *Cardiovascular Division, Department of Medicine, Brigham and Women's Hospital, Boston, MA, USA*

MICHAEL J. LANDZBERG, MD, *Department of Cardiology, Boston Adult Congenital Heart Service, Children's Hospital, Boston, MA; Division of Cardiology, Brigham and Women's Hospital, Boston, MA; Harvard Medical School, Boston, MA*

MARZIA LEACCHE, MD, *Vanderbilt Heart and Vascular Institute, Nashville, TN, USA*

STAMATIOS LERAKIS, MD, *Division of Cardiology, Department of Internal Medicine, Emory University Hospital, Atlanta, GA, USA*

LEONARD S. LILLY, MD, *Cardiovascular Division, Department of Medicine, Harvard Medical School, Brigham and Women's Hospital, Boston, MA, USA*

ALI MAHAJERIN, MD, *Division of Cardiovascular Medicine, Beth Israel Deaconess Medical Center, Boston, MA, USA*

KEVIN C. MAKI, PhD, *Provident Clinical Research & Consulting, Inc., Glen Ellyn, IL, USA*

SYLVIA C.W. MCKEAN, MD, FACP, *Department of Medicine, BWH/Faulkner Hospitalist Service, Harvard Medical School and Brigham and Women's Hospital, Boston, MA, USA*

DALTON S. MCLEAN, MD, *Division of Cardiology, Department of Internal Medicine, Emory University Hospital, Atlanta, GA, USA*

JUDITH L. MEADOWS, MD, *Cardiovascular Division, Department of Medicine, Brigham and Women's Hospital, Boston, MA, USA*

EMILE R. MOHLER III, MD, *Department of Vascular Medicine, University of Pennsylvania School of Medicine, Philadelphia, PA, USA*

MARY P. MULLEN, MD, PhD, *Department of Cardiology, Boston Adult Congenital Heart Service, Children's Hospital, Boston, MA; Harvard Medical School, Boston, MA*

KIRAN MUSUNURU, MD, PhD, *Division of Cardiology, Johns Hopkins University School of Medicine, Baltimore, MD, USA*

BRAHMAJEE K. NALLAMOTHU, MD, *Division of Cardiovascular Medicine, University of Michigan, Ann Arbor, MI, USA*

STEPHEN J. NICHOLLS, MD, *Department of Cardiovascular Medicine, Center for Cardiovascular Diagnostics and Prevention, Heart and Vascular Institute, Cleveland Clinic Foundation, Cleveland, OH, USA*

PATRICK T. O'GARA, MD, *Cardiovascular Division, Department of Medicine, Brigham and Women's Hospital, Boston, MA, USA*

MIGUEL PORTOCARRERO, MD, *Division of Nephrology, University of Maryland Medical System, Baltimore, MD, USA*

PAOLO RAGGI, MD, *Division of Cardiology, Department of Radiology, Emory University School of Medicine, Atlanta, GA, USA; Department of Nephrology, Ospedale San Paolo, Milan, Italy*

CHARLES REASNER, MD, *Division of Endocrinology, Department of Medicine, University of Texas Health Science Center and Texas Diabetes Institute, San Antonio, TX, USA*

THORSTEN REFFELMANN, MD, *Department of Internal Medicine, Ernst Moritz Arndt University of Greifswald, Greifswald, Germany*

MARTYN R. RUBIN, PhD, *Provident Clinical Research and Consulting, Inc., Glen Ellyn, IL, USA*

FIDENCIO SALDANA, MD, *Cardiovascular Division, Department of Medicine, Harvard Medical School, Brigham and Women's Hospital, Boston, MA, USA*

ADAM C. SCHAFFER, MD, *Harvard Medical School, Brigham and Women's Hospital, Boston, MA, USA*

NICHOLAS SHAMMAS, MD, MS, *Midwest Cardiovascular Research Foundation, Davenport, IA, USA*

NATALIYA V. SOLENKOVA, MD, *Vanderbilt Heart and Vascular Institute, Nashville, TN, USA*

GARRICK C. STEWART, MD, *Department of Cardiovascular Medicine, Brigham and Women's Hospital, Boston, MA, USA*

PETER P. TOTH, MD, PhD, *Preventive Cardiology, University of Illinois College of Medicine, Peoria, IL, USA*

RAMANAN UMAKANTHAN, MD, *Vanderbilt Heart & Vascular Institute, Nashville, TN, USA*

MATTHEW R. WEIR, MD, *Division of Nephrology, University of Maryland Medical System, Baltimore, MD, USA*

I

CARDIOVASCULAR DISEASE RISK FACTORS

1

Cardiovascular Epidemiology and Characterization of Atherosclerotic Disease Risk Factors

Kevin C. Maki and Martyn R. Rubin

CONTENTS

Key Words: Cardiovascular disease; Causation; Cohort; Incidence; Relative risk; Risk factor.

From: *Contemporary Cardiology: Comprehensive Cardiovascular Medicine in the Primary Care Setting*
Edited by: Peter P. Toth, Christopher P. Cannon, DOI 10.1007/978-1-60327-963-5_1
© Springer Science+Business Media, LLC 2010

KEY POINTS

- Over 80 million people in the United States exhibit one or more forms of cardiovascular disease (CVD), and atherosclerotic CVD (mainly coronary heart disease and stroke) is, by far, the leading cause of death among men and women. More women die from CVD in the United States each year than men.
- Atherosclerotic CVD has become a worldwide pandemic. While CVD mortality has declined over the last several decades in developed countries, incidence and prevalence of atherosclerotic CVD are increasing in the developing world.
- Potentially modifiable factors account for a large percentage of the variation between and within populations in CVD risk, with population attributable risk fractions estimated at 90% or higher worldwide.
- Traditional CVD risk factors include dyslipidemia, elevated blood pressure, cigarette smoking, and diabetes mellitus. Lifestyle factors are very important in the atherothrombotic disease process and therapeutic lifestyle changes—including a diet low in saturated fat, cholesterol, and trans fats; regular physical activity; attainment and maintenance of a healthy body weight; and smoking cessation—remain central to preventive efforts.
- Numerous novel and emerging risk factors are under study. Improved understanding of the roles of these factors in the atherothrombotic disease process may aid in risk stratification and/or in identifying and testing novel targets for therapy.
- Presently, the greatest utility of nontraditional risk factors such as inflammatory markers or measures of subclinical CVD is for identifying those individuals with at least moderate risk for a CVD event for whom aggressive therapy may be warranted.

1.1. THE BURDEN OF ATHEROSCLEROTIC CARDIOVASCULAR DISEASE IN THE UNITED STATES

Atherosclerotic cardiovascular disease (CVD) encompasses a range of conditions resulting from atherosclerotic plaques in arterial beds including those in the heart (coronary heart disease or CHD), legs (peripheral arterial disease), aorta, carotid, cerebral and renal arteries. In the United States, lifetime risk for CVD (atherosclerotic and nonatherosclerotic) is approximately two in three for men and more than one in two for women *(1)*. According to the United States National Center for Health Statistics, the probability of dying from major CVD is 47%, which is greater than twice that for cancer (22%), the next leading cause of death *(1)*. In 2004, among women ≥65 years of age, the three leading causes of death were (1) diseases of the heart (primarily CHD), (2) cancer, and (3) stroke *(1)*. In men ≥65 years of age the leading causes of death were (1) diseases of the heart (primarily CHD), (2) chronic lower respiratory diseases, (3) cancer, and (4) stroke *(1)*.

In 2005, it was estimated that more than 80,000,000 people in the United States exhibited one or more forms of CVD, including CHD, high blood pressure (a major risk factor for atherosclerosis), history of stroke, heart failure, or congenital CVD *(1)*. Although surveys show that a majority of women feel more vulnerable to breast cancer *(2)*, CVD is by far the leading cause of death among women, and women are roughly six to eight times more likely to die from CVD than from breast cancer *(1)*. In fact, more women than men die each year from CVD, and women have also overtaken men in prevalence of CVD, with 42.7 and 37.9 million cases reported in women and men, respectively *(3)*.

1.2. CARDIOVASCULAR EPIDEMIOLOGY AND THE INVESTIGATION OF RISK FACTORS

Epidemiology is the study of the distributions and determinants of diseases in human populations. By studying characteristics of individuals who do and do not develop the disease or condition under study, epidemiologists are able to generate hypotheses about possible causal relationships, some of which may subsequently undergo evaluation in clinical intervention trials. Before the middle of the twentieth century, epidemiological methods had been employed mainly in the study of infectious disease outbreaks or "epidemics." In the latter half of the twentieth century, epidemiological methods were extended to the study of chronic diseases such as atherosclerotic CVD. These studies provided the foundation for the concept of CVD risk factors and ultimately led to large, randomized trials to evaluate strategies for primary and secondary CVD prevention.

Early studies compared CVD mortality rates between countries. For example, in the 1950s, Ancel Keys and colleagues documented that annual mortality from CVD per population unit (e.g., per 100,000 persons) varied by as much as 10-fold between countries *(4, 5)*. Autopsy studies showed that among individuals who died from accidents or in wars, those from countries with high CVD mortality rates had more fatty streaks and atherosclerotic lesions in their coronary arteries *(6)*. Other investigations showed that various factors were associated with higher CVD mortality rates, such as higher average levels of blood cholesterol and blood pressure and greater prevalence of cigarette smoking *(7, 8)*.

Immigration studies showed that people who migrated from countries with low CVD mortality rates to countries with high CVD mortality rates and adopted the lifestyle patterns of their new home showed changes in levels of blood cholesterol and blood pressure. For example, the Japan–Honolulu–San Francisco Study showed that people who migrated from Japan (where CVD mortality was low) to the United States (where CVD mortality was high) showed increases in blood pressure and cholesterol levels *(9)*. Furthermore, the degree to which these changes occurred and the subsequent risk for a CVD event depended on the degree to which the immigrants had adopted dietary and other lifestyle habits similar to those common in the United States *(10)*.

1.3. THE FRAMINGHAM HEART STUDY

The Framingham Heart Study, initiated in 1948, was one of the earliest large-scale investigations in cardiovascular epidemiology, and its findings helped to provide the foundation for the idea that variation in CHD rates within a population could be predicted by several "risk factors." The investigators measured characteristics of a group of roughly 5,000 residents in the town of Framingham, MA, and followed them (and eventually their offspring) over decades to determine what characteristics were associated with CVD events later in life. The Framingham study showed that many factors were associated with increased CVD incidence and that these were often identifiable years or decades before clinical events, suggesting the potential for prevention through risk factor modification. The enormous success of the Framingham Heart Study paved the way for later studies in the United States, and throughout the world that have confirmed and expanded their findings. More information about the history of cardiovascular epidemiology may be found at www.epi.umn.edu/cvdepi, including brief descriptions of many of the major population and intervention studies undertaken during the 1940s through the 1970s in the United States and elsewhere.

1.4. ATHEROSCLEROTIC CVD IS A WORLDWIDE PANDEMIC

A pandemic is a condition that occurs throughout a wide geographic area and affects a high proportion of the population. Despite extraordinary advances in options for prevention and treatment, CVD remains the leading cause of death worldwide. In fact, while mortality due to CVD has declined in developed countries, the rate of CVD-related mortality in developing countries has accelerated, likely due to increased urbanization and rising rates of obesity and other lifestyle-related risk factors *(11)*. The rising rates of CVD incidence and mortality in the developing world partly reflect declines in competing causes of death that shorten life expectancy. However, results from studies within and across populations strongly support the view that atherosclerotic CVD is largely a disease that is attributable to potentially modifiable lifestyle factors that promote biological changes (e.g., dyslipidemia, hypertension, obesity), which are injurious to the arterial system.

Data from the Nurses' Health Study (84,129 women) show that among female nurses living in the United States, those who demonstrate a "low-risk" profile, as indicated by abstinence from smoking, maintenance of a desirable body weight, regular exercise, healthy dietary habits, and moderate alcohol consumption, have a CHD event risk more than 80% lower than the remainder of the cohort who do not fit this "low-risk" profile *(3)*. In cohorts from the Multiple Risk Factor Intervention Trial and a large population study in Chicago, together comprising more than 366,000 men and women, a low risk factor burden, defined as blood pressure ≤120/80 mmHg, total cholesterol <200 mg/dL, absence of smoking, diabetes mellitus, and major electrocardiographic abnormalities, was associated with a 73–85% lower CVD mortality *(12)*.

1.5. DEVELOPMENT AND EVOLUTION OF THE ATHEROTHROMBOTIC PROCESS

Population and laboratory studies have provided a framework for understanding the evolution of atherothrombotic disease. A detailed description of this process is beyond the scope of this chapter, but will be described briefly (Fig. 1). The earliest stage atherosclerosis is the fatty streak, which can

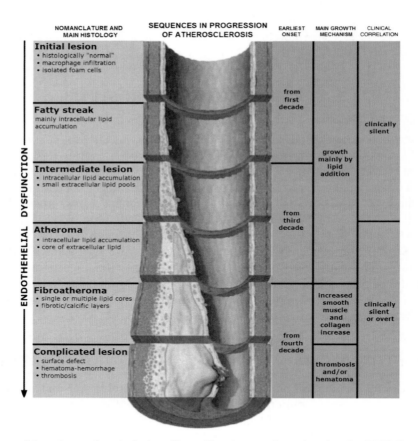

Fig. 1. Progression of the atherosclerotic lesion. Note: Fig. 1 was released under the GNU Free Documentation License. The GNU Free Documentation License is a copy license for free documentation, designed by the Free Software Foundation (FSF) for the GNU Project. It is similar to the GNU General Public License, giving readers the rights to copy, redistribute, and modify a work and requires all copies and derivatives to be available under the same license. The GFDL was designed for manuals, textbooks, other reference and instructional materials, and documentation that often accompanies GNU software.

often be found in the coronary arteries of children, particularly in countries with high CVD event rates. Fatty streak formation involves a process through which lipoproteins enter the arterial wall, undergo modification (e.g., oxidation), and are taken up by macrophages in an unregulated fashion, creating foam cells. Foam cells coalesce to form fatty streaks. The fatty streak can grow over time into a raised lesion with a connective tissue cap and a lipid-filled core. If sufficiently large, such lesions may impede blood flow and cause ischemia (e.g., exertional angina or claudication).

An acute clinical event (myocardial infarction or ischemic stroke) generally occurs when a plaque becomes unstable. Inflammatory processes are important in the development of plaque instability because inflammation can produce thinning of the connective tissue cap, enhancing the probability of fissure formation or frank rupture. Exposure of subendothelial connective tissue and other plaque components in a ruptured plaque activates platelets and can trigger the formation of an occlusive thrombus, disrupting blood flow to the affected organ. This process can be exacerbated by endothelial dysfunction because disruption of the normal endothelium increases vasoconstriction and platelet activation. Myocardial ischemia and infarction can trigger ventricular arrhythmia, which is often the proximal cause of sudden cardiac death.

Thus, the atherothrombotic process can be thought of as a "response to injury" and can be induced or accelerated by factors that enhance the entry of atherogenic lipoproteins into the arterial wall such as increased concentrations of cholesterol-containing atherogenic lipoproteins; factors that disrupt normal endothelial function such as elevated blood pressure, hyperglycemia, and toxins from cigarette smoking; factors that enhance inflammation such as cigarette smoking and increased adiposity; and factors that alter the balance between thrombosis and fibrinolysis such as blood viscosity and endothelial dysfunction. In addition, the susceptibility of the myocardium to electrical instability during an ischemic event can be influenced by factors such as sympathetic tone and myocardial fatty acid concentrations.

1.6. PREDICTION VERSUS CAUSATION

Early studies identified CVD risk factors that were strongly related to event risk, including dyslipidemia, hypertension, smoking, and diabetes mellitus. However, causation cannot be established solely on the basis of associations in observational studies. Noncausal associations can arise due to chance, bias, or confounding. A risk factor may also be associated with a disease because it reflects a process that is involved in the causal pathway, but is not itself causal. For example, an elevated level of C-reactive protein (CRP), a marker for peripheral inflammation, is associated with an increased risk for CVD events. However, a study of polymorphisms associated with increased CRP, but not with inflammation, showed that such polymorphisms were not themselves associated with increased ischemic CVD risk *(13)*. Thus, while CRP is a risk factor that is strongly associated with CVD events, it appears unlikely that the CRP molecule itself is involved in atherogenesis. Instead, an elevated level of CRP likely reflects inflammatory processes that are involved in atherosclerosis. Accordingly, there is a low probability that development of a pharmacological agent that blocks the biological actions of CRP will be effective for lowering CVD event risk *(14)*. In contrast, interventions that reduce inflammation in the vascular wall are promising targets for therapy.

The probability that a relationship between a risk factor and a disease is causal must be inferred from the totality of the evidence, including the strength and consistency of the relationship across studies and populations, dose–response, a biologically plausible mechanism to explain the association, appropriateness of the temporal relationship between the risk factor and the disease (i.e., the risk factor precedes the disease), and availability of confirmatory evidence from laboratory and clinical intervention studies. Epidemiological investigations have helped to establish the physiologic links between lifestyle patterns and biological changes (e.g., increases in blood pressure and circulating lipoproteins) pointing toward testable hypotheses regarding causal pathways and, therefore, targets for intervention.

Using hypercholesterolemia as an example, population studies showed a strong relationship between elevated blood cholesterol and CVD event and mortality rates. Dietary intervention studies showed that high intakes of saturated fats and cholesterol produced elevations in blood cholesterol. Animal studies indicated that raising the blood cholesterol level by feeding a diet high in saturated fat and cholesterol produced atherosclerosis. These observational and laboratory studies thus laid the foundation for clinical trials that have since demonstrated that lowering an elevated level of cholesterol carried by atherogenic lipoproteins reduces CVD event risk (15, 16).

Although atherosclerotic CVD can be thought of as a disease that results largely from behaviors that increase risk, it does not follow that efforts at prevention should be limited to lifestyle interventions. Some risk factors, once established, are resistant to modification through lifestyle changes. Moreover, some pharmacologic interventions to modify risk factors have been shown to be effective in the absence of substantial lifestyle changes and should not be denied to individuals who are unwilling to change their habits regarding diet, exercise, and/or smoking. On the other hand, clinicians often underestimate the importance of lifestyle in producing an adverse CVD risk factor profile and the potential for lifestyle changes to reduce the risk factor burden.

1.7. POPULATION ATTRIBUTABLE RISK FRACTION

The impact of a risk factor on the incidence of a disease in a population depends on two features: (1) the strength of the relationship between the risk factor and the disease (assuming a causal relationship) and (2) the prevalence of the risk factor. Thus, a causal factor that has a strong association with the disease outcome might, nevertheless, have only a minor influence on the population attributable risk fraction if it has a low prevalence. Conversely, a causal factor that produces a modest increase in risk can have a high population attributable risk fraction if it is very common. In the United States, the major established modifiable risk factors (dyslipidemia, hypertension, and smoking) have high population attributable risk fractions because they are both common and strongly related to CVD risk (17). The six major, established CVD risk factors are shown in Table 1.

The estimation of population attributable risk fraction is complicated by the fact that risk factors are often correlated with one another. For example, diabetes mellitus is a strong CVD risk factor, but it is also associated with other risk factors such as obesity; elevated triglycerides; depressed high-density lipoprotein cholesterol (HDL-C); small, dense low-density lipoprotein (LDL) particles; increased levels of inflammatory markers; and elevated blood pressure. Modification of some of the associated risk factors, particularly dyslipidemia and hypertension, is effective for reducing CVD event risk in patients with diabetes (18). In contrast, aggressive glycemic control, which reduces risks of microvascular complications, has not proven consistently effective for preventing CVD events, suggesting that the increased CVD event risk associated with diabetes is largely attributable to other risk factors and that hyperglycemia per se may play a smaller role than once believed (19).

CVD risk quantification methods recommended for clinical practice generally do not include factors such as obesity, physical inactivity, and poor diet, not because they lack predictive value, but because they are more distal in the causal pathway, exerting their influence mainly through changes in other risk factors that are used in the risk calculations. Nevertheless, these risk factors remain important targets for therapy (20) (Fig. 2).

Despite continued uncertainty and controversy about the relative importance of specific risk markers, it is clear that potentially modifiable factors account for a large percentage of the variation between and within populations in CVD risk. For example, results from INTERHEART (7), a study of risk factors for acute myocardial infarction across 52 countries, suggest that more than 90% of the population attributable risk for CHD in men and women can be explained by potentially modifiable risk factors. These results, together with those from many other investigations, strongly support the view that substantial potential exists for preventive efforts, both on a population basis and in clinical settings,

Table 1

Major Atherosclerotic Cardiovascular Disease Risk Factors—Excluding Atherogenic Lipoproteins[a]

Cigarette smoking
Hypertension
Systolic blood pressure ≥140 mmHg or diastolic blood pressure
 ≥90 mmHg or use of antihypertensive medication
Family history of premature CHD
CHD in a male first-degree relative[b] <55 years of age
CHD in a female first degree relative[b] <65 years of age
Age
≥45 years of age for men
≥55 years of age for women
High-density lipoprotein cholesterol <40 mg/dL
If ≥60 mg/dL, this counts as a "negative" risk factor, subtracting 1 from
 the total

[a]Atherogenic lipoprotein cholesterol levels (low-density lipoprotein and non-high-density lipoprotein cholesterol) are not included among the risk factors because the purpose of the National Cholesterol Education Program classification system is to determine the treatment goals for these variables. Diabetes is a coronary heart disease risk equivalent, so is not counted as a major risk factor in the ATP III classification system.

[b]First-degree relatives include parents, siblings, and children.

Adapted from the National Cholesterol Education Program Adult Treatment Panel III (NCEP ATP III) Classification System *(17)*.

although it should be emphasized that, at present, clinical outcomes data from randomized clinical trials are only available for a limited number of preventive strategies, most notably treatment of dyslipidemia, treatment of hypertension, and the use of aspirin.

Some of the interventions recommended in current guidelines, such as smoking cessation or those for physical activity, are unlikely to ever be tested in large-scale CVD event trials due to practical or ethical considerations. In such cases, observational studies and studies on the effects of the intervention on accepted risk factors (e.g., lipoprotein lipids, blood pressure) will remain the best guide to clinical practice. The science of CVD prevention is evolving rapidly, and the reader is referred to the frequently updated list of Scientific Statements and Practice Guidelines from the American Heart Association (AHA) for current recommendations, www.americanheart.org/presenter.jhtml?identifier=9181.

The remainder of this chapter will provide an overview of traditional and emerging risk factors for atherosclerotic CVD and explore some areas where controversies persist. The reader should also note that there is some variation with regard to the relationships between individual risk factors and the different manifestations of atherosclerotic CVD. For instance, hypertension is a stronger risk factor for stroke than for CHD, while cigarette smoking and diabetes are particularly strong correlates of peripheral arterial disease. The focus herein will be on risk factors for atherosclerotic CVD in general, and we will not attempt to differentiate the importance of individual risk factors for predicting specific clinical outcomes.

1.8. DYSLIPIDEMIA

Because atherosclerotic plaques contain a lipid core, hypercholesterolemia was investigated early on as a possible CVD precursor. High levels of cholesterol were found to be associated with increased risk, although later studies showed that this relationship was more complicated than was appreciated

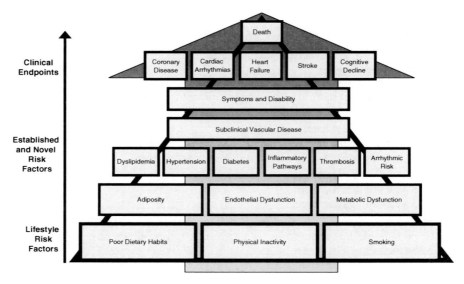

Fig. 2. The relations of lifestyle, established and novel risk factors, and cardiovascular disease. Assessment and treatment of dyslipidemia, hypertension, and diabetes are major foci of clinical care, practice guidelines, performance measures, and scientific research. These established cardiovascular risk factors are strongly influenced by lifestyle, including dietary behaviors, physical inactivity, smoking, and adiposity. Adiposity itself is largely a result of poor diet (excess calories) and inactivity. Lifestyle risk factors also influence disease risk via effects on other novel risk factors such as endothelial function, inflammation/oxidative stress, thrombosis/coagulation, arrhythmia, and other pathways. These basic lifestyle habits—poor diet, physical inactivity, and smoking—are thus the most proximal risk factors for cardiovascular disease *(20)*.

at first. Higher levels of cholesterol carried by HDL particles seemed to be protective. Furthermore, the circulating triglyceride was also found to correlate directly with risk, particularly in women.

Cholesterol and triglycerides are not water soluble, thus they are carried in the blood in lipoprotein particles. The three main classes of circulating lipoproteins in the fasting state are

- very low-density lipoproteins (VLDL),
- low-density lipoproteins (LDL), and
- high-density lipoproteins (HDL).

The triglyceride concentration in plasma correlates very strongly with the VLDL cholesterol concentration, which is the basis for the Friedewald equation that is used for calculation of LDL cholesterol (LDL cholesterol = total cholesterol – HDL cholesterol – triglycerides/5).

1.8.1. Measures of Atherogenic Lipoprotein Burden

Although treatment guidelines have traditionally focused on an elevated level of LDL cholesterol as the primary target for therapy, results from recent population and clinical intervention studies have shown that other markers, including apolipoprotein B, non-HDL cholesterol, and LDL particle number, are each better predictors of event risk than LDL cholesterol *(21, 22)*. The apolipoprotein B concentration reflects the total number of circulating atherogenic particles because each VLDL and LDL particle contains one molecule of apolipoprotein B. Unless the individual has very high triglycerides, nearly all of the apolipoprotein B is carried by VLDL and LDL particles in the fasting state, and <1% is carried by chylomicron remnants that contain a truncated 48 amino acid form of apolipoprotein B rather than the 100 amino acid form of hepatic origin.

Non-HDL cholesterol is calculated as the difference between the total and HDL cholesterol concentrations and represents the cholesterol carried by all atherogenic lipoprotein particles (mainly VLDL and LDL). Apolipoprotein B and non-HDL cholesterol levels are highly correlated. While apolipoprotein B may be a slightly better predictor of CVD events than non-HDL cholesterol, it appears unlikely that the modest increase in predictive ability will justify the incremental expense and complexity of running an additional test. Non-HDL cholesterol can be easily calculated from the standard laboratory lipoprotein profile, and fasting is not required to obtain an accurate non-HDL cholesterol concentration. Until recently, it was not widely recognized that each 1 mg/dL increment in VLDL cholesterol is associated with roughly the same increase in CHD event risk as a 1 mg/dL increment in LDL cholesterol, whether or not triglycerides are elevated, accounting for the superior predictive value of non-HDL cholesterol over LDL cholesterol (23) (Fig. 3).

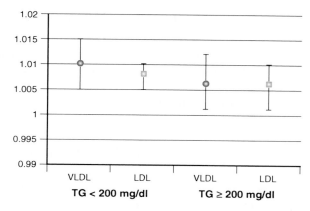

Fig. 3. Risk of coronary heart disease incidence for very low-density lipoprotein (VLDL) and low-density lipoprotein (LDL) cholesterol, as continuous variables, by triglyceride (TG) levels, adjusted for age, gender, study, smoking status, systolic blood pressure, and prevalent diabetes (at baseline) (23).

Results from population studies suggest that each 1% increment in HDL cholesterol is associated with a 2–3% reduction in CHD risk. Data from clinical trials indicate that lowering an elevated non-HDL cholesterol level by 1% produces a reduction in CHD event risk of 1.0–1.5% over 5–6 years, or roughly half the reduction that might be expected based on population studies (24). While not conclusive, findings from observational studies, such as those of individuals with genetic mutations that result in lower LDL and non-HDL cholesterol throughout life, suggest that maintaining a low burden of atherogenic lipoproteins over an extended period may reduce risk to a greater extent than has been demonstrated to date in clinical trials (25).

1.8.2. Measures of Antiatherogenic Lipoproteins

Low HDL cholesterol is strongly linked with increased CVD risk. Each 1% decrement in HDL cholesterol is associated with a 2–3% increase in CHD risk (26). Moreover, as was the case for atherogenic lipoproteins (apolipoprotein B), the concentration of apolipoprotein AI, a measure of the number of HDL particles, is a stronger predictor of CHD risk than the HDL cholesterol concentration (27). HDL concentration also appears to play an important role in the difference between men and women in CVD risk. Before puberty, boys and girls have similar levels of HDL cholesterol, but the level drops in boys as testosterone level increases. The mean difference between men and women in HDL cholesterol concentration (~10 mg/dL lower in men) accounts for a large fraction of the difference between the sexes in CVD risk.

Evidence from clinical trials supports the view that increases in HDL cholesterol or apolipoprotein AI levels contribute to the reduction in risk associated with lipid-altering therapies *(28)*. However, since changes in HDL cholesterol in clinical intervention studies are nearly always associated with changes in other lipid and non-lipid risk factors (non-HDL cholesterol and triglycerides), the quantitative role of changes in HDL cholesterol or particle number in risk reduction has not been fully defined. In addition, HDL cholesterol can be raised through a variety of mechanisms and it is not certain that all would produce the same benefit with regard to CVD event risk. For this reason, HDL cholesterol is a secondary target of therapy and current guidelines do not assign specific treatment goals for the HDL cholesterol level.

1.8.3. Ratios of Atherogenic to Antiatherogenic Lipoproteins

Because atherogenic and antiatherogenic lipoproteins are both strong predictors of CVD risk, it is not surprising that their ratios, such as total/HDL cholesterol and apolipoprotein B/apolipoprotein AI, are better predictors than their components. The main objection to the use of such a ratio in clinical practice is that it is not certain that changes in the numerator and denominator that produce equivalent changes in the ratio will produce equivalent changes in CVD risk.

1.8.4. Triglycerides and LDL Particle Size

An elevated level of triglycerides is associated with increased CVD risk, particularly in women. However, an increased triglyceride concentration is also associated with higher concentrations of triglyceride-rich lipoproteins (VLDL and chylomicron remnants), lower levels of HDL cholesterol, and increased levels of small, dense LDL particles. Much of the risk associated with elevated triglycerides is likely secondary to increased levels of atherogenic particles (particularly VLDL) and reduced levels of antiatherogenic particles (HDL). It remains a matter of controversy as to whether lowering triglycerides will have any benefits beyond those derived from changing the levels of atherogenic (chylomicron remnants, VLDL, LDL) and antiatherogenic (HDL) particle numbers.

One argument in favor of a potential benefit from lowering triglyceride level beyond that reflected by changes in non-HDL cholesterol level is that the triglyceride level is an important determinant of LDL particle size. Individuals seem to have a threshold for triglyceride level below which they will exhibit a predominance of large, buoyant LDL particles (pattern A) and above which they will exhibit a predominance of small, dense particles (pattern B) *(29)*. This threshold varies between individuals, but falls in the range of 100–250 mg/dL for most of the population. Thus, lowering the triglyceride level from 600 to 250 mg/dL will have no effect on LDL size for most people because the threshold for conversion from pattern B to pattern A will not be breached. However, lowering the triglyceride concentration from 250 to 100 mg/dL will cause most individuals to convert to pattern A.

Small, dense LDL particles may be more atherogenic than larger LDL and VLDL particles for a variety of reasons, including greater ease of entry into the subendothelial space, enhanced interaction with subendothelial proteoglycans, and greater susceptibility to oxidation *(30)*. According to this model, a gradient of atherogenicity exists with large VLDL at one end, followed by small VLDL particles, then large LDL particles, and finally small LDL particles at the most atherogenic end of the spectrum. At present the existence and/or steepness of this gradient remains uncertain, so the emphasis remains on achievement of LDL and non-HDL cholesterol goals, with triglyceride and HDL cholesterol concentrations included in the guidelines as secondary targets of therapy. However, a recent analysis from the Pravastatin or Atorvastatin Evaluation and Infection Therapy–Thrombolysis in Myocardial Infarction (PROVE IT–TIMI) 22 Trial showed that an on-treatment triglyceride level <150 mg/dL was independently associated with a lower risk of a recurrent CHD event in a group of subjects with a history of an acute coronary syndrome *(31)*. This relationship remained significant after adjustment for LDL-C and non-HDL-C, supporting the notion that triglycerides per se may be an important target for intervention. One theory advanced as a possible explanation is that elevated triglycerides are associated with changes in HDL and LDL particles that may alter their atherogenicity, rendering HDL particles less protective (less effective at promoting reverse cholesterol transport) and LDL particles more atherogenic (as discussed above).

1.8.5. Lipoprotein (a)

Lipoprotein (a) is a subspecies of LDL particles that contain a protein [apoprotein (a)] that varies in length depending on the number of repeating segments (kringles) that are expressed. Apoprotein (a) is similar in structure to plasminogen and, as a result, increased levels of lipoprotein (a) in circulation may interfere with the function of plasminogen by competing for its binding site *(32)*.

Many studies have suggested that an elevated level of lipoprotein (a) is a risk factor for CVD, with values >30 mg/dL (75 nmol/L) considered to be of concern. Current US guidelines do not recommend screening routinely for lipoprotein (a), but such screening may be reasonable in cases where an individual has a strong family history of CVD, particularly if this history is not clearly associated with traditional risk factors. Lipoprotein (a) is highly heritable and identification of a value >30 mg/dL in a patient with a strong family history of CVD may warrant more aggressive management of other risk factors, especially reducing levels of atherogenic lipoproteins.

1.9. HYPERTENSION

The Seventh Joint National Committee on Prevention, Evaluation and Treatment of High Blood Pressure defines hypertension as a systolic blood pressure ≥140 mmHg or a diastolic blood pressure ≥90 mmHg or current use of antihypertensive medication. Persons with blood pressures <120 (systolic) and <80 (diastolic) mmHg are considered normal, whereas those with blood pressures between these categories are considered to have "prehypertension" *(33)*.

Intervention trials have shown that lowering blood pressure reduces risk for CHD and stroke. Beginning at a blood pressure of 115/75 mmHg, the risk for CVD doubles with each increment of 20 mmHg for systolic blood pressure and 10 mmHg for diastolic blood pressure. Treating hypertension to a goal of <140/90 mmHg (or <130/80 mmHg for those with diabetes or renal disease) has been shown to reduce CVD morbidity and mortality. Each 5 mmHg reduction in systolic blood pressure is associated with reductions of 14% for mortality from stroke and 9% for mortality from CHD *(34)*.

Evidence of end-organ damage such as left ventricular hypertrophy, glomerular filtration rate <60 mL/min, or microalbuminuria are associated with greater CVD morbidity and mortality at any level of blood pressure (Fig. 4). Left ventricular hypertrophy has been shown to regress with aggressive blood pressure management and lifestyle interventions such as sodium restriction, weight loss, and increased physical activity enhance regression. Although not conclusive, the balance of the available data support the view that greater left ventricular hypertrophy regression is associated with improved outcomes *(35)*.

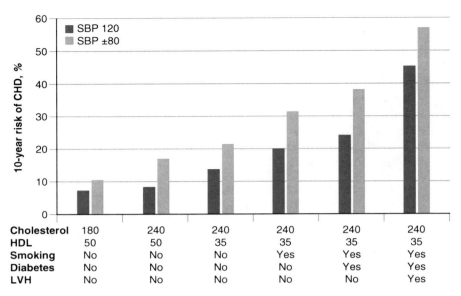

Fig. 4. Ten-year risk for coronary heart disease by systolic blood pressure and presence of other risk factors *(33)*. Abbreviations: CHD = coronary heart disease, HDL = high-density lipoprotein cholesterol, LVH = left ventricular hypertrophy, SBP = systolic blood pressure.

1.10. SMOKING

Cigarette smoking is the last of the "big three" major modifiable CVD risk factors: dyslipidemia, hypertension, and cigarette smoking. Cigarette smoking (and to a lesser extent pipe and cigar smoking) has a number of adverse effects on the vascular system that promote the atherothrombotic process. Toxins from cigarette smoke damage the endothelium and enhance platelet aggregation, making thrombosis more likely. Smoking also induces insulin resistance, raises the triglyceride concentration, and lowers the HDL cholesterol level *(2)*.

Many investigations show a dose-dependent increase in risk associated with cigarette smoking, and being a current smoker of 20 cigarettes per day increases CVD event risk by two- to threefold relative to a never smoker. Although randomized trials of smoking cessation and CVD events are not feasible for ethical reasons, prospective investigations have shown lower CVD morbidity and mortality for former smokers compared with continuing smokers. A reduction in risk is evident within months after smoking cessation, and increasing intervals since quitting are associated with progressively lower CVD morbidity and mortality. Benefits from quitting are observed in former smokers even after many years of heavy smoking.

1.11. OVERWEIGHT, OBESITY, AND BODY FAT DISTRIBUTION

Overweight and obesity are very common in the United States and other developed countries. Data from the National Health and Examination Survey indicate that in 2003–2004 the prevalence of overweight (body mass index 25.0–29.9 kg/m^2) or obesity (body mass index $\geq$30.0 kg/m^2) in the United States was 66.3% among adults 20 years of age or older. Within this group, 29.3% were overweight and 37.0% obese.

Increased adiposity is associated with greater morbidity and mortality from CVD and also increases the probability of developing other risk factors such as dyslipidemia, hypertension, and diabetes. This is particularly true when increased adiposity is centrally distributed. Expanded visceral adipose depots (in the abdominal cavity—mainly omental and mesenteric) are particularly metabolically harmful because these have increased fatty acid turnover and contribute disproportionately to the fatty acids released into the circulation *(36)*. Expanded visceral adipose depots increase the release of free fatty acids that drain into the portal circulation. Thus, the impact of increased adiposity on the metabolic profile is partly dependent on the location of the expanded fat cells. Visceral adiposity is most metabolically harmful, upper body subcutaneous adiposity has an intermediate influence, and lower body subcutaneous fat has only a modest metabolic effect. Waist circumference is an indicator of both total and abdominal adiposities with >90% of the variance in waist girth explained by differences in total fat mass and visceral adipose tissue area *(37)*, whereas waist/hip ratio is an indication of the propensity of an individual to store body fat centrally.

Increased hepatic free fatty acid flux stimulates synthesis and secretion of triglyceride-rich VLDL particles. A rise in circulating VLDL triglyceride enhances exchange of triglyceride for cholesterol between VLDL and HDL particles, contributing to a decline in HDL cholesterol. Furthermore, since VLDL is the precursor to LDL, an increase in VLDL secretion can also lead to elevation in the LDL cholesterol concentration. When the circulating free fatty acid level is chronically elevated, resistance develops to the ability of insulin to stimulate glucose uptake in skeletal muscle, leading to the need for compensatory hyperinsulinemia to maintain normal glucose tolerance *(36)*. Hyperinsulinemia enhances renal sodium reabsorption and sympathetic activation, increasing fluid volume, heart rate, and cardiac output, thereby increasing risk for hypertension. Over time, chronic insulin resistance can lead to pancreatic beta-cell dysfunction and, consequently, glucose intolerance and diabetes mellitus.

Obesity has both environmental and genetic determinants. An individual with two obese parents has greater than an 80% probability of being obese in young adulthood. However, even among those with a genetic predisposition, obesity may not become manifest in the absence of an obesity-promoting lifestyle. For example, Pima Indians living in Arizona in the Gila River basin have a famously high prevalence of obesity, with more than 85% of male Pimas classified as obese by age 35 years *(38)*. However, Pima Indians living in mountainous areas in Mexico who live a traditional lifestyle characterized by high levels of physical activity and little consumption of processed foods have very little obesity *(38)*.

1.12. METABOLIC SYNDROME AND DIABETES MELLITUS

Type 2 diabetes mellitus and atherosclerotic CVD share a number of common risk factors. Several of these cluster together more often than would be predicted by chance, suggesting that they are metabolically linked. Over the years this group of interrelated risk factors has been referred to variously as syndrome X, the deadly quartet, the insulin resistance syndrome, and the cardiometabolic risk syndrome. The National Cholesterol Education Program Adult Treatment Panel III coined the term metabolic syndrome and proposed a set of criteria for its diagnosis *(39)*. Table 2 shows an updated definition for the NCEP definition of the metabolic syndrome.

Risks for both diabetes mellitus and atherosclerotic CVD increase progressively as the number of metabolic syndrome components increase. The underlying link between these conditions is thought to be resistance to the ability of insulin to promote glucose uptake and suppress free fatty acid release from adipose tissue. While increased adiposity is the most common cause of insulin resistance, it can occur in the absence of obesity and such "metabolically obese" individuals may have the metabolic syndrome without increased body mass index or waist circumference. The primary aim of creating a diagnostic category for the metabolic syndrome was to assist in targeting this group for more aggressive preventive measures, including therapeutic lifestyle changes (weight loss and increased physical activity), as well as other therapies as needed to manage the individual risk factors. In the Diabetes Prevention Program, a lifestyle intervention aimed at reducing body weight by 7% and increasing physical

Table 2
Criteria for Clinical Diagnosis of Metabolic Syndrome *(39)*

Any three or more components	*Cutpoints*
Elevated waist circumference[a,b]	≥40 in. (102 cm) in men
	≥35 in. (88 cm) in women
Elevated triglycerides	≥150 mg/dL (1.7 mmol/L)
	or
	On drug treatment for elevated triglycerides[c]
Reduced HDL-C	<40 mg/dL (0.9 mmol/L) in men
	<50 mg/dL (1.1 mmol/L) in women
	or
	Drug treatment for reduced HDL-C[c]
Elevated blood pressure	≥130 mmHg systolic blood pressure
	or
	≥85 mmHg diastolic blood pressure
	or
	Antihypertensive drug treatment in a patient with a history of hypertension
Elevated fasting glucose	≥100 mg/dL (5.6 mmol/L)
	or
	Drug treatment for elevated glucose

[a]To measure waist circumference, locate top of right iliac crest. Place a measuring tape in a horizontal plane around the abdomen at the level of iliac crest. Before reading the tape measure, ensure that tape is snug but does not compress the skin and is parallel to the floor. Measurement is made at the end of a normal expiration.

[b]Some US adults of non-Asian origin (e.g., white, black, Hispanic) with marginally increased waist circumference, e.g., 94–102 cm (37–39 in.) in men and 80–88 cm (31–35 in.) in women, may have strong genetic contribution to insulin resistance and should benefit from changes in lifestyle habits, similar to men with categorical increases in waist circumference. Lower waist circumference cutpoint, e.g., ≥90 cm (35 in.) in men and ≥80 cm (31 in.) in women, appears to be appropriate for Asian Americans.

[c]Fibrates and nicotinic acid are the most commonly used drugs for elevated triglyceride and reduced HDL cholesterol. Patients taking one of these drugs are presumed to have high triglycerides and low HDL cholesterol.

activity to 150 min/week reduced new-onset diabetes by 58% over an average follow-up period of 3.3 years among individuals with impaired glucose tolerance *(40)*.

1.12.1. Diabetes Mellitus

Diabetes mellitus (type 1 or 2) is considered a CHD risk equivalent because CVD event rates among individuals with diabetes are similar to those of people with a prior CHD event. The presence of diabetes increases risk for a CVD event by two- to eightfold and mortality is higher among those with diabetes after a CVD event *(18, 41)*. The increase in relative risk for CVD associated with diabetes is larger for women than men *(3)*.

Because the prevalence of obesity in the United States roughly doubled between 1980 and 2005, the incidence and prevalence of type 2 diabetes have been increasing, and this is expected to continue well into the future *(42)*. Data from clinical trials show that intensive glycemic control is effective for reducing microvascular complications (e.g., retinopathy, neuropathy, nephropathy) in patients with type 1 or 2 diabetes mellitus *(19)*. Aggressive glycemic control has not been consistently demonstrated to reduce macrovascular complications in type 2 diabetes, but other preventive measures (lipid management, blood pressure control, and use of aspirin) have proven effective for reducing CVD events in patients with diabetes *(43–46)*. Thus, while adequate glycemic control remains an important goal of therapy, aggressive risk factor management is central to efforts to reduce CVD morbidity and mortality in those with diabetes.

1.13. DIET AND PHYSICAL ACTIVITY

Throughout this chapter, emphasis has been placed on the importance of lifestyle in driving adverse changes in risk factors that, in turn, promote the atherothrombotic process. Lifestyle modification plays a critical role in preventive efforts and favorable changes in diet and physical activity habits simultaneously improve multiple risk factors *(47)*. Table 3 summarizes the lifestyle recommendations from the AHA Nutrition Committee.

Table 3
American Heart Association Diet and Lifestyle Recommendations for Cardiovascular Risk Reduction *(47)*

Balance calorie intake and physical activity to achieve or maintain a healthy body weight
Consume a diet rich in vegetables and fruits
Choose whole-grain, high-fiber foods
Consume fish, especially oily fish, at least twice per week
Limit intake of saturated fat to <7% of energy, trans fat to <1% of energy, and cholesterol to <300 mg/day by

- Choosing lean meats and vegetable alternatives
- Selecting fat-free (skim), 1% fat, and low-fat dairy products
- Minimizing intake of partially hydrogenated fats

Minimize intake of beverages and foods with added sugars
Choose and prepare foods with little or no salt
Consume alcohol in moderation, if at all
Follow these diet and lifestyle recommendations when food is eaten outside the home

1.13.1. Dietary Factors

In addition to maintenance of a healthy body weight, the recommendations from the AHA emphasize consumption of fruits, vegetables, nuts, legumes, whole grains, and dietary fiber. Population studies show that higher intakes of these foods are associated with reduced CVD risk, although the mechanisms responsible for these relationships are not fully understood and are under active investigation *(47)*. The recommendations also include consumption of oily varieties of fish, which contain the long-chain omega-3 fatty acids eicosapentaenoic and docosahexaenoic acid. Both population studies and clinical trials have shown that greater intake of these fatty acids is associated with reduced CVD mortality *(48)*. The benefits of omega-3 fatty acids may derive, at least in part, from incorporation of these fatty acids into myocardial membranes, which appears to reduce susceptibility to arrhythmias, particularly those triggered by ischemia *(49)*. Reducing added sugars and salt helps with maintenance of normal body weight and blood pressure, and lowering intakes of saturated fats, trans fats, and cholesterol to levels below those in the typical American diet helps to maintain normal levels of cholesterol and atherogenic lipoproteins.

Vitamin D status has also recently emerged as a risk factor for CVD events. Data from cohort studies suggest that low circulating levels of 25-hydroxyvitamin D are associated with greater risks for cardiovascular events and mortality, although it is uncertain whether increasing vitamin D status through greater dietary intake and/or sun exposure will reduce CVD risk *(50, 51)*. Given the strength and consistency of this relationship across several studies and the high prevalence of vitamin D insufficiency in the United States and elsewhere, this appears to be a promising area for investigation with substantial public health implications.

1.13.2. Alcohol Consumption

A consistent association has been observed between moderate alcohol consumption and reduced CVD morbidity and mortality in many populations and this relationship holds true for both wine and other types of alcoholic beverages *(52)*. Alcohol raises HDL cholesterol in a dose–response manner and has effects on platelet function and inflammatory markers that may help to explain this association *(53)*. At higher intakes, alcohol has a number of adverse effects, including raising levels of triglycerides and blood pressure. At higher levels of alcohol intake, increases in morbidity and mortality from other causes offset any cardiovascular benefits *(52)*. Alcohol is not recommended for CVD prevention because it is potentially addictive; but for patients who do consume alcohol, the recommendation is to limit intake to no more than two drinks per day for men and one drink per day for women (a drink is 12 oz beer, 4 oz of wine, 1.5 oz of spirits).

1.13.3. Physical Activity

Regular physical activity is associated with lower risks for CVD, obesity, diabetes, hypertension, osteoporosis, and cancers of the breast and colon *(47)*. Regular activity, particularly if at least some of it is vigorous, has been demonstrated to improve levels of blood pressure, blood lipids (triglyceride and HDL cholesterol levels), insulin resistance, adiposity, as well as biomarkers of inflammation and hemostasis *(54)*.

Among adults >18 years of age who responded to the 2006 National Health and Nutrition Examination Survey, 62% reported no vigorous physical activity lasting >10 min per session *(55)*. Less than half of the US population meets current recommendations for physical activity of ≥ 30 min, ≥ 5 days/week *(55)*. The prevalence of sedentary lifestyle increases with age, is higher in women than men, and is especially high in minority (African American and Hispanic) subsets of the population *(54)*.

1.14. INFLAMMATORY MARKERS

As described earlier, the atherothrombotic process is essentially a "response to injury" in the arterial wall in which inflammation plays a central role. Given the central role of inflammation in atherothrombosis, it is not surprising that various biological markers for inflammation are associated with increased CVD event risk. For a variety of reasons, many of these are poorly suited for use in clinical practice, but some do have potential clinical applications, particularly CRP and lipoprotein-associated phospholipase A2 (Lp-PLA2). General screening for elevations in inflammatory markers is not recommended. The greatest utility of these markers in clinical practice is likely to be for identifying those individuals with at least moderate risk for a CVD event for whom the clinician is not certain whether more aggressive therapy, particularly lipid-altering therapy, is warranted *(56, 57)*.

Because of significant intraindividual variation, the measurement of high sensitivity CRP (hs-CRP) should be completed on at least two separate occasions, and the results averaged. Results may be categorized as follows based on population tertiles:

- Low:<1.0 mg/L
- Average: 1.0–3.0 mg/L
- High: >3.0 mg/L

The high tertile for hs-CRP is associated with a relative risk for a CVD event that is roughly twofold that of the lowest tertile and does appear to add predictive value beyond that of traditional risk markers *(58, 59)*. It should be noted that noncardiovascular causes can produce hs-CRP elevation and other causes such as infection or trauma should be considered if the value is >10 mg/L.

The Justification for the Use of Statins in Prevention: An Intervention Trial Evaluating Rosuvastatin (JUPITER) study evaluated whether rosuvastatin (20 mg/day), compared with placebo, would decrease the rate of occurrence of first major cardiovascular events in otherwise healthy individuals with elevated hs-CRP ($\geq$2.0 mg/L) and LDL-C <130 mg/dL *(60)*. Rosuvastatin therapy reduced LDL-C by 50% and hs-CRP by 37%. The trial was stopped early because the rosuvastatin group showed reductions of $\sim$50% in several cardiovascular endpoints relative to the placebo group. The JUPITER results provide clear evidence that those with elevated hs-CRP are at increased CHD risk and that rosuvastatin therapy lowers this risk. However, JUPITER did not answer the question of whether hs-CRP reduction per se should be a target of therapy. An additional outstanding question is the mechanisms that account for the increased risk associated with elevated hs-CRP. Is hs-CRP elevation reflecting vascular inflammation, dysregulation of adipose tissue resulting in the release of proinflammatory cytokines, greater hepatic sensitivity to inflammatory stimuli, or does hs-CRP itself promote some aspect of the atherothrombotic process? Results from genetic studies indicate that polymorphisms associated with elevated hs-CRP are not themselves predictive of cardiovascular disease risk, suggesting that hs-CRP itself is not raising risk, but instead that acquired hs-CRP elevation is a marker for some process that is proatherogenic and/or prothrombotic *(13, 14)*.

Lp-PLA2 is an enzyme that is secreted by macrophages in the arterial intima and may therefore serve as a marker specific for an inflammatory process in the arterial wall *(61)*. Lp-PLA2 hydrolyzes oxidized phospholipids on lipoprotein particles in the subendothelial space. It is carried by lipoproteins in plasma and preferentially associates with LDL particles, especially small, dense, electronegative LDL particles, although some Lp-PLA2 is carried by HDL and triglyceride-rich lipoproteins *(61)*.

Compared to CRP, the Lp-PLA2 level in circulation is much more stable, with an intraindividual coefficient of variation of 10%, versus >40% for hs-CRP *(62)*. Approximate population tertiles for Lp-PLA2 mass concentrations are as follows *(63)*:

- Low: <200 ng/mL
- Average: 200–260 ng/mL
- High: >260 ng/mL

Like hs-CRP, an elevated concentration of Lp-PLA2 is associated with an increase in CVD event risk after adjustment for other risk factors. Compared to the bottom tertile, an Lp-PLA2 concentration in the top two tertiles is associated with a hazard ratio for a cardiovascular event of $\sim$1.5–2.0 *(61)*. The combination of increased Lp-PLA2 and hs-CRP appears to increase risk beyond that associated with elevation of either in isolation *(56)*.

1.15. MEASURES OF SUBCLINICAL CVD

Like testing for inflammatory markers, tests for subclinical atherosclerotic CVD have the greatest utility for patients at intermediate risk and can help the clinician to decide whether more aggressive risk factor intervention is warranted. In various studies, a positive test for subclinical atherosclerosis has been shown to provide predictive information above and beyond that available from traditional global risk scoring *(64)*. The cost associated with many tests for subclinical disease such as electron beam computed tomography for coronary calcium scoring, carotid intima-media thickness, or screening graded exercise testing is high. Summarizing the various recommendations for their application in clinical practice is beyond the scope of this chapter, although the use of calcium scoring to assess coronary plaque burden and ankle-brachial index as an indicator of peripheral arterial disease will be discussed briefly.

1.15.1. Coronary Calcium

In 2007, an American College of Cardiology Foundation/AHA Clinical Expert Consensus document included recommendation for use of coronary artery calcium scoring in CVD risk assessment *(65)*. In a secondary analysis of four reports summarized in the document, annual CHD event rates (death or myocardial infarction) were 0.4, 1.3, and 2.4% for the first, second, and third tertiles, respectively, of coronary calcium among individuals with an intermediate Framingham risk score (10–20% 10-year risk). The tertile cutpoints for coronary calcium score were <100, 100–399, and ≥400. Thus, the recommendations of the consensus panel were to give consideration to measurement of coronary calcium in patients whose Framingham risk score indicates a 10–20% 10-year CHD event risk and to treat such patients as having a CHD risk equivalent if they display a coronary calcium score ≥400. However, a low score (even a score of 0) is not sufficient reason to forego risk factor modification. (Global risk assessment using the Framingham risk score will be covered in detail in the next chapter.) Later follow-up studies have provided further support for the use of coronary calcium testing in CVD risk assessment. Coronary calcium has been reported to be an independent predictor of mortality after accounting for other CVD risk factors *(66)* and a strong predictor of CVD event risk across racial and ethnic subgroups *(67)*.

1.15.2. Ankle-Brachial Index

The use of the ankle-brachial index to assess suspected peripheral arterial disease is simple and inexpensive to perform. A value <0.9 is diagnostic of lower extremity arterial disease and a CHD risk equivalent *(17)*. Intensive risk factor modification is warranted in such patients.

1.16. HEMOSTATIC VARIABLES

A number of variables associated with the balance between thrombosis and fibrinolysis are associated with CVD event risk including fibrinogen, plasminogen activator inhibitor-1, tissue plasminogen activator, and others. At present these generally remain research tools and are not recommended for clinical risk assessment *(68)*.

1.17. NONMODIFIABLE RISK FACTORS

A number of factors that cannot be modified are associated with increased CVD event risk including age, family history of CVD, and race/ethnicity. Although age and family history cannot be altered, they are important for risk stratification. In addition, a strong family history of premature CVD may prompt investigation for nontraditional risk markers such as elevated levels of Lp-PLA2 or lipoprotein (a). The prevalence of some risk factors varies by race/ethnicity, and the clinician should be aware of these differences. For example, hypertension is particularly common among African Americans, and diabetes is more common among Hispanic Americans, compared with non-Hispanic whites. However, the available evidence suggests that the relationships between risk factors and CVD event risk do not vary markedly by race/ethnicity.

1.18. PSYCHOSOCIAL FACTORS

A number of psychosocial factors have been associated with increased risk for CVD, including low social support, depression, personality traits (e.g., type A personality, locus of control), perceived stress, life change events, and others *(69)*. This is a promising area for research aimed at identification of high-risk individuals and has generated a number of testable hypotheses; however, methods for identification and management have generally not been incorporated into guidelines for prevention of CVD. In addition, low educational attainment and low socioeconomic status have also been shown to predict higher CVD risk. The available data suggest that the higher risk in these subgroups can be largely accounted for by greater prevalence and severity of established risk CVD factors *(70)*.

1.19. SLEEP APNEA, SLEEP QUANTITY AND QUALITY

It has been known for some time that sleep apnea is associated with increased CVD risk. Central or obstructive sleep apnea is strongly associated with a number of conditions that are CVD risk factors such as obesity, diabetes, and hypertension. The AHA/American College of Cardiology Foundation has recently released a Scientific Statement on sleep apnea and CVD *(71)*.

Even in the absence of apnea, lower sleep quantity and quality have been found to correlate with a number of risk factors, including obesity, insulin resistance, hypertension, and inflammation *(71)*. A recent analysis from the Coronary Artery Risk Development in Young Adults study showed that incident coronary calcification over an average follow-up period of 5 years was associated with low sleep duration *(72)*. Each additional hour of sleep per night measured by actigraphy was associated with a 33% reduction in the incidence of new coronary calcium. While the clinical implications of these findings are unclear at present, they represent an important area for additional research since sleep quantity and quality are potentially modifiable risk factors.

1.20. CONCLUSIONS—TRANSLATING RISK FACTOR IDENTIFICATION INTO PREVENTION

Application of epidemiological methods of investigation has contributed tremendously to the understanding of atherosclerotic CVD disease etiology and led to the identification and testing of numerous preventive measures. Population studies continue to play an important role in advancing the field of preventive cardiology. Investigation of risk factors and interactions between risk factors remains a source of intense scientific inquiry.

Some once promising interventions, based on observations from population studies, have proven to be ineffective or otherwise not lived up to expectations after testing in randomized clinical trials. Among these are the use of B vitamins for reduction of homocysteinemia, antioxidant vitamins, postmenopausal sex hormone therapy, and intensive glycemic control in those with type 2 diabetes. On the other hand, interventions for treating dyslipidemia, hypertension, and the use of aspirin and omega-3 fatty acids have proven effective. New techniques for evaluating genetic determinants of risk and response to intervention, as well as investigation of new potential targets for therapy such as vascular inflammation, vitamin D status, and sleep quality, suggest that the coming decades will provide more, and more effective, means through which the scourge of atherosclerotic CVD can be brought under control.

REFERENCES

1. Rosamond W, Flegal K, Furie K, et al. Heart disease and stroke statistics—2008 update: a report from the American Heart Association Statistics Committee and Stroke Statistics Subcommittee. *Circulation*. 2008;117:e25–e146.
2. Meagher EM. Cardiovascular disease in women: the management of dyslipidemia. In: Davidson MH, Toth PP, Maki KC, eds. *Therapeutic Lipidology*. Totowa, NJ: Humana Press; 2007:349–368.
3. Mosca L, Banka CL, Benjamin EJ, et al. Evidence-based guidelines for cardiovascular disease prevention in women: 2007 update. *Circulation*. 2007;115:1481–1501.
4. Keys A. Coronary heart disease in seven countries. *Nutrition*. 1970;13:250–252.
5. Steinberg D. Thematic review series: the pathogenesis of atherosclerosis. An interpretive history of the cholesterol controversy: part II: the early evidence linking hypercholesterolemia to coronary disease in humans. *J Lipid Res*. 2005;46:179–190.
6. Epstein FH. Contribution of epidemiology to understanding coronary heart disease. In: Marmot M, Elliott P, eds. *Coronary Heart Disease Epidemiology from Aetiology to Public Health*. New York, NY: Oxford University Press; 1992:20–32.
7. Yusuf S, Hawken S, Ounpuu S, et al. Effect of potentially modifiable risk factors associated with myocardial infarction in 52 countries (the INTERHEART study): case-control study. *Lancet*. 2004;364:937–952.
8. Brown BG, Stukovsky KH, Zhao XQ. Simultaneous low-density lipoprotein-C lowering and high-density lipoprotein-C elevation for optimum cardiovascular disease prevention with various drug classes, and their combinations: a meta-analysis of 23 randomized lipid trials. *Curr Opin Lipidol*. 2006;17:631–636.
9. Shaper AG, Elford J. Regional variations in coronary heart disease in Great Britain: risk factors and changes in environment. In: Marmot M, Elliott P, eds. *Coronary Heart Disease Epidemiology from Aetiology to Public Health*. New York, NY: Oxford University Press; 1992:127–139.
10. Robertson TL, Kato H, Gordon T, et al. Epidemiologic studies of coronary heart disease and stroke in Japanese men living in Japan, Hawaii and California. Coronary heart disease risk factors in Japan and Hawaii. *Am J Cardiol*. 1977;39:244–249.
11. Yusuf S, Reddy S, Ounpuu S, Anand S. Global burden of cardiovascular diseases: part I: general considerations, the epidemiologic transition, risk factors, and impact of urbanization. *Circulation*. 2001;104:2746–2753.
12. Winkleby MA, Feldman HA, Murray DM. Joint analysis of three U.S. community intervention trials for reduction of cardiovascular disease risk. *J Clin Epidemiol*. 1997;50:645–658.
13. Zacho J, Tybjaerg-Hansen A, Jensen JS, Grande P, Sillesen H, Nordestgaard BG. Genetically elevated C-reactive protein and ischemic vascular disease. *N Engl J Med*. 2008;359:1897–1908.
14. Schunkert H, Samani NJ. Elevated C-reactive protein in atherosclerosis—chicken or egg? *N Engl J Med*. 2008;359:1953–1955.
15. O'Regan C, Wu P, Arora P, Perri D, Mills EJ. Statin therapy in stroke prevention: a meta-analysis involving 121,000 patients. *Am J Med*. 2008;121:24–33.
16. Mills EJ, Rachlis B, Wu P, Devereaux PJ, Arora P, Perri D. Primary prevention of cardiovascular mortality and events with statin treatments: a network meta-analysis involving more than 65,000 patients. *J Am Coll Cardiol*. 2008;52:1769–1781.
17. National Cholesterol Education Panel. Third report of the National Cholesterol Education Program (NCEP) Expert Panel on detection, evaluation, and treatment of high blood cholesterol in adults (Adult Treatment Panel III). Final report. Bethesda, MD: National Heart, Lung, and Blood Institute, National Institutes of Health; 2002
18. Buse JB, Ginsberg HN, Bakris GL, et al. Primary prevention of cardiovascular diseases in people with diabetes mellitus: a scientific statement from the American Heart Association and the American Diabetes Association. *Circulation*. 2007;115:114–126.
19. Skyler JS, Bergenstal R, Bonow RO, et al. Intensive glycemic control and the prevention of cardiovascular events: implications of the ACCORD, ADVANCE, and VA Diabetes Trials. A position statement of the American diabetes association and a scientific statement of the American College of cardiology foundation and the American heart association. *Circulation*. 2009;119:351–357.
20. Mozaffarian D, Wilson PW, Kannel WB. Beyond established and novel risk factors: lifestyle risk factors for cardiovascular disease. *Circulation*. 2008;117:3031–3038.
21. Pischon T, Girman CJ, Sacks FM, Rifai N, Stampfer MJ, Rimm EB. Non-high-density lipoprotein cholesterol and apolipoprotein B in the prediction of coronary heart disease in men. *Circulation*. 2005;112:3375–3383.
22. Mora S, Szklo M, Otvos JD, et al. LDL particle subclasses, LDL particle size, and carotid atherosclerosis in the Multi-Ethnic Study of Atherosclerosis (MESA). *Atherosclerosis*. 2007;192:211–217.
23. Liu J, Sempos CT, Donahue RP, Dorn J, Trevisan M, Grundy SM. Non-high-density lipoprotein and very-low-density lipoprotein cholesterol and their risk predictive values in coronary heart disease. *Am J Cardiol*. 2006;98: 1363–1368.

24. Maki KC, Galant R, Davidson MH. Non-high-density lipoprotein cholesterol: the forgotten therapeutic target. *Am J Cardiol.* 2005;96:59 K–64 K.

25. Cohen JC, Boerwinkle E, Mosley TH Jr, Hobbs HH. Sequence variations in PCSK9, low LDL, and protection against coronary heart disease. *N Engl J Med.* 2006;354:1264–1272.

26. Gordon DJ, Probstfield JL, Garrison RJ, et al. High-density lipoprotein cholesterol and cardiovascular disease. Four prospective American studies. *Circulation.* 1989;79:8–15.

27. Toth PP. High-density lipoprotein and cardiovascular risk. *Circulation.* 2004;109:1809–1812.

28. Davidson MH, Ose L, Frohlich J, et al. Differential effects of simvastatin and atorvastatin on high-density lipoprotein cholesterol and apolipoprotein A-I are consistent across hypercholesterolemic patient subgroups. *Clin Cardiol.* 2003;26:509–514.

29. Davidson MH, Bays HE, Stein E, Maki KC, Shalwitz RA, Doyle R. Effects of fenofibrate on atherogenic dyslipidemia in hypertriglyceridemic subjects. *Clin Cardiol.* 2006;29:268–273.

30. Packard CJ. Triacylglycerol-rich lipoproteins and the generation of small, dense low-density lipoprotein. *Biochem Soc Trans.* 2003;31:1066–1069.

31. Miller M, Cannon CP, Murphy SA, et al. Impact of triglyceride levels beyond low-density lipoprotein cholesterol after acute coronary syndrome in the PROVE IT-TIMI 22 trial. *J Am Coll Cardiol.* 2008;51:724–730.

32. Koschinsky ML. Lipoprotein(a) and atherosclerosis: new perspectives on the mechanism of action of an enigmatic lipoprotein. *Curr Atheroscler Rep.* 2005;7:389–395.

33. Chobanian AV, Bakris GL, Black HR, et al. Seventh report of the Joint National Committee on prevention, detection, evaluation, and treatment of high blood pressure. *Hypertension.* 2003;42:1206–1252.

34. Whelton PK, He J, Appel LJ, et al. Primary prevention of hypertension: clinical and public health advisory from The National High Blood Pressure Education Program. *JAMA.* 2002;288:1882–1888.

35. Anderson KM, Odell PM, Wilson PW, Kannel WB. Cardiovascular disease risk profiles. *Am Heart J.* 1991;121:293–298.

36. Wajchenberg BL. Subcutaneous and visceral adipose tissue: their relation to the metabolic syndrome. *Endocr Rev.* 2000;21:697–738.

37. Pouliot MC, Després JP, Lemieux S, et al. Waist circumference and abdominal sagittal diameter: best simple anthropometric indexes of abdominal visceral adipose tissue accumulation and related cardiovascular risk in men and women. *Am J Cardiol.* 1994;73:460–468.

38. Maki KC. Dietary factors in the prevention of diabetes mellitus and coronary artery disease associated with the metabolic syndrome. *Am J Cardiol.* 2004;93:12C–17C.

39. Grundy SM, Cleeman JI, Daniels SR, et al. Diagnosis and management of the metabolic syndrome: an American Heart Association/National Heart, Lung, and Blood Institute Scientific Statement. *Circulation.* 2005;112:2735–2752.

40. Knowler WC, Barrett-Connor E, Fowler SE, et al. Reduction in the incidence of type 2 diabetes with lifestyle intervention or metformin. *N Engl J Med.* 2002;346:393–403.

41. Eckel RH, Kahn R, Robertson RM, Rizza RA. Preventing cardiovascular disease and diabetes: a call to action from the American Diabetes Association and the American Heart Association. *Circulation.* 2006;113:2943–2946.

42. Ogden CL, Carroll MD, Curtin LR, McDowell MA, Tabak CJ, Flegal KM. Prevalence of overweight and obesity in the United States, 1999–2004. *JAMA.* 2006;295:1549–1555.

43. Gerstein HC, Miller ME, Byington RP, et al. Effects of intensive glucose lowering in type 2 diabetes. *N Engl J Med.* 2008;358:2545–2559.

44. Patel A, MacMahon S, Chalmers J, et al. Intensive blood glucose control and vascular outcomes in patients with type 2 diabetes. *N Engl J Med.* 2008;358:2560–2572.

45. Duckworth W, Abraira C, Moritz T, et al. Glucose control and vascular complications in veterans with type 2 diabetes. *N Engl J Med.* 2009;360:129–139.

46. Holman RR, Paul SK, Bethel MA, Neil HA, Matthews DR. Long-term follow-up after tight control of blood pressure in type 2 diabetes. *N Engl J Med.* 2008;359:1565–1576.

47. Lichtenstein AH, Appel LJ, Brands M, et al. Diet and lifestyle recommendations revision 2006: a scientific statement from the American Heart Association Nutrition Committee. *Circulation.* 2006;114:82–96.

48. Kris-Etherton PM, Harris WS, Appel LJ. American Heart Association. Nutrition Committee. Fish consumption, fish oil, omega-3 fatty acids, and cardiovascular disease. *Circulation.* 2002;106:2747–2757.

49. Reiffel JA, McDonald A. Antiarrhythmic effects of omega-3 fatty acids. *Am J Cardiol.* 2006;98:50i–60i.

50. Dobnig H, Pilz S, Scharnagl H, et al. Independent association of low serum 25-hydroxyvitamin d and 1,25-dihydroxyvitamin d levels with all-cause and cardiovascular mortality. *Arch Intern Med.* 2008;168:1340–1349.

51. Giovannucci E, Liu Y, Hollis BW, Rimm EB. 25-hydroxyvitamin D and risk of myocardial infarction in men: a prospective study. *Arch Intern Med.* 2008;168:1174–1180.

52. Corrao G, Bagnardi V, Zambon A, La Vecchia C. A meta-analysis of alcohol consumption and the risk of 15 diseases. *Prev Med.* 2004;38:613–619.

53. Mascitelli L, Pezzetta F. Anti-inflammatory effects of alcohol. *Arch Intern Med*. 2003;163:2393.
54. Thompson PD, Buchner D, Pina IL, et al. Exercise and physical activity in the prevention and treatment of atherosclerotic cardiovascular disease: a statement from the Council on Clinical Cardiology (Subcommittee on Exercise, Rehabilitation, and Prevention) and the Council on Nutrition, Physical Activity, and Metabolism (Subcommittee on Physical Activity). *Circulation*. 2003;107:3109–3116.
55. Lloyd-Jones D, Adams R, Carnethon M, et al. Heart disease and stroke statistics—2009 update. A report from the American Heart Association Statistics Committee and Stroke Statistics Subcommittee. *Circulation*. 2009;119:480–486.
56. Pearson TA, Mensah GA, Alexander RW, et al. Markers of inflammation and cardiovascular disease: application to clinical and public health practice: a statement for healthcare professionals from the Centers for Disease Control and Prevention and the American Heart Association. *Circulation*. 2003;107:499–511.
57. Davidson MH, Corson MA, Alberts MJ, et al. Consensus panel recommendation for incorporating lipoprotein-associated phospholipase A2 testing into cardiovascular disease risk assessment guidelines. *Am J Cardiol*. 2008;101:51F–57F.
58. Ridker PM, Rifai N, Rose L, Buring JE, Cook NR. Comparison of C-reactive protein and low-density lipoprotein cholesterol levels in the prediction of first cardiovascular events. *N Engl J Med*. 2002;347:1557–1565.
59. Ridker PM. Clinical application of C-reactive protein for cardiovascular disease detection and prevention. *Circulation*. 2003;107:363–369
60. Ridker PM, Danielson E, Fonseca FA, et al. Rosuvastatin to prevent vascular events in men and women with elevated C-reactive protein. *N Engl J Med*. 2008;359:2195–2207.
61. Sudhir K. Clinical review: lipoprotein-associated phospholipase A2, a novel inflammatory biomarker and independent risk predictor for cardiovascular disease. *J Clin Endocrinol Metab*. 2005;90:3100–3105.
62. Lerman A, McConnell JP. Lipoprotein-associated phospholipase A2: a risk marker or a risk factor? *Am J Cardiol*. 2008;101:11F–22F.
63. Lanman RB, Wolfert RL, Fleming JK, et al. Lipoprotein-associated phospholipase A2: review and recommendation of a clinical cut point for adults. *Prev Cardiol*. 2006;9:138–143.
64. Greenland P, Smith SC Jr, Grundy SM. Improving coronary heart disease risk assessment in asymptomatic people: role of traditional risk factors and noninvasive cardiovascular tests. *Circulation*. 2001;104:1863–1867.
65. Greenland P, Bonow RO, Brundage BH, et al. ACCF/AHA 2007 clinical expert consensus document on coronary artery calcium scoring by computed tomography in global cardiovascular risk assessment and in evaluation of patients with chest pain: a report of the American College of Cardiology Foundation Clinical Expert Consensus Task Force (ACCF/AHA Writing Committee to Update the 2000 Expert Consensus Document on Electron Beam Computed Tomography). *Circulation*. 2007;115:402–426.
66. Budoff MJ, Shaw LJ, Liu ST, et al. Long-term prognosis associated with coronary calcification: observations from a registry of 25,253 patients. *J Am Coll Cardiol*. 2007;49:1860–1870.
67. Detrano R, Guerci AD, Carr JJ, et al. Coronary calcium as a predictor of coronary events in four racial or ethnic groups. *N Engl J Med*. 2008;358:1336–1345.
68. Koenig W. Cardiovascular biomarkers: added value with an integrated approach? *Circulation*. 2007;116:3–5.
69. Frasure-Smith N, Lespérance F. Recent evidence linking coronary heart disease and depression. *Can J Psychiatry*. 2006;51:730–737.
70. Thombs BD, de Jonge P, Coyne JC, et al. Depression screening and patient outcomes in cardiovascular care: a systematic review. *JAMA*. 2008;300:2161–2171.
71. Somers VK, White DP, Amin R, et al. Sleep apnea and cardiovascular disease: an American Heart Association/American College of Cardiology Foundation Scientific Statement from the American Heart Association Council for High Blood Pressure Research Professional Education Committee, Council on Clinical Cardiology, Stroke Council, and Council on Cardiovascular Nursing. In collaboration with the National Heart, Lung, and Blood Institute National Center on Sleep Disorders Research (National Institutes of Health). *Circulation*. 2008;118:1080–1111.
72. King CR, Knutson KL, Rathouz PJ, Sidney S, Liu K, Lauderdale DS. Short sleep duration and incident coronary artery calcification. *JAMA*. 2008;300:2859–2866.

2 Arterial Hypertension

Daniel A. Duprez

CONTENTS

Key Words: Angiotensin; Beta-blocker; Blood pressure; Isolated systolic hypertension; Hypertensive nephropathy.

KEY POINTS

- High blood pressure is one of the most important cardiovascular risk factors.
- The general cutpoint for hypertension is 140/90 mmHg.
- In diabetes mellitus and chronic kidney disease, the BP goal should be lower than 130/80 mmHg.
- Prehypertension is a cardiovascular risk factor.
- The pathogenesis of essential hypertension is a heterogeneous process and several systems are involved in the changes of cardiovascular hemodynamics.

From: *Contemporary Cardiology: Comprehensive Cardiovascular Medicine in the Primary Care Setting*
Edited by: Peter P. Toth, Christopher P. Cannon, DOI 10.1007/978-1-60327-963-5_2
© Springer Science+Business Media, LLC 2010

- In more than 90% of patients, elevated blood pressure is due to essential hypertension, in which genetic and environmental factors are involved.
- Interpretation of blood pressure values is dependent on whether they are measured in the office, at home, or during a 24-h ambulatory BP recording.
- In the evaluation of hypertension, other risk factors have to be taken into consideration.
- Treatment of hypertension is not only lowering blood pressure but the main aim is to reduce the risk for CV morbidity and mortality as well to preserve renal function.
- Antihypertensive treatment should be focused on lifestyle changes and personalized blood pressure lowering therapy in the context of other concomitant morbid conditions.
- Several landmark trials have shown that there can be a difference in cardiovascular and renal outcome, depending on how blood pressure is lowered.
- Age is not a contraindication to lowering blood pressure.

2.1. INTRODUCTION

High blood pressure (BP) is a very important cardiovascular (CV) risk factor and is often labeled the "silent killer" because arterial hypertension will lead to serious CV events such as ischemic heart disease, stroke, and heart failure. Moreover, uncontrolled essential hypertension also leads to renal insufficiency, which accelerates the process of blood pressure elevation *(1, 2)*. There is a shift regarding diagnosis and treatment of arterial hypertension. With aging, systolic hypertension is becoming a more important risk factor than diastolic hypertension and is more difficult to control.

2.2. DEFINITION

Hypertension is now defined on the basis of systolic (SBP) and diastolic (DBP) blood pressure levels and classified into stages on the basis of the degree of elevation. The generally recognized cutpoint for hypertension is an average office BP of 140/90 mmHg or greater, which has been obtained by a recommended standard technique with an accurate manometer and has been confirmed on at least one other occasion. This general definition has been modified for the classification of hypertension in specific high-risk populations such as diabetes mellitus and chronic kidney disease (CKD).

Throughout middle and old age, BP is strongly and directly related to vascular and overall mortality, without any evidence of a threshold down to at least 115/75 mmHg. Normal BP is widely considered to being less than 120/80 mmHg. Alternate definitions for hypertension exist for BP measurements made with home BP and ambulatory BP monitoring. Home BPs of more than 135/85 mmHg generally correlate well with office BPs of 140/90 mmHg or greater. Awake ambulatory BPs of more than 140/90 mmHg and sleep averaged BPs of more than 125/75 mmHg are now considered to be sufficient for the diagnosis of hypertension. Although pulse pressure (PP), the difference between SBP and DBP in mmHg, has been used to characterize CV risk in hypertension, it does not yet contribute to the definition of the hypertensive status.

Prehypertension is now considered to be a CV risk factor *(3)*. It is defined as an SBP between 120 and 139 mmHg systolic and a DBP of 80–89 mmHg. These subjects are at very high risk to develop arterial hypertension.

2.3. EPIDEMIOLOGY OF HYPERTENSION

Hypertension is considered to be the most common reversible or treatable CV risk factor. When defined as a BP of 140/90 mmHg, it affects 50 million residents of the United States, with an estimated one billion people worldwide. The population attributable risk due to elevated BP is large and present in all ethnic groups and regions of the world. It is not then surprising that hypertension has been identified as a condition that accounts for a substantial portion of total global disease burden *(4)*. From a clinical perspective, there is one generally accepted cardinal principle that describes the hypertensive state and that has served to define the importance of hypertension to world health. The presence of an elevated uncontrolled BP over time will lead to progression in the severity or stage of hypertension, the development or worsening of target organ damage, and increased CV morbidity and mortality. Given the relationship of hypertension to stroke, myocardial infarction, heart failure, and other vascular disease, the control of high BP will have a profound impact on individual well-being and national healthcare costs.

Elevated BP demonstrates a consistent, strong, and graded relationship with multiple CV events including CV death, myocardial infarction, stroke, heart failure, and renal dysfunction. The risk of CV mortality has been observed to double with each 20/10 mmHg increase in BP from 115/75 mmHg in adults aged from 40 to 69 years of age. This relationship between SBP and DBP elevation and CVD mortality is best described by the Prospective Studies Collaboration, a meta-analysis that found 120,000 deaths among one million participants in 61 cohorts *(4)*. Individuals with preexisting vascular disease were excluded from this meta-analysis. During 12.7 million person-years at risk, there were about 56,000 vascular deaths (12,000 strokes, 34,000 ischemic heart disease, 10,000 other vascular) that occurred in adults between 40 and 89 years of age. Throughout middle age, as BP increases, each difference of 20 mmHg in the usual SBP (usual BP at the start of each decade) and/or approximately equivalent 1 mmHg usual difference in DBP was associated with a more than twofold increase in the stroke death rate. Because stroke is much more common in old age than in middle age, the absolute annual differences in stroke death associated with a given BP difference were greater in old patients. In addition, each 20 mmHg difference in usual SBP was associated with a twofold difference in the death rate from ischemic heart disease. All of the proportional differences found in vascular mortality were reduced by half in the 80–89 year age group. Age-specific associations for men and women were similar. Perhaps the most striking finding of this meta-analysis was that relatively small reductions in mean SBP would be associated with large absolute reductions in premature deaths and disabling strokes. Thus a 2-mmHg lower mean SBP could lead to a 7% lower risk of ischemic heart disease death and a 10% lower risk of stroke death. Unfortunately, a gap continues to exist between hypertension and awareness and control worldwide *(5)*.

2.4. MECHANISMS OF HYPERTENSION

The pathogenesis of essential hypertension is a heterogeneous process and involves several systems resulting in altered cardiovascular hemodynamics. Arterial blood pressure is the product of cardiac output (stroke volume × heart rate) × total peripheral vascular resistance.

2.4.1. Hemodynamics

The blood pressure required to supply the different organs and tissues with blood through the circulatory bed is provided by the pumping action of the heart (cardiac output) and arterial tone (total peripheral vascular resistance). Each of these primary components is determined by the interaction of a complex series of factors. Arterial hypertension has been attributed to abnormalities in nearly every one of these factors *(6)*. In recent years there has been more attention devoted to pulse pressure, which is the difference between SBP and DBP and is a simple parameter conferring information about arterial stiffness *(7)*.

An increase in arterial tone has traditionally been viewed as the hallmark for an elevated BP. Although some have suggested that an increase in cardiac output with a normal vascular resistance is the initial hemodynamic abnormality in patients with hypertension, the chronic hypertensive state usually is associated with an increase in total systemic vascular resistance. This increase in resistance is generally attributed to an increase in vascular tone. Multiple mechanisms possibly contribute to this increase in systemic vascular resistance: activation of the sympathetic nervous system and the renin–angiotensin–aldosterone system (RAAS), endothelial dysfunction, electrolyte changes, and alterations in the release of endothelial relaxing factor.

2.4.2. Renal

The relationship between the development or pathogenesis of hypertension and the kidney is complex. The kidney, through a variety of distinct mechanisms, can cause or contribute to the development and progression of hypertension. On the other hand, hypertension per se can contribute to progressive renal structural and vascular damage, which in turn may contribute to a worsening or perpetuation of the hypertensive state. Renal functional and structural changes can promote sodium retention. Excessive sodium reabsorption can lead to plasma volume expansion, an increase in cardiac output and ultimately an increase in total peripheral resistance and BP. These mechanisms most certainly contribute to the BP elevation, which accompanies CKD and some cases of primary hypertension *(8)*. Several other renal factors have received attention as potential contributors to this vicious cycle that is characterized by development of hypertension and progressive renal damage. Inappropriate or excessive activation of the RAAS in relationship to the sodium/volume balance may contribute to BP elevation, especially in the setting of renal parenchymal disease.

2.4.3. Neurohumoral Factors

Many factors are now implicated in the development of hypertensive vascular disease, and the RAAS appears to be one of the most significant. Angiotensin II, the principal effector peptide of the RAAS, has far-reaching effects on vascular structure, growth, and fibrosis, and is a key regulator of vascular remodeling and inflammation *(9)*. The RAAS is an important contributor to the regulation of BP, water and salt balance, and tissue growth. It functions both as a circulating endocrine system and as a tissue paracrine/autocrine system, most notably in the heart, brain, kidney, and vasculature. Aldosterone is the major mineralocorticoid hormone secreted by the adrenal cortex. Identification of mineralocorticoid receptors in the heart, vasculature, and brain has raised speculation that aldosterone may directly mediate its detrimental effects in these target organs, independent of angiotensin II and the regulatory role of aldosterone in kidney function and BP.

2.4.4. Baroreflexes

The arterial baroreflex is known to represent a mechanism of fundamental importance for short-term BP homeostasis in daily life. Reduced baroreflex sensitivity appears to characterize not only patients with established hypertension, but also normotensive offspring of hypertensive parents.

2.4.5. Aging

Available evidence suggests that the incidence of systolic hypertension is increasing in individuals over 50 years of age. There are multiple mechanisms involved. These include an altered vascular resistance, the classical hallmark of high BP, as well as changes in arterial stiffness and wave reflection, which occur in the conduit arteries, mainly the aorta and its principal branches *(10)*.

2.5. ETIOLOGY OF HYPERTENSION

The specific set of events that lead to progressive elevation of BP and the development of hypertension remains unknown. Depending on the clinical setting, 93–95% of hypertensives have no known cause for their hypertension. For that reason, most hypertension states were originally classified as "essential" hypertension.

2.5.1. Essential or Primary Hypertension

Although the pathogenesis of essential or primary hypertension is uncertain, as previously noted, specific mechanisms appear to be involved in the development of primary hypertension: altered regulation of the sympathetic nervous system, abnormalities of the renin–angiotensin–aldosterone system, salt sensitivity, as well as other vascular and hormonal factors. In addition to these multiple physiologic abnormalities, diet, environment, other lifestyle factors, and most certainly genetics frequently play a role in the development of hypertension. Thus, the etiology of primary hypertension is very complex and includes a mosaic of interrelated factors, which may affect total peripheral resistance and result in the development of primary hypertension. Irrespective of the exact etiologic mechanisms whereby patients develop hypertension, most patients seem to progress along a similar hemodynamic cascade, which involves an early increase in cardiac output, followed by a subsequent rise in total peripheral resistance.

There still, however, is a possibility that our concept of primary hypertension is flawed and that we are dealing with multiple distinct clinical syndromes. The majority of patients who develop primary hypertension do so between 20 and 50 years of age. Most cases are diagnosed as part of routine examinations and generally in the absence of overt target organ damage at initial presentation.

Patients with primary hypertension are generally asymptomatic. Although some patients report symptoms related to hypertension such as headache, dizziness, fatigue, palpitations, and chest discomfort, these symptoms and their level of intensity generally do not correlate well with BP level. Thus, primary hypertension has no consistent signs or symptoms, except for the elevated BP itself. A specific type of headache has, however, been reported to occur with elevated BP. Hypertensive headache is a clinical entity, which has been described as a diffuse morning headache and is generally associated with more severe stages of hypertension in some circumstances. These headaches may actually be associated with sleep apnea complicating arterial hypertension, rather than the BP itself.

2.5.2. Secondary Hypertension

Secondary causes of hypertension are uncommon and account for less than 5% of all cases of high BP in unselected hypertensive populations. Although infrequent, secondary forms of hypertension account for many cases of drug-resistant hypertension. As a result of this finding, higher prevalence rates of secondary hypertension have been noted in specialized hypertension clinics. Secondary hypertension is usually associated with specific organ and/or vascular abnormalities, a metabolic abnormality, or endocrine disorder. The diagnosis of these specific hypertensive conditions is important because of the potential for a permanent cure, or improvement in control of hypertension. If left undiagnosed, secondary hypertension may lead to progressive target organ damage, as well as CV and renal complications.

In secondary hypertension, the elevated BP may be the major presenting manifestation of an underlying process, or elevated BP may simply be one component of a complex group of signs and symptoms in a patient with a systemic disease. Secondary causes of hypertension are often nonspecific in their presentation, and laboratory tests and/or imaging studies are required for screening and confirmation of the diagnosis. Nevertheless, there are some well-recognized clinical presentations and clinical clues that deserve mention and that should raise a clinician's suspicion of a secondary cause of hypertension.

The documented early (less than age 30 years) or late (more than age 50 years) onset of hypertension is thought to raise the possibility of secondary forms of hypertension. In pediatric populations, congenital renal or endocrine causes of secondary hypertension are more likely to result in elevated BP. Fibromuscular dysplasia of the renal artery(s) characteristically occurs in young white women, generally without a strong family history of hypertension. The most common cause of secondary hypertension in older patients, with associated vascular disease, is atherosclerotic renal artery stenosis. In obese patients, obstructive sleep apnea and Cushing's disease should be considered as potential causes of secondary hypertension.

A thorough search for secondary causes of hypertension is not considered cost effective in most patients with hypertension. Expanded workups should be considered with compelling clinical or laboratory evidence for a specific secondary cause, or when a patient presents with drug-resistant or refractory hypertension, or hypertensive crisis and should be referred to a hypertension specialty clinic. Causes of secondary hypertension are listed in Table 1.

Table 1
Secondary Causes of Hypertension

Chronic kidney disease (renal parenchymal disease)
Renovascular hypertension
Atherosclerosis
Fibromuscular dysplasia
Renal artery aneurysm
Systemic vasculitis
Renin-secreting tumor
Primary hyperaldosteronism
Aldosterone-producing adenoma
Idiopathic hyperaldosteronism
Glucocorticoid-remediable hyperaldosteronism
Pheochromocytoma
Cushing's disease/syndrome
Coarctation of the aorta
Hypothyroidism
Sleep apnea

2.5.3. Chronic Kidney Disease (CKD)—Renal Parenchymal Hypertension

CKD, or renal parenchymal disease, is the most common form of secondary hypertension. Hypertension occurs in more than 80% of patients with chronic renal failure and is a major factor causing their increased CV morbidity and mortality seen in CKD. Any type of CKD, including acute or chronic glomerulonephritis, may be associated with hypertension. Hypertension is frequently the presenting feature of adult polycystic kidney disease. Clinically, affected patients may experience abdominal pain and hematuria, and the renal or associated hepatic cysts may be palpable on physical examination. CKD should be suspected when the estimated glomerular filtration rate (eGFR) is less than or equal to 60 mL/min or when 1+ or greater proteinuria and/or specific urinary sediment abnormalities are noted on urine analysis. The diagnosis can be confirmed either by the direct measurement of glomerular filtration rate (GFR) or collection for a creatinine clearance showing a value of less than 60 mL/min. Proteinuria should be confirmed by a 24-h urine, which should demonstrate a total protein excretion of more than 150 mg, or by a spot urine specimen showing microalbuminuria defined as a urine albumin-to-urine creatinine ratio between 30 and 300 mg/g.

In patients with mild or moderate renal insufficiency, stringent BP control is imperative to reduce the progression to end-stage renal disease and to reduce the excessive CV risk associated with CKD.

2.5.4. Renovascular Hypertension

Renovascular hypertension may be the most common form of potentially curable hypertension (11). Current estimates indicate that is seen in 1–2% of a hypertensive population in general medical practice. There are two major causes: atheromatous disease and fibromuscular dysplasia of the renal artery, and each is associated with a distinct clinical presentation.

Renovascular hypertension is frequently associated with resistance to a multiple drug antihypertensive regimen. It is not surprising, therefore, that up to 30% of patients referred to some specialized hypertension clinics are found to have renovascular hypertension. Several clinical clues occurring alone or in combination may point to the diagnosis of renovascular hypertension:

1. New-onset or drug-resistant hypertension before age 30 or after age 50
2. Accelerated or malignant hypertension
3. Lateralizing epigastric or upper quadrant systolic–diastolic abdominal bruit noted in a hypertensive patient
4. Progressive worsening of renal function in response to an ACE-inhibitor
5. Diffuse atherosclerotic vascular disease in the setting of severe hypertension
6. Unexplained pulmonary edema (flash pulmonary edema) generally associated with progressive renal insufficiency and occurring during antihypertensive therapy for renin-dependent hypertension

Other mechanisms can also contribute to the development of progressive hypertension in the setting of renovascular hypertension. Long-standing or accelerated hypertension can promote the development of structural changes such as arteriolar nephrosclerosis in a contralateral kidney in the case of unilateral renal artery stenosis. Associated renal parenchymal damage may also contribute further to BP elevation, and renal impairment.

The most common cause of renovascular hypertension is atherosclerotic renal artery stenosis, which generally affects the proximal renal arteries. Atherosclerotic renal artery stenosis is progressive and may lead to worsening hypertension, renal artery occlusion, ischemic nephropathy, and renal failure. The majority of these cases with atherosclerotic renal artery disease occur in the setting of other coronary, cerebrovascular, or peripheral vascular disease. Fibromuscular dysplasia of the renal arteries is the most frequent cause of renovascular hypertension in young women (those under 50 years old). This disease occurs rarely in males, but may on occasion be seen in males with strong family histories of fibromuscular dysplasia.

The clinical suspicion and even the confirmed diagnosis of renovascular hypertension will frequently present clinicians with difficult diagnostic and therapeutic dilemmas. Individualized treatment decisions are currently required for the effective management and treatment of renovascular hypertension. The diagnostic evaluation and therapeutic strategy for patients with suspected renovascular hypertension is predicated on several factors, including the severity of hypertension, the presence of associated renal failure or insufficiency, the type of renal artery lesion, the location of the stenotic lesion, the presence of concomitant CVD, a patient's general health status, and the ability of a patient to tolerate multiple antihypertensive medications.

Patients with clinical presentations suggestive of renovascular hypertension can be screened with noninvasive studies, and, if results are positive, confirmation of the diagnosis can be made with renal arteriography. If the index of suspicion for renovascular hypertension is high, renal arteriography can be performed in the absence of noninvasive tests. Noninvasive testing is frequently employed to diagnose or confirm the anatomical site of a renal artery lesion, or to examine the functional significance of a renal artery stenosis.

Intensive medical therapy for renovascular hypertension is generally required for BP control and involves the use of an ACE-inhibitor, in conjunction with multiple other medications. Treatment frequently involves the use of a calcium channel blocker (CCB), judicious use of diuretics, and occasionally the use of a sympathetic inhibitor. Renal function and serum potassium should be monitored regularly, as they can deteriorate with ACE inhibition or BP reduction alone. ACE-inhibitors should be withdrawn with moderate deterioration (>30%) in renal function and/or if a patient becomes hyperkalemic. Angiotensin receptor blockers (ARBs) should be substituted in those patients who develop an ACE-I cough or those who develop mild hyperkalemia with ACE inhibition.

Medical management of renovascular hypertension includes intensive treatment of associated CV risk factors, with concomitant aggressive lipid lowering, smoking cessation, and the use of low-dose aspirin. Percutaneous renal artery angioplasty and stenting or surgical revascularization of the renal arteries should be considered in the setting of drug-resistant and worsening hypertension, in patients who develop progressive renal failure in response to medical therapy, and finally in those with high-grade bilateral renal artery stenosis. Preservation of renal function is currently the leading cited indication for intervention in patients with renal artery stenosis and renovascular hypertension. BP can now be frequently controlled with potent multidrug antihypertensive regimens. Revascularization, however, may prevent renal artery occlusion, progressive ischemic nephropathy, and renal atrophy. Percutaneous and surgical procedures are not without risk. Patient selection and timing may be crucial to limit complications and to maximize outcomes.

2.5.5. Primary Hyperaldosteronism

Primary hyperaldosteronism, or Conn's syndrome, is characterized by hypokalemia, hypertension, very low plasma or suppressed renin activity (PRA), and excessive aldosterone secretion *(12)*. Aldosterone binds with the mineralocorticoid receptor in the distal nephron and contributes to salt and water homeostasis and maintenance of plasma volume through this interaction. Excessive production of the hormone promotes an exaggerated renal Na^+–K^+ exchange, which usually results in hypokalemia. The diagnosis of primary hyperaldosteronism should be considered in any patient with severe refractory hypertension. Traditionally, it was thought that 1–2% of patients with hypertension had primary hyperaldosteronism. The syndrome has been reported to be more common in females and may present with mild, moderate, or resistant hypertension. Patients are generally asymptomatic, though symptoms such as muscle cramps, weakness, and paresthesias attributable to hypokalemia may predominate. Polyuria and polydipsia have also been reported. Many patients with primary hyperaldosteronism will present with severe, persistent, or refractory diuretic-induced hypokalemia. The best clinical clues to the diagnosis in patients with hypertension is either unprovoked hypokalemia with a serum K^+ less than 3.5 mmol/L in the absence of diuretic therapy, or the development of more profound hypokalemia during diuretic therapy with a serum K^+ less than 3.0 mmol/L. Laboratory testing is frequently required to differentiate between secondary hyperaldosteronism associated with diuretic use, renovascular hypertension, and renin-secreting tumors. The most utilized confirmatory test is the urine aldosterone excretion rate, which involves the 24-h collection of urine, under conditions of a high-salt load. Adrenal computed tomography (CT) scans with 3-mm cuts should be used to localize adenomas or neoplasm. Control of BP and hypokalemia can be obtained with antihypertensive regimens based on spironolactone, eplerenone, or, on occasion, with amiloride. Multiple medications will be frequently required. Unilateral adrenalectomy is highly effective for reversing the metabolic consequences of hyperaldosteronism in patients with aldosterone-producing adenoma.

2.5.6. Pheochromocytoma

Pheochromocytomas are rare catecholamine-producing tumors that originate from chromaffin cells of the adrenergic system. The majority of these tumors are benign and are located in the adrenal gland, but others can develop as functioning paragangliomas in a variety of extra-adrenal sites. Pheochromocytomas generally secrete both norepinephrine and epinephrine, though norepinephrine is usually the predominant amine *(13)*.

Classic clinical presentations are characterized by hypertension, palpitations, headache, and hyperhidrosis. The hypertension can be severe and sustained (55%) or paroxysmal (45%). Pounding headaches, palpitations, and diaphoresis are prominent features of the syndrome and may occur together in a paroxysmal attack. Postural hypotension may occasionally be present as a result of low or constricted plasma volume. Hypertension associated with panic attacks as well as other causes of neurogenic hypertension, including the BP elevations, sometimes seen with sympathomimetic agents, and obstructive sleep apnea, can be confused with pheochromocytoma. Plasma-free metanephrines, if available, are a preferred screening test for excluding or confirming the diagnosis of pheochromocytoma. Twenty-four-hour urine collections for metanephrine (100% sensitive) are also useful for screening for the tumor. The accuracy of the 24-h urine metanephrine may be improved by indexing urinary metanephrine levels by urine creatinine levels. Patients with a suspicion of pheochromocytoma should be referred to a specialized center and to emergency rooms in case of a hypertensive crisis.

2.6. COMPLICATED MANAGEMENT PROBLEMS IN HYPERTENSION

2.6.1. Resistant Hypertension

Resistant hypertension or "hard-to-treat" hypertension is becoming an increasingly common problem with the national guidelines focusing on lower goal BPs (14). True drug-resistant hypertension is relatively rare, but treatment failure is relatively common, frequently being secondary to nonadherence, socioeconomic factors, and lifestyle issues. Resistant hypertension is generally defined as the failure to achieve a therapeutic target of less than 140/90 mmHg in most hypertensive patients, or less than 130/80 mmHg in diabetics or patients with CKD on a well-designed three-drug antihypertensive medical regimen combined with intensive lifestyle modification. In most cases, resistant hypertension is now defined on the basis of a persistently high SBP level. Before embarking on an expanded workup to determine the cause of drug-resistant hypertension, clinicians should be careful to rule out "pseudoresistance" secondary to BP measurement artifacts or errors and "white-coat" hypertension. Out-of-office measurements, including home BPs, or 24-h ambulatory BP monitoring (ABPM) may be required to establish a patient's actual BP. The absence of target organ damage in the setting of prolonged resistant or refractory hypertension should raise a clinician's suspicion regarding pseudoresistance. Patients with resistant hypertension are older and commonly present with obesity, unrestricted or excessive dietary salt intake, and the clinical syndrome of sleep apnea. Common causes of resistant hypertension are summarized in Table 2.

Current approaches to correction of drug resistance focus on evaluation and correction of potential contributing causes, the development of a more effective drug regimen, and identifying any unrecognized secondary causes of hypertension. Volume expansion plays a key role in drug resistance, and it cannot be adequately assessed with a clinical exam. Treatment should include a strong emphasis on lifestyle changes including weight loss, exercise, dietary, and salt restriction, all of which should be monitored. New multidrug antihypertensive regimens should incorporate the more potent vasodilator antihypertensive agents such as calcium channel blockers (CCBs) or direct-acting vasodilators with adequate diuretic therapy, especially if intense vasoconstriction is suspected as the physiologic cause or culprit. Recent data indicate that aldosterone antagonists may be effective when added to existing antihypertensive regimens even in the absence of primary aldosterone (15). Consultation with a hypertension specialist should be considered if target BP cannot be achieved.

2.6.2. Hypertensive Emergencies and Urgencies

Hypertensive emergencies and urgencies present infrequently in medical practice. When they do occur, they require prompt evaluation and intervention. A hypertensive emergency can be defined as

Table 2
Causes of Resistant Hypertension

Poor adherence to medical regimen
Improper BP measurement
Improper cuff size
Poor adherence to lifestyle changes
Obesity and weight gain
Heavy alcohol intake
Stress or office hypertension
Pseudoresistance in the elderly
Volume overload
Excess sodium intake
Pseudotolerance
Progressive CKD
Drug-induced or other causes
Inadequate doses of antihypertensive medication
Inappropriate combinations of antihypertensive medications
Drug interactions
Nonsteroidal anti-inflammatory drugs
Cocaine, amphetamines, other illicit drugs
Sympathomimetics (decongestants, anorectics)
Oral contraceptives, adrenal steroids
Cyclosporine and tacrolimus
Erythropoietin
Licorice ingestion
Unsuspected secondary hypertension
Sleep apnea

a sudden and/or severe elevation in BP that causes or contributes to pathologic disturbances in the central nervous system, the heart, the vascular system, or the kidneys, and that requires prompt BP reduction in order to maintain the integrity of the CV system.

Hypertensive emergencies are true medical emergencies that require prompt recognition and thoughtful management in order to reduce the morbidity and mortality associated with severe hypertension. BP reduction typically is begun within minutes to hours of diagnosis and is frequently required to prevent worsening of an underlying clinical condition (16).

The term "hypertensive urgency" refers to a clinical presentation of severe hypertension where the SBP is usually more than 200 mmHg and/or the DBP is usually more than 120 mmHg. These patients are generally asymptomatic and do not have evidence of acute target organ damage. BP lowering may occur over hours to days in the absence of acute target organ damage or serious comorbid disease.

The presence of severe hypertension alone is not sufficient to make the diagnosis of hypertensive emergency. The diagnosis of hypertensive emergencies ultimately depends on the clinical presentation rather than on the absolute level of the BP. Thus, these cases usually present with severe hypertension complicated by some cardiac, renal, neurologic, hemorrhagic, or obstetric manifestation. Hypertensive encephalopathy, acute aortic dissection, and pheochromocytoma crisis are well-recognized hypertensive emergencies. Some cases of accelerated or malignant hypertension, acute left ventricular failure, cerebral infarction, head injury, scleroderma, and acute myocardial infarction can also present as hypertensive emergencies. Other causes for an acute symptomatic rise in BP include medications, noncompliance, and poorly controlled chronic hypertension. The clinical history and physical examination should be highly focused in an attempt to determine the cause of a patient's severe hypertension and should attempt to exclude other clinical presentations that may mimic hypertensive emergencies or urgencies such as panic attack or postictal hypertension.

The choice of an appropriate oral or parenteral antihypertensive medication for treatment of severe hypertension depends upon the type of hypertensive emergency, the presence of associated target organ damage, and the specific hemodynamic properties and side effects of the emergency or urgency. When possible, clinicians should opt for a gradual controlled reduction of BP and avoid antihypertensive agents or methods that have been associated with rapid or precipitous reductions in BP.

Catastrophic side effects including acute myocardial infarction, cortical blindness, stroke, and death have been reported with rapid or precipitous reduction in BP in patients presenting with hypertensive urgency or emergency. Treatment of hypertensive emergency needs to be tailored to each individual patient and presentation. Prompt and rapid reduction of BP under continuous surveillance is essential in patients who are symptomatic and have acute end-organ damage. Parenteral therapy, typically in a monitored bed in the intensive care unit, is recommended for the treatment of most hypertensive emergencies. Sodium nitroprusside is the "gold standard" for treating hypertensive emergencies, and the agent to which other parenteral agents are measured. Nitroprusside is metabolized to thiocyanate and cyanide, and may accumulate in patients receiving high doses, or prolonged infusions especially with CKD. Repeated intravenous injections ("mini bolus" of 10–20 mg) of the combined alpha- and beta-adrenergic receptor-blocking agent labetalol can produce a prompt but gradual reduction of arterial BP without the induction of a reflex tachycardia.

Hypertensive urgencies are usually treated with oral antihypertensive medications. Single oral agents or combinations of antihypertensive medications have been used to lower BP in this setting. Clinicians should avoid using short-acting oral or sublingual nifedipine in the treatment of hypertensive urgency and emergency, especially in those patients with known or suspected coronary artery disease.

2.7. BLOOD PRESSURE MEASUREMENT

2.7.1. Office Blood Pressure Measurement

The most common reason for an outpatient physician visit is for the diagnosis and treatment of hypertension. Standardized BP measurement is the basis for the diagnosis, management, treatment, epidemiology, and research of hypertension, and the decisions affecting these aspects of hypertension will be influenced, for better or worse, by the accuracy of measurement. Accurate BP measurement is well described by the Joint National Committee on Prevention, Detection, Evaluation and Treatment of High Blood Pressure (JNC VII) *(17)*, the World Health Organization–International Society of Hypertension (WHO/ISH) *(18)*, and the American Heart Association (AHA) *(19)*. All of these guidelines are a synthesis of the methodology used in all the important epidemiologic and treatment trials of hypertension. Factors important in this methodology include (1) resting for 5 min, (2) sitting with back supported and feet on the floor, (3) arm supported at heart level, (4) appropriate-size cuff applied, (5) use of the Korotkoff Phase I sound for SBP and Phase V for DBP, and (6) using the mean of two or more BP measurements as the patient's BP. Failure to conform to all of these recommendations can result in significant errors in auscultated BP and misdiagnosis and mistreatment of the hypertensive patient.

Certain groups of people merit special consideration for BP measurement. These include children; the elderly, who often have isolated systolic hypertension or autonomic failure with postural hypotension; obese people in whom the inflatable bladder may be too small for the arm size, leading to "cuff hypertension"; patients with arrhythmias in whom BP measurement may be difficult and the mean of a number of measurements may have to be estimated; pregnant women in whom the disappearance of sounds (Phase V) is the most accurate measurement of diastolic pressure, except when sounds persist to zero, when the fourth phase of muffling of sounds should be used; and any individual during exercise.

Bilateral measurements should be made on first consultation, and, if persistent differences greater than 20 mmHg for systolic or 10 mmHg for diastolic pressure are present on consecutive readings, the patient should be referred to a CV center for further evaluation with simultaneous bilateral measurement and the exclusion of arterial disease. The second option for accurate BP measurement is the use of validated automated BP devices. The automated BP measuring devices use a proprietary oscillometric method. Each of these devices needs to be independently validated and then calibrated to each patient. Rarely, they do not sense BP accurately, but more commonly fail if the cardiac rhythm is very irregular (e.g., atrial fibrillation). It is interesting to note that even with auscultatory BP measurement in elderly patients with atrial fibrillation, considerable observer variability is seen. It is critically important that if an automated BP-measuring device is used, it must have passed a recognized validation protocol.

2.7.2. Home BP

Home BP monitoring has become popular in clinical practice, and several automated devices for home BP measurement are now recommendable. Home BP is generally lower than clinic BP, and similar to daytime ambulatory BP. Home BP measurement eliminates the white-coat effect and provides a high number of readings, and it is considered more accurate and reproducible than clinic BP. It can improve the sensitivity and statistical power of clinical drug trials and may have a higher prognostic value than clinic BP. Home monitoring may improve compliance and BP control and reduce costs of hypertension management (20). Home BP provides an opportunity for additional monitoring of BP levels and its variability.

2.7.3. Ambulatory BP

Ambulatory blood pressure (ABPM) provides automated measurements of brachial-artery pressure over a 24-h period while patients are engaging in their usual activities. This method has been used for more than 30 years in clinical research on hypertension. These studies demonstrated that BP has a highly reproducible circadian profile, with higher values when the patient is awake and mentally and physically active, much lower values during rest and sleep, and an early-morning surge lasting 3–5 h during the transition from sleep to wakefulness. In a patient with hypertension, 24-h BP monitoring has substantial appeal. It yields multiple BP readings during all of the patient's activities, including sleep, and gives a far better representation of the "BP burden" than what might be obtained in a few minutes in the doctor's office (21).

Several prospective clinical studies, as well as population-based studies, have indicated that the incidence of CV events is predicted by BP as measured conventionally or with ambulatory methods, even after adjustment for a number of established risk factors (22, 23).

In clinical practice, measurements are usually made at 20–30-min intervals in order not to interfere with activity during the day and with sleep at night. Measurements can be made more frequently when indicated. Whatever definition of daytime and nighttime is used, at least two thirds of SBPs and DBPs during the daytime and nighttime periods should be acceptable. If this minimum requirement is not met, the ABPM should be repeated. A diary card may be used to record symptoms and events that may influence ABPM measurements, in addition to the time of drug ingestion, meals, and going to and arising from bed. If there are sufficient measurements, editing is not necessary for calculating average 24-h, daytime, and nighttime values, and only grossly incorrect readings should be deleted from the recording. Normal ranges for ABPM are average daytime ABPM of less than 135/85 mmHg and average nighttime ABPM less than 120/70 mmHg, but even lower values are advocated, particularly in high-risk groups such as diabetic patients (Table 3).

ABMP is accepted as being of benefit in patients with the conditions listed in Table 4. ABPM has a number of advantages: it provides a profile of BP away from the medical environment, thereby allowing identification of individuals with a white-coat response, and it shows BP behavior over a 24-h

Table 3
**Recommended Levels of Normality for Ambulatory Blood
Pressure Monitoring in Adults**

	Blood pressure value (mmHg)		
	Optimal	Normal	Abnormal
Awake	<130/80	<135/85	>140/90
Asleep	<115/65	<120/70	>125/75

Table 4
**Recommendations for the Use of Ambulatory Blood
Pressure Monitoring in Clinical Practice**

Indication	JNC VII	WHO/ISH
White-coat hypertension	Yes	Yes
Labile hypertension	Yes	Yes
Resistant hypertension	Yes	Yes
Hypotensive episodes	Yes	Yes
Postural hypotension	Yes	No

period during usual daily activities, rather than when the individual is sitting in the artificial circumstances of a clinic or office. It can indicate the duration of decreased BP over a 24-h period. ABPM can identify patients with blunted or absent BP reduction at night—the nondippers—who are at greater risk for organ damage and CV morbidity. It can demonstrate a number of patterns of BP behavior that may be relevant to clinical management, such as white-coat hypertension, isolated systolic hypertension, and masked hypertension.

Self-monitoring of the BP at home and at work can be used to assess whether there is a large disparity between the office and out-of-office BPs before ambulatory monitoring is considered. It is likely that many patients whose self-monitored BP is apparently normal will have elevated ambulatory BP and would benefit from antihypertensive therapy. For those whose ambulatory BP is truly normal (<130/80 mmHg) despite an elevated office BP and in whom there is no evidence of other CV risk factors or target organ disease, avoidance of unnecessary drug therapy would be a clear benefit of the monitoring procedure.

2.8. EVALUATION OF HYPERTENSION

Following the confirmation of hypertension, a targeted history and physical examination and limited laboratory evaluation should be performed (24, 25). The standard hypertensive workup includes an assessment of CV risk and the identification of hypertensive target organ damage, and is designed to rule out secondary hypertension. This examination should include information regarding a patient's habits and lifestyle, which could contribute to his or her hypertension.

The identification of other CV risk factors or concomitant disorders may affect prognosis and guide treatment. The major CV risk factors and types of hypertension-associated target organ damage are listed in Table 5. The medical history and physical examination are also the most important components of a pretreatment evaluation in differentiating between primary and secondary hypertension. The medical history should include detailed questioning which focuses on the following medical information.

Table 5
Cardiovascular Risk Factors

Hypertension
Cigarette smoking
Obesity (BMI > 30 kg/m^2)
Physical inactivity
Dyslipidemia
Diabetes mellitus
Microalbuminuria or estimated GFR (glomerular filtration rate) <60 mL/min
Age (>55 years for men, >65 years for women)
Family history of premature CVD (men <55 years or women <65 years)
Target organ damage
Left ventricular hypertrophy
Angina or prior myocardial infarction
Coronary atherosclerosis
Prior coronary revascularization
Heart failure
Mild cognitive impairment
Stroke or transient ischemic attack
Chronic kidney disease
Peripheral arterial disease
Retinopathy

Family history of hypertension:

1. Family history of premature CVD, diabetes, or dyslipidemia
2. Estimated duration of hypertension, current and previous hypertension stage, and drug therapy
3. Home BP measurements
4. Medical history, clinical signs, and symptoms of CV or renal disease
5. Medical history, clinical signs, and symptoms of comorbid disease, which may affect selection of drug therapy (asthma, chronic obstructive pulmonary disease [COPD])
6. Complete medication history including prescription, over-the-counter (OTC) medications, herbal remedies, and drug allergies
7. History of drug and alcohol abuse

The importance of the medication history cannot be overemphasized. A variety of drugs can elevate BP and interfere with the effect of antihypertensive medications. Corticosteroids, cyclosporine, tacrolimus, and oral contraceptives are well-recognized causes of BP elevation. Ephedrine, sympathomimetics, and amphetamine-like agents, available in OTC cough and sinus preparations, can increase peripheral resistance and interfere with BP control. Commonly used drugs such as nonsteroidal anti-inflammatory drugs (NSAIDs) can also cause hypertension or interfere with the effect of a variety of antihypertensive medications.

The initial physical examination should include the following:

1. Vital signs, including body mass index (BMI)
2. Sitting and standing BP and heart rate
3. BP measurement in the contralateral arm
4. Examination of optic fundi, neck, heart, lungs, and abdomen
5. Auscultation of the neck and abdomen for bruits
6. Palpation of peripheral pulses, and extremity check for edema
7. Neurological examination

A limited laboratory evaluation is recommended at the time of initial diagnosis. This should include a complete blood cell count, serum chemistry (including Na, K, Ca, glucose, and uric acid), a complete lipid profile, and urinalysis. Recent trends have focused on better baseline assessment of renal function in hypertensive patients. Although not mandatory in most hypertensive patients, a measurement of urinary albumin excretion or albumin/creatinine ratio may be useful in diagnosing renal disease or establishing future CV risk. A positive result could affect the intensity and type of antihypertensive therapy. Many reference laboratories now routinely calculate the estimated glomerular filtration rate (eGFR), which can be used to identify or exclude CKD (chronic kidney disease), or to monitor the effect of antihypertensive therapy on renal function.

Additional laboratory and imaging tests may be required to quantify CV risk, to characterize target organ damage, or to screen for secondary hypertension in some complicated patients. Given the high frequency of additional CV risk factors in hypertension, clinicians may want to use a risk assessment tool for determining a patient's 10-year risk for developing coronary heart disease (CHD). Such risk assessments may be useful for estimating global CV risk and in modifying patient behavior. Given the higher than expected frequency of hyperlipidemia with hypertension, clinicians could elect to use the risk-scoring calculator developed by The National Cholesterol Education Program (NCEP). The NCEP now recommends using a modification of the Framingham risk prediction model to estimate CV risk and adjust therapy in patients with dyslipidemia (26). The risk factors included in this Framingham calculation of 10-year risk are age, total cholesterol, high-density lipoprotein cholesterol, SBP, treatment for hypertension, and cigarette smoking. This modification of the Framingham point score does not account for all risk factors for CHD and should only be used in conjunction with NCEP guidelines. Separate NCEP Framingham risk calculators are available for men and women. Other risk factor calculators could be used for those patients who present without dyslipidemia.

2.9. TREATMENT

The stated goal for the treatment of hypertension is to prevent CV morbidity and mortality associated with high BP. Such a goal now requires the treatment of all identified reversible risk factors accompanying hypertension to maximize CV event reduction. The clinical goal is to lower BP to below 140/90 mmHg while controlling other CV risk factors. Further reductions in BP to a level less than 130/80 mmHg have been recommended in hypertensive patients with diabetes or renal disease. Reduction in BP to less than 130/80 mmHg can also be pursued with due regard in other populations, especially high-risk patients. Nondrug therapy should be employed in the management of all stages of hypertension and should also be implemented in individuals with prehypertension as a preventive strategy. New guidelines for diagnosis and treatment of hypertension—JNC VIII—are expected in 2011. The most recent ESH/ISH Guidelines for Diagnosis and Treatment of Hypertension were published in 2007 (25).

The use of drug therapy is generally predicated on the stage of hypertension, the presence of high CV risk, comorbid conditions, and the documentation of target organ damage. For example, patients with prehypertension and specific comorbid conditions, such as diabetes mellitus or hypertensive nephropathy, may benefit from early drug therapy.

Lifestyle modification may prevent or delay the onset of sustained hypertension, lower BP, and reduce the number of BP medications necessary for control in patients with established hypertension. Comprehensive lifestyle modification has been well studied and includes the following interventions:

1. Weight reduction in those who are overweight or obese
2. Adoption of a Dietary Approaches to Stop Hypertension (DASH) diet—a low-fat diet rich in fruits, vegetables, and low-fat dairy products
3. Reduce sodium intake to 100 mmol/day (2.4 g sodium or 6 g sodium chloride)

4. Limit alcohol intake to ~1 oz/day (24 oz of beer per day, 8 oz of wine per day, or 2 oz of 100 proof whiskey per day)
5. Regular aerobic exercise
6. Stop smoking and modify other known CV risk factors

Adherence to one or several of these lifestyle modifications can result in a substantial fall in BP and aid in the management of hypertension. In general, weight loss and dietary changes have been observed to have the most dramatic effect on BP reduction (27), a 1,600 mg sodium DASH eating plan has been shown to have effects on BP reduction similar to single-drug therapy (28). Adoption of healthy lifestyles in both prehypertension and hypertension is critical for the prevention of future CVD.

Although the JNC VII guideline recommends the use of pharmacologic therapy in patients with BPs greater than or equal to 140/90 mmHg, many clinicians continue to initiate a 3- to 6-month trial of comprehensive lifestyle modification in highly motivated patients who have uncomplicated Stage I hypertension. Drug therapy should be considered if BP remains greater than or equal to 140/90 mmHg after 3–6 months or if the patient is noncompliant with nondrug therapy.

Multiple drug classes, with different mechanisms of action and different side effects, are available for the treatment of hypertension (24, 25). Table 6 summarizes the oral antihypertensive drugs. Several classes of antihypertensives, including diuretics, calcium antagonists, ACEIs, and angiotensin receptor antagonists, are suitable for the initiation and maintenance of antihypertensive therapy. Beta-blockers and alpha-blockers are less favored by many clinicians and guidelines as first-line therapy.

The selection of a specific medication for initial treatment of hypertension is complex and may depend on a variety of factors, including age and race, comorbid CV and non-CVD, and target organ damage. Potential drug–drug interactions with a patient's existing medical regimen may further limit therapeutic options. Repeated clinical observations have suggested that diuretics and CCBs may be more effective in standard doses in older patients and African Americans, while beta-blockers and ACEIs appear to be more effective in younger and Caucasian populations. Gender has not been found to be a reliable predictor for drug response. For the majority of patients without a compelling indication for another class of an antihypertensive medication, a low dose of a thiazide diuretic is frequently recommended as the first choice of therapy. Table 7 summarizes the preferential antihypertensive drugs in case of specific target organ damage or specific populations.

On average, no more than 50% of a hypertensive population will be controlled by a single antihypertensive medication. In the Antihypertensive and Lipid-Lowering Treatment to Prevent Heart Attack Trial (ALLHAT), in a population of older hypertensives with Stage I and II hypertension and high CV risk, BP was lowered to less than 140/90 mmHg in 66% of the population at 5 years. A total of 63% of the ALLHAT cohort were taking two or more medications at the end of the trial (29).

Physicians have been notably reluctant to change or to add medications in those patients whose BPs are not at recommended goals. This phenomenon, which is commonly seen in the management of hypertension, is now referred to as "clinical inertia." Clinical inertia is defined as the failure of healthcare providers to initiate or intensify therapy when indicated (30). Many physicians are still inclined to practice sequential monotherapy substituting individual agents in order to identify the most effective antihypertensive medication for a given patient and to limit the number of antihypertensive medications that a patient takes. The preferred strategy for the management of hypertension involves the use of multiple medications and utilizing the additive benefits of agents in combination. It is well recognized that the skillful use of two or more agents in combination can improve hypertension control rates to well above 80%.

In this chapter the different classes of antihypertensive drugs will be discussed in relation to subclasses with side effects and target population. Recently, a new class of antihypertensive drugs, the direct renin inhibitors (DRI), has been introduced and the first DRI, aliskiren, is now available for clinical use.

Table 6
Oral Antihypertensive Drugs

Drug	Trade name	Usual dose range, total mg/day (frequency/day)	Selected side effects and comments
Diuretics (partial list)			Short term: increases cholesterol and glucose levels; biochemical abnormalities; decreases potassium, sodium, and magnesium levels, increases uric acid and calcium levels; rare: blood dyscrasias, photosensitivity, pancreatitis, hyponatremia
Chlorthalidone (G)	Hygroton	12.5–50 (1)	
Hydrochlorothiazide (G)	HydroDIURIL, Microzide, Esidrix	12.5–50 (1)	
Indapamide	Lozol	1.25–5 (1)	(Less or no hypercholesterolemia)
Metolazone	Mykrox	0.5–1.0 (1)	
	Zarxolyn	2.5–10 (1)	
Loop diuretics			
Bumetanide (G)	Bumex	0.5–4 (2–3)	(Short duration of action, no hypercalcemia)
Ethacrynic acid	Edecrin	25–100 (2–3)	(Only nonsulfonamide diuretic, ototoxicity)
Furosemide (G)	Lasix	40–240 (2–3)	(Short duration of action, no hypercalcemia)
Torsemide	Demadex	5–100 (1–2)	
Potassium-sparing agents			
Amiloride hydrochloride (G)	Midamor	5–10 (1)	Hyperkalemia
Spironolactone (G)	Aldactone	25–100 (1)	(Gynecomastia)
Triamterene (G)	Dyrenium	25–100 (1)	
Adrenergic inhibitors			
Peripheral agents			
Guanadrel sulfate	Hylorel	10–75 (2)	(Postural hypotension, diarrhea)
Fanethidine monosulfate	Ismelin	10–150 (1)	(Postural hypotension, diarrhea)
Reserpine (G)	Serpasil	0.05–0.25 (1)	(Nasal congestion, sedation, depression, activation of peptic ulcer)
Central alpha-agonist			Sedation, dry mouth, bradycardia, withdrawal hypertension
Clonidine hydrochloride (G)	Catapres	0.2–1.2 (2–3)	(More withdrawal)
Guanabenz acetate (G)	Wytensin	8–32 (2)	
Guanfacine hydrochloride (G)	Tenex	1–3 (1)	(Less withdrawal)
Methyldopa (G)	Aldomet	500–3,000 (2)	(Hepatic and "autoimmune" disorders)

(Continued)

Table 6
(Continued)

Drug	Trade name	Usual dose range, total mg/day (frequency/day)	Selected side effects and comments
Alpha-blockers			Can elevate HDL
Doxazosin mesylate	Cardura	1–16 (1)	
Prazosin hydrochloride (G)	Minipress	2–30 (2–3)	
Terazosin hydrochloride	Hytrin	1–20 (1)	
Beta-blockers			Bronchospasm, bradycardia, heart failure; may mask insulin-induced hypoglycemia; less serious: impaired peripheral circulation, insomnia, fatigue, decreased exercise tolerance, hypertriglyceridemia (except agents with intrinsic sympathomimetic activity), reduced HDL, impaired glyceric control
Acebutolol	Sectral	200–800 (1)	
Atenolol (G)	Tenormin	25–100 (1–2)	
Betaxolol hydrochloride	Kerlone	5–20 (1)	
Bisoprolol fumarate	Zebeta	2.5–10 (1)	
Carteolol hydrochloride	Cartrol	2.5–10 (1)	
Metoprolol tartrate (G)	Lopressor	50–300 (2)	
Metoprolol succinate	Toprol XL	50–300 (1)	
Nadolol	Corgard	40–320 (1)	
Penbutolol sulfate	Levatol	10–20 (1)	
Pindolol (G)	Visken	10–60 (1)	
Propranolol hydrochloride (G)	Inderal	40–480 (2)	
	Inderal LA	40–480 (1)	
Timolol maleate (G)	Blocadren	20–60 (2)	
Nebivolol	Bystolic	2.5–5–10 (1)	Postural hypotension, bronchospasm
Combined alpha and beta-blockers			
Carvedilol	Coreg	12.5–50 (2)	
Labetalol hydrochloride (G)	Normodyne, Trandate	200–1,200 (2)	
Direct vasodilators			
Hydralazine hydrochloride (G)	Apresoline	50–300 (2)	Headaches, fluid retention, tachycardia (Lupus syndrome)
Minoxidil	Loniten	5–100 (1)	(Hirsutism)

Calcium antagonists			
Nondihydropyridine			Conduction defects, worsening of systolic dysfunction, gingival hyperplasia (Nausea, headache)
Diltiazem hydrochloride	Cardizem SR	120–360 (2)	
	Cardizem CD, Dilacor XR, Tiazac	120–360 (1)	
Verapamil hydrochloride	Isoptin Sr, Calan SR	90–480 (2)	
	Verelan, Covera-HS	120–480 (1)	
Dihydropyridines			Edema of the ankle, flushing, headache, gingival hypertrophy
Amlodipine besylate	Norvasc	2.5–10 (1)	
Felodipine	Plendil	2.5–10 (1)	
Isradipine	DynaCirc	5–20 (2)	
	DynaCirc CR	5–20 (1)	
Nicardipine hydrochloride	Cardene SR	60–90 (2)	
Nifedipine	Procardia XL, Adalat CC	30–120 (1)	
Nisoldipine	Sular	20–60 (1)	
Angiotensin-converting enzyme inhibitors			Common: cough; rare: angioedema, hyperkalemia, rash, loss of taste, leukopenia
Benazepril hydrochloride	Lotensin	5–40 (1–2)	
Captopril (G)	Capoten	25–150 (2–3)	
Enalapril maleate	Vasotec	5–40 (1–2)	
Fosinopril sodium	Monopril	10–40 (1–2)	
Lisinopril	Prinivil, Zestril	5–40 (1)	
Moexipril hydrochloride	Univasc	7.5–15 (2)	
Quinapril hydrochloride	Accupril	5–80 (1–2)	
Ramipril	Altace	1.25–20 (1–2)	
Trandolapril	Mavik	1–4 (1)	
Angiotensin II receptor blockers			Angioedema (very rare); hyperkalemia
Losartan potassium	Cozaar	25–100 (1–2)	
Valsartan	Diovan	80–320 (1)	

(Continued)

Table 6
(Continued)

Drug	Trade name	Usual dose range, total mg/day (frequency/day)	Selected side effects and comments
Irbesartan	Avapro	150–300 (1)	
Telmisartan	Micardis	20–80 (1)	
Olmesartan	Benicar	20–40 (1)	
Candesartan	Atacand	8–32 (1–2)	
Direct renin inhibitor	Tekturna	150–300 (1)	Angioedema (very rare); hyperkalemia
Combination formulations			
Enalapril maleate/felodipine	Lexxel	5/5 (1)	Angioedema (very rare); hyperkalemia; edema from the CCB component
Trandolapril/verapamil	Tarka	2/180, 1–4/240 (1)	
Amlodipine/benazepril hydrochloride	Lotrel	2.5–10/10–20	
Amlodipine/valsartan	Exforge	5–160/10–160/5–320/ 10–320	

Table 7
Antihypertensive Therapy in Function of Target Organ Damage

Heart
Left ventricular hypertrophy: ACE-I, ARB, CA
Previous myocardial infarction: BB, ACE-I, ARB
Coronary artery disease—angina pectoris: BB, CCB
Heart failure: diuretics, BB, ACE-I, ARB, antialdosterone antagonists
Left ventricular dysfunction: ACE-I
Atrial fibrillation:
    Permanent: BB, nondihydropyridine CCB
    Recurrent: ACE-I, ARB
Tachyarrhythmias: BB

Noncoronary atherosclerosis
Poststroke: any antihypertensive drug
Peripheral artery disease: CCB

Kidney
Microalbuminuria/proteinuria: ACE-I, ARB
Renal dysfunction: ACE-I, ARB
End-stage renal disease: ACE-I, ARB

Special groups
Isolated hypertension (elderly): diuretics, CA
Metabolic syndrome: ACE-I, ARB, CCB
Diabetes mellitus: ACE-I, ARB
Pregnancy: methyldopa, CCB, BB
Glaucoma: BB
ACE-I-induced cough: ARB

ACE-I = angiotensin-converting enzyme inhibitors, ARB = angiotensin II receptor blockers, BB = beta-blockers, CCB = calcium channel blockers, CA = calcium antagonists.

2.9.1. Diuretics

It has been well documented that diuretics are effective antihypertensive drugs. Hydrochlorothiazide at a dose of 12.5 mg or 25 mg/day is the most frequently used diuretic. Chlorthalidone is also very effective. Diuretics cause salt and water depletion. The most important side effects are hypokalemia, hyperuricemia, impotence, and risk for diabetes in the long term. Thiazides are less effective in conditions of renal impairment (eGFR < 30 mL/min). In these cases furosemide can be used as an alternative therapy. Thiazides can be combined with a potassium-sparing diuretic like triamterene or spironolactone. Aldosterone antagonists, spironolactone and eplerenone, are potassium-sparing diuretics but should be considered in a category of a RAAS blocker, because of their ancillary cardiovascular protective effects beyond their diuretic effect. Electrolytes need to be monitored for hyperkalemia. Gynecomastia is a side effect, especially with spironolactone use. In patients on diuretic therapy, renal function should be monitored.

2.9.2. Beta-blockers

Beta-blockers can be categorized into nonselective (propranolol), cardio-selective (metoprolol, atenolol), with intrinsic sympathomimetic activity (pindolol), or with an alpha-blocking effect (labetolol, carvedilol). Most of the beta-blockers are metabolized by the liver, while atenolol is cleared by the kidney. Therefore, caution should be taken when atenolol is used in cases of renal impairment and dosing needs to be adapted. Beta-blockers are indicated in hypertensive patients with angina, postmyocardial infarction, and postrevascularization either with balloon angioplasty or coronary bypass grafting. Beta-blockers should be avoided in patients with asthma, chronic obstructive pulmonary disease, or heart block.

2.9.3. ACE-inhibitors

ACE-inhibitors block the RAAS by inhibiting the angiotensin-converting enzyme, leading to less conversion of angiotensin I to angiotensin II. ACE-inhibitors are indicated in hypertensive patients with diabetes mellitus, impaired renal function, microalbuminuria or proteinuria, postmyocardial infarction, coronary artery disease, heart failure, and poststroke. Angioedema is the most severe side effect but very rare. The most frequent side effect is cough. Hyperkalemia is sometimes found if renal function is not monitored. ACE-inhibitors are contraindicated during pregnancy.

2.9.4. Angiotensin II Receptor Blockers

Angiotensin II receptor blockers (ARB) block the RAAS by blocking the angiotensin II type 1 receptor. ARBs are indicated in hypertensive patients with diabetes, impaired renal function, microalbuminuria or proteinuria, postmyocardial infarction, and heart failure. Side effects are rare. Hyperkalemia is sometimes found if renal function is not monitored. ARBS are contraindicated during pregnancy. ARBs have a role in patients who are intolerant to ACE-inhibitors.

2.9.5. Direct Renin Inhibitors

The RAAS blockers (ACE-I and ARB) further activate the RAAS, leading to an increase of plasma renin activity and plasma renin concentration. After decades of research, an oral renin inhibitor, aliskiren, has been developed *(31)*. Aliskiren is the first orally active direct renin inhibitor and is an effective and well-tolerated antihypertensive agent when used in monotherapy or in combination with other antihypertensive agents in patients with mild to moderate hypertension. In contrast with ACE-I and ARBs, aliskiren reduces plasma renin activity. A number of clinical trials with aliskiren are ongoing or completed and provide us with objective evidence regarding the clinical importance of direct renin inhibition in the treatment of cardiovascular disease.

2.9.6. Calcium Channel Blockers

Calcium channel blockers (CCB) are categorized in two groups: dihydropyridines and nondihydropyridines. The nondihydropyridines are verapamil and diltiazem and their slow-releasing preparations. The dihydropyridines are nifedipine (short- and long-acting), nisoldipine, nicardipine, amlodipine, felodipine, and isradipine. They are effective in lowering blood pressure. The most frequent side effects of the dihydropyridines are flushing and ankle edema. Ankle edema can be avoided by administrating the long-acting calcium antagonist at bedtime. The nondihydropyridines have an effect on the sinus node and AV conduction. So, attention needs to be paid in cases of low heart rate or heart block. CCBs also have a negative inotropic effect and, therefore, one needs to be cautious about their use in the presence of heart failure.

2.9.7. Alpha-1 Blockers

Alpha-1 blockers (doxazosin, terazosin) are used in case of prostate hypertrophy. One of the side effects is orthostatic hypotension. In the ALLHAT trial doxazosin was stopped because of an increased number of cardiovascular events.

2.9.8. Central Alpha-2 Agonists and Other Centrally Acting Drugs

The most frequently used in this category are clonidine and methyldopa. Methyldopa is still the most preferred antihypertensive agent during pregnancy because of its extensive record of safety over years. Clonidine is used less these days because of its side effects such as dry mouth, sleepiness, and, last but not the least, its risk for rebound phenomena when stopping it abruptly.

2.9.9. Direct Vasodilators

In cases of severe hypertension, direct vasodilators such as hydralazine and minoxidil can be used. They cause reflex tachycardia and, by stimulating RAAS, they will lead to sodium and fluid retention. Therefore, when hydralazine or minoxidil is used, diuretics should simultaneously be used. Hydralazine and nitrates have been very effective in heart failure in cases of hypertensive cardiomyopathy.

2.10. GUIDELINES FOR TREATMENT OF HYPERTENSION

2.10.1. Joint National Committee VII Guidelines

The therapeutic recommendations in JNC VII are in great part predicated on the findings of ALL-HAT *(29)*. In the meantime, several landmark trials (discussed in the next section) with antihypertensive drugs have not been incorporated into these recommendations. The new highlights are:

1. In those older than age 50, SBP greater than or equal to 140 mmHg is a more important CVD risk factor than DBP.
2. CVD risk doubles for each increment of 20/10 mmHg beginning at 115/75 mmHg.
3. Even those who are normotensive at 55 years of age will have a 90% lifetime risk of developing hypertension.
4. Individuals with prehypertension now defined as SBP 120–139 mmHg or DBP 80–89 mmHg require health-promoting lifestyle modifications to prevent the progressive rise in BP and CVD.
5. In uncomplicated primary hypertension, thiazide diuretics should be used in drug treatment for most, either alone or combined with drugs from other classes. With the evidence we have now, it seems that ACE-I together with dihydropyridines would be more effective in reducing cardiovascular morbidity and mortality.
6. High-risk conditions that are generally defined by concomitant CVD are now recognized as compelling indications for the use of other antihypertensive drug classes (ACEIs, ARBs, beta-blockers, and CCBs).
7. Two or more antihypertensive medications will be required to achieve goal BP (<140/90 mmHg or <130/80 mmHg) for many patients with primary hypertension and those with diabetes and CKD.
8. In patients whose BP is more than 20 mmHg above the SBP goal or more than 10 mmHg above the DBP goal, initiation of therapy using two antihypertensive agents, one of which usually will be a thiazide diuretic, should be considered.
9. Hypertension will be controlled only if patients are motivated to stay on their treatment.

These themes were in part designed to correct persistent and prevalent misperceptions surrounding the treatment of hypertension, including the following: that most cases of hypertension can be controlled with one antihypertensive medication, that DBP is a better indicator than SBP for advancing or intensifying antihypertensive therapy, and that the age-related increase in SBP is normal. A stated goal of JNC VII was to present clinicians with a streamlined, clear, and concise guideline for the classification and management of hypertension. As a result, the classification of hypertension, the integration of CV risk into the treatment paradigm, and treatment recommendations were simplified. Figure 1 shows a simplified algorithm.

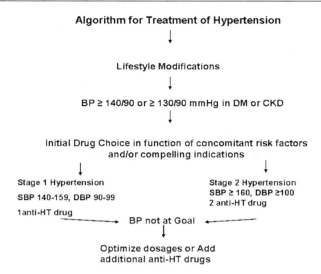

Fig. 1. Treatment of arterial hypertension (simplified from JNC VII). DM = diabetes, CKD = chronic kidney disease, anti-HT = antihypertensive.

2.11. RECENT LANDMARK HYPERTENSION TRIALS: IMPLICATIONS FOR EVIDENCE-BASED MEDICINE

A new series of trials has been completed, and several other trials started in efforts to further elucidate the effects of ACEIs, ARBs, CCBs, and other BP-lowering drugs on mortality and major CV morbidity in several populations of patients, including those with hypertension, diabetes mellitus, CHD, or renal disease.

The overview of placebo-controlled trials of ACEIs revealed 30% reductions in stroke, 20% in CHD, and 21% in major CV events. The overview of placebo-controlled trials of calcium antagonists showed 39% reductions in stroke and 28% in major CV events. In the overview of trials comparing BP-lowering strategies of different intensity, there were reduced risks of stroke (20%), CHD (19%), and major CV events (15%) with more intensive therapy *(32)*. Several landmark trials in hypertension treatment have been published, providing more evidence-based medicine data regarding optimal treatment of hypertension to reduce CV morbidity and mortality.

2.11.1. Intervention as a Goal in Hypertension Treatment

The Intervention as a Goal in Hypertension Treatment (INSIGHT) study was a prospective, randomized, double-blind trial in 6,321 patients, aged 55–80 years with hypertension (BP greater than or equal to 150/95 mmHg, or greater than or equal to 160 mmHg systolic) *(33)*. Patients had at least one additional CV risk factor. Patients were randomly assigned to nifedipine 30 mg in a long-acting gastrointestinal transport system (GITS) formulation, or co-amilozide (hydrochlorothiazide 25 mg plus amiloride 2.5 mg). Dose titration was by dose doubling, and addition of atenolol 25–50 mg or enalapril 5–10 mg. The primary outcome was CV death, myocardial infarction, heart failure, or stroke. Analysis was done by intention to treat. Primary outcomes occurred in 200 (6.3%) of the patients in the nifedipine group and in 182 (5.8%) in the co-amilozide group (18.2 versus 16.5 events per 1,000 patient-years; relative risk 1.10 [95% CI 0.91–1.34], $p = 0.35$). Overall mean BP dropped from 173/99 to 138/82 mmHg. There was an 8% excess of withdrawals from the nifedipine group because of peripheral edema, but serious adverse events were more frequent in the co-amilozide group ($p = 0.02$). Deaths were mainly nonvascular (nifedipine 176 versus co-amilozide 172; $p = 0.81$). Nifedipine once daily and co-amilozide were equally effective in preventing overall CV or cerebrovascular complications.

2.11.2. European Lacidipine Study on Atherosclerosis

The European Lacidipine Study on Atherosclerosis (ELSA) study was a randomized, double-blind trial in 2,334 patients with hypertension that compared the effects of a 4-year treatment based on either lacidipine or atenolol on an index of carotid atherosclerosis, the mean of the maximum intima-media thickness (IMT) in the far walls of the common carotids and bifurcations (CBMmax) *(34)*. The yearly IMT progression rate was 0.0145 mm/year in the atenolol-treated and 0.0087 mm/year in the lacidipine-treated patients (completers, 40% reduction; $p = 0.0073$). Patients with plaque progression were significantly less common, and patients with plaque regression were significantly more common in the lacidipine group. Clinic BP reductions were identical in both treatments, but 24-h ambulatory SBP/DBP changes were greater with atenolol (10/9 mmHg) than with lacidipine (7/5 mmHg). No significant difference between treatments was found in any CV events, although the relative risk for stroke, major CV events, and mortality showed a trend favoring lacidipine. The greater efficacy of lacidipine on carotid IMT progression and number of plaques per patient, despite a smaller ambulatory BP reduction, indicates an antiatherosclerotic action of lacidipine independent of its antihypertensive action.

2.11.3. Comparison of Amlodipine Versus Enalapril to Limit Occurrences of Thrombosis

The Comparison of Amlodipine versus Enalapril to Limit Occurrences of Thrombosis (CAMELOT) study was a double-blind, randomized, multicenter 24-month trial comparing amlodipine or enalapril with placebo in 1991 patients with angiographically documented coronary artery disease (CAD > 20% stenosis by coronary angiography) and DBP less than 100 mmHg *(35)*. A substudy of 274 patients measured atherosclerotic progression by intravascular ultrasound (IVUS). Patients were randomized to receive amlodipine 10 mg, enalapril 20 mg, or placebo. IVUS was performed at baseline and study completion. The primary efficacy parameter was the incidence of CV events for amlodipine versus placebo. Other outcomes included comparisons of amlodipine versus enalapril and enalapril versus placebo. CV events included CV death, nonfatal myocardial infarction, resuscitated cardiac arrest, coronary revascularization, hospitalization for angina pectoris, hospitalization for congestive heart failure, fatal or nonfatal stroke or transient ischemic attack, and new diagnosis of peripheral vascular disease. The IVUS substudy normalized endpoint was change in atheroma volume. Baseline BP averaged 129/78 mmHg for all patients; it increased by 0.7/0.6 mmHg in the placebo group and decreased by 4.8/2.5 mmHg and 4.9/2.4 mmHg in the amlodipine and enalapril groups, respectively ($p < 0.001$ for both versus placebo). CV events occurred in 151 (23.1%) placebo-treated patients, in 110 (16.6%) amlodipine-treated patients (hazard ratio [HR], 0.69; 95% CI, 0.54–0.88, $p = 0.003$), and in 136 (20.2%) enalapril-treated patients (HR, 0.85; 95% CI, 0.67–1.07, $p = 0.16$). Primary endpoint comparison for enalapril versus amlodipine was not significant (HR, 0.81; 95% CI, 0.63–1.04, $p = 0.10$). The IVUS substudy showed a trend toward less progression of atherosclerosis in the amlodipine group versus placebo ($p = 0.12$), with significantly less progression in the subgroup with SBPs greater than the mean ($p = 0.02$). Compared with baseline, IVUS showed progression in the placebo group ($p < 0.001$), a trend toward progression in the enalapril group ($p = 0.08$), and no progression in the amlodipine group ($p = 0.31$). For the amlodipine group, correlation between BP reduction and progression was $r = 0.19$, $p = 0.07$. Administration of amlodipine to patients with CAD and normal BP resulted in a reduction of adverse CV events. Directionally similar, but smaller and nonsignificant treatment effects were observed with enalapril. For amlodipine, IVUS showed evidence of slowing atherosclerosis progression.

2.11.4. Controlled Onset Verapamil Investigation of CV Endpoints

The Controlled Onset Verapamil Investigation of CV Endpoints (CONVINCE) trial was a randomized trial, double-blind, actively controlled multicenter, international clinical trial designed to test the hypothesis of equivalence of two antihypertensive drug regimens, beginning either with controlled-onset, extended-release verapamil or the investigator's preselected choice of either atenolol or hydrochlorothiazide in reducing CV events *(36)*. A total number of 16,602 hypertensive patients were enrolled with one or more additional CV risk factors. The primary objective was to compare the two regimens in preventing acute myocardial infarction, stroke, or CVD-related death. Major secondary outcomes included (1) an expanded CVD endpoint (hospitalization for angina, cardiac revascularization or transplant, heart failure, transient ischemic attacks or carotid endarterectomy, accelerated or malignant hypertension, or renal failure in addition to primary outcome); (2) all cause mortality; (3) cancer; (4) hospitalization for bleeding (excluding hemorrhagic stroke); and (5) incidence of primary endpoints occurring between 6:00 a.m. and noon. The overall results did not differ significantly by treatment group, and the prespecified equivalence criteria were not met. In addition, treatment differences for the major endpoints were consistent for four geographical regions defined a priori—United States, Canada, Western Europe, and "other countries."

2.12. VALSARTAN ANTIHYPERTENSIVE LONG-TERM USE EVALUATION (VALUE) TRIAL

The Valsartan Antihypertensive Long-term Use Evaluation (VALUE) trial was designed to test the hypothesis that for the same BP control, valsartan would reduce cardiac morbidity and mortality more than amlodipine in hypertensive patients at high CV risk *(37, 38)*. A total number of 15,245 patients, aged 50 years or older with treated or untreated hypertension and high risk of cardiac events participated in a randomized, double-blind, parallel-group comparison of therapy based on valsartan or amlodipine. Duration of treatment was event driven and the trial lasted until at least 1,450 patients had reached a primary endpoint, defined as a composite of cardiac mortality and morbidity. Patients from 31 countries were followed up for a mean of 4.2 years. BP was reduced by both treatments, but the effects of the amlodipine-based regimen were more pronounced, especially in the early period (BP 4.0/2.1 mmHg lower in amlodipine than valsartan group after 1 month; 1.5/1.3 mmHg after 1 year; $p < 0.001$ between groups). The primary composite endpoint occurred in 810 patients in the valsartan group (10.6%, 25.5 per 1,000 patient-years) and 789 in the amlodipine group (10.4%, 24.7 per 1,000 patient-years; HR 1.04, 95% CI 0.94–1.15, $p = 0.49$). The main outcome of cardiac disease did not differ between the treatment groups. Unequal reductions in BP might account for differences between the groups in cause-specific outcomes. The findings emphasized the importance of prompt BP control in hypertensive patients at high CV risk. The VALUE trial was designed to test whether, for the same achieved BPs, regimens based on valsartan or amlodipine would have differing effects on CV endpoints in high-risk hypertension. But inequalities in BP favoring amlodipine throughout the multiyear trial limited the comparison of outcomes.

2.13. ANGLO-SCANDINAVIAN CARDIAC OUTCOMES TRIAL (ASCOT)

The apparent shortfall in prevention of CHD noted in early hypertension trials has been attributed to potential metabolic disadvantages of the diuretic and beta-blocker therapy. For a given reduction in BP, some suggested that newer agents would confer advantages over diuretics and beta-blockers. The aim of the Anglo-Scandinavian Cardiac Outcomes Trial (ASCOT) was to compare the effect on nonfatal myocardial infarction and fatal CHD of combinations of atenolol with a thiazide versus amlodipine with perindopril. The ASCOT was a multicenter, prospective, randomized controlled trial in 19,257 patients with hypertension who were aged 40–79 years and had at least three other CV risk factors *(39)*. Patients were assigned either amlodipine 5–10 mg, adding perindopril 4–8 mg as required (amlodipine-based regimen; $n = 9,639$), or atenolol 50–100 mg, adding bendroflume-thiazide 1.25–2.5 mg and potassium as required (atenolol-based regimen; $n = 9,618$). The primary endpoint was nonfatal myocardial infarction (including silent myocardial infarction) and fatal CHD. Analysis was by intention to treat. The study was stopped prematurely by the DSMI after 5.5 years' median follow-up and accumulated in total 106,153 patient-years of observation. Though not significant, compared with the atenolol-based regimen, fewer individuals on the amlodipine-based regimen had a primary endpoint (429 versus 474; unadjusted HR 0.90, 95% CI 0.79–1.02, $p = 0.1052$), fatal and nonfatal stroke (327 versus 422; 0.77, 0.66–0.89, $p = 0.0003$), total CV events and procedures (1,362 versus 1,602; 0.84, 0.78–0.90, $p < 0.0001$), and all cause mortality (738 versus 820; 0.89, 0.81–0.99, $p = 0.025$). The incidence of developing diabetes was less on the amlodipine-based regimen (567 versus 799; 0.70, 0.63–0.78, $p < 0.0001$). The amlodipine-based regimen prevented more major CV events and induced less diabetes than the atenolol-based regimen.

2.13.1. Conduit Artery Function Evaluation (CAFE) Trial

Different BP-lowering drugs could have different effects on central aortic pressures and, thus, CV outcome despite similar effects on brachial BP. The Conduit Artery Function Evaluation (CAFE) study, a substudy of ASCOT, examined the impact of two different BP-lowering regimens (atenolol thiazide-based versus amlodipine–perindopril-based therapy) on derived central aortic pressures and hemodynamics. The CAFE study recruited 2,199 patients in five ASCOT centers *(40)*. Radial artery applanation tonometry and pulse wave analysis were used to derive central aortic pressures and hemodynamic indexes on repeated visits for up to 4 years. Most patients received combination therapy throughout the study. Despite similar brachial SBPs between treatment groups (Δ 0.7 mmHg; 95% CI, 0.4–1.7; $p = 0.2$), there were substantial reductions in central aortic pressures with the amlodipine regimen (central aortic SBP, Δ 4.3 mmHg; 95% CI, 3.3–5.4; $p < 0.0001$; central aortic PP, Δ 3.0 mmHg; 95% CI, 2.1–3.9; $p < 0.0001$). Cox proportional hazards modeling showed that central PP was significantly associated with a post-hoc-defined composite outcome of total CV events/procedures and development of renal impairment in the CAFE cohort (unadjusted, $p < 0.0001$; adjusted for baseline variables, $p < 0.05$). BP-lowering drugs can have substantially different effects on central aortic pressures and hemodynamics despite a similar impact on brachial BP. Moreover, central aortic PP may be a determinant of clinical outcomes, and differences in central aortic pressures may be a potential mechanism to explain the different clinical outcomes between the two BP treatment arms in ASCOT.

2.14. TRIAL OF PREVENTION OF HYPERTENSION (TROPHY)

Prehypertension is considered a precursor of Stage I hypertension and a predictor of excessive CV risk. The Trial of Preventing Hypertension (TROPHY) studied whether pharmacologic treatment of prehypertension prevents or postpones Stage I hypertension *(41)*. Participants with repeated measurements of systolic pressure of 130–139 mmHg and diastolic pressure of 89 mmHg or lower, or systolic pressure of 139 mmHg or lower and diastolic pressure of 85–89 mmHg, were randomly assigned to receive 2 years of candesartan or placebo, followed by 2 years of placebo for all. When a participant reached the study endpoint of Stage I hypertension, treatment with antihypertensive agents was initiated. Both the candesartan group and the placebo group were instructed to make changes in lifestyle to reduce BP throughout the trial. A total of 409 participants were randomly assigned to candesartan and 400 to placebo. Data on 772 participants (391 in the candesartan group and 381 in the placebo group; mean age, 48.5 years; 59.6% men) were available for analysis. During the first 2 years, hypertension developed in 154 participants in the placebo group and 53 of those in the candesartan group (relative risk reduction, 66.3%; $p < 0.001$). After 4 years, hypertension had developed in 240 participants in the placebo group and 208 of those in the candesartan group (relative risk reduction, 15.6%; $p < 0.007$). Over a period of 4 years, Stage I hypertension developed in nearly two thirds of patients with untreated prehypertension (the placebo group). Treatment of prehypertension with candesartan appeared to be well tolerated and reduced the risk of incident hypertension during the study period. Thus, treatment of prehypertension appears to be feasible. However, we need to learn who should be treated, for how many years, and with which drug and at what dose. For now, a healthy lifestyle is the foundation for all therapies in persons with prehypertension. This is still true even after the lessons of the TROPHY study.

2.15. ACCOMPLISH TRIAL

The optimal combination drug therapy for hypertension is not established, although current US guidelines recommend inclusion of a diuretic. The ACCOMPLISH trial hypothesized that treatment with the combination of an angiotensin-converting enzyme (ACE) inhibitor and a dihydropyridine calcium channel blocker would be more effective in reducing the rate of cardiovascular events than treatment with an ACE-inhibitor plus a thiazide diuretic (42). In a randomized, double-blind trial, we assigned 11,506 patients with hypertension who were at high risk for cardiovascular events to receive treatment with either benazepril plus amlodipine or benazepril plus hydrochlorothiazide. The primary endpoint was the composite of death from cardiovascular causes, nonfatal myocardial infarction, nonfatal stroke, hospitalization for angina, resuscitation after sudden cardiac arrest, and coronary revascularization. The trial was terminated early after a mean follow-up of 36 months, when the boundary of the prespecified stopping rule was exceeded. Mean blood pressures after dose adjustment were 131.6/73.3 mmHg in the benazepril–amlodipine group and 132.5/74.4 mmHg in the benazepril–hydrochlorothiazide group. There were 552 primary-outcome events in the benazepril–amlodipine group (9.6%) and 679 in the benazepril–hydrochlorothiazide group (11.8%), representing an absolute risk reduction with benazepril–amlodipine therapy of 2.2% and a relative risk reduction of 19.6% (hazard ratio, 0.80, 95% confidence interval [CI], 0.72–0.90; $p < 0.001$). For the secondary endpoint of death from cardiovascular causes, nonfatal myocardial infarction, and nonfatal stroke the hazard ratio was 0.79 (95% CI, 0.67–0.92; $p = 0.002$). Rates of adverse events were consistent with those observed from clinical experience with the study drugs. In conclusion, the benazepril–amlodipine combination was superior to the benazepril–hydrochlorothiazide combination in reducing cardiovascular events in patients with hypertension who were at high risk for such events.

2.16. HYVET

Whether the treatment of patients with hypertension who are 80 years of age or older is beneficial is unclear. It has been suggested that antihypertensive therapy may reduce the risk of stroke, despite possibly increasing the risk of death. In the HYVET trial 3,845 patients who were 80 years of age or older and had a sustained systolic blood pressure of 160 mmHg or more were randomly assigned to either the diuretic indapamide (sustained release, 1.5 mg) or matching placebo (43). The angiotensin-converting enzyme inhibitor perindopril (2 or 4 mg), or matching placebo, was added if necessary to achieve the target blood pressure of 150/80 mmHg. The primary endpoint was fatal or nonfatal stroke. The active-treatment group (1,933 patients) and the placebo group (1,912 patients) were well matched (mean age, 83.6 years; mean blood pressure while sitting, 173.0/90.8 mmHg); 11.8% had a history of cardiovascular disease. Median follow-up was 1.8 years. At 2 years, the mean blood pressure while sitting was 15.0/6.1 mmHg lower in the active-treatment group than in the placebo group. In an intention-to-treat analysis, active treatment was associated with a 30% reduction in the rate of fatal or nonfatal stroke (95% confidence interval [CI], 1–51; $p = 0.06$), a 39% reduction in the rate of death from stroke (95% CI, 1–62; $p = 0.05$), a 21% reduction in the rate of death from any cause (95% CI, 4–35; $p = 0.02$), a 23% reduction in the rate of death from cardiovascular causes (95% CI, 1–40; $p = 0.06$), and a 64% reduction in the rate of heart failure (95% CI, 42–78; $p < 0.001$). Fewer serious adverse events were reported in the active-treatment group (358 versus 448 in the placebo group; $p = 0.001$). The results of the HYVET trial provide evidence that antihypertensive treatment with indapamide (sustained release), with or without perindopril, in persons 80 years of age or older is beneficial.

2.17. ON TARGET

In patients who have vascular disease or high-risk diabetes without heart failure, angiotensin-converting enzyme (ACE) inhibitors reduce mortality and morbidity from cardiovascular causes, but the role of angiotensin-receptor blockers (ARBs) in such patients is unknown. The ON TARGET trial was a comparison between the ACE-inhibitor ramipril, the ARB telmisartan, and the combination of the two drugs in patients with vascular disease or high-risk diabetes (44). After a 3-week, single-blind run-in period, patients underwent double-blind randomization, with 8,576 assigned to receive 10 mg of ramipril per day, 8,542 assigned to receive 80 mg of telmisartan per day, and 8,502 assigned to receive both drugs (combination therapy). The primary composite outcome was death from cardiovascular causes, myocardial infarction, stroke, or hospitalization for heart failure. Mean blood pressure was lower in both the telmisartan group (a 0.9/0.6 mmHg greater reduction) and the combination-therapy group (a 2.4/1.4 mmHg greater reduction) than in the ramipril group. At a median follow-up of 56 months, the primary outcome had occurred in 1,412 patients in the ramipril group (16.5%), as compared with 1,423 patients in the telmisartan group (16.7%; relative risk, 1.01; 95% confidence interval [CI], 0.94–1.09). As compared with the ramipril group, the telmisartan group had lower rates of cough (1.1% versus 4.2%, $p < 0.001$) and angioedema (0.1% versus 0.3%, $p = 0.01$) and a higher rate of hypotensive symptoms (2.6% versus 1.7%, $p < 0.001$); the rate of syncope was the same in the two groups (0.2%). In the combination-therapy group, the primary outcome occurred in 1,386 patients (16.3%; relative risk, 0.99; 95% CI, 0.92–1.07); as compared with the ramipril group, there was an increased risk of hypotensive symptoms (4.8% versus 1.7%, $p < 0.001$), syncope (0.3% versus 0.2%, $p = 0.03$), and renal dysfunction (13.5% versus 10.2%, $p < 0.001$). The results showed that telmisartan was equivalent to ramipril in patients with vascular disease or high-risk diabetes and was associated with less angioedema. The combination of the two drugs was associated with more adverse events without an increase in benefit. This study is very helpful in the establishment of new hypertension guidelines.

In conclusion, diagnosis and treatment of arterial hypertension remains a challenge. Since the JNC VII guidelines were published, there has been a large number of new landmark trials that provide significant new insights into how hypertension can be managed in the most efficacious manner possible.

2.18. CASE STUDIES

2.18.1. Case Study 1—Hypertensive Emergency

A 52-year-old white women presents to the emergency room with complaints of severe headache with a severity of 9/10, blurred vision, and shortness of breath. She smokes about a half pack cigarettes/day. She has a family history of arterial hypertension and stroke. She is 3 year postmenopausal. Her blood pressure was measured the past years sporadically and varied between 135 and 160 mmHg systolic and 85 and 95 mmHg diastolic. However, the patient was reluctant to take antihypertensive medication beyond salt restriction and dietary advice, which was not followed very well.

Physical examination in the emergency room revealed:

Blood pressure right arm: 226/118 mmHg; blood pressure left arm: 230/120 mmHg
Pulse: 66 bpm
BMI: 29.2 kg/m^2
Physical exam: alert and awake
Head and neck: no carotid bruits, no jugular vein distension
Heart: prominent S2, regular rhythm, no bruit
Lung: few basilar crackles
Abdomen: no bruits over renal arteries
Extremities: decreased pulses at both tibial arteries 3+/4
Neurological exam: normal
Optic fundi: retinal bleedings

2.18.1.1. Laboratory Data (Initial Tests)

Sodium 138 mEq/L (136–145)
Potassium 4.1 mEq/L (3.5–5.0)
Chloride 110 mEq/L (98–110)
Calcium 9.2 mEq/L (8.8–10.0)
Blood urea nitrogen 23.0 mg/dL (8.0–22.0)
Creatinine 1.3 mg/dL (0.5–1.2)
eGFR 46 mL/min/1.73 m^2
Glucose 118 mg/dL (70–110)

2.18.1.2. Issues and Discussion Points

2.18.1.2.1. What Is the Difference Between a Hypertensive Emergency and Urgency?   Hypertensive emergencies require prompt recognition and thoughtful management in order to reduce the morbidity and mortality associated with severe hypertension. BP reduction typically is begun within minutes to hours of diagnosis and is frequently required to prevent worsening of an underlying clinical condition.

The term "hypertensive urgency" refers to a clinical presentation of severe hypertension where the SBP is usually more than 200 mmHg and/or the DBP is usually more than 120 mmHg. These patients are generally asymptomatic and do not have evidence of acute target organ damage. BP lowering may occur over hours to days in the absence of acute target organ damage or serious comorbid disease.

2.18.1.2.2. How Would You Manage This Hypertensive Emergency Case?   Treatment of hypertensive emergency needs to be tailored to each individual patient and presentation. Prompt and rapid reduction of BP under continuous surveillance is essential in patients who are symptomatic and have acute end-organ damage. Parenteral therapy, typically in a monitored bed in the intensive care unit, is recommended for the treatment of most hypertensive emergencies. Sodium nitroprusside is the "gold standard" for treating hypertensive emergencies and the agent to which other parenteral agents are measured.

Repeated intravenous injections ("mini bolus" of 10–20 mg) of the combined alpha- and beta-adrenergic receptor-blocking agent labetalol can produce a prompt but gradual reduction of arterial BP without the induction of a reflex tachycardia. Repeated intravenous injections ("mini bolus" of 10–20 mg) of the combined alpha- and beta-adrenergic receptor-blocking agent labetalol can produce a prompt but gradual reduction of arterial BP without the induction of a reflex tachycardia. This patient received a sodium nitroprusside infusion and also a bolus of furosemide because of the development of acute heart failure.

2.18.1.2.3. Which Tests Do You Perform in Cases of Hypertensive Emergency/Urgency? The patient needs an extensive workup with a blood exam (CBC, basic metabolic panel consisting of electrolytes, renal parameters, glucose, lipid profile, and thyroid function). A urine evaluation for microalbuminuria or proteinuria is mandatory as well for cell casts. An ECG is done to rule out rhythm abnormalities, myocardial ischemia, and left ventricular hypertrophy. An echocardiogram provides information about myocardial and valvular function. Depending upon clinical symptoms and physical examination findings, ancillary tests will be performed to rule secondary causes of secondary hypertension.

2.18.1.2.4. Which Chronic Antihypertensive Therapy? In addition to the nitroprusside infusion and intravenous furosemide during the first 24 h, a beta-blocker (metoprolol) was started together with the calcium antagonist amlodipine at bedtime (evening dosing of this medication reduces lower extremity edema compared to giving it in the morning). An ACE-inhibitor was also started in a low dose beyond oral furosemide. A renal panel and electrolytes were checked during follow-up. The patient was provided extensive information to quit smoking. Because of the presence of hypercholesterolemia and hypertension, statin therapy was started. The patient was also started on aspirin therapy as well because during the workup, the patient was diagnosed with peripheral arterial disease.

2.18.2. Case Study 2—Chronic Poorly Controlled Hypertension with Patient Referred to a Hypertension Specialist

A 61-year-old African-American male with arterial hypertension for 25 years is referred to a hypertension specialist clinic because of resistant hypertension. He feels tired and has COPD. He quit smoking about 1 year ago. He has received several antihypertensive medications to lower his blood pressure including hydrochlorothiazide, chlorthalidone, nadolol, atenolol, metoprolol, alpha-methyldopa, clonidine, nifedipine, felodipine, captopril, and hydralazine in different combinations and at several doses. However, blood pressure never reached goal, especially systolic blood pressure, which varied between 140–160 mmHg despite different antihypertensive regimen and between 85 and 95 mmHg for the diastolic blood pressure.

Family history: mother died from a stroke at age 63 years and father died from sudden cardiac death at age 59 years. Multiple siblings have hypertension.

Physical examination:

Blood pressure right arm: 158/90 mmHg; Blood pressure left arm: 154/92 mmHg
Pulse: 74 bpm
BMI: 28.7 kg/m^2
Head and neck: bruit at right common carotid artery, no jugular vein distension
Heart: systolic murmur 1/6 left parasternal border
Lung: decreased breath sounds
Abdomen: no bruits over renal arteries
Extremities: decreased pulses at both dorsal and tibial posterior arteries
Neurological exam: normal

2.18.2.1. LABORATORY TESTS

Sodium 137 mEq/L (136–145)
Potassium 3.7 mEq/L (3.5–5.0)
Chloride 107 mEq/L (98–110)
Calcium 9.2 mEq/L (8.8–10.0)
Blood urea nitrogen 25.0 mg/dL (8.0–22.0)
Creatinine 1.32 mg/dL (0.5–1.2)

eGFR 71 mL/min/1.73 m^2
Glucose 114 mg/dL (70–110)
Total cholesterol 248 mg/dL (<200)
LDL-cholesterol 147 mg/dL (<130)
HDL-cholesterol 39 mg/dL (>40)
Triglycerides 156 mg/dL (<150)
Albuminuria/creatinine ratio (μg/mg) 32

2.18.2.2. ISSUES AND DISCUSSION POINTS

2.18.2.2.1. What Is Resistant Hypertension?   Resistant or "hard-to-treat" hypertension is generally defined as the failure to achieve a therapeutic target of less than 140/90 mmHg in most hypertensive patients, or less than 130/80 mmHg in diabetics or patients with chronic kidney disease, on a well-designed three-drug antihypertensive medical regimen combined with intensive lifestyle modification diuretic therapy. In most cases, resistant hypertension is now defined on the basis of a persistently high systolic blood pressure level.

2.18.2.2.2. Which Antihypertensive Treatment Plan Do You Establish?   The antihypertensive regimen for this patient was constructed on the following basis: African-American hypertensive patients react very well to diuretics and calcium antagonists. Therefore, we recommended hydrochlorothiazide 25 mg/day and amlodipine 10 mg at bedtime. Because of his extensive COPD and prediabetes he was not given a beta-blocker. The patient was continued on lisinopril 20 mg/day. Resistant hypertensive patients respond very well to aldosterone antagonists. This patient was given spironolactone 12.5 mg/day and was followed-up with electrolytes and renal function indices within 1 week. Arterial blood pressure after 1 week was 148/82 mmHg. Because it is known that African Americans have endothelial dysfunction and often have a decreased synthesis of nitric oxide, we added isosorbide dinitrate 30 mg/day in the morning. It is known that nitrates effectively lower central aortic blood pressure more than peripheral pressure and have a beneficial effect on systolic blood pressure. As a consequence blood pressure decreased to 135/78 mmHg. The patient also received statin therapy and aspirin (81 mg/day).

2.18.2.2.3. Should We Go for a Tailored Antihypertensive Therapy?   There is a change in the concept that arterial hypertension is an expression of an already-existing vascular disease in which endothelial dysfunction is often the beginning detrimental factor. When arterial hypertension is diagnosed, there are often concomitant risk factors and target organ damage such as microalbuminuria, left ventricular hypertrophy, and carotid artery disease. Many hypertensive patients have type 2 diabetes or the metabolic syndrome. Therefore, the choice of antihypertensive therapy needs to be directed not only by the blood pressure lowering effect, but also by its capacity to reduce insulin resistance or to provide renal protection.

2.18.2.2.4. Should We Titrate Antihypertensive Therapy to a Maximum Dose or Start Earlier with Combination Therapy?   Several studies have shown that combination therapy is more effective in controlling arterial blood pressure than uptitrating to the maximal dose of an antihypertensive medication and if the goal is not reached to add an additional blood pressure lowering pill. The advantage to start with combination therapy is that the dose of each blood pressure lowering medication can be kept at a lower dose and, consequently, there is a lower risk for side effects. The simplicity of combination therapy favors fewer pills and a greater potential for therapeutic adherence as well as less expense. Moreover, we need to realize that the majority of hypertensive patients need lipid-lowering therapy and a large group also requires treatment for diabetes.

2.18.2.2.5. Do Efficacy and Adverse Effects of Hypertension Treatment Differ by Race?

Randomized trials demonstrate that antihypertensive medications can control hypertension and prevent complications in African Americans and Caucasians. Meta-analyses have shown that African Americans demonstrate reduced blood pressure responses to monotherapy with β(beta)-blockers, angiotensin-converting enzyme inhibitors, or angiotensin-receptor blockers, compared with diuretics or calcium channel blockers. These differences are usually eliminated by adding adequate doses of a diuretic.

There is also evidence that a DASH (Dietary Approaches to Stop Hypertension) and salt-reducing diet can have a more significant blood pressure reducing effect in African Americans compared with Caucasians.

The combination of isosorbide dinitrate with hydralazine has shown a significant effect in risk reduction in cardiovascular morbidity and mortality in heart failure in an African-American population who were already treated with the standard therapy for heart failure.

REFERENCES

1. Cohn JN. Arteries, myocardium, blood pressure and cardiovascular risk towards a revised definition of hypertension. *J Hypertens.* 1998;16:2117–2124.
2. Lloyd-Jones DM, Leip EP, Larson MG, Vasan RS, Levy D. Novel approach to examining first cardiovascular events after hypertension onset. *Hypertension.* 2005;45:39–45.
3. Giles TD, Berk BC, Black HR, et al. Expanding the definition and classification of hypertension. *J Clin Hypertens.* 2005;7:505–512.
4. Lewington S, Clarke R, Quizilbash N, Peto R, Collins R. Age-specific relevance of usual blood pressure to vascular mortality: a meta-analysis of individual data for one million adults in 61 prospective studies. *Lancet.* 2002;360:1903–1913.
5. Hajjar I, Kotchen TA. Trends in prevalence, awareness, treatment, and control of hypertension in the United States, 1988–2000. *JAMA.* 2003;290:199–206.
6. Freis ED. Studies in hemodynamics and hypertension. *Hypertension.* 2001;38:1–5.
7. Duprez DA, Kaiser DR, Whitwam W, et al. Determinants of radial artery pulse wave analysis in asymptomatic individuals. *Am J Hypertens.* 2004;17:647–653.
8. Guyton AC. Dominant role of the kidneys and accessory role of whole-body autoregulation in the pathogenesis of hypertension. *Am J Hypertens.* 1989;2:575–585.
9. Duprez DA. Role of the renin–angiotensin–aldosterone system in vascular remodeling and inflammation: a clinical review. *J Hypertension.* 2006;24:983–991.
10. Pepe S, Lakatta EG. Aging hearts and vessels: masters of adaptation and survival. *Cardiovasc Res.* 2005;66:190–193.
11. Textor SC, Wilcox CS. Renal artery stenosis: a common, treatable cause of renal failure. *Annu Rev Med.* 2001;52:421–442.
12. Williams JS, Williams GH, Raji A, et al. Prevalence of primary hyperaldosteronism in mild to moderate hypertension without hypokalaemia. *J Hum Hypertens.* 2006;20:129–136.
13. Lenders JW, Pacak K, Walther MM, et al. Biochemical diagnosis of pheochromocytoma, which test is best. *JAMA.* 2002;287:1427–1434.
14. Calhoun DA, Jones D, Textor S, et al. Resistant hypertension: diagnosis, evaluation, and treatment: a scientific statement from the American Heart Association Professional Education Committee of the Council for High Blood Pressure Research. *Circulation.* 2008;117:e510–e526.
15. Calhoun D. Use of aldosterone antagonists in resistant hypertension. *Prog Cardiovasc Dis.* 2006;48:387–396.
16. Elliott-William J. Clinical features in the management of selected hypertensive emergencies. *Prog Cardiovasc Dis.* 2006;48:316–325.
17. Joint National Committee on Prevention, Detection, Evaluation, and Treatment of High Blood Pressure. Seventh report of the Joint National Committee on prevention, detection, evaluation, and treatment of high blood pressure. *JAMA.* 2003;289:2560–2572.
18. World Health Organization–International Society of Hypertension Guidelines for the Management of Hypertension. Guidelines subcommittee. *J Hypertens.* 1999;17:151–183.
19. American Heart Association. Recommendations for human blood pressure determination by sphygmomanometers. Report of a special task force appointed by the steering committee. *Hypertension.* 1988;11:210A–222A.

20. O'Brien E, Asmar R, Beilin L, et al. On behalf of the European Society of Hypertension Working Group on blood pressure monitoring. Practice guidelines of the European Society of hypertension for clinic, ambulatory and self blood pressure measurement. *J Hypertension.* 2005;23:697–701.

21. Pickering TG, Shimbo D, Haas D. Ambulatory blood-pressure monitoring. *N Engl J Med.* 2006;354:2368–2374.

22. Clement DL, De Buyzere M, De Bacquer DA, et al. Prognostic value of ambulatory blood-pressure recordings in patients with treated hypertension. *N Engl J Med.* 2003;348:2407–2415.

23. White WB. Ambulatory blood-pressure monitoring in clinical practice. *N Engl J Med.* 2003;348:2377–2378.

24. Chobanian AV, Bakris GL, Black HR, et al. National High Blood Pressure Education Program Coordinating Committee. The Seventh Report of the Joint National Committee on prevention, detection, evaluation, and treatment of high blood pressure. The JNC 7 report. *JAMA.* 2003;289:3560–3572.

25. Mancia G, De Backer G, Dominiczak A, et al. ESH-ESC practice guidelines for the management of arterial hypertension: ESH-ESC task force on the management of arterial hypertension. *J Hypertens.* 2007;25:1751–1762.

26. Expert Panel on Detection, Evaluation, and Treatment of High Blood Cholesterol in Adults. Executive summary of the third report of the National Cholesterol Education Program (NCEP) expert panel on detection, evaluation, and treatment of high blood cholesterol in adults (Adult Treatment Panel III). *JAMA.* 2001;285:2486–2497.

27. He J, Whelton PK, Appel LJ, Charleston J, Klag MJ. Long-term effects of weight loss and dietary sodium reduction on incidence of hypertension. *Hypertension.* 2000;35:544–549.

28. Sacks FM, Svetkey LP, Vollmer WM, et al. For the DASH-Sodium Collaborative Research Group. Effects on blood pressure of reduced dietary sodium and the dietary approaches to stop hypertension (DASH) diet. *N Engl J Med.* 2001;344:3–10.

29. Officers ALLHAT. Coordinators for the ALLHAT Collaborative Research Group. Major outcomes in high-risk hypertensive patients randomized to angiotensin-converting enzyme inhibitor or calcium channel blocker vs diuretic. The antihypertensive and lipid-lowering treatment to prevent heart attack trial (ALLHAT). *JAMA.* 2002;288:2981–2997.

30. Moser M. Physician or clinical inertia: what is it? Is it really a problem? And what can be done about it. *J Clin Hypertens.* 2009;11:1–4.

31. Duprez DA. Aliskiren: the next innovation in renin-angiotensin-aldosterone system blockade. *Aging Health.* 2009;5:269–279.

32. Blood Pressure Lowering Treatment Trialists' Collaboration. Effects of ACE inhibitors, calcium antagonists, and other blood-pressure-lowering drugs. *Lancet.* 2000;356:1955–1964.

33. Brown MJ, Palmer CR, Castaigne A, et al. Morbidity and mortality in patients randomized to doubleblind treatment with a long-acting calcium-channel blocker or diuretic in the International Nifedipine GITS study: intervention as a goal in hypertension treatment (INSIGHT). *Lancet.* 2000;356:366–372.

34. Zanchetti A, Bond G, Hennig M, et al. Calcium antagonist slows down progression of asymptomatic carotid atherosclerosis. Principal results of the European Lacidipine study on atherosclerosis (ELSA), a randomised, double-blind, long-term trial. *Circulation.* 2002;106:2422–2427.

35. Nissen SE, Tuczu EM, Libby P, et al. Effect of antihypertensive agents on cardiovascular events in patients with coronary artery disease and normal blood pressure. The CAMELOT Study: a randomized controlled trial. *JAMA.* 2004;292:2217–2226.

36. Black HR, Elliott WJ, Grandits G, et al. Principal results of the Controlled ONset Verapamil INvestigation of Cardiovascular Endpoints (CONVINCE) trial. *JAMA.* 2003;289:2073–2082.

37. Julius S, Kjelden SE, Weber M, et al. Outcomes in hypertensive patients at high cardiovascular risk treated with regimens based on valsartan or amlodipine: the VALUE randomised trial. *Lancet.* 2004;363:2022–2031.

38. Weber MA, Julius S, Kjeldsen SE, et al. Blood pressure dependent and independent effects of antihypertensive treatment on clinical events in the VALUE trial. *Lancet.* 2004;363:2049–2051.

39. Dahlöf B, Sever PS, Poulter NR, et al. Prevention of cardiovascular events with an antihypertensive regimen of amlodipine adding perindopril as required versus atenolol adding bendroflumethiazide as required, in the Anglo-Scandinavian cardiac outcomes trial-blood pressure lowering arm (ASCOT-BPLA): a multicentre randomised controlled trial. *Lancet.* 2005;366:895–906.

40. Williams B, Lacy PS, Thom SM, et al. Differential impact of blood pressure-lowering drugs on central aortic pressure and clinical outcomes. *Circulation.* 2006;113:1213–1215.

41. Julius S, Nesbitt SD, Egan BM, et al. Feasibility of treating prehypertension with an angiotensin receptor blocker. *N Engl J Med.* 2006;354:1685–1697.

42. Jamerson K, Weber MA, Bakris GL, et al. Benazepril plus amlodipine or hydrochlorothiazide for hypertension in high-risk patients. *N Engl J Med.* 2008;359:2417–2428.

43. Beckett NS, Peters R, Fletcher AE, et al. Treatment of hypertension in patients 80 years of age or older. *N Engl J Med.* 2008;358:1887–1898.

44. ONTARGET Investigators, Yusuf S, Teo KK, Pogue J, et al. Telmisartan, ramipril, or both in patients at high risk for vascular events. *N Engl J Med.* 2008;358:1547–1559.

3   Management of Dyslipidemia

Peter P. Toth

CONTENTS

Key Words: Cholesterol; Chylomicron; Fibrate; Lipoproteins; Triglyceride; Statin.

KEY POINTS

- Dyslipidemia is a highly heterogeneous class of metabolic disorders. The etiologies of dyslipidemias depend upon specific metabolic backgrounds (e.g., insulin resistance, thyroid dysfunction) as well as abnormalities in the gastrointestinal absorption of cholesterol and lipids and mutations in cell surface receptors and enzymes in pathways regulating lipid metabolism.
- Dyslipidemia is a widely prevalent risk factor for CAD and all forms of atherosclerotic disease. It is associated with elevations in serum LDL-C, non-HDL-C, lipoprotein(a), and triglycerides, and low levels of HDL-C.
- When making the diagnosis of dyslipidemia, it is important to rule out and treat secondary causes of dyslipidemia, such as alcoholism, thyroid dysfunction, metabolic syndrome, diabetes mellitus, and nephrotic syndrome, among others.
- A complete 10–12-h fasting lipoprotein profile should be performed on patients undergoing screening for dyslipidemia.
- The diagnosis of dyslipidemia requires comprehensive, global cardiovascular risk evaluation with 10-year Framingham risk estimation. Target levels for LDL-C and non-HDL-C are risk stratified. An HDL-C <40 mg/dL is a categorical risk factor for CAD.
- Dyslipidemia is a *modifiable* risk factor.
- LDL-C reduction is the primary goal of lipid-modifying therapy.
- Lifestyle modification is the first-line therapy for all patients with dyslipidemia. However, based on specific individual circumstances, health care providers may deem it essential to initiate lifestyle modi-

From: *Contemporary Cardiology: Comprehensive Cardiovascular Medicine in the Primary Care Setting*
Edited by: Peter P. Toth, Christopher P. Cannon, DOI 10.1007/978-1-60327-963-5_3
© Springer Science+Business Media, LLC 2010

fication simultaneous with pharmacologic intervention, as in patients with an acute coronary syndrome or patients with established coronary artery disease.

- In patients with low HDL-C, therapeutic interventions should be made to increase the level of this lipoprotein as much as possible.
- Dyslipidemia can be treated with statins, fibrates, niacin, thiazolidenediones, ezetimibe, bile acid-binding resins, omega-3 fish oils, and combinations thereof.
- The treatment of dyslipidemia in both the primary and secondary prevention settings should always be done in tandem with the aggressive identification and management of all risk factors patients present, including hypertension, diabetes mellitus, obesity, cigarette smoking, as well as nephropathy and chronic kidney disease.

3.1. INTRODUCTION

An estimated 16 million adults in the United States have coronary heart disease (CHD), which accounts for more deaths than any single cause or group of causes of death in the United States *(1)*. Atherosclerosis is a complex, multifactorial disease. Over the course of the past five decades, numerous prospective observational cohort studies have established beyond any doubt that risk for atherosclerotic disease is driven by a number of risk factors, which include dyslipidemia, hypertension, insulin resistance and diabetes mellitus, obesity, cigarette smoking, and age *(2–6)*. The greater the burden of risk factors, the higher the likelihood for developing such manifestations of atherosclerosis as coronary artery disease (CAD), carotid artery disease, and peripheral arterial disease. Atherosclerotic disease is unequivocally associated with increased risk for myocardial infarction, stroke, renal artery disease and renal insufficiency, claudication and lower extremity amputation, and death. Progressive accumulation of lipid in arterial walls is a cardinal structural manifestation of atherosclerotic disease. Arresting this process of lipid infiltration and retention is an important goal in modern cardiovascular medicine.

Dyslipidemia is characterized by abnormalities in serum levels of a variety of lipoproteins. Dyslipidemia is frequently described as "mixed," in that it simultaneously involves abnormalities in multiple components of the lipid profile. Dyslipidemia is highly prevalent in industrialized nations. Dyslipidemia is the product of suboptimal diet, obesity, sedentary lifestyle, as well as abnormalities in metabolism and genetic background. Hundreds of polymorphisms in the genes regulating lipid biosynthetic enzymes, serum lipases, and cell surface receptors give rise to many patterns of dyslipidemia, which require highly individualized approaches to therapy. The role of lipid modification therapy in both the primary and secondary prevention settings is one of the most intensively studied issues in modern medicine. Aggressive, sustained lipid management reduces risk for cardiovascular morbidity and mortality. Dyslipidemia is a modifiable risk factor and can be treated with a variety of strategies, including lifestyle modification measures and pharmacologic therapy using drugs such as statins, fibrates, niacin, and combinations thereof. This chapter will review principles of lipid metabolism and dyslipidemia management.

3.2. LIPOPROTEIN METABOLISM AND ATHEROGENESIS

3.2.1. Low-Density Lipoprotein and Very Low-Density Lipoprotein

Cholesterol and lipids such as phospholipids, triglycerides, and cholesterol esters serve diverse purposes in biological systems. Lipids are an important source of energy, are critical structural components of cell membranes, and function in a variety of cellular signaling pathways. Derangements in cholesterol and lipid metabolism induce the development and progression of atherosclerosis. Cholesterol, monoglycerides, free fatty acids, and phospholipids arising from both dietary and biliary sources are absorbed from micelles in the intestinal lumen via a series of translocators located within the brush border of jejunal enterocytes (Fig. 1). Absorbed cholesterol and lipid are assimilated with

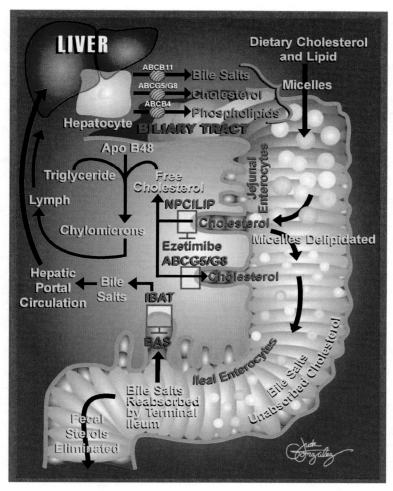

Fig. 1. Micelle formation and lipid and bile acid transport in the gastrointestinal tract. Dietary and biliary sources of cholesterol and lipid are solubilized in micelles in the gastrointestinal lumen. Hepatocytes use a variety of adenosine 5′-triphosphate (ATP)-binding membrane cassette (ABC) transport proteins along their canalicular surface to transport cholesterol (ABCG5/G8), bile salts (ABCB11), and phospholipids (ABCB4) from the cytosol into the biliary tract where these species can assimilate through a combination of saponification and thermodynamic driving forces to form micelles. Micelles move down the GI tract and deliver cholesterol and lipid (triglycerides and phospholipids) to specific translocases along the intestinal epithelium for absorption and systemic distribution. Cholesterol and plant sterols (e.g., beta-sitosterol) can be taken up by the Niemann–Pick C1-like 1 protein expressed along the jejunal brush border. This transporter is inhibited by ezetimibe. Once absorbed, the cholesterol can either be packaged into chylomicrons with triglycerides and apoprotein B48 and transported via the lymphatics to the central circulation, or transported back into the gut lumen via the activity of ABCG5/G8. Bile salts are reabsorbed in the terminal ileum by the ileal apical sodium bile acid cotransporter. This transporter facilitates the reentry of bile salts into the portal circulation and, ultimately, the hepatic bile salt pool. The bile acid sequestration agents interrupt this uptake process and restrict the enterohepatic recirculation of bile salts and promote their fecal elimination.

apoprotein B48 (apoB48) to form chylomicrons. Chylomicrons are released into the lymphatic system and ultimately transported to the central circulation via the thoracic duct. The triglycerides in chylomicrons are hydrolyzed by lipoprotein lipase, and this reaction produces chylomicron remnant particles, which are taken up by receptors along the hepatocyte surface. The liver secretes very low-density lipoprotein (VLDL), a lipoprotein enriched with triglycerides, cholesterol, and apoprotein B100 (apoB100). As the triglycerides in VLDL are hydrolyzed by lipoprotein lipase, the size of the lipoprotein particle decreases, yielding intermediate-density lipoprotein and then low-density lipoprotein (LDL) particles. LDL particles are concentrated with cholesterol and cholesterol esters and relatively depleted of triglycerides. LDL is not secreted directly from hepatocytes; rather, it is a by-product of VLDL metabolism. As the VLDL is progressively converted to LDL, it releases constituents from its surface coat (apoproteins A-I, A-II, and phospholipids) that are used to form high-density lipoprotein (HDL) in serum. HDL particles can also be directly secreted from jejunal enterocytes as well as hepatocytes.

Serum VLDL remnant particles and LDL function as delivery vehicles of cholesterol to peripheral tissues, including blood vessel walls. These lipoproteins are atherogenic because they can traverse the endothelial cell barrier. In the setting of an atherogenic milieu, endothelial cells become dysfunctional. The connections (gap junctions) between cells can loosen, thereby weakening the sieving or filtering capacity of the endothelial barrier. Endothelial cells express a variety of adhesion molecules (vascular cell adhesion molecule-1, intercellular adhesion molecule-1, and selectins) that promote the binding, rolling, and transmigration across defective gap junctions along the endothelial layer. This promotes the influx of proinflammatory cells such as T cells, mast cells, and monocytes. Monocytes can transform into macrophages when exposed to monocyte colony-stimulating factor. Macrophages resident within the subendothelial space exposed to LDL oxidized by enzymes such as lipoxygenase or myeloperoxidase upregulate the expression of scavenger receptors (SR-A, CD-36) on their surface and actively take up excessive amounts of cholesterol. The macrophages become progressively more loaded with lipid, culminating in foam cell and fatty streak development, events that contribute to the development of atheromatous plaque formation. The activation of macrophages also promotes an inflammatory response with the elaboration of cytokines, interleukins, C-reactive protein, cell mitogens, matrix metalloproteinases, and reactive oxygen species that facilitate lesion progression and instability (7).

LDL and VLDL remnants not taken up by peripheral tissues can be cleared from the circulation by hepatic LDL receptors. Therapies targeted at the upregulation of hepatic LDL receptors are antiatherogenic by virtue of their ability to reduce circulating levels of atherogenic lipoproteins.

3.2.2. High-Density Lipoprotein

A low level of HDL-C (i.e., <40 mg/dL in men and <50 mg/dL in women) constitutes an independent risk factor for the development of CAD and for CV morbidity and mortality (8). In patients with low HDL-C, therapeutic effort should be made to raise the level of this lipoprotein as much as possible. HDL-C plays an important role in modulating atherogenesis, although the mechanisms for its antiatherogenic effects are incompletely understood.

HDL-C constitutes 20–30% of total serum cholesterol and plays several critical roles in maintaining a healthy vasculature. HDL particles appear to protect the vasculature from progressive injury and atherogenesis in a number of ways including inhibiting the expression of endothelial cell adhesion molecules and selectins, stimulating endothelial cell nitric oxide and prostacyclin production, inhibiting endothelial cell apoptosis, decreasing platelet aggregability, and reducing LDL oxidation, among other functions (8). HDL promotes cellular export of cholesterol, or reverse cholesterol transport (RCT), a series of enzymatic reactions in which systemic cholesterol is delivered back to the liver for elimination as bile salts or biliary cholesterol (Fig. 2) (10). Reverse cholesterol transport has been validated in both animal and human studies (11–13). HDL particles can carry up to 75 different proteins, and the specific protein cargo depends on metabolic conditions and influences its functionality. These proteins include apoproteins, lipid-modifying enzymes (e.g., lecithin cholesteryl acyltransferase, cholesteryl ester transfer protein), immunity factors (complement proteins), redox active

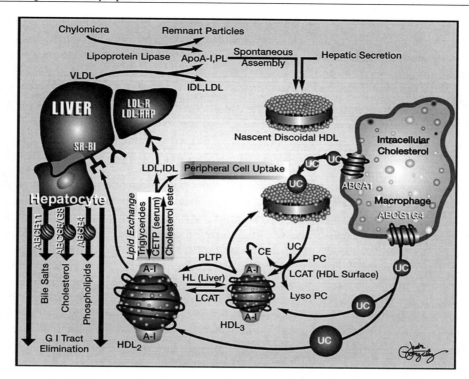

Fig. 2. Metabolism of HDL and reverse cholesterol transport. In order to deliver peripheral cholesterol back to the liver or steroidogenic organs (adrenals, placenta, ovaries, testes), apoA-I and nascent discoidal (nd) HDL interact with macrophages within the subendothelial space of blood vessel walls. ApoA-I and ndHDL are high-affinity cholesterol acceptors that bind to ABCA1 and promote cholesterol mobilization and externalization. HDL undergoes a series of cell receptor- and serum enzyme-dependent maturation reactions (i.e., "HDL speciation"). Externalized cholesterol is esterified by LCAT. The cholesterol esters are compartmentalized within the hydrophobic core of HDL particles. As the particles become more enriched with cholesterol ester, they become larger and rounder, forming in turn, HDL_3 and then the larger HDL_2. These spherical species can also promote cholesterol mobilization from macrophages by interacting with ABCG1. HDL can interact directly with a number of hepatocyte receptors. The cholesterol ester in HDL can be delivered back to the liver via an "indirect pathway" for RCT, which depends upon CETP and the LDL and LDL-RRP receptors. The "direct pathway" for RCT depends upon SR-BI, which binds and selectively delipidates HDL particles and then releases the lipid-poor HDL back into the circulation to begin another cycle of RCT. Reproduced with permission from (9). ABCA1 and G/1G4 = ATP-binding membrane cassette transporters A1 and G1/G4, ApoA-I = apoprotein A-I, ApoE = apoprotein E, CE = cholesteryl ester, CETP = cholesterol ester transfer protein, HL = hepatic lipase, IDL = intermediate-density lipoprotein, LCAT = lecithin: cholesteryl acyltransferase, LDL = low-density lipoprotein, LDL-R = low-density lipoprotein receptor, LDL-RRP = low-density lipoprotein receptor-related protein, lysoPC = lysophosphatidylcholine, PC = phosphatidylcholine, PGN = proteoglycans, PL = phospholipid, PLTP = phospholipid transfer protein, SR-BI = scavenger receptor BI, Trigly = triglyceride, UC = unesterified cholesterol, VLDL = very low-density lipoprotein.

enzymes (paraoxonase, platelet-activating factor acetyl hydrolase, glutathione peroxidase), and acute phase reactants (serum amyloid A), among many others *(14, 15)*.

With few exceptions, in prospective epidemiologic and case–control studies conducted throughout the world, high HDL-C levels have been found to be protective against the development of CAD *(4, 16–18)*. For instance, patients with familial hypoalphalipoproteinemia (low HDL) have increased risk for premature CAD, while patients with familial hyperalphalipoproteinemia are relatively resistant to atherosclerotic disease. In contrast to LDL, which promotes cholesterol delivery to and uptake by vessel wall macrophages, HDL extracts excess cellular cholesterol and delivers it back to the liver for elimination through the gastrointestinal tract through RCT. Recent studies suggest that among the elderly, low HDL may be a better predictor of risk for CAD, stroke, and disability than LDL *(19)*. An HDL >60 mg/dL is a negative risk factor. To summarize, the higher the level of serum HDL, the lower the risk for CAD, though there is never a guarantee that even patients with very high serum levels of HDL-C will not have or develop CAD.

3.2.3. Triglycerides

Recent meta-analyses show that hypertriglyceridemia is an independent risk factor for CVD, and there is increasing clinical trial evidence of the benefit of treating elevated TG in patients with dyslipidemia *(20, 21)*. Hypertriglyceridemia is a feature of the metabolic syndrome and occurs in patients with a variety of other clinical conditions, including familial combined hyperlipidemia, chylomicronemia, and dysbetalipoproteinemia, as well as in patients with diabetes mellitus, lipoprotein lipase-deficiency, and hepatic lipase-deficiency states. Among patients with CAD and a history of an acute syndrome on statin therapy, hypertriglyceridemia is associated with a higher incidence of morbidity and mortality compared to patients who are normotriglyceridemic *(22)*. Hypertriglyceridemia can arise from excess fat in the diet, impaired capacity to metabolize triglyceride, or increased endogenous biosynthesis of triglyceride. Hypertriglyceridemia is highly correlated with insulin resistance and hepatic steatosis. In the setting of insulin resistance, insulin becomes relatively ineffective at inhibiting hormone-sensitive lipase, an enzyme in visceral adipocytes that hydrolyzes triglycerides to free fatty acids. The portal circulation and hepatic parenchyma become flooded with excess fatty acid. In the liver, the fatty acid can be reassimilated into triglyceride and packaged into VLDL (resulting in hypertriglyceridemia), oxidized as fuel by mitochondria (beta-oxidation), or shunted toward gluconeogenesis (potentiating hyperglycemia). If these systems are overwhelmed, then the excess triglyceride is deposited in the hepatic parenchyma leading to steatosis. When triglycerides are severely elevated (>500 mg/dL), patients are vulnerable to the development of pancreatitis.

A substantial part of the toxicity attributable to triglycerides is because they impair the normal flow of lipoprotein metabolism. As triglycerides increase in serum, there is increased transfer of triglyceride mass from VLDL into LDL and HDL particles by the enzyme cholesteryl ester transfer protein. This TG enrichment renders these lipoproteins more vulnerable to lipolysis by hepatic lipase, generating small, dense LDL and increased catabolism of HDL particles, resulting in an atherogenic lipid profile. Consequently, as triglycerides progressively increase, LDL particle number increases, particle size decreases, and serum levels of HDL particles decrease. All of these changes are associated with increased risk for atherosclerotic disease. Small LDL particles may be more atherogenic by virtue of their smaller size and increased permeability into vessel walls, decreased clearance from the circulation because of reduced affinity for the LDL receptor on the surface of hepatocytes, and increased vulnerability to oxidative modification.

3.3. DYSLIPIDEMIA

Dyslipidemia is associated with elevations in serum low-density lipoprotein cholesterol (LDL-C) and non-high-density lipoprotein cholesterol (non-HDL-C) and low levels of high-density lipoprotein cholesterol (HDL-C). Non-HDL-C is a sensitive measure of the atherogenic lipoprotein burden in serum; includes VLDL, IDL, LDL, and lipoprotein(a); and is calculated by subtracting HDL-C from total cholesterol (non-HDL-C + TC – HDL-C). Dyslipidemia is a highly heterogeneous class of metabolic disorders whose etiology can depend upon poor diet and excessive gastrointestinal absorption of cholesterol and lipids, mutations in cell surface receptors, abnormalities in the production or activity of lipolytic enzymes in serum and within cells, and alterations in apoprotein metabolism.

Of tantamount importance to this discussion is the fact that dyslipidemia is a *modifiable risk factor*. The management of dyslipidemia in the context of both primary and secondary prevention must be coupled with the aggressive identification and management of all risk factors, including hypertension, diabetes mellitus, obesity, cigarette smoking, established atherosclerotic disease, as well as nephropathy and chronic kidney disease. A comprehensive assessment of risk factor burden for CHD is indicated in patients with dyslipidemia as the intensity of treatment is dependent on risk stratification (Table 1). Risk stratification is performed by evaluating a patient's cardiovascular risk factor burden (number of risk factors) and, if two or more risk factors are present, calculation of the Framingham risk score. Based on the National Cholesterol Education Program Adult Treatment Panel III (NCEP-ATP III) *(24)*, for persons categorized as low risk (0–1 risk factors), the LDL-C goal is <160 mg/dL, while for those with moderate risk (2+ risk factors and a 10-year risk <10%), the LDL-C goal is <130 mg/dL. For those with moderately high risk (2+ risk factors and a 10-year risk of 10–20%), the LDL-C goal is <130 mg/dL with an optional goal of <100 mg/dL. For high-risk persons with CHD or CHD risk equivalents and a 10-year risk >20%, the LDL-C goal is <100 mg/dL with an optional goal of <70 mg/dL if they meet criteria for "very high risk" (Table 1) *(23)*. Among patients with multiple risk factors and no history of CAD or a CAD risk equivalent, it is important to calculate the Framingham risk score so as to differentiate moderate, moderately high, and high risk. An electronic version of a Framingham risk calculator for men and women can be downloaded at

Table 1
Low-Density Lipoprotein Cholesterol Goals and Thresholds for Initiating Lifestyle Change and Pharmacologic Intervention. Based on *(23)*

Risk category[a,b]	LDL goal	LDL level Initiate TLC	LDL level Consider drug therapy
CHD or CHD risk equivalents (10-year risk >20%)	<100 mg/dL (optional goal <70)[c]	≥100 mg/day	≥130 mg/dL (100–129 mg/dL, drug optional)
		All patients regardless of LDL	≥100 mg/day[d] (<100 mg/dL, drug optional)
2+ Risk factors (10-year risk 10–20%)	<130 mg/dL (optional goal <100)	≥130 mg/day	≥130 mg/dL
		All patients regardless of LDL	(>100 mg/dL, drug optional[d])
2+ Risk factors (10-year risk ≤10%)	130 mg/dL	≥130 mg/dL	≥160 mg/dL
0–1 Risk factor	160 mg/dL	≥160 mg/dL	≥190 mg/dL (160–189 mg/dL, LDL-lowering drug optional)

[a]CHD risk equivalents include diabetes mellitus, peripheral vascular disease, carotid artery disease, and abdominal aortic aneurysm.

[b]Risk factors included in Framingham risk evaluation are age, systolic blood pressure, total cholesterol, HDL-C, and smoking status.

[c]The optional goal of <70 mg/dL is particularly targeted at patients who are "very high" risk, i.e., patients with a recent acute coronary syndrome, poorly controlled diabetics with multiple risk factors, etc.

[d]When initiating statin therapy in these patients, the goal for LDL-C reduction should be 30–40% from baseline.

www.nhlbi.nih.gov/guidelines/cholesterol. Patients with CAD or CAD risk equivalents (symptomatic carotid artery disease, abdominal aortic aneurysm, diabetes mellitus, peripheral arterial disease, or a 10-year Framingham risk score > 20%) are high risk by definition. Examples of very high-risk patients include patients with CAD who have had a recent acute coronary syndrome (ACS), who still smoke, or who have multiple poorly controlled components of the metabolic syndrome (defined below) (see Table 2).

At any level of risk, LDL-C is the primary target of lipid-lowering therapy. Among patients with a serum triglyceride level >200 mg/dL, non-HDL-C is the secondary target of therapy. The risk-stratified target is the LDL-C target plus 30 mg/dL. The NCEP-ATP III major risk factors are outlined in Table 3. An LDL-C <100 mg/dL is defined as "optimal" for patients without evidence of atherosclerotic disease. Once HDL-C exceeds 60 mg/dL, it is protective against atherosclerosis and is defined as a negative risk factor (it constitutes a −1 in Framingham risk scoring). Triglycerides are considered

Table 2
Who Is the High-Risk Patient?

CHD
History of MI
Unstable angina
Stable angina
Angioplasty or bypass surgery
Clinically significant myocardial ischemia

CHD risk equivalents
Peripheral arterial disease
Abdominal aortic aneurysm
Carotid artery disease (e.g., TIA, stroke, >50% obstruction of a carotid artery)
Diabetes mellitus
2+ Risk factors with >20% 10-year risk for CHD

Very high risk + established CVD
Multiple major risk factors (especially diabetes)
Severe and poorly controlled risk factors (especially continued cigarette smoking)
Multiple risk factors of the metabolic syndrome (especially TG ≥ 200 mg/dL + non-HDL-C ≥ 130 mg/dL with HDL-C < 40 mg/dL)
Acute coronary syndromes (unstable angina or acute MI)

CHD = coronary heart disease, CVD = cardiovascular disease, HDL-C = high-density lipoprotein cholesterol, MI = myocardial infarction, TG = triglycerides, TIA = transient ischemic attack.
Adapted from *(25)*, with permission from *(26)*.

Table 3
National Cholesterol Education Program Risk Factors

Negative
HDL-C >60 mg/dL

Positive
Cigarette smoking
HDL <40 mg/dL
Hypertension (blood pressure >140/90 mmHg or use of antihypertensive agents)
Family history of premature coronary artery disease (CAD in male first-degree relative <55 years; CAD in female first-degree relative <65 years)
Age (men ≥ 45 years, women ≥ 55 years)

normal if less than 150 mg/dL. For patients with very high serum HDL-C, it cannot be assumed that the HDL-C will counteract all other risk factors. A Framingham risk score should still be calculated for these patients with LDL-C and non-HDL-C targets determined through risk stratification. When making the diagnosis of dyslipidemia, it is also important to rule out and treat secondary causes of dyslipidemia, such as thyroid dysfunction, alcoholism, insulin resistance and diabetes mellitus, use of HIV antiretroviral agents, and nephrotic syndrome, among others.

3.4. THERAPEUTIC LIFESTYLE CHANGE

Lifestyle modification is the first-line therapy for all patients with dyslipidemia. Therapeutic lifestyle change (TLC) constitutes front-line therapy and involves the use of interventions to reduce CHD risk, including physical activity, modified dietary intake, smoking cessation, weight management, blood pressure control, and stress management. The NCEP-ATP III guidelines outline TLC as a multifaceted lifestyle approach for atherogenic lipid lowering and raising serum levels of HDL-C. The recommendations for TLC include a reduction in saturated fat intake to <7% of total calories and cholesterol to <200 mg/day, weight reduction, increased physical activity, therapeutic options for enhancing LDL lowering such as the use of plant stanols/sterols (2 g/day), and increased viscous (soluble) fiber (10–25 g/day) to reduce cholesterol absorption (24). The recommended distribution of calories from other nutrients includes 15% protein, 50–60% carbohydrates, 10% polyunsaturated fat, and 20% monounsaturated fat (Table 4). Reductions in saturated fat and increased ingestion of mono- and polyunsaturated fats are associated with reductions in serum LDL-C.

Table 4
Dietary Recommendations for Therapeutic Lifestyle Change

Dietary component	Recommendation allowance
Polyunsaturated fat	Up to 10% of total calories
Monounsaturated fat	Up to 20% of total calories
Total fat	25–35% of total calories
Carbohydrate	50–60% of total calories
Dietary fiber	20–30 g/day
Protein	Approximately 15% of total calories
Dietary cholesterol	<200 mg/day

The NCEP-ATP III guidelines also recommend that patients who smoke achieve smoking cessation. Smoking is associated with endothelial cell dysfunction as well as increased levels of oxidized LDL-C and reduced serum HDL-C (27). Patients should be encouraged to exercise for 20–30 min five times weekly. Exercise facilitates weight loss, which helps to relieve visceral adiposity and insulin resistance. These changes are associated with reduced serum triglycerides and elevations in HDL-C.

Therapeutic lifestyle change is a particularly important intervention in patients with the metabolic syndrome. In the United States, it is estimated that 35–40% of adults have the metabolic syndrome, a cluster of lipid and nonlipid disorders (8, 28). The metabolic syndrome is characterized by a set of five risk factors including abdominal obesity, elevated blood pressure, triglycerides, fasting glucose, and low HDL-C (Table 5). The diagnosis of metabolic syndrome is made when a patient has any three or more of these defining clinical features. Metabolic syndrome develops secondary to the effects of insulin resistance and obesity. Although the metabolic syndrome significantly increases risk for atherosclerotic disease and diabetes mellitus, it is not defined as a CAD risk equivalent. The Framingham risk score should be calculated on all of these patients and LDL and non-HDL goals should be defined by risk stratification. If triglycerides remain elevated (200–499 mg/dL) after the LDL

Table 5
NCEP-ATP III Criteria for Diagnosing the Metabolic
Syndrome[a]

Risk factor	Defining level
Abdominal obesity	
Men	Waist >40 in.
Women	Waist >35 in.
Triglycerides	≥150 mg/dL
HDL-C	
Men	40 mg/dL
Women	50 mg/dL
Blood pressure	≥130/≥85 mmHg
Fasting glucose	≥100 mg/dL

[a]Patients having any three of the above five risk factors meet
criteria for the diagnosis of the metabolic syndrome (24).

goal has been reached, then consideration should be given to the addition of a triglyceride-lowering drug. If triglycerides are >500 mg/dL, aggressive management to reduce them is the first priority of therapy in order to reduce risk for pancreatitis. Patients with severe hypertriglyceridemia should be treated aggressively with triglyceride-lowering medication and a very low-fat diet with ≤15% of calories derived from fat.

The NCEP-ATP III guidelines do not define target levels for HDL; however, it is recommended that an effort be made to raise low HDL (<40 mg/dL in men, <50 mg/dL in women) through lifestyle modification and drug therapy. The European Consensus Panel on HDL and the US Expert Group on HDL suggest that HDL be raised to >40 mg/dL in patients at high risk or with metabolic syndrome (29, 30). The American Diabetes Association recommends that HDL be raised to >40 mg/dL in diabetic men and >50 mg/dL in diabetic women.

3.5. PHARMACOLOGIC MANAGEMENT

If target goals are not achieved with intensified TLC, the NCEP-ATP III guidelines recommend that drug treatment be initiated. The general approach is to start an LDL-lowering drug therapy and evaluate the response after 6 weeks. If the LDL-C goal is not achieved, LDL-lowering therapy is intensified with the use of a higher dose or with combination drug therapy (24). Several options exist for the pharmacologic management of dyslipidemia (Table 6). The intensity of pharmacologic intervention depends upon a given individual's risk-stratified NCEP-ATP III targets for LDL-C and non-HDL-C.

Table 6
Pharmacologic Agents for Dyslipidemia Management and Their
Effects on Lipid Fractions

Agent	Lipid fraction		
	LDL-C	HDL-C	TC
Statins	18–5% ↓	5–15% ↑	7–30% ↓
Fibric acids	5–20% ↓	10–20% ↑	20–50% ↓
Nicotinic acid	5–25% ↓	15–35% ↑	20–50% ↓
Bile and sequestrants	15–30% ↓	3–5% ↑	No change
Ezetimibe	18–20% ↓	1–4% ↑	8% ↓

3.5.1. Statins

The statins are reversible, competitive 3-hydroxy-3-methylglutaryl coenzyme A (HMG-CoA) reductase inhibitors. HMG-CoA reductase is the rate-limiting step of cholesterol biosynthesis. Statins are recognized as first-line therapy for the treatment of dyslipidemia as they provide the most potent means currently available by which to reduce serum levels of LDL-C. A large number of statin outcome trials have established that lowering LDL-C results in significant reductions in multiple "hard" cardiovascular endpoints, including myocardial infarction, stroke, and death in both primary (31, 32) and secondary cohorts (33, 34) as well as in patients with hypertension (35), diabetes mellitus (36), or heightened inflammation (37) as measured by serum levels of high-sensitivity C-reactive protein levels (see Table 7 and 8 for overview). Statins benefit both men and women as well as the elderly (39). In addition, statin therapy is associated with reduced frequency and severity of angina pectoris as well as claudication (33) need for coronary and peripheral revascularization (37) and slows or even reverses atheromatous plaque progression. As a rule of thumb, when it comes to LDL-C reduction and intensity of statin therapy, lower LDL-C levels are associated with better reductions in cardiovascular endpoints (40–42) (Fig. 2) and higher likelihood of coronary plaque regression (43, 44) and patients given more intensive doses of statins generally do better than patients given less intensive doses (45, 46). In an analysis of 14 prospective randomized statin trials by the Cholesterol Treatment Trialists Collaboration, for every 39 mg/dL (1 mmol/L) reduction in serum LDL-C with statin therapy over a mean 5-year follow-up, there was a 12% reduction in all-cause mortality, a 19% reduction in coronary mortality, a 24% reduction in myocardial infarction or coronary death, a 24% reduction in need for revascularization, and a 17% reduction in fatal/nonfatal stroke (Fig. 3) (47). Among diabetic patients in these 14 trials, similar reductions in these endpoints were observed (48). For patients admitted to hospital with an ACS, it is standard care to initiate statin therapy irrespective of baseline lipid profile. If a patient has CHD or a CHD risk equivalent and the LDL-C is below 100 mg/dL on no medication, it is recommended that the patient's LDL-C be reduced at least 30% below baseline with statin therapy (49). Of considerable importance is the observation in both primary and secondary prevention studies that statins are safe and have a very large benefit-to-risk ratio (50–52). Despite the safety and therapeutic benefit of statin therapy, approximately 50% of patients discontinue their statin after only 6 months (53). Patients should be carefully counseled on each visit about the importance of remaining compliant on statin therapy.

In addition to reducing cholesterol biosynthesis, the statins augment the clearance of atherogenic apoB100-containing lipoproteins (VLDL, VLDL remnants, and LDL) by upregulating the expression of the LDL receptor on the surface of hepatocytes. By reducing hepatic VLDL secretion, they also decrease serum levels of triglycerides. These drugs stimulate apoA-I expression and hepatic HDL secretion secondary to weak peroxisomal proliferator-activated receptor-α (PPAR-α) agonism (54).

The statins may exert benefit distinct from their ability to alter circulating levels of lipoproteins through their "pleiotropic effects." Statins inhibit the posttranslational modification and activation of small G-proteins (rho and ras) by blocking the production of isoprenoids such as farnesyl-pyrophosphate and geranylgeranyl-pyrophosphate. This is associated with reductions in the production of a large number of atherogenic stimuli (C-reactive protein, reactive oxygen species, tissue factor, interleukins, adhesion molecules, monocyte chemoattract protein-1, angiotensin II receptor, and endothelin-1), decreased platelet reactivity and smooth cell proliferation, and a reversal of endothelial dysfunction, among other effects. Consequently, statins appear to modulate inflammation, oxidative status, vasodilation, thrombotic tendency, and the capacity of a variety of cell types in vessel walls to interact and drive atherogenesis (55).

Table 7
Prospective randomized statin trials in both primary and secondary prevention

Study	Drug	Design	Outcomes
Primary prevention studies			
AFCAPS/TexCAPS[1]	Lovastatin, 20–40 mg/day vs. placebo	6,605 men and women	40% reduction in fatal and nonfatal MI; 37% reduction in first ACS; 33% reduction in coronary revascularizations; and unstable angina reduced by 32%
ASCOT[2]	Atorvastatin 10 mg/day vs. placebo	10,305 hypertensive men (n=8463) and women (n=1942) with treated high BP and no previous CAD	36% reduction in total CHD/nonfatal MI; 27% reduction in fatal and nonfatal stroke; total coronary event reduced by 29%; fatal and nonfatal stroke reduced by 27%
CARDS[3]	Atorvastatin 10 mg/day vs. placebo	2,838 patients with type 2 diabetes mellitus and 1 CHD risk factor(s)	37% reduction of major cardiovascular events; 27% of total mortality; 13.4% reduction of acute CVD events; 36% reduction of acute coronary events; 48% reduction of stroke
Heart Protection Study[4]	Simvastatin 40 mg/day vs. placebo	20,536 high-risk (previous CHD, other vascular disease, hypertension among men aged > 65 years, or diabetes)	25% reduction in all-cause and coronary death rates and in strokes; need for revascularisation reduced by 24%; fatal and nonfatal stroke reduced by 25%; nonfatal MI reduced by 38%; coronary mortality reduced by 18%; all cause mortality reduced by 13%; cardiovascular event rate reduced by 24%
PROSPER[5]	Pravastatin 40 mg/day vs. placebo	5804 men (n=2,804) and women (n=3,000) aged 70–82 years	15% reduction in combined endpoint (fatal/nonfatal MI or stroke); 19% reduction in total/nonfatal CHD; no effect on stroke (but 25% reduction in TIA)
WOSCOPS[6]	Pravachol therapy 40 mg/day vs. placebo	6,595 men	CHD death of nonfatal MI reduced by 31%; CVD death reduced by 32%; total mortality 22% reduction
Secondary prevention studies			
4S[7]	Simvastatin 20 mg/day vs. placebo	4,444 patients with angina pectoris or history of MI	Coronary mortality reduced by 42%; myocardial revascularization reduction of 37%; all cause mortality reduced by 30%; nonfatal major coronary event reduced by 34%; fatal and nonfatal stroke reduced by 30%
AVERT[8]	Atorvastatin 80 mg/day vs. angioplasty + usual care	341 patients with stable CAD	36% reduction in ischemic event; delayed time to first ischemic event reduced by 36%
CARE[9]	Pravastatin 40 mg/day vs. placebo	3,583 men and 576 women with history of MI	Death from CHD or nonfatal MI reduced by 24%;death from CHD reduced by 20%; nonfatal MI reduced by23%; fatal MI reduced by 37%; CABG or PTCA reduced by 27%

Trial	Comparison	Population	Results
IDEAL[10]	Atorvastatin 80 mg/day vs. simvastatin 20–40 mg/day	8,888 men and women with CHD	Major cardiac events reduced by 13%, nonfatal MI reduced by 17%, revascularization reduced by 23%, peripheral arteril disease reduced by 24%
JUPITER[11]	Rosuvastatin 20 mg/day vs. placebo	17,802 men (> 50 years) and women (> 60 years) with no history of CAD or DM, entry LDL < 130 mg/dL and CRP > 2.0 mg/L	44% reduction in primary endpoint of major coronary events; 65% reduction in nonfatal MI; 48% reduction in nonfatal stroke; 46% reduction in need for revascularization; 20% reduction in all cause mortality
LIPID[12]	Pravachol 40 mg/day vs. placebo	9,014 patients	Coronary mortality reduced by 24%; stroke reduced by 19%; fatal CHD or nonfatal MI reduced by 24% fatal or nonfatal MI reduced by 29%
LIPS[13]	Fluvastatin 40 mg/day vs. placebo	1,667 men and women aged 18–80 years post-angioplasty for CAD	22% lower rate of major coronary events (e.g., cardiac deaths, nonfatal MI, or reintervention procedure)
MIRACL[14]	Atorvastatin 80 mg/day vs. placebo	3,086 patients with ACS	Reduction in composite endpoint by 16%; ischemia reduced by 26%; stroke reduced by 50%
PROVE IT[15]	Atorvastatin 80 mg/day vs. pravastatin 40 mg/day	4,162 patient with ACS	16% reduction of composite endpoint; 14% reduction in CHD death, MI, or revascularization; revascularizations reduced by 14%; unstable angina reduced by 29%
REVERSAL[16]	Atorvastatin 80 mg/day vs. pravastatin 40 mg/day	654 patients with CAD	Atheroma: atorvastatin – 0.4%, pravastatin 2.7%, difference of – 3.1%, p = 0.02
TNT[17]	Atorvastatin 10 mg/day vs. 80 mg/day	10,003 patients with CHD and LDL cholesterol 130– 250 mg/dL	22% reduction in composite endpoint; MI reduced by 22%; stroke reduced by 25%

(Continued)

Abbreviations: ACS, acute coronary syndrome; CABG, coronary artery bypass grafting; CAD, coronary artery disease; CHD, coronary heart disease; LDL, low-density lipoprotein; MI, myocardial infarction;, PTCA, percutaneous transluminal coronary angioplasty. Trial acronyms: AFCAPS/TexCAPS, The Air Force/Texas Coronary Atherosclerosis Prevention Study: Implications for Preventive Cardiology in the General Adult US Population; ASCOT, Anglo-Scandinavian Cardiac Outcomes Trial-Lipid Lowering Arm; CARDS, Collaborative Atorvastatin Diabetes Study; PROSPER, Pravastatin in elderly individuals at risk of vascular disease; WOSCOPS,West of Scotland Coronary Prevention Study; 4S, The Scandinavian Simvastatin Survival Study; AVERT, Atorvastatin versus Revascularization Treatment Investigators; CARE, Cholesterol and Recurrent Events Trial; IDEAL, Incremental Decrease in End Points Through Aggressive Lipid Lowering Study; JUPITER, The Justification for the Use of Statins in Prevention: an Intervention Trial Evaluating Rosuvastatin; LIPID, Long-Term Intervention with Pravastatin in Ischemic Disease; LIPS, Lescol Intervention Prevention Study; MIRACL, Myocardial Ischemia Reduction with Aggressive Cholesterol Lowering Study; PROVE IT, Pravastatin or Atorvastatin Evaluation and Infection Therapy Study; REVERSAL, The REVERSing Atherosclerosis with Aggressive Lipid Lowering Study; TNT, Treating to New Targets Trial.

Table 7
(Continued)

[1] Whitney E. The Air Force/Texas Coronary Atherosclerosis Prevention Study: implications for preventive cardiology in the general adult US population. *Curr Atheroscler Rep.* 1999;1:38–43.

[2] Sever PS, et al. Prevention of coronary and stroke events with atorvastatin in hypertensives patients who have average or lower-than-average cholesterol concentrations, in the Anglo-Scandinavian Cardiac Outcomes Trial-Lipid Lowering Arm (ASCOT-LLA): a multicentre randomized controlled trial. *Lancet.* 2003, 361: 1149–1158.

[3] Colhoun HM, et al. Primary prevention of cardiovascular disease with atorvastatin in type 2 diabetes in the Collaborative Atorvastatin Diabetes Study (CARDS): multicentre randomised placebo-controlled trial. *Lancet.* 2004;364:685–696.

[4] Heart Protection Study Collaborative Group. MRC/BHF Heart Protection Study of cholesterol lowering with simvastatin in 20536 high-risk individuals: a randomized placebo-controlled trial. *Lancet.* 2002;360:7–22.

[5] Shepherd J, et al. Pravastatin in elderly individuals at risk of vascular disease (PROSPER): a randomized controlled trial. *Lancet.* 2002;360:1623–1630.

[6] Shepherd J, Cobbe SM, Ford I, et al. Prevention of coronary heart disease with pravastatin in men with hypercholesterolemia. *N Engl J Med.* 1995;333:1301–1307.

[7] Scandinavian Simvastatin Survival Study Group. Randomised trial of choslesterol lowering in 4444 patients with coronary heart disease: the Scandinavian Simvastatin Survival Study (4S). *Lancet.* 1994;344:1383–1389.

[8] Pitt B, et al. Aggressive lipid-lowering therapy compared with angioplasty in stable coronary artery disease. Atorvastatin versus Revascularization Treatment Investigators. *N Engl J Med.* 1999;341:70–76.

[9] Sacks FM, et al. The effect of pravastatin on coronary events after myocardial infarction in patients with average cholesterol levels. *N Engl J Med.* 1996;335: 1001–1009.

[10] Pedersen, TR, et al. High-dose atorvastatin vs usual-dose simvastatin for secondary prevention after myocardial infarction: the IDEAL study: a randomized controlled trial. *JAMA.* 2005;294(19):2437–2445.

[11] Ridker, PM, et al. Rosuvastatin to prevent vascular events in men and women with elevated C-reactive protein. *N Engl J Med.* 2008;359:2195–2207.

[12] The LIPID Study Group. Design features and baseline characteristics of the LIPID (Long-Term Intervention with Pravastatin in Ischemic Disease) Study: a randomized trial in patients with previous acute myocardial infarction and/or unstable angina pectoris. *Am J Cardiol.* 1995;76:474–479.

[13] Serruys PW, et al. Fluvastatin for prevention of cardiac events following successful first percutaneous coronary intervention. A randomized controlled trial. *JAMA.* 2002;287:3215–3222.

[14] Schwartz GG, et al. Effects of atorvastatin on early recurrent ischemic events in acute coronary syndromes: the MIRACL Study: a randomized controlled trial. *JAMA.* 2001;285:1711–1718.

[15] Cannon CP, et al. Intensive versus moderate lipid lowering with statins after acute coronary syndromes. *N Engl J Med.* 2004;350:1495–1504.

[16] Nissen S, et al. Aggressive lipid-lowering therapy and regression of coronary atheroma. *JAMA.* 2004, 292:1–3.

[17] LaRosa JC, et al. Intensive lipid lowering with atorvastatin in patients with stable coronary disease. *N Engl J Med.* 2005;352:1425–1435.

Table 8
Recommendations to Health Professionals Regarding Muscle and Statin Safety

Patient monitoring
1. Routine CK levels in asymptomatic patients are not recommended
2. Obtain baseline CK in high-risk patients (renal dysfunction, liver disease, polypharmacy)
3. Consider CK levels in patients with muscle-related symptoms
4. Rule out other etiologies in other symptomatic patients or those with elevated CK levels (hypothyroidism, trauma, seizures, infection, strenuous physical activity)
5. Exacerbating factors should be considered (concomitant medications and herbal remedies), such as use of red rice yeast that contains lovastatin

Management of muscle symptoms
1. If intolerable muscle symptoms develop, discontinue statin regardless of CK levels and rechallenge only after patient becomes asymptomatic
2. If muscle symptoms are tolerable and CK elevation is mildly elevated (<10 times upper limit of normal) then statin may be continued and muscle symptoms can be used as guide to stop or continue treatment
3. If muscle symptoms are tolerable and CK elevation is moderate to severe, then discontinue statin therapy and weigh risk and benefits
4. If muscle symptoms are tolerable and CK elevation is associated with elevated creatinine or need for IV hydration, then discontinue therapy

CoA = coenzyme A, HMG-CoA =3-hydroxy-3-methylglutaryl-coenzyme A, PP = pyrophosphate, CK = creatinine kinase.

Reprinted with permission from *(38)*.

Statins are used to target the reduction of elevated LDL and to improve the lipid profile. Statins have clinically relevant differences in efficacy, pharmacokinetics, and safety profiles. Therefore, the specific choice of a statin should be dictated by the magnitude of LDL-C reduction required (baseline versus risk-stratified NCEP-ATP III target). The specific statin and dose are chosen based on the patient's level of risk (low, moderate, moderately high, high, or very high) and the percentage of LDL-lowering needed *(52)*. The LDL-C reducing capacity of the statins is as follows: rosuvastatin (Crestor), 45–63% (5–40 mg daily); atorvastatin (Lipitor) 26–60% (10–80 mg daily); simvastatin (Zocor) 26–47% (10–80 mg daily); lovastatin (Mevacor) 21–42% (10–80 mg daily); fluvastatin (Lescol) 22–36% (10–20 mg daily); and pravastatin (Pravachol) 22–34% (10–80 mg daily). Each doubling of the statin dose yields an additional 6% reduction, on average, in serum LDL-C (the so-called "rule of 6s"). In general, statin therapy provides dose-dependent reductions in serum triglyceride levels (typically 10–25%) and elevations in serum HDL-C (2–14%). Atorvastatin has a tendency to be less effective at raising HDL-C as the dose is titrated to higher levels. In patients with high baseline triglycerides (>300 mg/dL), the statins increase HDL-C significantly more than in patients who are normotriglyceridemic. For instance, simvastatin and rosuvastatin can raise HDL-C up to 18 and 22%, respectively, in these patients. One of the reasons for this has to do with the fact that as triglycerides increase in serum, HDL particles become progressively more loaded with triglyceride via the action of cholesterol ester transfer protein. This renders the HDL particle more vulnerable to lipolysis and eventual catabolism by the enzyme hepatic lipase. As triglycerides rise, HDL thus has a tendency to decrease. Statins help to prevent this by reducing serum concentrations of triglyceride.

The statins also differ in their pharmacokinetic profiles. Due to their relatively short half-lives (1–4 h), lovastatin, pravastatin, fluvastatin, and simvastatin should be taken in the evening so as to intercept the peak activity of HMG-CoA-reductase, which occurs around midnight. Atorvastatin and rosuvastatin can be taken at any time during the day because of their long half-lives (approximately 19 h). The coadministration of cytochrome P450 3A4 inhibitors (azole-type antifungals [ketoconazole, itraconazole], HIV protease inhibitors, macrolide antibiotics [erythromycin, clar-

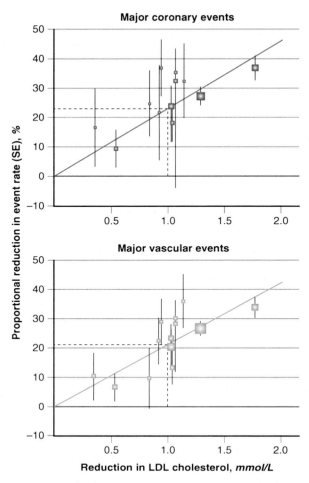

Fig. 3. Relation between proportional reduction in incidence of major coronary events and major vascular events and mean absolute LDL cholesterol reduction at 1 year. Each square represents a single trial plotted against mean absolute LDL cholesterol reduction at 1 year, with vertical lines above and below corresponding to one standard error of unweighted event rate reduction. For each outcome, the regression line represents the weighted event rate reduction per mmol/L (39 mg/dL) of LDL-C reduction. Reproduced with permission from *(47)*.

ithromycin], nefazadone, greater than 1 qt of grapefruit juice daily, and cyclosporine) with simvastatin, lovastatin, and atorvastatin should be avoided as these statins are dependent on this P450 isozyme for metabolism. Concomitant administration can lead to increased risk for toxicity. The dose of Zocor should not exceed 20 mg daily in patients receiving verapamil or amiodarone.

Statins do not completely eliminate the risk of CVD-related events as they frequently do not normalize all of the components of the lipid profile *(56)*. Statin therapy is often insufficient in achieving adequate risk reduction for many patients with CHD, who require the use of combination therapy to achieve their risk-stratified NCEP target goals. As the initial priority of pharmacologic therapy in the management of CVD is to achieve the goal for LDL-C, an LDL-lowering drug such as a statin, but adjuvant therapies with other drugs can and should be provided as indicated, especially in high-risk and very high-risk patients (Table 9) *(24)*. In patients unable to achieve their LDL-C target with TLC and statin therapy, consideration should be given to combination therapy such as the addition of ezetimibe or a bile acid-binding resin.

Table 9
How to Treat Very High-Risk Patients to Their LDL-C Goal of <70 mg/dL

Consider intensive therapy for all patients admitted to the hospital with ACS

- Measure LDL-C within 24 h of admission to determine drug choice and regimen
  Initiate statin therapy regardless of baseline LDL-C to obtain at least a 30–40% reduction in LDL-C
- In patients with high baseline LDL-C:
  Use (or switch to) a more powerful statin (e.g., atorvastatin, rosuvastatin)
  If monotherapy is unsuccessful, try combination therapy with statin + ezetimibe, statin +
  colesevelam, statin + ezetimibe and colesevelam, or statin + niacin; choice of combinations
  dictated by specific features of lipid profile
- In patients with LDL-C <100 mg/dL after standard-dose statin therapy:
  Use low dose of a more powerful statin or uptitrate standard regimen
  When triglycerides are elevated (≥200 mg/dL), use statin therapy to achieve a non-HDLC level of
  30 mg/dL above the LDL-C goal
- When HDL-C is low and/or triglycerides are elevated, consider combination therapy with statin +
  niacin or statin + fenofibrate, and combinations thereof as indicated

Reproduced with permission from *(57)*.

3.5.1.1. STATIN MYOPATHY

The statins have a very favorable benefit-to-risk ratio with respect to liver, muscle, and renal safety concerns. Statin-associated myotoxicity, including skeletal muscle necrosis that may result in life-threatening rhabdomyolysis, is a concern with high-dose statin therapy. However, statin-induced myopathy and rhabdomyolysis are relatively rare events (1 in 1,000 and 1 in 10,000, respectively) *(58–60)*. Myopathy is a general term for any muscle symptom or pathology, whereas myalgia is defined as muscle symptoms without creatine kinase (CK) elevation. Myositis is defined as muscle symptoms with an elevation in CK, and rhabdomyolysis is defined as muscle symptoms associated with marked CK elevations, typically >10 times the upper limit of normal (ULN) with an elevation in serum creatinine requiring intravenous hydration therapy *(61, 62)*. Drug interactions, muscle injury, thyroid dysfunction, age, renal and hepatic function, abuse of illegal drugs (e.g., heroin), and possibly serum electrolyte disturbances can increase the risk for statin myalgia and myopathy *(50)*.

In the Heart Protection Study *(63)*, the largest clinical trial of statin therapy to date, five cases (0.05%) of nonfatal rhabdomyolysis (muscle symptoms plus creatine kinase >40 times ULN) were reported in patients receiving simvastatin 40 mg compared with three cases (0.03%) in patients receiving placebo. While the risk of rhabdomyolysis is <0.1% (approximately two cases/100,000 patients receiving therapy/year), patients must be counseled about the possibility as well as warning signs for rhabdomyolysis (escalating muscle pain, proximal weakness, brownish-red discoloration of urine suggesting presence of myoglobin). Muscle metabolism can be adversely impacted by statin therapy in several ways, including changes in fatty acid oxidation, autoimmune phenomena, reduced coenzyme Q_{10} biosynthesis, and increased myocyte protein (actin, myosin) degradation via the activity of atrogin-1 and the ubiquitin–proteasome pathway, among other pathways *(50)*.

Statins can induce myalgia. However, myalgias in general are common throughout the population. Among the 20,536 patients in the Heart Protection Study *(63)* randomized to either placebo or simvastatin 40 mg daily, the incidence of myalgia was identical in the two groups of patients. If a patient is experiencing significant myalgia or muscle weakness, a serum creatine kinase (CK) level can be obtained. Table 10 and Fig. 4 outline clinical management strategies for patients with risk factors for muscle toxicity or those who develop muscle complaints and elevation in CK levels. Statins should be discontinued in patients who develop intolerable muscle complaints in the absence of exacerbating factors or other etiologies *(50)*. However, prior to statin discontinuation, especially in high-risk

Table 10
The National Lipid Association Statin Safety Assessment Task Force Recommendations to Healthcare
Professionals Regarding the Liver and Statin Safety

1. Obtain transaminase levels prior to initiating statins. If abnormal, investigate to determine the etiology
2. The available evidence does not support routine monitoring of liver biochemical tests. Until there is a
    change in the FDA-approved prescribing information for statins, it is appropriate to continue to measure
    transaminase levels before starting therapy, 12 weeks later, after a dose increase, and periodically
    thereafter
3. The clinician should be alert to signals of potential hepatotoxicity. Evidence for hepatotoxicity includes
    jaundice, hepatomegaly, increased indirect bilirubin level, and elevated prothrombin time (rather than
    simple elevations in liver transaminase levels)
4. The preferred biochemical test to ascertain significant liver injury is fractionated bilirubin. In the
    absence of biliary obstruction, it is a more accurate prognosticator of liver injury than isolated
    transaminase levels
5. Should the clinician identify objective evidence of significant liver injury in a patient receiving a statin,
    the statin should be discontinued. Other etiologies should be sought and, if indicated, the patient should
    be referred to a specialist
6. For an isolated asymptomatic transaminase level 1–3 times ULN, there is no need to discontinue the
    statin
7. An isolated asymptomatic transaminase level >3 times ULN during a routine evaluation of a patient on a
    statin should be repeated and, if still elevated, other etiologies should be ruled out. Consideration should
    be given to continuing the statin, reducing its dose, or discontinuing it based on clinical judgment
8. Patients with chronic liver disease including nonalcoholic fatty liver disease may safely receive statins

Reproduced with permission from *(38)*.

patients, patients should be thoroughly examined and evaluated. Patients frequently complain of statin-induced myalgia when in fact they are experiencing arthralgia from osteoarthritis, may have sustained muscle or tendon injury unrelated to statin therapy, or have injured muscle from exertion or direct impact. Statins are contraindicated in pregnant and nursing women.

Analysis from the TNT and PROVE-IT-TIMI trials demonstrated that adverse events were unrelated to statin dose or to the degree of LDL lowering *(46, 64)*. One exception to this is simvastatin, which at a dose of 80 mg daily is associated with a higher risk for myopathy compared to other statins *(65, 66)*. As myalgia and myopathy are leading reasons cited by patients for statin discontinuation, managing dyslipidemia with optimal statin therapy without adversely affecting patient safety remains an important clinical challenge and goal.

3.5.1.2. STATIN HEPATOTOXICITY

Statins are associated with asymptomatic elevations in serum transaminase levels. The elevation of alanine aminotransferase (ALT) and aspartate aminotransferase (AST) >3 times ULN can be seen with all statins and is dose related *(67)*. It is postulated that ALT and AST are released in response to statin therapy as a result of hepatocyte injury, altered cell membrane integrity, or as an adaptive response to enzyme induction. Other possible mechanisms include disruption of surface transport proteins, cytolytic T-cell activation, apoptosis (programmed cell death) of hepatocytes, mitochondrial disruption, or impaired prenylation of proteins.

There is no evidence that minor asymptomatic elevations of ALT and AST precede acute liver failure, nor is there support for routine monitoring for acute liver failure *(68)*. Although rare, liver injury can occur with the use of statin therapy. Hepatotoxicity is defined as an ALT elevation ≥3 times the upper limit of normal (ULN) on two occasions at least 1 month apart. The average risk of this on statin therapy approximates 1%, but risk increases as a function of dose. Mild elevations in serum transaminases are relatively common and they tend to spontaneously resolve. If transaminitis or hepa-

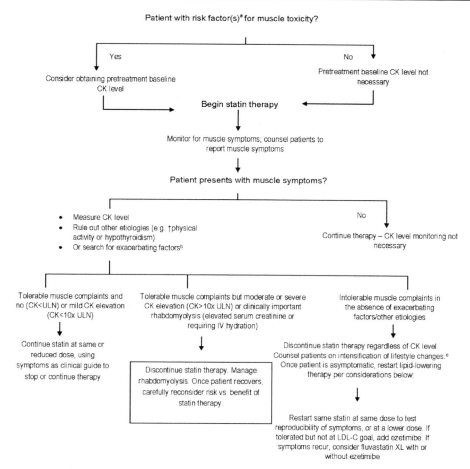

Fig. 4. Clinical algorithm for the management and diagnosis of statin myopathy. [a]Risk factors for muscle toxicity include advanced age and frailty, small body frame, deteriorating renal function, infection, untreated hypothyroidism, interacting drugs, perioperative periods, and alcohol abuse. [b]Common etiologies for elevated CK levels/muscle toxicity: increased physical activity, trauma, falls, accidents, seizure, shaking chills, hypothyroidism, infections, carbon monoxide poisoning, polymyositis, dermatomyositis, alcohol abuse, and drug abuse (cocaine, amphetamines, heroin, or PCP). [c]Patient counseling regarding intensification of therapeutic lifestyle changes (reduced intake of saturated fats and cholesterol, increased physical activity, weight control) should be an integral part of management in all patients with statin-associated intolerable muscle symptoms. Reproduced with permission from (50). CK = creatine kinase, LDL-C = low-density lipoprotein cholesterol, ULN = upper limit of normal.

totoxicity (jaundice, elevated prothrombin time, increased indirect bilirubin, or hepatomegaly) develops, statin therapy should be discontinued until transaminase levels normalize and a different statin can be started at a lower dose. The incidence of liver failure on statin therapy approximates to the background incidence for the population as a whole. The National Lipid Association's recommendations on monitoring for statin-induced hepatotoxicity are summarized in Table 10.

3.5.2. Ezetimibe

Ezetimibe is a selective cholesterol absorption inhibitor that blocks cholesterol absorption at the intestinal brush border (69, 70). Ezetimibe blocks cholesterol absorption by binding to the Niemann–

Pick C1-like 1 (NPC1L1) protein, a sterol transporter that translocates cholesterol and phytosterols (plant sterols) from the intestinal lumen into the jejunal enterocyte *(69–71)*. As monotherapy, ezetimibe reduces levels of LDL-C by approximately 20%, whereas in combination with statins, it has an additive LDL-C-lowering effect *(70, 72, 73)*. Ezetimibe also decreases triglycerides by up to 8% and raises HDL-C by 1–4%. Ezetimibe does not decrease the absorption of bile acids, steroid hormones (ethinyl estradiol, progesterone) or fat-soluble vitamins such as vitamin A, D, E, or α- and β-carotenes. Ezetimibe can be used as primary therapy for LDL-C reduction in statin-intolerant patients.

Ezetimibe remains a primary adjunct to statins in reducing elevated LDL-C. Fixed-dose ezetimibe is also available in combination with increasing doses of simvastatin (Vytorin; 10/10; 10/20; 10/40; 10/80 mg daily). Ezetimibe can also be safely used in combination with other statins. Vytorin dosed at 10/20, 10/40, or 10/80 mg, and LDL-C is reduced by 51, 57, and 59% *(74)*. Ezetimibe therapy equates to approximately three statin titration steps ("rule of 6s"). Vytorin at the 10/20 mg dose helps 82% of high-risk patients reach the LDL-C <100 mg/dL, and at the 10/40 mg dose 52% of patients reach the LDL-C goal of <70 mg/dL *(74)*. The risk of hepatotoxicity with ezetimibe is nearly identical to placebo (0.5% versus 0.3%) and there is no documented evidence of increased risk for myopathy. The addition of ezetimibe to a statin regimen substantially reduces the likelihood of having to titrate the statin. This is a viable alternative for patients who do not tolerate moderate to high doses of statins or who refuse to comply with such doses. The efficacy of ezetimibe for reducing risk for cardiovascular morbidity and mortality in patients with established CAD is being evaluated in the IMProved Reduction of Outcomes: Vytorin Efficacy International (IMPROVE-IT) Trial *(75)*.

3.5.3. Bile Acid-Binding Resins

The bile acid sequestration agents (BASA) are orally administered anion exchange resins that bind bile acids in the gastrointestinal tract and prevent them from being reabsorbed into the enterohepatic circulation. These drugs reduce serum LDL-C by two mechanisms: (1) increased catabolism of cholesterol secondary to the upregulation of 7-α-hydroxylase, the rate-limiting enzyme for the conversion of cholesterol into bile acids; and (2) increased expression of LDL receptors on the hepatocyte surface, which augments the clearance of apoB100-containing lipoproteins from plasma.

The clinical benefit of bile acid sequestrants has been demonstrated in several clinical trials, including the Lipid Research Clinics-Coronary Primary Prevention Trial *(76)* and the Familial Atherosclerosis Treatment Study *(77)*. At maximum doses, the BASA can reduce serum LDL-C by 15–30% and increase HDL-C by 3–5%. It is recommended that these drugs be used in conjunction with a statin whenever possible because BASA therapy increases HMG-CoA reductase activity in the liver, which leads to increased hepatic biosynthesis of cholesterol, thereby offsetting the effects of the BASA over time. Combination therapy with statin and colesevelam hydrochloride has been shown to significantly lower LDL-C levels by up to 34% in patients with hypercholesterolemia *(78–80)*. The BASA are contraindicated in patients with baseline triglycerides >400 mg/dL since they can exacerbate hypertriglyceridemia.

There are currently three different BASA available. These include cholestyramine (Questran; 4–24 g daily in two to three divided doses daily), colestipol (Colestid; 5–30 g in two to three divided doses daily), and colesevelam (Welchol; 1,250 mg two to three times daily). The development of constipation, flatulence, and bloating is relatively frequent, though colesevelam has the most favorable side-effect profile of the three available BASA. Increasing water and soluble fiber ingestion ameliorates some of the difficulty with constipation. The BASA bind negatively charged molecules in a nonspecific manner. Consequently, they can decrease the absorption of warfarin, phenobarbital, thiazide diuretics, digitalis, β-blockers, thyroxine, statins, fibrates, and ezetimibe. These medications should be taken 1 h before or 4 h after the ingestion of BASA. The BASA can reduce the absorption of fat-soluble vitamins.

Colesevelam hydrochloride (HCl) has also been demonstrated to reduce hemoglobin A_{1c} (Hgb A_{1c}) in subjects with type 2 diabetes mellitus by approximately 0.4–0.6% *(81–83)*. The exact mechanism of action by which BASA decrease glucose levels is not yet fully characterized, though it is believed they impact activity of the nuclear transcription factor, farnesoid X receptor-alpha. This leads to alterations in luminal bile acid composition, increases in the incretins cholecystokinin and glucagon-like peptide-1, effects related to hepatocyte nuclear factor 4-alpha *(84)* and reduced gluconeogenesis *(85)* or increased hepatic glycogen synthesis, potentially mediated through enhanced insulin sensitivity *(86)*. It is not known whether the glucose-lowering effects of colesevelam HCl reduces risk for microvascular disease in patients with diabetes mellitus; however, any manner by which serum glucose can be safely lowered is likely beneficial *(87)*.

3.5.4. Fibrates

Fibrates are an important class of drugs for the management of combined dyslipidemia as fibrate–statin combination therapy can be used to promote reductions in LDL-C and triglycerides and simultaneous increases in HDL-C. The fibrates are fibric acid derivatives that exert a number of effects on lipoprotein metabolism. These agents reduce serum triglycerides by 25–50% and raise HDL-C by 10–20%. Fibrates activate lipoprotein lipase by reducing levels of apoprotein CIII (an inhibitor of this enzyme) and increasing levels of apoprotein CII (an activator of lipoprotein lipase). This stimulates the hydrolysis of triglycerides in chylomicrons and VLDL. Fibrates increase HDL-C by two mechanisms. First, the fibrates are PPAR-α agonists and stimulate hepatic expression of apoproteins A-I and A-II. Second, by activating lipoprotein lipase, surface coat mass (phospholipids and apoproteins) derived from VLDL is ultimately used to assimilate HDL in serum. In some patients, fibrate therapy may be associated with an increase in serum LDL-C (the so-called "β" effect) secondary to increased enzymatic conversion of VLDL to LDL. This effect may diminish over time as the patient increases the expression of hepatic LDL receptors but may also be countered with concomitant LDL-C-lowering therapy with either statins or ezetimibe.

Gemfibrozil (Lopid) therapy is associated with reductions in cardiovascular events. The Helsinki Heart Study was a primary prevention trial in 4,081 men 40–55 years of age with a non-HDL cholesterol level >200 mg/dL and compared gemfibrozil therapy (600 mg po bid) to placebo *(88)*. The group treated with gemfibrozil experienced an overall 34% reduction in first-time CAD-related events. Among subjects with triglycerides >200 mg/dL and HDL <42 mg/dL, risk decreased nearly 72%, though this was not statistically significant. In the Veterans Affairs High-Density Lipoprotein Intervention Trial (VA-HIT), men with CAD and mean LDL-C 111 mg/dL, HDL-C 31 mg/dL, and triglyceride 161 mg/dL were randomized to receive either gemfibrozil (600 mg po bid) or placebo over a 5-year follow-up period. The treatment group experienced a 6% elevation in HDL, no change in LDL, and a 31% decrease in triglycerides *(89)*. Among patients treated with gemfibrozil, there was a 22% ($p = 0.006$) reduction in the composite endpoint of all-cause mortality and nonfatal myocardial infarction. Treatment with gemfibrozil reduced the risk of stroke and transient ischemic attacks by 31 and 59%, respectively, and decreased the need for carotid endarterectomy by 65%. The diabetic patients in VA-HIT derived the greatest benefit from gemfibrozil therapy, with reductions of 32% in the combined endpoint, 40% in stroke, and 41% in CHD death *(90)*. The VA-HIT trial was the first to demonstrate a reduction in cardiovascular and cerebrovascular events with an antilipidemic medication independent of changes in serum LDL-C. Most of the benefit of gemfibrozil therapy in this trial was attributed to HDL-C elevation and pleiotropic effects of fibrate therapy.

The Bezafibrate Infarction Prevention (BIP) trial was a secondary prevention trial that compared therapy with bezafibrate (400 mg/day) to placebo in 3,122 men and women with a documented history of CHD *(91)*. Patients were followed for an average of 6.2 years and the primary endpoints in the BIP trial were fatal or nonfatal myocardial infarction and sudden death. Mean lipid parameters in study subjects included LDL 148 mg/dL, HDL 34.6 mg/dL, and triglycerides 145 mg/dL. The patients given bezafibrate experienced a 5% reduction in LDL-C, a 12% increase in HDL, and a 22% decrease in triglyceride (TG). In the cohort, as a whole, bezafibrate therapy reduced risk for the primary composite endpoint by only 7.3%, which was not significant. However, in a post hoc analysis, among patients with a baseline serum triglyceride >200 mg/dL and HDL <35 mg/dL, bezafibrate therapy reduced the composite endpoint by 41%. If baseline HDL levels were ≥35 mg/dL among patients with hypertriglyceridemia, the primary endpoint was reduced 35.9% ($p = 0.33$), which was not statistically significant. In the Fenofibrate Intervention and Event Lowering in Diabetes (FIELD) trial, fenofibrate therapy was shown to decrease the risk of nonfatal MI (24%) and revascularization (21%), and to reduce the progression of microvascular disease, with a 31% reduction in need for photocoagulation therapy for proliferative retinopathy, a 38% reduction in lower extremity amputation, and a 14% reduction in albuminuria in patients with type 2 diabetes mellitus *(92)*.

Fibrates have been shown to exert many of the same pleiotropic effects as statins and reduce atheromatous plaque progression in native coronary vessels and in coronary venous bypass grafts *(93–96)*. Based on the studies discussed above, the optimal clinical scenarios to prescribe fibrates include hypertriglyceridemia and in patients with high triglycerides and low HDL-C. Like the statins, fibrates are associated with a low incidence of myopathy and mild elevations in serum transaminases. Fibrate therapy can increase the risk for cholelithiasis and can raise prothrombin times by displacing warfarin from albumin-binding sites. The periodic monitoring of serum transaminases (6–12 weeks after initiating therapy and twice annually thereafter) is recommended. The three most commonly used fibrates are gemfibrozil (Lopid; 600 mg twice daily), fenofibrate (Tricor; 54 or 160 mg daily), and fenofibric acid (Trilipix; 45 and 135 mg daily). Trilipix is the only fibrate that is approved by the Food and Drug Administration for use in combination with a statin. Bezafibrate is available in Europe and is dosed at 400 mg daily. As gemfibrozil significantly reduces the glucuronidation of statins, which decreases their elimination, there is an increased risk for myopathy/rhabdomyolysis and hepatotoxicity *(97, 98)*. When used in combination with gemfibrozil, the doses for simvastatin and rosuvastatin should not exceed 10 mg daily. A general consideration for the use of fibrate combination therapy is that fenofibrate and fenofibric acid are safer choices, as neither drug adversely impacts the glucuronidation of statins. The efficacy of fenofibrate used in combination with simvastatin compared to simvastatin monotherapy is being tested prospectively in patients with diabetes mellitus in the Action to Control Cardiovascular Risk in Diabetes Trial (http://www.nhlbi.nih.gov/health/prof/heart/other/accord/).

3.5.5. Niacin

Niacin, or nicotinic acid, is a form of vitamin B_3, one of the water-soluble B complex vitamins. Niacin is a potent lipid-modifying agent with broad-spectrum effects, which include reduction of LDL-C, TG, and lipoprotein a (Lp[a]) as well as increasing HDL-C. Evidence of niacin's efficacy in reducing CV events was first demonstrated in the Coronary Drug Project, which demonstrated a 26% reduction in risk of nonfatal myocardial infarction and a 24% reduction in stroke compared to placebo in over 3,900 subjects with established CAD *(99)*.

In patients with metabolic syndrome, niacin stimulates hepatic biosynthesis of apoA-I and HDL *(100)*. Niacin appears to block HDL particle uptake and catabolism by hepatocytes without adversely impacting rates of reverse cholesterol transport. This helps to increase circulating levels of HDL. Niacin reduces hepatic VLDL and triglyceride secretion according to two mechanisms: (1) it decreases the flux of fatty acids from adipose tissue to the liver by inhibiting hormone-sensitive lipase activity; and (2) it inhibits triglyceride formation within hepatocytes by inhibiting diacylglycerol acyltransferase. Niacin also reduces serum LDL-C concentrations by increasing the catabolism of apoB and increases LDL particle size and decreases LDL particle number. Consequently, niacin beneficially impacts all components of the lipoprotein profile.

Niacin is often added to a statin in patients with combined hyperlipidemia, especially if the HDL is low or Lp(a) is high. As demonstrated in the HDL-Atherosclerosis Treatment Study (HATS), combination therapy with high-dose niacin (2–4 g with simvastatin) reduced cardiovascular morbidity and mortality by up to 90% compared to placebo, along with evidence of atheromatous plaque stabilization over a 3-year follow-up period *(101)*. When added to statin therapy in patients with established CAD, extended-release niacin adjuvant therapy is associated with stabilization of carotid intima media thickness (CIMT, a surrogate of atherosclerosis), whereas those patients receiving statin monotherapy experienced significant progression despite having a mean baseline LDL-C of 90 mg/dL *(102)*. In an open-label extension of this trial it was shown that CIMT regression was highly correlated with the magnitude of HDL-C elevation on combination statin–niacin therapy *(103)*.

Niacin should be started at a low dose and gradually titrated upward based on the results of follow-up lipid panels. When evaluated as a function of dose (500–2,000 mg daily), extended-release niacin (ER niacin, Niaspan) induces the following changes in serum lipid levels: LDL-C, 3–16% reduction; triglycerides, 5–32% reduction; HDL-C, 10–24% elevation. It is recommended that Niaspan be the preferred formulation for niacin use as it has the highest available purity, is the best tolerated, and has very low rates of hepatotoxicity *(104)*.

The clinical use of niacin has been limited by cutaneous flushing, a well-recognized associated adverse effect. Niacin-associated flushing has been attributed as the major reason for discontinuation of therapy, estimated at rates as high as 25–40% *(105, 106)*. The flushing is prostaglandin mediated and a number of studies have established that moderate doses of prostaglandin inhibitors can reduce the cutaneous flushing response. Extended-release niacin has been demonstrated to result in reduced flushing including decreased incidence, intensity, and duration as a monotherapy and in statin combination therapy *(107–109)*. Measures to reduce flushing include the use of consistent dosing and dosing with meals. Limiting fat intake for 2–3 h before taking niacin also helps as fat is a source of arachidonic acid, the substrate for cyclooxygenase. The use of aspirin has been found to be beneficial in control of niacin-related flushing, with higher doses of aspirin demonstrating greater efficacy compared to lower-dose aspirin (80 or 160 mg compared to 325 mg) *(110)*. It can also be advantageous to grind the aspirin and suspend it in clear juice. This provides a much more robust, sudden absorption of aspirin and can provide a more substantial level of inhibition of cyclooxygenase. Taking niacin with applesauce can also reduce flushing, possibly because of the pectin, which further slows rates of niacin absorption. ER niacin is also currently available as combination formulations with lovastatin (Advicor; 500/20, 1,000/20, and 2,000/40 mg) and simvastatin (Simcor; 500/20, 750/20, 1,000/20), and the two drugs induce additive changes in the levels of serum lipoproteins.

Ongoing research will provide additional information on the benefit of niacin therapy on CVD mortality and morbidity. The Atherothrombosis Intervention in Metabolic Syndrome with Low HDL/High Triglycerides and Impact on Global Health Outcomes (AIM-HIGH) study is comparing the effects of extended-release niacin and simvastatin. This US–Canadian multicenter, randomized study will enroll up to 3,300 patients with established vascular disease and atherogenic dyslipidemia with follow-up extending through 2010. A number of outcome measures including CHD death, nonfatal myocardial infarction, ischemic stroke, or hospitalization for high-risk acute coronary syndrome will be explored.

A large number of drugs are currently in development that target serum HDL-C elevation or augmentation in the functionality of HDL particles *(111)*. It will be at least 5–8 years before these drugs have been studied enough to attain regulatory approval. In the meantime, currently available drugs such as ER niacin, statins, and fibrates can be used to increase HDL-C. Raising low serum levels of HDL-C can be extremely challenging. Figure 5 outlines a variety of approaches that can be used in the setting of specific lipid profiles. The target of 40 mg/dL is used as any value less than this is considered abnormal. The attainment of 40 mg/dL is often not possible in patients with very low HDL-C since currently available drugs do not always target the molecular lesions that are leading to either inadequate production of HDL-C or increased rates of its catabolism.

Lifestyle modification is a first step in managing low HDL-C (<40 mg/dL). Weight loss and aerobic exercise are important means by which to raise HDL-C since they both relieve insulin resistance.

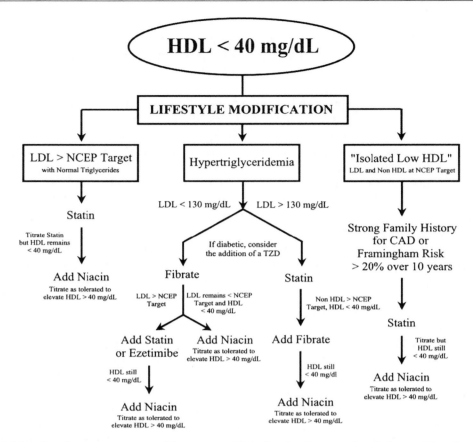

Fig. 5. Algorithm for the management of low-serum high-density lipoprotein cholesterol levels. Reproduced with permission from *(112)*. HDL-C = high-density lipoprotein cholesterol, LDL-C = low-density lipoprotein cholesterol, NCEP = National Cholesterol Education Program, TZD = thiazolidinedione.

Smoking cessation can yield elevations of 15–20%. Cigarette smoking can block the maturation of HDL and promote insulin resistance by stimulating visceral adipocytes to produce tumor necrosis factor-alpha. Carbohydrate restriction is also associated with increases in serum HDL-C. If LDL-C is elevated above NCEP-ATP III targets and TG are normal, statin therapy can be used followed by combination statin/niacin therapy as tolerated to elevate HDL-C >40 mg/dL. If hypertriglyceridemia is present and LDL-C <130 mg/dL, fibrate therapy can be used and then combined with statin or ezetimibe or niacin therapy to achieve the HDL-C goal of >40 mg/dL. In the presence of hypertriglyceridemia (TG >150 mg/dL) and elevated LDL-C (>130 mg/dL), statin therapy alone or in combination with fibrate or niacin regimens can be utilized. In isolated low HDL-C, where a strong family history for CAD exists or the 10-year Framingham risk is > 20%, statin monotherapy followed by combination statin/niacin therapy can be used. Niacin therapy has the greatest capacity for raising HDL-C and newer formulations of extended-release niacin have improved side-effect profiles. In many patients with low HDL-C, however, combination therapy is usually needed. Because many patients with CVD have low HDL-C as their primary lipid abnormality, especially persons with insulin resistance and/or the metabolic syndrome, treating low HDL-C is essential for decreasing risk of CHD and CHD-related events *(8)*. In patients with diabetes mellitus, the thiazolidenediones (pioglitazone, rosiglitazone) can be used to relive insulin resistance, increase HDL-C, and reduce triglycerides and non-HDL-C *(113)*.

3.5.6. Fish Oils

The cardiovascular benefits of omega-3 fatty acids contained in fish oils, namely, eicosapentaenoic acid (EPA) and docosahexaenoic acid (DHA), have been demonstrated as monotherapy as well as in combination with statins *(114–116)*. The American Heart Association guidelines for secondary prevention of CVD recommend consumption of omega-3 FAs in the form of oily fish twice weekly or 1 g/day of EPA and DHA in capsule form, with up to 4 g/day for patients needing TG lowering *(115)*. Ingestion of EPA and DHA lowers tissue levels of arachidonic acid by inhibiting its synthesis and by taking its place in membrane phospholipids. In addition, the same enzyme systems that convert arachidonic acid into eicosanoids can utilize EPA to produce eicosanoids that are typically less active than those made from arachidonic acids. As a result, when EPA and DHA are added to the diet, the eicosanoid balance shifts to a less inflammatory, less thrombotic, and less vasoconstrictive state *(56)*.

A number of clinical trials including the Gruppo Italiano per lo Studio della Sopravvivenza nell'Infarto Miocardio (GISSI) Prevenzione trials have established the effect of omega-3 FA on CVD mortality *(117)*. In the GISSI trial, use of omega-3 FA (850 mg highly purified EPA + DHA per day) demonstrated a significant reduction in mortality (28%) in 11,323 patients surviving a recent (<3 months) myocardial infarction. An even greater reduction (47%) was noted for risk of sudden death; the difference was seen within 6 months of the start of EPA+DHA *(117)*. The treatment benefit was sustained throughout the 3.5-year follow-up without serious side effects such as bleeding. Additional evidence of the benefits of omega-3 FA was demonstrated in the Japan EPA Lipid Intervention Study (JELIS) in which nearly 19,000 Japanese men and women with hypercholesterolemia were prospectively randomized to statin therapy with or without 1,800 mg/day of EPA *(118)*. The combination therapy resulted in an additional 19% reduction in major coronary events at 4.6 years of follow-up compared to statin monotherapy. There were no differences between the statin-only- and statin+EPA-treated patients for LDL-C (26% reduction at 5 years for both groups); however, HDL-C was increased by 3% with statin only and by 5% with statin + EPA, leading the investigators to conclude that the EPA helped prevent CHD events through a cholesterol-independent mechanism *(118)*. In the United States, an omega-3 FA ethyl ester is available at a dosage of 4.0 g/day in capsule form with an indication for TG lowering in patients with very high triglyceride levels (≥500 mg/dL) (Lovaza). The availability of this product eliminates concerns about purity (heavy metal contaminants such as mercury) and standardization of dosage that are raised with nonprescription omega-3 supplements.

3.6. CASE STUDIES

3.6.1. Case 1: Heterozygous Familial Hypercholesterolemia

J.D. is a 26-year-old Caucasian male who presents to clinic concerned about his risk for heart disease. His father and two paternal uncles all sustained myocardial infarctions in their early to mid-forties. His paternal grandfather died suddenly of a "heart attack" at age 47. J.D. does not want to suffer a similar fate as he knows that when it comes to family history, history repeats itself. The patient has no symptoms of myocardial ischemia. He runs 3 miles five times weekly. He is on no medications, and his personal past medical history is completely unremarkable. He does not smoke and occasionally drinks one or two glasses of wine. J.D. has a normal physical examination with no xanthomas or infiltrative lipid dermatitis. His blood pressure is 110/70 mmHg, pulse 56 bpm, and respiratory rate 16 per minute. His fasting lipid profile reveals a total cholesterol of 376 mg/dL, LDL-C 300 mg/dL, triglyceride 70 mg/dL, and HDL-C 62 mg/dL. His Framingham risk score is 1%. The patient by risk scoring is low risk, but based on his family history and the fact that he meets criteria for heterozygous familial hypercholesterolemia, he has substantial risk. The patient is advised that it is extremely important that his LDL-C be lowered aggressively. His markedly elevated LDL-C likely stems from a loss of function mutation in the gene for the LDL receptor, resulting in impaired LDL-C clearance from blood. If this is not addressed, he will remain at risk for the development of premature CAD, just like his father and paternal uncles.

The patient is counseled to begin rosuvastatin at 20 mg daily. He understands that statin therapy is associated with risk for skeletal muscle and liver toxicity. After 6 weeks of therapy, his LDL-C decreases to 165 mg/dL. The rosuvastatin is then titrated to 40 mg daily with LDL-C decreasing to 148 mg/dL. Colesevelam is added at three tablets twice daily. After 2 months, LDL-C decreases to 113 mg/dL. The patient understands that an optimal LDL-C is <100 mg/dL, a level he would like to try and attain. Ezetimibe is added to his regimen and after 6 weeks of this three-drug combination therapy, his LDL-C decreases to 97 mg/dL. He is tolerating his medications without adverse side effect. J.D. understands that his exercise regimen, attention to diet, and pharmacologic therapy must be lifelong if he is to effectively prevent the development of premature CAD.

3.6.2. Case 2: Severe Hypertriglyceridemia

S.Y. is a 41-year-old African-American female who presents to clinic as a new patient. She just moved to town. She notes that she had an episode of pancreatitis 3 years ago. She was told at the time to take gemfibrozil and to eat a low-fat diet because she had severe hypertriglyceridemia. She was uncomfortable at the time with taking a lipid-lowering medication, but did her best to adhere to a low-fat diet as prescribed by a dietitian. She read in a health magazine that pancreatitis causes pancreatic injury and can result in diabetes mellitus, a disease she wishes to avoid at all costs.

Apart from her history of pancreatitis and hypertriglyceridemia, S.Y.'s past medical history is unremarkable. Her father died of an MI at age 47, while her mother is alive and well at age 59. She has no siblings. She does not smoke, and since her episode of pancreatitis strictly avoids alcohol. Blood pressure is 130/78, pulse 80 bpm, and respiratory rate is 14 per minute. Her physical examination is normal with waist circumference of 26 in. A fasting lipid profile shows serum triglyceride to be 4,000 mg/dL with HDL-C 32 mg/dL, and LDL-C not calculable because her triglycerides exceed 400 mg/dL. Fasting blood sugar is 89 mg/dL, and her serum electrolytes, renal indices, liver functions, and thyroid profile were all normal.

S.Y. is counseled about the need to normalize her triglycerides as she remains at substantial risk for recurrence of pancreatitis. She understands that she likely has a significant functional lipoprotein lipase deficiency resulting in severely elevated serum triglyceride levels. She is started on a combination of fenofibric acid 135 mg/dL and Lovaza 4.0 g daily. She is also referred to a dietitian to intensify her dietary restriction of saturated and trans fat. After 8 weeks of this therapy, her triglycerides decrease to 750 mg/dL and HDL-C is 43 mg/dL. She is walking 2.5 miles daily and has severely curtailed her diet. She is willing to take additional medication to lower her triglycerides into a safer range. She is advised to begin the pancreatic lipase inhibitor, orlistat (Xenical), a drug that reduces the absorption of fat within the gastrointestinal tract, with each meal. She understands that this drug can induce the formation of oily, fatty stools with risk for sudden onset diarrhea. After 8 additional weeks, her triglycerides decrease to 210 mg/dL, her HDL-C is 58 mg/dL, and her LDL-C is 120 mg/dL. She is tolerating her pharmacologic regimen. She understands that she must continue her pharmacologic regimen and lifestyle modification lifelong in order to prevent recurrent pancreatitis as well as atherosclerotic disease from her severe baseline dyslipidemia.

3.7. CONCLUSION

Dyslipidemia remains a major risk factor for CVD and is a leading cause of morbidity and mortality. The treatment of dyslipidemia with lifestyle modification and pharmacologic intervention is associated with significant CVD risk reduction. While LDL-C remains the primary target for CVD risk reduction, there is growing recognition of the importance of targeting low HDL and elevated TG and non-HDL-

C as part of the management of dyslipidemia. As dyslipidemia is a modifiable risk factor, aggressive lipid management for cardiovascular protection is, therefore, crucial to any clinical effort directed at reducing risk for cardiovascular events in both the primary and secondary prevention settings.

REFERENCES

1. Lloyd-Jones D, Adams R, Carnethon M, et al. Heart disease and stroke statistics—2009 update: a report from the American Heart Association Statistics Committee and Stroke Statistics Subcommittee. *Circulation.* 2009;119:480–486; Erratum appears in *Circulation.* 2009;119(3):e182.
2. Stamler J, Wentworth D, Neaton JD. Is relationship between serum cholesterol and risk of premature death from coronary heart disease continuous and graded? Findings in 356,222 primary screenees of the Multiple Risk Factor Intervention Trial (MRFIT). *JAMA.* 1986;256:2823–2828.
3. Castelli WP. Cholesterol and lipids in the risk of coronary artery disease—the Framingham Heart Study. *Can J Cardiol.* 1988;4(Suppl A):5A–10A.
4. Assmann G, Cullen P, Schulte H. The Munster Heart Study (PROCAM). Results of follow-up at 8 years. *Eur Heart J.* 1998;19(Suppl A):A2–A11.
5. Goldbourt U, Holtzman E, Neufeld HN. Total and high density lipoprotein cholesterol in the serum and risk of mortality: evidence of a threshold effect. *Br Med J (Clin Res Ed).* 1985;290:1239–1243.
6. Verschuren WM, Jacobs DR, Bloemberg BP, et al. Serum total cholesterol and long-term coronary heart disease mortality in different cultures. Twenty-five-year follow-up of the seven countries study. *JAMA.* 1995;274:131–136.
7. Libby P. Inflammation in atherosclerosis. *Nature.* 2002;420:868–874.
8. Toth PP. When high is low: raising low levels of high-density lipoprotein cholesterol. *Curr Cardiol Rep.* 2008;10:488–496.
9. Toth PP, Gotto AM. High-density lipoprotein cholesterol. In: Gotto AM, Toth PP, eds. *Comprehensive Management of High Risk Cardiovascular Patients.* New York, NY: Informa Healthcare; 2006:295–339.
10. Armani A, Toth PP. SPARCL: the glimmer of statins for stroke risk reduction. *Curr Atheroscler Rep.* 2007;9:347–351.
11. Fielding CJ, Fielding PE. Molecular physiology of reverse cholesterol transport. *J Lipid Res.* 1995;36:211–228.
12. Navab M, Anantharamaiah GM, Reddy ST, et al. Oral D-4F causes formation of pre-beta high-density lipoprotein and improves high-density lipoprotein-mediated cholesterol efflux and reverse cholesterol transport from macrophages in apolipoprotein E-null mice. *Circulation.* 2004;109:3215–3220.
13. Cuchel M, Rader DJ. Macrophage reverse cholesterol transport: key to the regression of atherosclerosis? *Circulation.* 2006;113:2548–2555.
14. Heinecke JW. The HDL proteome: a marker—and perhaps mediator—of coronary artery disease. *J Lipid Res.* 2009;50(Suppl):S167–S171.
15. Vaisar T, Pennathur S, Green PS, et al. Shotgun proteomics implicates protease inhibition and complement activation in the antiinflammatory properties of HDL. *J Clin Invest.* 2007;117:746–756.
16. Castelli WP. Cholesterol and lipids in the risk of coronary artery disease—the Framingham Heart Study. *Can J Cardiol.* 1988;4:5A–10A.
17. Castelli WP, Doyle JT, Gordon T, et al. HDL cholesterol and other lipids in coronary heart disease. The cooperative lipoprotein phenotyping study. *Circulation.* 1977;55:767–772.
18. Gordon DJ, Probstfield JL, Garrison RJ, et al. High-density lipoprotein cholesterol and cardiovascular disease. Four prospective American studies. *Circulation.* 1989;79:8–15.
19. Sacco RL, Benson RT, Kargman DE, et al. High-density lipoprotein cholesterol and ischemic stroke in the elderly: the Northern Manhattan Stroke Study. *JAMA.* 2001;285:2729–2735.
20. Sarwar N, Danesh J, Eiriksdottir G, et al. Triglycerides and the risk of coronary heart disease: 10,158 incident cases among 262,525 participants in 29 Western prospective studies. *Circulation.* 2007;115:450–458.
21. Toth PP, Dayspring TD, Pokrywka GS. Drug therapy for hypertriglyceridemia: fibrates and omega-3 fatty acids. *Curr Atheroscler Rep.* 2009;11:71–79.
22. Miller M, Cannon CP, Murphy SA, Qin J, Ray KK, Braunwald E. Impact of triglyceride levels beyond low-density lipoprotein cholesterol after acute coronary syndrome in the PROVE IT-TIMI 22 trial. *J Am Coll Cardiol.* 2008;51: 724–730.
23. Grundy SM, Cleeman JI, Merz CN, et al. Implications of recent clinical trials for the National Cholesterol Education Program Adult Treatment Panel III guidelines. *Circulation.* 2004;110:227–239. [erratum appears in Circulation. 2004 Aug 10;110(6):763]
24. Expert Panel on Detection EaToHBCiA. Executive summary of the third report of the National Cholesterol Education Program (NCEP) Expert Panel on Detection, Evaluation, and Treatment of High Blood Cholesterol in Adults (Adult Treatment Panel III). *JAMA.* 2001;285:2486–2497.

25. Sarnak MJ, Levey AS, Schoolwerth AC, et al. Kidney disease as a risk factor for development of cardiovascular disease: a statement from the American Heart Association Councils on kidney in cardiovascular disease, high blood pressure research, clinical cardiology, and epidemiology and prevention. *Hypertension.* 2003;42:1050–1065.

26. Toth PP. Intensive LDL-C lowering: which patients benefit? *Fam Pract Recertification.* 2007;29(8):24–37.

27. Brischetto CS, Connor WE, Connor SL, Matarazzo JD. Plasma lipid and lipoprotein profiles of cigarette smokers from randomly selected families: enhancement of hyperlipidemia and depression of high-density lipoprotein. *Am J Cardiol.* 1983;52(7):675–680.

28. Ford ES. Prevalence of the metabolic syndrome defined by the International Diabetes Federation among adults in the US [see comment]. *Diabetes Care.* 2005;28:2745–2749.

29. Chapman MJ, Assmann G, Fruchart JC, Shepherd J, Sirtori C. Raising high-density lipoprotein cholesterol with reduction of cardiovascular risk: the role of nicotinic acid—a position paper developed by the European Consensus Panel on HDL-C. *Curr Med Res Opin.* 2004;20:1253–1268.

30. Sacks FM. The role of high-density lipoprotein (HDL) cholesterol in the prevention and treatment of coronary heart disease: expert group recommendations. *Am J Cardiol.* 2002;90:139–143.

31. Downs JR, Clearfield M, Weis S, et al. Primary prevention of acute coronary events with lovastatin in men and women with average cholesterol levels: results of AFCAPS/TexCAPS. Air Force/Texas Coronary Atherosclerosis Prevention Study. *JAMA.* 1998;279:1615–1622.

32. Influence of pravastatin and plasma lipids on clinical events in the West of Scotland Coronary Prevention Study (WOSCOPS). *Circulation.* 1998;97:1440–1445.

33. Randomised trial of cholesterol lowering in 4444 patients with coronary heart disease: the Scandinavian Simvastatin Survival Study (4S). *Lancet.* 1994;344:1383–1389.

34. Prevention of cardiovascular events and death with pravastatin in patients with coronary heart disease and a broad range of initial cholesterol levels. The Long-Term Intervention with Pravastatin in Ischaemic Disease (LIPID) Study Group. *N Engl J Med.* 1998;339:1349–1357.

35. Sever PS, Dahlof B, Poulter NR, et al. Prevention of coronary and stroke events with atorvastatin in hypertensive patients who have average or lower-than-average cholesterol concentrations, in the Anglo-Scandinavian Cardiac Outcomes Trial—Lipid Lowering Arm (ASCOT-LLA): a multicentre randomised controlled trial. *Lancet.* 2003;361: 1149–1158.

36. Colhoun HM, Betteridge DJ, Durrington PN, et al. Primary prevention of cardiovascular disease with atorvastatin in type 2 diabetes in the Collaborative Atorvastatin Diabetes Study (CARDS): multicentre randomised placebo-controlled trial. *Lancet.* 2004;364:685–696.

37. Ridker PM, Danielson E, Fonseca FA, et al. Rosuvastatin to prevent vascular events in men and women with elevated C-reactive protein. *N Engl J Med.* 2008;359:2195–2207.

38. McKenney JM, Davidson MH, Jacobson TA, Guyton JR. National Lipid Association Statin Safety Assessment Task F. Final conclusions and recommendations of the National Lipid Association Statin Safety Assessment Task Force. *Am J Cardiol.* 2006;97:17.

39. Shepherd J, Blauw GJ, Murphy MB, et al. Pravastatin in elderly individuals at risk of vascular disease (PROSPER): a randomised controlled trial. *Lancet.* 2002;360:1623–1630.

40. Cannon CP, Braunwald E, McCabe CH, et al. Intensive versus moderate lipid lowering with statins after acute coronary syndromes. *N Engl J Med.* 2004;350:1495–1504.

41. Cannon CP. The IDEAL cholesterol: lower is better. *JAMA.* 2005;294:2492–2494.

42. Toth PP. Low-density lipoprotein reduction in high-risk patients: how low do you go? *Curr Atheroscler Rep.* 2004;6:348–352.

43. Nissen SE, Nicholls SJ, Sipahi I, et al. Effect of very high-intensity statin therapy on regression of coronary atherosclerosis: the ASTEROID trial. *JAMA.* 2006;295:1556–1565.

44. Nissen SE, Tuzcu EM, Schoenhagen P, et al. Effect of intensive compared with moderate lipid-lowering therapy on progression of coronary atherosclerosis: a randomized controlled trial. *JAMA.* 2004;291:1071–1080.

45. Cannon CP, Steinberg BA, Murphy SA, Mega JL, Braunwald E. Meta-analysis of cardiovascular outcomes trials comparing intensive versus moderate statin therapy. *J Am College Cardiol.* 2006;48:438–445.

46. LaRosa JC, Grundy SM, Waters DD, et al. Intensive lipid lowering with atorvastatin in patients with stable coronary disease. *N Engl J Med.* 2005;352:1425–1435.

47. Baigent C, Keech A, Kearney PM, et al. Efficacy and safety of cholesterol-lowering treatment: prospective meta-analysis of data from 90,056 participants in 14 randomised trials of statins. *Lancet.* 2005;366:1267–1278.

48. Kearney PM, Blackwell L, Collins R, et al. Efficacy of cholesterol-lowering therapy in 18,686 people with diabetes in 14 randomised trials of statins: a meta-analysis. *Lancet.* 2008;371:117–125.

49. Grundy SM, Cleeman JI, Merz CN, et al. Implications of recent clinical trials for the National Cholesterol Education Program Adult Treatment Panel III guidelines. *Circulation.* 2004;110:227–239.

50. Toth PP, Harper CR, Jacobson TA. Clinical characterization and molecular mechanisms of statin myopathy. *Expert Rev Cardiovasc Ther.* 2008;6:955–969.

51. Toth PPCC. Implications of recent statin trials for primary care practice. *J Clin Lipidol.* 2007;1:182–190.
52. Toth PP, Davidson MH. High-dose statin therapy: benefits and safety in aggressive lipid lowering. *J Fam Prac.* 2008;57:S29–S36.
53. Jackevicius CA, Mamdani M, Tu JV. Adherence with statin therapy in elderly patients with and without acute coronary syndromes. *JAMA.* 2002;288:462–467.
54. Fruchart JC. Peroxisome proliferator-activated receptor-alpha activation and high-density lipoprotein metabolism. *Am J Cardiol.* 2001;88:24N–29N.
55. Liao JK, Laufs U. Pleiotropic effects of statins. *Annu Rev Pharmacol Toxicol.* 2005;45:89–118.
56. Jones P, Beyond LDL-C. Importance of triglycerides and non-HDL as an independent cardiovascular disease risk factor. *J Am Acad Phys Assist.* 2008;11:S7–S19.
57. Toth PP. Why do patients at highest CV risk receive the least treatment? The danger of doing too little. *Res Staff Phys.* 2007;53:s1–s7.
58. Alsheikh-Ali AA, Maddukuri PV, Han H, Karas RH. Effect of the magnitude of lipid lowering on risk of elevated liver enzymes, rhabdomyolysis, and cancer: insights from large randomized statin trials. [see comment]. *J Am Coll Cardiol.* 2007;50:409–418.
59. Jacobson TA. The safety of aggressive statin therapy: how much can low-density lipoprotein cholesterol be lowered? *Mayo Clin Proc.* 2006;81:1225–1231.
60. Jacobson T. Statin safety: lessons from new drug applications for marketed statins. *Am J Cardiol.* 2006;97(Suppl): 44C–51C.
61. Pasternak RC, Smith SC Jr., Bairey-Merz CN, et al. ACC/AHA/NHLBI clinical advisory on the use and safety of statins.[see comment]. *Stroke.* 2002;33:2337–2341.
62. McKenney JM, Davidson MH, Jacobson TA, Guyton JR, National Lipid Association Statin Safety Assessment Task Force. Final conclusions and recommendations of the National Lipid Association Statin Safety Assessment Task Force. *Am J Cardiol.* 2006;97:89C–94C.
63. Heart Protection Study Collaborative Group. MRC/BHF Heart Protection Study of cholesterol lowering with simvastatin in 20,536 high-risk individuals: a randomised placebo-controlled trial. Summary for patients in *Curr Cardiol Rep.* 2002;4(6):486–487; PMID: 123791690. *Lancet.* 2002;360:7–22.
64. Cannon CP, Braunwald E, McCabe CH, et al. Intensive versus moderate lipid lowering with statins after acute coronary syndromes. *N Engl J Med.* 2004;350:1495–1504; Erratum appears in *N Engl J Med.* 2006 Feb; 354(7):778.
65. de Lemos JA, Blazing MA, Wiviott SD, et al. Early intensive vs a delayed conservative simvastatin strategy in patients with acute coronary syndromes: phase Z of the A to Z trial. *JAMA.* 2004;292:1307–1316.
66. Nissen SE. High-dose statins in acute coronary syndromes: not just lipid levels. *JAMA.* 2004;292:1365–1367.
67. Puri P, Sanyal AJ. Why do lipid-lowering agents affect serum transaminase levels, are these drugs toxic to the liver, and can they precipitate liver failure? In: Toth PP, Sica DA, eds. *Clinical Challenges in Lipid Disorders.* Oxford: Atlas Publishing; 2008:189–201.
68. Sniderman AD. Is there value in liver function test and creatine phosphokinase monitoring with statin use? *Am J Cardiol.* 2004;94:30F–34F.
69. Altmann SW, Davis HR Jr, Zhu LJ, et al. Niemann-Pick C1 Like 1 protein is critical for intestinal cholesterol absorption. *Science.* 2004;303:1201–1204.
70. Bruckert E, Giral P, Tellier P. Perspectives in cholesterol-lowering therapy: the role of ezetimibe, a new selective inhibitor of intestinal cholesterol absorption. *Circulation.* 2003;107:3124–3128.
71. Kastelein JJ, Akdim F, Stroes ES, et al. Simvastatin with or without ezetimibe in familial hypercholesterolemia. *N Engl J Med.* 2008;358:1431–1443; Erratum appears in *N Engl J Med.* 2008;358(18):1977.
72. Davidson MH, McGarry T, Bettis R, et al. Ezetimibe coadministered with simvastatin in patients with primary hypercholesterolemia. *J Am Coll Cardiol.* 2002;40:2125–2134.
73. Jackevicius CA, Tu JV, Ross JS, Ko DT, Krumholz HM. Use of ezetimibe in the United States and Canada. *N Engl J Med.* 2008;358:1819–1828.
74. Ballantyne CM, Abate N, Yuan Z, King TR, Palmisano J. Dose-comparison study of the combination of ezetimibe and simvastatin (Vytorin) versus atorvastatin in patients with hypercholesterolemia: the Vytorin Versus Atorvastatin (VYVA) study. *Am Heart J.* 2005;149:464–473.
75. Cannon CP, Giugliano RP, Blazing MA, et al. Rationale and design of IMPROVE-IT (IMProved Reduction of Outcomes: Vytorin Efficacy International Trial): comparison of ezetimbe/simvastatin versus simvastatin monotherapy on cardiovascular outcomes in patients with acute coronary syndromes. *Am Heart J.* 2008;156: 826–832.
76. The lipid research clinics coronary primary prevention trial results. I. Reduction in incidence of coronary heart disease. *JAMA.* 1984;251:351–364.
77. Brown G, Albers JJ, Fisher LD, et al. Regression of coronary artery disease as a result of intensive lipid-lowering therapy in men with high levels of apolipoprotein B. *N Engl J Med.* 1990;323:1289–1298.

78. Davidson MH, Toth P, Weiss S, et al. Low-dose combination therapy with colesevelam hydrochloride and lovastatin effectively decreases low-density lipoprotein cholesterol in patients with primary hypercholesterolemia. *Clin Cardiol.* 2001;24:467–474.

79. Knapp HH, Schrott H, Ma P, et al. Efficacy and safety of combination simvastatin and colesevelam in patients with primary hypercholesterolemia. *Am J Med.* 2001;110:352–360.

80. Hunninghake D, Insull W Jr, Toth P, Davidson D, Donovan JM, Burke SK. Coadministration of colesevelam hydrochloride with atorvastatin lowers LDL cholesterol additively. *Atherosclerosis.* 2001;158:407–416.

81. Zieve FJ, Kalin MF, Schwartz SL, Jones MR, Bailey WL. Results of the glucose-lowering effect of WelChol study (GLOWS): a randomized, double-blind, placebo-controlled pilot study evaluating the effect of colesevelam hydrochloride on glycemic control in subjects with type 2 diabetes. *Clin Thera.* 2007;29:74–83.

82. Goldberg RB, Fonseca VA, Truitt KE, Jones MR. Efficacy and safety of colesevelam in patients with type 2 diabetes mellitus and inadequate glycemic control receiving insulin-based therapy. *Arch Int Med.* 2008;168:1531–1540.

83. Fonseca VA, Rosenstock J, Wang AC, Truitt KE, Jones MR. Colesevelam HCl improves glycemic control and reduces LDL cholesterol in patients with inadequately controlled type 2 diabetes on sulfonylurea-based therapy. *Diabetes Care.* 2008;31:1479–1484.

84. Bays HE, Cohen DE. Rationale and design of a prospective clinical trial program to evaluate the glucose-lowering effects of colesevelam HCl in patients with type 2 diabetes mellitus. *Curr Med Res Opin.* 2007;23:1673–1684.

85. Stayrook KR, Bramlett KS, Savkur RS, et al. Regulation of carbohydrate metabolism by the farnesoid X receptor.[see comment]. *Endocrinology.* 2005;146:984–991.

86. Musha H, Hayashi A, Kida K, et al. Gender difference in the level of high-density lipoprotein cholesterol in elderly Japanese patients with coronary artery disease. *Intern Med.* 2006;45:241–245.

87. Bays H, Jones PH. Colesevelam hydrochloride: reducing atherosclerotic coronary heart disease risk factors. *Vasc Heal Risk Manag.* 2007;3:733–742.

88. Manninen V, Elo MO, Frick MH, et al. Lipid alterations and decline in the incidence of coronary heart disease in the Helsinki Heart Study. *JAMA.* 1988;260:641–651.

89. Robins SJ, Collins D, Wittes JT, et al. Relation of gemfibrozil treatment and lipid levels with major coronary events: VA-HIT: a randomized controlled trial. *JAMA.* 2001;285:1585–1591.

90. Rubins HB, Robins SJ, Collins D, et al. Diabetes, plasma insulin, and cardiovascular disease: subgroup analysis from the Department of Veterans Affairs high-density lipoprotein intervention trial (VA-HIT). *Arch Intern Med.* 2002;162:2597–2604.

91. Secondary prevention by raising HDL cholesterol and reducing triglycerides in patients with coronary artery disease: the Bezafibrate Infarction Prevention (BIP) study. *Circulation.* 2000;102:21–27.

92. Keech A, Simes RJ, Barter P, et al. Effects of long-term fenofibrate therapy on cardiovascular events in 9795 people with type 2 diabetes mellitus (the FIELD study): randomised controlled trial. *Lancet.* 2005;366:1849–1861.

93. Ericsson CG, Hamsten A, Nilsson J, Grip L, Svane B, de Faire U. Angiographic assessment of effects of bezafibrate on progression of coronary artery disease in young male postinfarction patients. *Lancet.* 1996;347:849–853.

94. Frick MH, Syvanne M, Nieminen MS, et al. Prevention of the angiographic progression of coronary and vein-graft atherosclerosis by gemfibrozil after coronary bypass surgery in men with low levels of HDL cholesterol. Lopid coronary angiography trial (LOCAT) Study Group. *Circulation.* 1997;96:2137–2143.

95. Karpe F, Taskinen MR, Nieminen MS, et al. Remnant-like lipoprotein particle cholesterol concentration and progression of coronary and vein-graft atherosclerosis in response to gemfibrozil treatment. *Atherosclerosis.* 2001;157:181–187.

96. Effect of fenofibrate on progression of coronary-artery disease in type 2 diabetes: the Diabetes atherosclerosis intervention study, a randomised study. *Lancet.* 2001;357:905–910.

97. Prueksaritanont T, Zhao JJ, Ma B, et al. Mechanistic studies on metabolic interactions between gemfibrozil and statins. *J Pharmacol Exp Ther.* 2002;301:1042–1051.

98. Prueksaritanont T, Subramanian R, Fang X, et al. Glucuronidation of statins in animals and humans: a novel mechanism of statin lactonization. *Drug Metab Dispos.* 2002;30:505–512.

99. Canner PL, Berge KG, Wenger NK, et al. Fifteen year mortality in Coronary Drug Project patients: long-term benefit with niacin. *J Am Col Cardiol.* 1986;8:1245–1255.

100. Lamon-Fava S, Diffenderfer MR, Barrett PH, et al. Extended-release niacin alters the metabolism of plasma apolipoprotein (Apo) A-I and ApoB-containing lipoproteins. *c*the combination for the prevention of coronary disease. *N Engl J Med.* 2001;345:1583–1592.

101. Brown BG, Zhao XQ, Chait A, et al. Simvastatin and niacin, antioxidant vitamins, or the combination for the prevention of coronary disease. *N Engl J Med.* 2001;345(22):1583–1592.

102. Taylor AJ, Sullenberger LE, Lee HJ, Lee JK, Grace KA. Arterial biology for the investigation of the treatment effects of reducing cholesterol (ARBITER) 2: a double-blind, placebo-controlled study of extended-release niacin on atherosclerosis progression in secondary prevention patients treated with statins. *Circulation.* 2004;110:3512–3517.

103. Taylor AJ, Lee HJ, Sullenberger LE. The effect of 24 months of combination statin and extended-release niacin on carotid intima-media thickness: ARBITER 3. *Curr Med Res Opin.* 2006;22:2243–2250.
104. Mosca L, Appel LJ, Benjamin EJ, et al. Evidence-based guidelines for cardiovascular disease prevention in women. American Heart Association scientific statement. *Arterioscler Thromb Vasc Biol.* 2004;24:e29–e50.
105. Guyton JR, Bays HE. Safety considerations with niacin therapy. *Am J Cardiol.* 2007;99:22C–31C.
106. Birjmohun RS, Kastelein JJ, Poldermans D, Stroes ES, Hostalek U, Assmann G. Safety and tolerability of prolonged-release nicotinic acid in statin-treated patients. *Curr Med Res Opin.* 2007;23:1707–1713.
107. Cefali EA, Simmons PD, Stanek EJ, Shamp TR. Improved control of niacin-induced flushing using an optimized once-daily, extended-release niacin formulation. *Int J Clin Pharmacol Ther.* 2006;44:633–640.
108. Cefali EA, Simmons PD, Stanek EJ, McGovern ME, Kissling CJ. Aspirin reduces cutaneous flushing after administration of an optimized extended-release niacin formulation. *Int J Clin Pharmacol Ther.* 2007;45:78–88.
109. Rubenfire M, Impact of Medical Subspecialty on Patient Compliance to Treatment Study Group. Safety and compliance with once-daily niacin extended-release/lovastatin as initial therapy in the Impact of Medical Subspecialty on Patient Compliance to Treatment (IMPACT) study. *Am J Cardiol.* 2004;94:306–311.
110. Oberwittler H, Baccara-Dinet M. Clinical evidence for use of acetyl salicylic acid in control of flushing related to nicotinic acid treatment. *Int J Clin Prac.* 2006;60:707–715.
111. Toth PP. Novel therapies for increasing serum levels of HDL. *Endocrinol Metab Clin North Am.* 2009;38:151–170.
112. Toth PP. High-density lipoprotein and cardiovascular risk. *Circulation.* 2004;109:1809–1812.
113. Goldberg RB, Kendall DM, Deeg MA, et al. A comparison of lipid and glycemic effects of pioglitazone and rosiglitazone in patients with type 2 diabetes and dyslipidemia. *Diabetes Care.* 2005;28:1547–1554.
114. Harper CR, Jacobson TA. Usefulness of omega-3 fatty acids and the prevention of coronary heart disease. *Am J Cardiol.* 2005;96:1521–1529.
115. Kris-Etherton PM, Harris WS, Appel LJ. American Heart Association. Nutrition Committee. Fish consumption, fish oil, omega-3 fatty acids, and cardiovascular disease. *Circulation.* 2002;106:2747–2757; Erratum appears in *Circulation.* 2003;107(3):512.
116. Lee JH, O'Keefe JH, Lavie CJ, Marchioli R, Harris WS. Omega-3 fatty acids for cardioprotection. *Mayo Clin Proc.* 2008;83:324–332; Erratum appears in *Mayo Clin Proc.* 2008;83(6):730.
117. Marchioli R, Barzi F, Bomba E, et al. Early protection against sudden death by n-3 polyunsaturated fatty acids after myocardial infarction: time-course analysis of the results of the Gruppo Italiano per lo Studio della Sopravvivenza nell'Infarto Miocardico (GISSI)-Prevenzione. *Circulation.* 2002;105:1897–1903.
118. Yokoyama M, Origasa H, Matsuzaki M, et al. Effects of eicosapentaenoic acid on major coronary events in hypercholesterolaemic patients (JELIS): a randomised open-label, blinded endpoint analysis. *Lancet.* 2007;369:1090–1098; Erratum appears in *Lancet.* 2007;370(9583):220.

4 Obesity and Therapeutic Approaches to Weight Loss

Robert F. Kushner

CONTENTS

Key Words: Body mass index; Bariatric surgery; Mediterranean diet; Obesity; Orexigen; Weight loss.

KEY POINTS

- The etiology of obesity is multifactorial, brought about by an interaction between predisposing genetic and metabolic factors and a rapidly changing environment.
- The USPSTF recommends that clinicians screen all adult patients for obesity and offer intensive counseling and behavioral interventions.
- Assessment of the patient should include the evaluation of body mass index (BMI), waist circumference, and overall medical risk.
- Obesity is a risk factor for multiple cardiovascular diseases accounting for 13% of total CVD mortality.
- The primary goal of treatment is to improve obesity-related, co-morbid conditions and reduce the risk of developing future co-morbidities through lifestyle, pharmacologic, and surgical interventions, when indicated.
- The initial goal of weight loss therapy is to reduce body weight by approximately 10% from baseline.
- Lifestyle management incorporates the three essential components of obesity care: dietary therapy, physical activity, and behavior therapy.
- The combination of dietary modification and exercise is the most effective behavioral approach for treatment of obesity.

From: *Contemporary Cardiology: Comprehensive Cardiovascular Medicine in the Primary Care Setting*
Edited by: Peter P. Toth, Christopher P. Cannon, DOI 10.1007/978-1-60327-963-5_4
© Springer Science+Business Media, LLC 2010

- Adjuvant pharmacological treatments should be considered for patients with a BMI $\geq$30 kg/m^2 or with a BMI $\geq$27 kg/m^2 who also have concomitant obesity-related risk factors.
- Bariatric surgery can be considered for patients with severe obesity (BMI >40 kg/m^2) or those with moderate obesity (BMI >35 kg/m^2) associated with a serious medical condition.

4.1. THE BURDEN OF OBESITY

Weight gain and obesity are becoming the most significant chronic public health conditions of our generation, impacting the well-being, productivity, longevity, and economics of our society. Obesity, along with diet and physical inactivity, is estimated to be responsible for approximately 400,000 preventable deaths per year and is expected to soon rival cigarette smoking as the most important public health concern (1). More than one-third of US adults—over 72 million people—were obese in 2005–2006 (2), accounting for over 9% of total annual US medical expenditures (3). The etiology of obesity is multifactorial, brought about by an interaction between predisposing genetic and metabolic factors and a rapidly changing environment, one that favors excessive caloric intake while at the same time reducing opportunities to engage in a physically active lifestyle. The net result of the obesity epidemic is a significantly increased mortality overall, mortality from cardiovascular disease (CVD), from some cancers, and from diabetes and kidney disease (4). Furthermore, the younger the age at onset of obesity along with occurrence of obesity-related morbidity is likely to lead to an increased burden of disability within the obese older population (5). For all of these reasons, it is imperative that clinicians actively evaluate and manage patients with obesity. This chapter reviews the identification, evaluation, and medical management of the adult obese patient. A previously published 10-booklet Primer from the American Medical Association reviews that the assessment and treatment of obesity will be helpful to interested readers who want further information about the implementation of obesity care into their office practice (6).

4.2. ASSESSMENT OF THE OVERWEIGHT AND OBESE PATIENT AND IDENTIFICATION OF RISK

In 1998 the National Heart, Lung, and Blood Institute (NHLBI) published *The Clinical Guidelines on the Identification, Evaluation, and Treatment of Overweight and Obesity in Adults (7)*. The expert panel used evidence-based methodology to develop key recommendations for assessing and treating overweight and obese patients. *A Practical Guide to the Identification, Evaluation, and Treatment of Overweight and Obesity in Adults* was subsequently developed cooperatively by the NHLBI and North American Association for the Study of Obesity (NAASO) and published in 2000 (8). Both guidelines recommend proactive obesity care, beginning with identification, classification, and categorization of risk. More recently, the US Preventive Services Task Force reinforced this recommendation by concluding that clinicians should screen all adult patients for obesity and offer intensive counseling and behavioral interventions to promote sustained weight loss for obese adults (9).

A thorough obesity-focused history, physical examination, and laboratory evaluation based on the patient's risk factors should be completed prior to discussing and initiating treatment (10). Assessment of the patient should include the evaluation of body mass index (BMI), waist circumference (for BMI <35 kg/m^2), and overall medical risk.

BMI is calculated as weight (kg)/height (m^2), or more conveniently as weight (pounds)/height (inches)^2 × 703. For easy reference, Table1 shows the corresponding BMI based on height and weight. Table 2 is used to define classification of weight status and risk of disease. A desirable or healthy BMI is 18.5–24.9 kg/m^2, overweight is 25–29.9 kg/m^2, and obesity is $\geq$30 kg/m^2. Obesity is further sub-defined into class I (30.0–34.9 kg/m^2), class II (35.0–39.9 kg/m^2), and class III

Table 1
Body Mass Index (BMI)

BMI	19	20	21	22	23	24	25	26	27	28	29	30	31	32	33	34	35
Height (in.)							Body weight (pounds)										
58	91	96	100	105	110	115	119	124	129	134	138	143	148	153	158	162	167
59	94	99	104	109	114	119	124	128	133	138	143	148	153	158	163	168	173
60	97	102	107	112	118	123	128	133	138	143	148	153	158	163	168	174	179
61	100	106	111	116	122	127	132	137	143	148	153	158	164	169	174	180	185
62	104	109	115	120	126	131	136	142	147	153	158	164	169	175	180	186	191
63	107	113	118	124	130	135	141	146	152	158	163	169	175	180	186	191	197
64	110	116	122	128	134	140	145	151	157	163	169	174	180	186	192	197	204
65	114	120	126	132	138	144	150	156	162	168	174	180	186	192	198	204	210
66	118	124	130	136	142	148	155	161	167	173	179	186	192	198	204	210	216
67	121	127	134	140	146	153	159	166	172	178	185	191	198	204	211	217	223
68	125	131	138	144	151	158	164	171	177	184	190	197	203	210	216	223	230
69	128	135	142	149	155	162	169	176	182	189	196	203	209	216	223	230	236
70	132	139	146	153	160	167	174	181	188	195	202	209	216	222	229	236	243
71	136	143	150	157	165	172	179	186	193	200	208	215	222	229	236	243	250
72	140	147	154	162	169	177	184	191	199	206	213	221	228	235	242	250	258
73	144	151	159	166	174	182	189	197	204	212	219	227	235	242	250	257	265
74	148	155	163	171	179	186	194	202	210	218	225	233	241	249	256	264	272
75	152	160	168	176	184	192	200	208	216	224	232	240	248	256	264	272	279
76	156	164	172	180	189	197	205	213	221	230	238	246	254	263	271	279	287

BMI	36	37	38	39	40	41	42	43	44	45	46	47	48	49	50	51	52	53	54
58	172	177	181	186	191	196	201	205	210	215	220	224	229	234	239	244	248	253	258
59	178	183	188	193	198	203	208	212	217	222	227	232	237	242	247	252	257	262	267
60	184	189	194	199	204	209	215	220	225	230	235	240	245	250	255	261	266	271	276
61	190	195	201	206	211	217	222	227	232	238	243	248	254	259	264	269	275	280	285
62	196	202	207	213	218	224	229	235	240	246	251	256	262	267	273	278	284	289	295
63	203	208	214	220	225	231	237	242	248	254	259	265	270	278	282	287	293	299	304
64	209	215	221	227	232	238	244	250	256	262	267	273	279	285	291	296	302	308	314
65	216	222	228	234	240	246	252	258	264	270	276	282	288	294	300	306	312	318	324
66	223	229	235	241	247	253	260	266	272	278	284	291	297	303	309	315	322	328	334
67	230	236	242	249	255	261	268	274	280	287	293	299	306	312	319	325	331	338	344
68	236	243	249	256	262	269	276	282	289	295	302	308	315	322	328	335	341	348	354
69	243	250	257	263	270	277	284	291	297	304	311	318	324	331	338	345	351	358	365
70	250	257	264	271	278	285	292	299	306	313	320	327	334	341	348	355	362	369	376

(Continued)

Table 1
(Continued)

BMI	36	37	38	39	40	41	42	43	44	45	46	47	48	49	50	51	52	53	54
71	257	265	272	279	286	293	301	308	315	322	329	338	343	351	358	365	372	379	386
72	265	272	279	287	294	302	309	316	324	331	338	346	353	361	368	375	383	390	397
73	272	280	288	295	302	310	318	325	333	340	348	355	363	371	378	386	393	401	408
74	280	287	295	303	311	319	326	334	342	350	358	365	373	381	389	396	404	412	420
75	287	295	303	311	319	327	335	343	351	359	367	375	383	391	399	407	415	423	431
76	295	304	312	320	328	336	344	353	361	369	377	385	391	402	410	418	426	435	443

Table 2
Classification of Weight Status and Risk of Disease

		Risk of disease (relative to having a healthy weight and waist size)	
		Waist circumference[a]	
		35 in. or less (women)	More than 35 in. (women)
		40 in. or less (men)	More than 40 in. (men)
Underweight	BMI below 18.5		
Healthy weight	BMI 18.5–24.9		
Overweight	BMI 25.0–29.9	Increased	High
Obesity	BMI 30.0–34.9	High	Very high
Obesity	BMI 35.0–39.9	Very high	Very high
Extreme obesity	BMI 40 or more	Extremely high	Extremely high

[a]Measure waist circumference just above the iliac crest. An increased waist circumference may indicate increased disease risk even at a normal weight.

Adapted from National Institutes of Health, National Heart, Lung, and Blood Institute. *Clinical Guidelines on the Identification, Evaluation, and Treatment of Overweight and Obesity in Adults (7).* US Department of Health and Human Services, Public Health Service; 1998.

($\geq$40 kg/m^2). According to the Practical Guide, patients at very high absolute risk that trigger the need for intense risk factor modification and management include the following—established coronary heart disease; presence of other atherosclerotic diseases such as peripheral arterial disease, abdominal aortic aneurysm, or symptomatic carotid artery disease; type 2 diabetes; and sleep apnea. Other symptoms and diseases listed by organ system that are directly or indirectly related to obesity are displayed in Table 3.

Overall risk is independently associated with excess abdominal fat, which can be clinically defined as a waist circumference $\geq$102 cm ($\geq$40 in.) in men and $\geq$88 cm ($\geq$35 in.) in women. According to the Practical Guide (8), "To measure waist circumference, locate the upper hip bone and the top of the right iliac crest. Place a measuring tape in a horizontal plane around the abdomen at the level of the iliac crest. Before reading the tape measure, ensure that the tape is snug, but does not compress the skin, and is parallel to the floor. The measurement is made at the end of a normal expiration." Overweight persons with waist circumferences exceeding these limits should be urged more strongly to pursue weight reduction. The importance of measuring and documenting waist circumference in patients with a BMI <35 kg/m^2 is due to the independent contribution of abdominal fat to the development of co-morbid diseases, particularly the metabolic syndrome (11, 12). The clinical evaluation of obese adults is depicted in Fig. 1 (13).

4.2.1. Cardiovascular Disease

As seen in Table 3, obesity is a risk factor for multiple cardiovascular diseases. In a recent analysis of cause-specific excess deaths associated with BMI, 13% of total CVD mortality was associated with obesity (4). Obesity affects the cardiovascular system through multiple known and yet unrecognized mechanisms (14). The positive association between body weight and blood pressure is well established from multiple epidemiology studies and weight loss is the cornerstone for non-pharmacological management (15). The recently published Multi-Ethnic Study of Atherosclerosis (MESA) study showed that the strong relationship between obesity and an increased burden of CVD risk factors is similar in all racial/ethnic and sex groups (16). As a result of these accumulating risk factors, an increased

Table 3
Obesity-Related Organ Systems Review

Cardiovascular	*Respiratory*
Hypertension	Dyspnea
Congestive heart failure	Obstructive sleep apnea
Atrial fibrillation	Hypoventilation syndrome
Cor pulmonale	Pickwickian syndrome
Varicose veins	Asthma
Pulmonary embolism	
Coronary artery disease	
Endocrine	*Gastrointestinal*
Metabolic syndrome	Gastroesophageal reflux disease (GERD)
Type 2 diabetes	Non-alcoholic fatty liver disease (NAFLD)
Dyslipidemia	Cholelithiasis
Polycystic ovarian syndrome (PCOS)/androgenicity	Hernias
Amenorrhea/infertility/menstrual disorders	Colon cancer
Musculoskeletal	*Genitourinary*
Hyperuricemia and gout	Urinary stress incontinence
Immobility	Obesity-related glomerulopathy
Osteoarthritis (knees and hips)	End stage renal failure
Low back pain	Hypogonadism (male)
	Breast and uterine cancer
	Pregnancy complications
Psychological	*Neurologic*
Depression/low self-esteem	Stroke
Body image disturbance	Idiopathic intracranial hypertension
Social stigmatization	*Meralgia paresthetica*
Integument	
Striae distensae (stretch marks)	
Stasis pigmentation of legs	
Lymphedema	
Cellulitis	
Intertrigo, carbuncles	
Acanthosis nigricans/skin tags	

incidence of atrial fibrillation *(17)*, congestive heart failure *(18)*, and coronary artery disease *(19)* has been seen among the obese with higher BMI associated with a younger age of first non-ST segment elevation myocardial infarction (NSTEMI) *(20)*. In addition to traditional risk factors, perhaps the strongest association of obesity with an increased risk of CVD is occurrence of the metabolic syndrome. The constellation of non-traditional metabolic abnormalities associated with insulin resistance includes increased atherogenic lipoproteins (small dense LDL particles, apolipoprotein B), biomarkers of chronic inflammation (C-reactive protein, tumor necrosis factor-″, interleukin-6), a prothrombotic state (increased plasma plasminogen activator inhibitor (PAI)-1 and fibrinogen), endothelial dysfunction (decreased endothelium-dependent vasodilatation), hemodynamic changes (increased sympathetic nervous activity and renal sodium retention), hyperuricemia, and non-alcoholic fatty liver disease (NAFLD) *(21)*. Abdominal obesity in particular is more strongly correlated with this cluster of abnormalities *(22, 23)*.

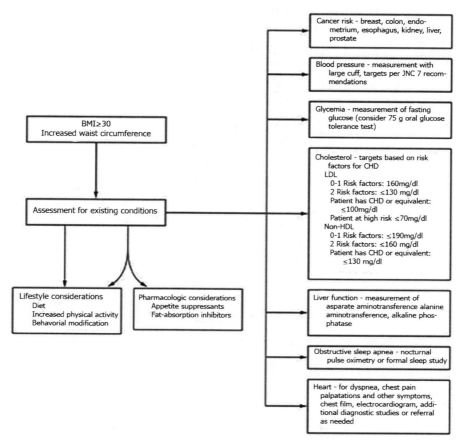

Fig. 1. Clinical evaluation of obese adults. All patients should be assessed for obesity-associated conditions through a history and physical examination. Cancer screening should be performed as recommended by the National Cancer Institute (www.cancer.gov/cancertopics/screening). The Seventh Report of the Joint National Committee (JNC 7) should be used to establish the goals of hypertension treatment (www.nhlbi.nih.gov/guidelines/hypertension). Guidelines from the National Cholesterol Education Program–Adult Treatment Panel III (NCEP–ATP III) should be used to establish acceptable levels of LDL cholesterol and non-HDL cholesterol (www.nhlbi.nih.gov/guidelines/cholesterol/index.htm). Patients at high risk (with a target of ≤70 mg/dL LDL cholesterol) have multiple major risk factors, including the metabolic syndrome, continued cigarette smoking, and, especially, diabetes (5). Reprinted from (13).

4.3. MEDICAL MANAGEMENT OF THE OVERWEIGHT AND OBESE PATIENT

4.3.1. The Goal of Therapy

Information obtained from the history, physical examination, and diagnostic tests is used to determine risk and to develop a treatment plan. The primary goal of treatment is to improve obesity-related co-morbid conditions and reduce the risk of developing future co-morbidities through nonpharmacologic, pharmacologic, and surgical interventions when indicated. The decision of how aggressively to treat patients and which modalities to use is determined by the patients' risk status, their expectations, and what resources are available. Table 4 provides a guide to selecting adjunctive treatments based on BMI category. Therapy for obesity always begins with lifestyle management and may include pharmacotherapy or surgery. The guidelines recommend setting an initial weight loss goal of 10% over

Table 4
A Guide to Selecting Treatment

BMI category	25–26.9	27–29.9	30–35	35–39.9	≥40
Treatment					
Diet, exercise, behavior therapy	With co-morbidities	With co-morbidities	+	+	+
Pharmacotherapy		With co-morbidities	+	+	+
Surgery				With co-morbidities	+

Source: NHLBI and NAASO *The Practical Guide: Identification, Evaluation, and Treatment of Overweight and Obesity in Adults.* US Department of Health and Human Services, Public Health Service, National Institutes of Health, National Heart, Lung, and Blood Institute. NIH Publication No. 00-4084, October, 2000.

6 months *(7)*. A recent meta-analysis of 80 weight loss clinical trials demonstrated that a mean weight loss of 5–8.5 kg (5–9%) was actually observed in clinical practice *(24)*.

4.4. LIFESTYLE MANAGEMENT

Lifestyle management incorporates the three essential components of obesity care: dietary therapy, physical activity, and behavior therapy.

Since obesity is fundamentally a disease of energy imbalance, all patients must understand how and when energy is consumed (diet), how and when energy is expended (physical activity), and how to incorporate this information into their daily life (behavior therapy).

In the current acute care office setting, there are limited evidence-based interventions shown to specifically improve health professionals' management of obesity *(25–27)*. Accordingly, a team approach to obesity care utilizing community and other office-based resources will be needed for effective management.

4.4.1. Diet Therapy

The NHLBI Guidelines recommend initiating treatment with a diet producing a calorie deficit of 500–1,000 kcal/day *(7)*. This translates into prescribing a diet containing 1,000–1,200 kcal/day for most women and between 1,200 and 1,600 kcal/day for men. The primary focus of diet therapy is on reducing overall consumption of calories and dietary sources of excessive fat and simple sugars. Since portion control is one of the most difficult strategies for patients to manage, use of pre-prepared products, called meal replacements, is a simple and convenient suggestion. Meal replacements are foods that are designed to take the place of a meal while at the same time providing nutrients and good taste within a known caloric limit *(28)*. Examples include frozen entrees, canned beverages, and bars. In a meta-analysis of six studies with a study duration ranging from 3 to 5 months, use of partial meal replacements resulted in a 7–8% weight loss *(29)*. Incorporation of meal replacements as a portion control strategy has also been successfully used in the Look AHEAD Study, where average weight loss among patients with type 2 diabetes was 8.6% of initial weight after 1 year of treatment *(30)*.

Beyond prescribing a calorie-controlled diet, an ongoing clinical and research question is the importance of the macronutrient diet content, such as low-carbohydrate, high-protein, or a Mediterranean dietary pattern.

In general, it is reasonable to vary the macronutrient composition of the diet depending on the patient's preference and medical condition.

The Institute of Medicine (IOM) Report published in 2002 recommends a broad range of acceptable macronutrient levels consisting of 45–65% of total calories from carbohydrates, 20–35% of total calories from fat, and 10–35% of total calories from protein *(31)*. Two meta-analyses of the effects of low-carbohydrate diets on weight loss and body composition have recently been published. Krieger et al. *(32)* found that short-term low-carbohydrate diets increase the loss of body weight, fat-free mass, fat mass, and percentage of body fat during weight reduction compared with traditional diets. Nordmann et al. *(33)* concluded that after 6 months, individuals assigned to low-carbohydrate diets lost more weight than those on low-fat diets, however, after 12 months, there was no significant difference between diets. A recent 2-year study demonstrated the effectiveness of a Mediterranean dietary pattern on weight loss along with improvement in the metabolic profile *(34)*. These and other studies *(35–37)* also suggest—two additional important factors—that increases in dietary protein may be more beneficial than carbohydrate restriction alone in terms of increasing satiety and that sustained adherence to the diet rather than diet type is likely to be the best predictor of weight loss outcome.

4.4.2. Physical Activity Therapy

Although exercise alone is only moderately effective for weight loss, the combination of dietary modification and exercise is the most effective behavioral approach for treatment of obesity. In contrast, the most important role of exercise appears to be in the maintenance of the weight loss *(38)*. Physical activity is beneficial for improved cardiorespiratory fitness, cardiovascular disease and cancer risk reduction, and improved mood and self-esteem. The recently released Physical Activity Guidelines for Americans recommends engaging in 2 h and 30 min/week of moderate intensity physical activity *(39)*. Focusing on simple ways to add physical activity into the normal daily routine, such as walking, using the stairs, doing home and yard work, and increasing recreational activity is a useful first step in counseling. Recommending that patients wear pedometers to monitor total accumulation of steps is a useful strategy and has been shown to increase physical activity and lead to significant reductions in BMI *(40)*. Studies have demonstrated that lifestyle activities are as effective as structured exercise programs in improving cardiorespiratory fitness *(41)* and weight loss *(42)*. The American College of Sports Medicine (ACSM) recommends that overweight and obese individuals progressively increase to a minimum of 150 min of moderate intensity physical activity per week as a first goal *(43)*. However, for long-term weight loss, higher amounts of exercise (e.g., 200–300 min/week or ≥2,000 kcal/week) are needed. The ACSM also recommends that resistance exercise supplements the endurance exercise program. Many patients would benefit from consultation with an exercise physiologist or personal trainer.

4.4.3. Behavioral Therapy

Implementing sustainable changes in the patient's diet and physical activity patterns is the most challenging feature of obesity care. Multiple behavioral modification theories and techniques have been applied to obesity with mostly modest outcomes. The most commonly used approaches include motivational interviewing *(44)*, transtheoretical model and stages of change *(45)*, and cognitive behavioral therapy (CBT) *(46)*. These techniques can be learned and used by physicians, but they do take time. In the setting of a busy practice, they are probably more reasonably applied by ancillary office staff such as a nurse clinician or registered dietician. Nonetheless, a few key behavioral principles should be utilized when possible. It is important to recognize that increasing knowledge by itself does not seem to be useful in promoting behavioral change.

CBT incorporates various strategies intended to help change and reinforce new dietary and physical activity behaviors *(47, 48)*. Strategies include self-monitoring techniques (e.g., journaling, weighing and measuring food, and activity), stress management, stimulus control (e.g., using smaller plates, not eating in front of the television or in the car), social support, problem solving, and cognitive restructuring, i.e., helping patients develop more positive and realistic thoughts about themselves. When recommending any behavioral lifestyle change, have the patient identify what, when, where, and how the behavioral change will be performed and have the patient and yourself keep a record of the anticipated behavioral change and follow-up progress at the next office visit. Among the behavioral strategies, self-monitoring of food records has repeatedly been shown to be a significant predictor of greater weight loss *(49, 50)*.

4.5. PHARMACOTHERAPY

Adjuvant pharmacological treatments should be considered for patients with a BMI ≥ 30 kg/m^2 or with a BMI ≥ 27 kg/m^2 who also have concomitant obesity-related risk factors or diseases and for whom dietary and physical activity therapy has not been successful (Table 4). Anti-obesity drugs require the implementation of lifestyle modification as a foundation for drug action due to the importance of the drug–behavior interaction. Whether the medication acts centrally to suppress appetite or peripherally to block the absorption of fat, patients must deliberately and consciously alter their behavior for weight loss to occur. In other words, for all anti-obesity drugs, the pharmacological action must be *translated* into behavior change. In a randomized trial by Wadden et al. *(51)*, evaluating the benefits of lifestyle modification in the pharmacologic treatment of obesity, investigators showed that the efficacy of sibutramine-induced mean weight loss at 1 year was significantly enhanced when subjects also attended a lifestyle support group (–10.8%) or lifestyle support group plus portion-controlled diet (–16.5%) versus sibutramine alone (–4.1%). Thus, when prescribing an anti-obesity medication, patients must be actively engaged in a lifestyle program that provides the strategies and skills needed to effectively use the drug.

There are several potential targets of pharmacological therapy for obesity, all based on the concept of producing a sustained negative energy (calorie) balance. Currently, there are only two categories of medication approved by the US Food and Drug Administration (FDA) for weight loss and maintenance of weight loss—appetite suppressants and gastrointestinal lipase inhibitors. Interested readers are referred to other recent comprehensive review articles on the pharmacological treatment of obesity *(52–55)*.

4.5.1. Centrally Acting Anorexiant Medications

Appetite-suppressing drugs, or anorexiants, effect *satiation*, the processes involved in the termination of a meal; *satiety*, the absence of hunger after eating; and *hunger*, a biological sensation that initiates eating. The target site for the actions of anorexiants is the ventromedial and lateral hypothalamic regions in the central nervous system. Their biological effect on appetite regulation is produced by variably augmenting the neurotransmission of three monoamines: norepinephrine, serotonin (5-hydroxytryptamine, 5-HT), and to a lesser degree, dopamine. The classical sympathomimetic adrenergic agents (benzphetamine, phendimetrazine, diethylpropion, mazindol, and phentermine) function by either stimulating norepinephrine release or blocking its reuptake. In contrast, sibutramine (Meridia^{TM}) functions as a serotonin and norepinephrine reuptake inhibitor (SNRI). Furthermore, unlike other previously FDA-approved anorexiants, sibutramine is not pharmacologically related to amphetamine and has no addictive potential. Sibutramine is the only drug in this class that is approved for long-term use. It produces a dose-dependent weight loss (available doses are 5, 10, and 15 mg capsules), with an average loss of about 5–9% of initial body weight at 12 months *(56)*. A meta-analysis on sibutramine efficacy reported a mean difference in weight loss (compared to placebo) of 3.43 kg (7.5 lb) at 6 months and 4.45 kg (9.8 lb) at 12 months *(57)*. The medication has been demonstrated to be useful in maintenance of weight loss for up to 2 years *(58)*.

The most commonly reported adverse events of sibutramine are headache, dry mouth, insomnia, and constipation. These are generally mild and well tolerated. The principal concern is a dose-related increase in blood pressure and heart rate that may require discontinuation of the medication. A dose of 10–15 mg/day causes an average increase in systolic and diastolic blood pressure of 2–4 mmHg and an increase in heart rate of 4–6 beats/min. For this reason, all patients should be monitored closely and seen back in the office within 1 month after initiating therapy. The risk of adverse effects on blood pressure is not greater in patients with controlled hypertension than in those who do not have hypertension *(59)*. Contraindications to sibutramine use include uncontrolled hypertension, congestive heart failure, symptomatic coronary heart disease, arrhythmias, or history of stroke.

4.5.2. Peripherally Acting Medication

Orlistat (Xenical^{TM}) is a synthetic hydrogenated derivative of a naturally occurring lipase inhibitor, lipostatin, produced by the mold *Streptomyces toxytricini*. Orlistat is a potent slowly reversible inhibitor of pancreatic, gastric, and carboxylester lipases and phospholipase A_2, which are required for the hydrolysis of dietary fat in the gastrointestinal tract into fatty acids and monoacylglycerols. The drug's activity takes place in the lumen of the stomach and small intestine by forming a covalent bond with the active serine residue site of these lipases *(60)*. Taken at a therapeutic dose of 120 mg tid, orlistat blocks the digestion and absorption of about 30% of dietary fat. The medication was approved by the FDA in 2007 for over-the-counter use at half the prescription dose, trade name Alli^{TM}.

A meta-analysis of clinical trials found that orlistat produced a weighted mean weight loss of 5.7 kg (12.6 lb) compared with 2.4 kg (5.3 lb) in the placebo group *(61)*. Pooled data have also shown that early weight loss (>5% of initial weight after 3 months) predicts weight loss at 18 months. In the longest published follow-up study, mean weight loss after 4 years for the orlistat-treated patients was 5.8 kg (12.8 lb) compared to 3.0 kg (6.6 lb) with placebo *(62)*. Since orlistat is minimally (<1%) absorbed from the gastrointestinal tract, it has no systemic side effects. Tolerability to the drug is related to the malabsorption of dietary fat and subsequent passage of fat in the feces. Six gastrointestinal tract adverse effects have been reported to occur in at least 10% of orlistat-treated patients: oily spotting, flatus with discharge, fecal urgency, fatty/oily stool, oily evacuation, and increased defecation. The events are generally experienced early, diminish as patients control their dietary fat intake, and infrequently cause patients to withdraw from clinical trials. Psyllium mucilloid is helpful in controlling the orlistat-induced GI side effects when taken concomitantly with the medication *(63)*. Serum concentrations of the fat-soluble vitamins D and E and β-carotene have been found to be significantly lower in some of the trials, although generally remain within normal ranges. The manufacturer's package insert for orlistat recommends that patients should take a vitamin supplement along with the drug to prevent potential deficiencies.

4.6. BARIATRIC SURGERY

Bariatric surgery can be considered for patients with severe obesity (BMI >40 kg/m^2) or those with moderate obesity (BMI >35 kg/m^2) associated with a serious medical condition. Weight loss surgical procedures are typically categorized as restrictive, restrictive–malabsorptive, and malabsorptive (Fig. 2) *(64, 65)*. Laparoscopic adjustable gastric banding (LAGB) is the commonly performed restrictive operation. The first banding device, the LAP-BAND^{TM}, was approved for use in the United States in 2001. The REALIZE^{TM} Band was recently approved in 2007. In these procedures, a prosthetic band is placed around the upper portion of the stomach creating a small gastric pouch and thus restricting storage capacity. Band diameter is adjusted by the subcutaneous injection or removal of saline solution in the band reservoir. Adjustment affects gastric outlet size and consequently volume and rate at which food can be consumed.

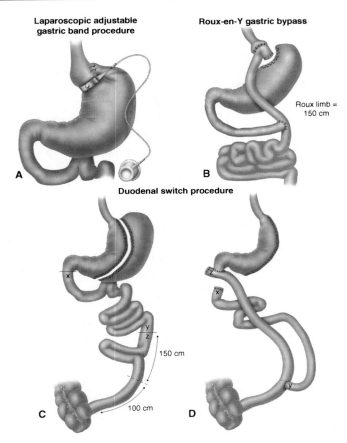

Fig. 2. (**a**) Laparoscopic adjustable gastric banding (LAGB). (**b**) Roux-en-Y gastric bypass (RYGB). (**c**) Biliopancreatic diversion (BPD). (**d**) Biliopancreatic diversion with duodenal switch (BPDDS). Kendrick and Dakin *(64)*, © 2006 Mayo Foundation for Medical Education and Research.

The Roux-en-Y gastric bypass (RYGB) is the most commonly performed and accepted restrictive–malabsorptive procedure. It involves formation of a 10–30-mL proximal gastric pouch by either surgically separating or stapling the stomach across the fundus. Outflow from the pouch is created by performing a narrow (10 mm) gastrojejunostomy. The distal end of jejunum is then anastomosed 50–150 cm below the gastrojejunostomy.

The biliopancreatic diversion (BPD) and biliopancreatic diversion with duodenal switch (BPDDS, a variation of the biliopancreatic diversion) are malabsorptive procedures. The BPD operation involves a subtotal gastrectomy, leaving a much larger gastric pouch compared with the RYGB. The small bowel is divided 250 cm proximal to the ileocecal valve and connected directly to the gastric pouch, producing a gastroileostomy. The remaining proximal limb (biliopancreatic conduit) is then anastomosed to the side of the distal ileum 50 cm proximal to the ileocecal valve. In the BPDDS procedure, the first portion of the duodenum is preserved. The distal small bowel is connected to the short stump of the duodenum, producing a 75–100 cm ileal-duodenal "common channel" for absorption of nutrients. The other end of the duodenum is closed, and the remaining small bowel is connected onto the enteral limb at about 75–100 cm from the ileocecal valve.

Although no recent randomized controlled trials compare weight loss after surgical and non-surgical interventions, available data from meta-analyses and large databases primarily obtained from observational studies suggest that bariatric surgery is the most effective weight loss therapy for those with clinically severe obesity *(66, 67)*. These procedures are generally effective in producing an average weight loss of approximately 30–35% of total body weight that is maintained in nearly 60% of patients at 5 years. An abundance of data supports the positive impact of bariatric surgery on obesity-related morbid conditions including diabetes mellitus, hypertension, obstructive sleep apnea, dyslipidemia, and non-alcoholic fatty liver disease *(68)*. In general, mean weight loss is greatest with the malabsorptive procedures, followed by the restrictive–malabsorptive, then the restrictive procedures. However, the greater weight loss with the BPD and BPDDS procedures is also associated with an increased surgical mortality rate and nutritional complications. The restrictive–malabsorptive procedures produce a predictable increased risk for micronutrient deficiencies of vitamin B_{12}, iron, folate, calcium, and vitamin D based on surgical anatomical changes. The patients require lifelong supplementation with these micronutrients *(69)*.

4.7. CASE STUDY

SC is a 52-year-old post-menopausal woman with a BMI of 30 kg/m^2 who is frustrated about the 15 lb weight gain and change in body shape (increased waist circumference) that occurred over the past 5 years. She has developed hypertension, stress urinary incontinence, and GERD. She tries to follow a healthy diet but is unable to control her body weight. She turns to you for help.

The initial goal of treatment is to educate SC about the importance of balancing caloric intake with caloric expenditure. SC should track her dietary intake recording the types, portions, and calories of foods and beverages consumed. She should also set a goal of engaging in 150 min/week of moderate intensity physical activity. By helping SC become more calorie conscious, she will feel in control of her body weight and learn to self-regulate her diet and physical activity.

4.8. CASE STUDY

AK is a 42-year-old severely obese man with a BMI of 42 kg/m^2. He has a 10 year history of type 2 diabetes treated with insulin, obstructive sleep apnea treated with nightly CPAP, hypertension, and mixed hyperlipidemia. He has experienced a progressive weight gain since childhood and has been unable to control his body weight despite enrollment in several commercial weight loss programs.

AK should consider weight loss surgery as a treatment for his obesity and obesity-related co-morbid conditions. He will need to be evaluated by the bariatric surgical team consisting of a registered dietician, clinical psychologist, and bariatric surgeon. Along with the surgical team, AK will need to have his medical conditions stabilized to reduce peri-operative risk and be prepared for the dietary and behavioral changes necessary for success. AK will require lifelong follow-up after the surgery to monitor for nutritional deficiencies and for weight relapse.

4.9. CONCLUSION

Obesity is a serious and highly prevalent disease associated with increased morbidity and mortality. Assessment and evaluation of obesity by BMI and risk classification should be part of the patient encounter. Treatment modalities should include diet, physical activity and behavior therapy for all patients, and use of pharmacotherapy or surgery in those selected as reasonable candidates. Primary treatment should be directed at controlling obesity-related co-morbidities and achieving an initial modest 10% weight loss for obese patients.

REFERENCES

1. Makdad AH, Marks JS, Stroup DF, Gerberding JL. Actual causes of death in the United States, 2000. *JAMA.* 2004;291:1238–1245.
2. Ogden CL, Carroll MD, McDowell MA, Flegal KM. Obesity among adults in the United States—no significant change since 2003–2004. *NCHS Data Brief.* 2007;1 (Nov):1–6.
3. Finkelstein EA, Fiebelkorn IC, Wang G. National medical spending attributable to overweight and obesity: how much, and who's paying? *Health Affairs.* 2003;W3:219–226.
4. Flegal KM, Graubard BI, Williamson DF, Gail MH. Cause-specific excess deaths associated with underweight, overweight, and obesity. *JAMA.* 2007;298:2028–2037.
5. Alley DE, Chang VW. The changing relationship of obesity and disability, 1988–2004. *JAMA.* 2007;298:2020–2027.
6. Kushner RF. *Roadmaps for Clinical Practice: Case Studies in Disease Prevention and Health Promotion—Assessment and Management of Adult Obesity: A Primer for Physicians.* Chicago, IL: American Medical Association; 2003. Available at: www.ama-assn.org/ama/pub/category/10931.html. Accessed November 5, 2008.
7. National Heart, Lung, and Blood Institute (NHLBI). Clinical guidelines on the identification, evaluation, and treatment of overweight and obesity in adults. The evidence report. *Obes Res.* 1998;6(Suppl 2):51S–210S.
8. National Heart, Lung, and Blood Institute (NHLBI) and North American Association for the Study of Obesity (NAASO). *Practical Guide to the Identification, Evaluation, and Treatment of Overweight and Obesity in Adults.* Bethesda, MD: National Institutes of Health. NIH Publication number 00–4084, Oct 2000.
9. Preventive Services US, Task F. Screening for obesity in adults: recommendations and rationale. *Ann Intern Med.* 2003;139:930–932.
10. Kushner RF, Roth JL. Assessment of the obese patient. *Endocrinol Metab Clin North Am.* 2003;32(4):915–934.
11. National Institutes of Health. *Third Report of the National Cholesterol Education Program Expert Panel on Detection, Evaluation, and Treatment of High Blood Cholesterol in Adults (Adult Treatment Panel III).* Bethesda, MD: National Institutes of Health. NIH Publication 01–3670, 2001.
12. Grundy SM, Brewer B, Cleeman JI, Smith SC, Lenfant C. Definition of metabolic syndrome. Report of the National Heart, Lung, and Blood Institute/American Heart Association conference on scientific issues related to definition. *Circulation.* 2004;109:433–438.
13. Eckel RH. Nonsurgical management of obesity in adults. *N Engl J Med.* 2008;358:1941–1950.
14. Poirier P, Giles TD, Bray GA, et al. Obesity and cardiovascular disease: pathophysiology, evaluation, and effect of weight loss. An update of the 1997 American Heart Association scientific statement on obesity and heart disease from the obesity committee of the council on nutrition, physical activity, and metabolism. *Circulation.* 2006;113:898–918.
15. Harsha DW, Bray GA. Weight loss and blood pressure control (pro). *Hypertension.* 2008;51:1420–1425.
16. Burke GL, Bertoni AG, Shea S, et al. The impact of obesity on cardiovascular disease risk factors and subclinical vascular disease. The multi-ethnic study of atherosclerosis. *Arch Intern Med.* 2008;168:928–935.
17. Wang TJ, Parise H, Levy D, et al. Obesity and the risk of new-onset atrial fibrillation. *JAMA.* 2004;292:2471–2477.
18. Kenchaiah S, Evans JC, Levy D, Wilson PWR, Benjamin EJ, Larson MG, Kannel WB, Vasan RS, et al. Obesity and the risk of heart failure. *N Engl J Med.* 2002;347:305–313.
19. Peeters A, Barendregt JJ, Willekens F, et al. Obesity in adulthood and its consequences for life expectancy: a life-table analysis. *Ann Intern Med.* 2003;138:24–32.
20. Madala MC, Franklin BA, Chen AY, et al. Obesity and age of first non-ST-segment elevation myocardial infarction. *J Am Coll Card.* 2008;52:979–985.
21. Van Gaal LF, Mertens IL, De Block CE. Mechanisms linking obesity with cardiovascular disease. *Nature.* 2006;444:16–18.
22. Zhu SK, Wang ZM, Heshka S, Heo M, Faith MS, Heymsfield SB. Waist circumference and obesity-associated risk factors among whites in the third national health and nutrition examination survey: clinical action thresholds. *Am J Clin Nutr.* 2002;76:743–749.
23. Janssen I, Katzmarzyk PT, Ross R. Waist circumference and not body mass index explains obesity-related health risk. *Am J Clin Nutr.* 2004;79:379–384.
24. Franz MJ, VanWormer JJ, Crain AL, et al. Weight-loss outcomes: a systematic review and meta-analysis of weight-loss clinical trials with a minimum of 1-year follow-up. *J Am Diet Assoc.* 2007;107:1755–1767.
25. Dansinger ML, Tatsioni A, Wong JB, Chung M, Balk EM. Meta-analysis: the effect of dietary counseling for weight loss. *Ann Intern Med.* 2007;147:41–50.
26. McQuigg M, Brown J, Broom J, et al. Counterweight Project Team. Empowering primary care to tackle the obesity epidemic: the Counterweight Programme. *Eur J Clin Nutr.* 2005;59(Suppl 1):S93–S100.
27. Moore H, Summerbell CD, Greenwood DC, et al. Improving management of obesity in primary care: cluster randomized trial. *BMJ.* 2005;327:1085–1089.

28. Bowerman S. The role of meal replacements in weight control. In: Bessesen DH, Kushner R, eds. *Evaluation & Management of Obesity*. Philadelphia, PA: Hanley & Belfus, Inc.; 2002:53–58.

29. Heymsfield SB, van Mierlo CAJ, van der Knaap HCM, Frier HI. Weight management using meal replacement strategy: meta and pooling analysis from six studies. *Int J Obes*. 2003;27:537–549.

30. The Look AHEAD, Research G. Reduction in weight and cardiovascular disease risk factors in individuals with type 2 diabetes. One-year results of the Look AHEAD trial. *Diabetes Care*. 2007;30:1374–1383.

31. National Research Council. *Dietary Reference Intakes for Energy, Carbohydrate, Fiber, Fat, Fatty Acids, Cholesterol, Protein, and Amino Acids*. Washington, DC: National Academy Press; 2002.

32. Krieger JW, Sitren HS, Daniels MJ, Langkamp-Henken B. Effects of variation in protein and carbohydrate intake on body mass and composition during energy restriction: a meta-analysis. *Am J Clin Nutr*. 2006;83:260–274.

33. Nordmann AJ, Nordmann A, Briel M, et al. Effects of low-carbohydrate vs low-fat diets and weight loss and cardiovascular risk factors. A meta-analysis of randomized controlled trials. *Arch Intern Med*. 2006;166:285–293.

34. Shai I, Schwarzfuchs D, Henkin Y, Shahar DR, et al. Weight loss with a low-carbohydrate, Mediterranean, or low-fat diet. *N Engl J Med*. 2008;359:229–241.

35. Adam-Perrot A, Clifton P, Brouns F. Low-carbohydrate diets: nutritional and physiological aspects. *Obes Rev*. 2006;7:49–58.

36. Dansinger ML, Gleason JA, Griffith JL, Selker HP, Schaefer EJ. Comparison of the Atkins, Ornish, weight watchers, and zone diets for weight loss and heart disease risk reduction. A randomized trial. *JAMA*. 2005;293:43–53.

37. Alhassan S, Kim S, Bersamin A, King AC, Gardner CD. Dietary adherence and weight loss success among overweight women: results from the A to Z weight loss study. *Int J Obes*. 2008;32:985–991.

38. Anderson JW, Kontz EC, Frederich RC, et al. Long-term weight-loss maintenance: a meta-analysis of US studies. *Am J Clin Nutr*. 2001;74:579–584.

39. 2008 Physical Activity Guidelines for Americans. www.health.gov/paguidelines.

40. Bravata DM, Smith-Spangler C, Sundaram V, et al. Using pedometers to increase physical activity and improve health. A systematic review. *JAMA*. 2007;298:2296–2304.

41. Dunn AL, Marcus BH, Kampert JB, Garcia ME, et al. Comparison of lifestyle and structured interventions to increase physical activity and cardiorespiratory fitness. A randomized trial. *JAMA*. 1999;281:327–334.

42. Anderson RE, Wadden TA, Bartlett SJ, Zemel B, Verde TJ, Franckowiak SC. Effects of lifestyle activity vs structured aerobic exercise in obese women. A randomized trial. *JAMA*. 1999;281:335–340.

43. Jakacic JM, Clark K, Coleman E, et al. Appropriate intervention strategies for weight loss and prevention of weight regain for adults. *Med Sci Sports Exerc*. 2001;33:2145–2156.

44. WR Miller and S Rollnick, eds. *Motivational Interviewing. Preparing People for Change*. 2nd ed. New York, NY: The Guilford Press; 2002.

45. Prochasea JO, DiClimente CC. Toward a comprehensive model of change. In: Miller WR, ed. *Treating Addictive Behaviors*. New York, NY: Plenum; 1986:3–27.

46. Wadden TA, Crerand CE, Brock J. Behavioral treatment of obesity. *Psychiatr Clin N Am*. 2005;28:151–170.

47. Foreyt JP, Poston WSC. What is the role of cognitive-behavior therapy in patient management? *Obes Res*. 1998;6 (Suppl 1):18S–22S.

48. Wadden TA, Foster GD. Behavioral treatment of obesity. *Med Clin North Am*. 2000;84:441–462.

49. Hollis JF, Gullion CM, Stevens VJ, et al. Weight loss during the intensive intervention phase of the weight-loss maintenance trial. *Am J Prev Med*. 2008;35:118–126.

50. Wadden TA, Berkowitz RI, Womble LG, et al. Randomized trial of lifestyle modification and pharmacotherapy for obesity. *N Engl J Med*. 2005;353:2111–2120.

51. Wadden TA, Berkowitz RI, Sarwer DB, et al. Benefits of lifestyle modification in the pharmacologic treatment of obesity. A randomized trial. *Arch Intern Med*. 2001;161:218–227.

52. Yanovski S, Yanovski JA. Obesity. *N Engl J Med*. 2002;346:591–602.

53. Haddock CK, Poston WSC, Dill PL, Foreyt JP, Ericsson M. Pharmacotherapy for obesity: a quantitative analysis of four decades of published randomized clinical trials. *Int J Obes*. 2002;26:262–273.

54. Padwal R, Li SK, Lau DCW. Long-term pharmacotherapy for overweight and obesity: a systematic review and meta-analysis of randomized controlled trials. *Int J Obes*. 2003;27:1437–1446.

55. Kushner RF. Anti-obesity drugs. *Expert Opin Pharmacother*. 2008;9:1339–1350.

56. Arterburn DE, Crane PK, Veenstra DL. The efficacy and safety of sibutramine for weight loss. A systematic review. *Arch Intern Med*. 2004;164:994–1003.

57. Shekelle PG, Morton SC, Maglione M, et al. Pharmacological and surgical treatment of obesity. Summary evidence report/technology assessment No. 103. AHRQ publication No. 04-E028-1. Rockville, MD: Agency for Healthcare Research and Quality; July 2004.

58. James WPT, Astrup A, Finer N, et al. Effect of sibutramine on weight maintenance after weight loss: a randomized trial. *Lancet*. 2000;356:2119–2125.

59. Hazenberg BP. Randomized, double-blind, placebo-controlled, multicenter study of sibutramine in obese hypertensive patients. *Cardiology.* 2000;94:152–158.
60. Lucas KH, Kaplan-Machlis B. Orlistat—a novel weight loss therapy. *Ann Pharmacother.* 2001;35:314–328.
61. Rucker D, Padwal R, Li SK, et al. Long term pharmacotherapy for obesity and overweight: updated meta-analysis. *BMJ.* 2007;335:1194–1199.
62. Torgerson JS, Hauptman J, Boldrin MN, Sjostrom L. XENical in the prevention of diabetes in Obese Subjects (XEN-DOS) Study. *Diabetes Care.* 2004;27:155–161.
63. Cavaliere H, Floriano I, Medeiros-Neto G. Gastrointestinal side effects of orlistat may be prevented by concomitant prescription of natural fibers (psyllium mucilloid) . *Int J Obes.* 2001;25:1095–1099.
64. Kendrick ML, Dakin GF. Surgical approaches to obesity. *Mayo Clin Proc.* 2006;8(Suppl):S18–S24.
65. Crookes PF. Surgical treatment of morbid obesity. *Annu Rev Med.* 2006;57:243–264.
66. Buchwald H, Avidor Y, Braunwald E, et al. Bariatric surgery: a systematic review and meta-analysis. *JAMA.* 2004;292:1724–1737.
67. Maggard MA, Shugarman LR, Suttorp M, et al. Meta-analysis: surgical treatment of obesity. *Ann Intern Med.* 2005;142:547–559.
68. Sjostrom L, Narbro K, Sjostrom CD, et al. Effects of bariatric surgery on mortality in Swedish obese subjects. *N Engl J Med.* 2007;357:741–752.
69. Kushner RF. Micronutrient deficiencies and bariatric surgery. *Curr Opin Endocrinol Diabetes.* 2006;13:405–411.

5 Inflammatory Markers and Novel Risk Factors

Stephen J. Nicholls

CONTENTS

Key Words: C-reactive protein; Interleukins; Inflammation; Lipoprotein-associated phospholipase A_2; Myeloperoxidase.

KEY POINTS

- Many patients with established coronary heart disease have no identifiable major cardiovascular risk factor.
- Emerging insights into the pathological events that promote formation and progression of atherosclerosis highlight potential biomarkers for risk stratification.
- High-sensitivity C-reactive protein (CRP) independently predicts cardiovascular risk in large cohorts and is likely to identify patients more likely to benefit from statin therapy.
- The role of lipoprotein-associated phospholipase A_2 (Lp-PLA$_2$) and myeloperoxidase (MPO) in the pathogenesis of plaque formation and rupture is likely to underscore their ability to predict cardiovascular risk.
- The role of thrombosis precipitating acute ischemia is consistent with the finding that multiple biomarkers reflecting increased thrombotic and decreased fibrinolytic activity predict cardiovascular events.
- A number of markers of renal impairment predict risk beyond that observed due to associated lipid and blood pressure abnormalities.
- Increasing evidence suggests that markers of systemic oxidative stress and factors that are likely to act as anti-oxidants predict risk.
- A panel of biomarkers that reflect the activity of multiple pathological pathways promoting atherosclerosis may provide incremental risk factor stratification.

From: *Contemporary Cardiology: Comprehensive Cardiovascular Medicine in the Primary Care Setting*
Edited by: Peter P. Toth, Christopher P. Cannon, DOI 10.1007/978-1-60327-963-5_5
© Springer Science+Business Media, LLC 2010

5.1. INTRODUCTION

Atherosclerotic cardiovascular disease is the leading cause of morbidity and mortality in the Western world. The escalation in global prevalence of abdominal adiposity and its associated metabolic risk factors has fueled speculation that cardiovascular disease will become the leading cause of mortality worldwide by 2020 *(1)*. Increasing interest has focused on the development of new systemic biomarkers to assist in the prediction of cardiovascular risk. This should facilitate more effective use of therapeutic strategies developed for cardiovascular prevention.

5.2. TRADITIONAL PREDICTION OF CARDIOVASCULAR RISK

Population studies have identified a number of clinical characteristics associated with an elevated prospective risk of developing coronary heart disease *(2)*. These factors include age, male gender, family history of premature CVD, hypercholesterolemia, hypertension, diabetes mellitus, smoking, obesity and low levels of high-density lipoprotein cholesterol (HDL-C). As a result, risk prediction algorithms have been developed that take into account the presence or absence of the totality of these factors in order to estimate the 10-year prospective cardiovascular risk *(3)*. Using such approaches, it has been possible to stratify patients as low (<10%), intermediate (10–20%) and high (>20%) risk. The use of risk prediction algorithms has been employed by guidelines for use of lipid-modifying therapies *(4)*.

However, it has become apparent that these approaches to risk prediction are limited. Conventional risk prediction algorithms may fail to predict the prospective risk of coronary heart disease in 25–50% of subjects *(5)*. Furthermore, in a pooled analysis of more than 120,000 subjects enrolled in 14 clinical trials of patients with established CHD, it was reported that up to 20% of subjects did not have a single traditional risk factor *(6)*. These findings suggest that evaluation of additional clinical factors will be required in order to achieve more effective prediction of cardiovascular risk.

5.3. DISEASE PATHOLOGY AND RELEVANCE TO NOVEL BIOMARKERS

As the factors that promote the pathogenesis of atherosclerotic cardiovascular disease continue to be elucidated, they identify not only targets for the development of new therapies but also potential markers of increased cardiovascular risk. In particular, it has become increasingly apparent that atherosclerosis is a chronic inflammatory process, with evidence of activation of a range of inflammatory cascades observed at all stages of the disease process *(7)*. In the earliest stages, prior to the development of atherosclerotic plaque, dysfunction of the endothelial layer is accompanied by an increase in expression of proinflammatory adhesion molecules [vascular cell adhesion molecule-1 (VCAM-1), intercellular adhesion molecule-1 (ICAM-1) and chemokines (monocyte chemoattractant protein-1 [MCP-1])]. These factors promote adhesion of circulating monocytes to the endothelial layer and their subsequent migration into the artery wall.

Within the vessel wall, monocytes undergo a morphological change to become macrophages. Uptake of oxidized LDL by macrophages forms foam cells, the cellular hallmark of atherosclerotic plaque. The foam cell subsequently plays a pivotal role in the ongoing development of atheroma, via its ability to elaborate a host of proinflammatory and proliferative factors, leading to ongoing accumulation of leukocytes and smooth muscle cells within the artery wall. As a result, a developing lesion that contains foam cells, inflammatory material and smooth muscle cells under a collagenous fibrous cap represents the mature atherosclerotic plaque.

The translation of atherosclerosis to acute ischemia is typically promoted by rupture of the fibrous cap. Elaboration of matrix metalloproteinases by macrophages within the atherosclerotic plaque results in a breakdown of collagen and elastin within the fibrous cap, creating a milieu that promotes cap rupture. Upon exposure of circulating blood to plaque components including lipid, inflammatory and necrotic material, activation of a number of thrombotic pathways leads to clot formation, with ensuing luminal compromise and ischemia. As a result, it has become clear that inflammatory, oxidative and thrombotic events are critical for the development and subsequent progression of atherosclerotic disease. Accordingly, it is possible that these pathways may identify novel markers that can enhance prediction of cardiovascular risk.

5.4. EMERGING INFLAMMATORY MARKERS

5.4.1. C-Reactive Protein

C-reactive protein (CRP) is a circulating pentraxin, largely produced by the liver in response to cytokine stimulation, and is a major component of the acute phase response. While its predominant role appears to be involved in the innate immune response, increasing evidence suggests that CRP may also participate in the promotion of atherosclerosis. CRP is also produced by smooth muscle cells within atherosclerotic plaque and CRP receptors have been identified on the surface of neutrophils and endothelial cells (8–10). The ability to localize CRP at the level of the artery wall (8–10) and reports that CRP promotes expression of cellular adhesion molecules and chemokines, activates thrombotic pathways and inhibits nitric oxide synthesis (10) support a potential role in the pathogenesis of atherosclerosis. This is further supported by reports that CRP transgenic mice demonstrate increased thrombus formation in response to arterial injury (11).

A large number of population cohorts have demonstrated that levels of high-sensitivity CRP independently predict the risk of developing a first vascular event (12–15). In the Physician's Health Study of more than 22,000 apparently healthy middle-aged males, those subjects with a CRP in the highest quartile had a threefold greater risk of myocardial infarction and a twofold greater risk of stroke (15). CRP has also been reported to predict the risk of a first event in women, with both the Women's Health Study and Nurse's Healthy Study demonstrating that CRP independently predicts cardiovascular risk, after controlling for traditional risk factors (14). In particular, elevated CRP levels predict risk at all levels of LDL-C and measures of global risk (12–15). As a result, it was estimated that measurement of CRP would reclassify the 10-year predicted risk in as many as 40% of women (12–15).

The ability of CRP levels to predict prospective cardiovascular risk has also been reported in many studies of subjects with an established diagnosis of coronary heart disease. In cohorts of subjects with stable or unstable coronary disease and in patients undergoing percutaneous coronary intervention or bypass grafting, elevated CRP levels are associated with an elevated risk of future cardiovascular events (16–23).

However, other investigators have suggested that the link between CRP and cardiovascular risk is relatively modest. In fact, some authors have suggested that the presence of an isolated elevation of CRP is uncommon, with some additional risk factor identified in up to 80% of subjects (24). While associations have been reported, it has yet to be unequivocally demonstrated that CRP plays a direct role in the pathogenesis of plaque formation and progression. This is further complicated by the observation that it is difficult to exclude contaminants such as endotoxin from CRP samples used in laboratory studies (25). Furthermore, some groups have suggested that the ability of CRP to predict the risk of a first vascular event is not as strong as previously reported. In a case-control analysis of a prospective study from Reykjavik, it was demonstrated that while CRP did predict the risk of an adverse cardiovascular outcome, this was not particularly strong with an odds ratio of 1.45 (95% confidence interval 1.25–1.68) (26).

Nevertheless, on the basis of findings from a large number of cohorts and use of well-validated and inexpensive assays, the Centers for Disease Control and American Heart Association recommended use of CRP in the assessment of subjects is deemed to be intermediate risk on the basis of conventional algorithms *(27)*. Using this approach, risk can be classified as low (<1 mg/L), intermediate (1–3 mg/L) and high (>3 mg/L) on the basis of CRP testing *(27)*. Ongoing exploration has endeavored to evaluate the risk prediction ability of incorporating CRP values in addition to assessment of traditional risk factors. Early studies of the role of the Reynold's risk score demonstrate a superior risk prediction role, resulting in reclassification of 40–50% of intermediate risk subjects into higher and lower risk categories *(28)*.

Additional interest in CRP has come from its ability to identify the likelihood of clinical benefit with therapeutic interventions. Increasing data suggest that statins can lower CRP levels in a manner that is independent of their LDL-C lowering properties *(29–31)*. Post-hoc analyses of placebo-controlled trials demonstrated the ability of CRP levels to identify those subjects likely to benefit from statin therapy. In the secondary prevention setting of the Cholesterol and Recurrent Events (CARE) Study, the presence of an elevated CRP at baseline predicted a greater reduction in clinical events with pravastatin, regardless of the baseline LDL-C *(23)* (Fig. 1). A similar finding was subsequently reported in the primary prevention setting in the Air Force/Texas Coronary Atherosclerosis Prevention Study (AFCAPS/TexCAPS) *(32)*. More recently, lowering CRP levels were reported to independently predict the benefit of high-dose atorvastatin on atheroma progression in the Reversal of Atherosclerosis with Aggressive Lipid Lowering (REVERSAL) Study *(33)* and clinical events in the Pravastatin or Atorvastatin Evaluation and Infection Therapy-Thrombolysis in Myocardial Infarction 22 (PROVE IT-TIMI 22) Study *(34)*.

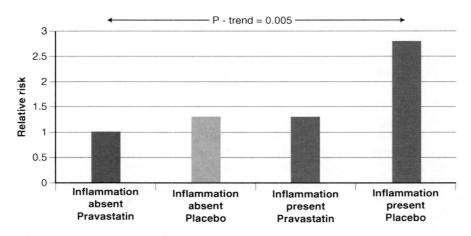

Fig. 1. Relative risk of recurrent coronary events among post-myocardial infarction patients according to the presence or absence of evidence of inflammation (both CRP and serum amyloid A levels above the ninetieth percentile) and by randomization to placebo or pravastatin in patients participating in the CARE study. Copied with permission from *(23)*.

The benefit of statin therapy in subjects with elevated CRP levels was further demonstrated in the Justification for the Use of Statins in Primary Prevention: An Intervention Trial Evaluating Rosuvastatin (JUPITER) Study *(35)*. Seventeen thousand eight hundred and two individuals with an LDL-C less than 130 mg/dL were identified on the basis of a CRP of 2 mg/L or higher and treated with rosuvastatin 20 mg daily or placebo for a median of 1.9 years. Lowering of LDL-C by 50% and CRP by 37% with rosuvastatin was associated with a 44% reduction in the combination of myocardial infarction, stroke, arterial revascularization, hospitalization for unstable angina and cardiovascular mortality ($p < 0.00001$), and a 20% reduction in all-cause mortality ($p = 0.02$). These findings provided further support for the importance of inflammation influencing cardiovascular risk. While no subjects with normal CRP levels were enrolled in the study, the findings suggest that evidence of inflammation does identify a patient who is likely to benefit from use of statin therapy, even in the setting of apparently normal LDL-C levels. The relative contribution of LDL-C and CRP lowering to the clinical benefit remains to be determined by ongoing analysis. While no specific CRP lowering therapy has been evaluated in clinical trials of cardiovascular prevention, it appears that the presence of an elevated CRP does identify a subject, with evidence of systemic inflammation and increased cardiovascular risk, who is likely to derive benefit from a more intensive approach to risk reduction strategies.

5.4.2. Myeloperoxidase

Myeloperoxidase (MPO) is leukocyte-derived member of the heme peroxidase superfamily. MPO is stored in azurophilic granules of circulating neutrophils, monocytes and some macrophages found within tissues such as atherosclerotic plaque. The major oxidant products of MPO-catalyzed pathways have been demonstrated to play an important role in the generation of lipid hydroperoxides, conversion of LDL to a high uptake form, reduced bioavailability of nitric oxide, endothelial cell apoptosis and platelet activation. More recently, MPO has been implicated as a pivotal factor involved in the oxidation and inactivation of apoA-I and the generation of dysfunctional HDL particles, possibly leading to reduced capacity for reverse cholesterol transport. As a result of these effects, it is likely that MPO plays a role in promoting each stage of atherosclerosis from endothelial dysfunction to formation and rupture of atherosclerotic plaque (36).

A number of lines of evidence from human studies further implicates the role of MPO in cardiovascular disease. MPO and its oxidant products have been localized within atherosclerotic plaque specimens (37–39). This is supported by the observation of relative protection from cardiovascular disease in individuals with genetic forms of MPO deficiency (20–42). More recently, an increasing number of studies have reported an association between systemic MPO levels and prospective cardiovascular risk. In asymptomatic patients evaluated with serial carotid ultrasound measurements, accelerated progression of lumenal stenoses was observed in association with elevated MPO levels (43). This relationship between MPO and progression of subclinical disease is supported by nested case-control reports from the European Prospective Investigation into Cancer and Nutrition (EPIC-Norfolk) cohort, which demonstrated a direct relationship between increasing baseline MPO levels and prospective risk of cardiovascular events during 8 years of follow-up, a finding that was independent of the presence of traditional risk factors (44).

In symptomatic patients with stable CAD presenting for diagnostic coronary angiography, the extent of angiographic disease has been reported to be associated with both the systemic MPO levels (45, 46) and the MPO content per leukocyte (47). A number of reports have demonstrated the ability of MPO levels to predict prospective clinical risk in patients with acute ischemic syndromes. In a study of 604 sequential patients evaluated in the emergency room for acute chest pain of suspected cardiac etiology, MPO levels predicted the diagnosis of myocardial infarction and acute coronary syndromes and independently predicted likelihood of experiencing a major adverse cardiovascular event during the next 6 months. These findings were also found in patients whose troponin levels were persistently within normal limits during their hospitalization, suggesting that MPO levels correlate with outcome even in the absence of evidence of myocardial necrosis (48) (Fig. 2). An MPO level less than the upper limit of normal (650 pmol/L) appears to predict a lower incidence of cardiovascular events (48). MPO levels were also found to be the most accurate predictor of future ischemic events in patients with an acute coronary syndrome who were enrolled in the c7E3 Anti-Platelet Therapy in Unstable Refractory (CAPTURE) angina (49) and Treat Angina with Aggrastat and determine Cost of Therapy with an Invasive or Conservative Strategy (TACTICS-TIMI 18) (50) trials.

Beyond its relationship with outcome in patients with clinical ischemia, MPO also plays a prognostic role in the setting of myocardial infarction and heart failure. MPO levels predict outcome in patients with evidence of myocardial infarction, regardless of the presence of ventricular dysfunction

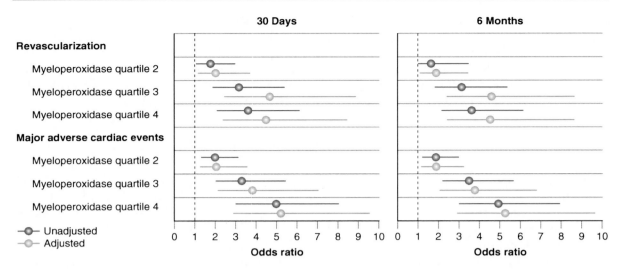

Fig. 2. Risk of revascularization and major adverse cardiac events among patients presenting to the emergency room for evaluation of acute chest pain of suspected cardiac etiology, who were persistently negative for troponin T, according to baseline myeloperoxide levels. Copied with permission from *(48)*.

or cardiogenic shock *(51, 52)*, and predict the presence of occult left ventricular systolic dysfunction, augmenting the role of BNP levels *(53)*, and also are elevated in patients with overt clinical heart failure *(54)*. These findings are consistent with reports that MPO plays an important role in the promotion of ventricular remodeling in murine models of chronic coronary artery ligation and ischemia-reperfusion *(55, 56)*.

5.4.3. Lipoprotein-Associated Phospholipase A₂

Lipoprotein-associated phospholipase A_2 (Lp-PLA$_2$), also known as platelet activating factor acetylhydrolase (PAF-AH), is a member of a family of intracellular and systemic enzymes that hydrolyze the sn-2 fatty acid bond of phospholipids, resulting in the generation of oxidized fatty acids and lysophospholipids. Produced by leukocytes, Lp-PLA$_2$ circulates in association with lipoproteins, predominantly on LDL particles. Considerable controversy has focused on the relative role of Lp-PLA$_2$ in atherosclerosis. The products of Lp-PLA$_2$ activity upregulate activation of inflammatory pathways involved in formation and propagation of atherosclerotic plaque. Lp-PLA$_2$ is found within matured and ruptured, but not early, plaques and colocalizes with foam cells and macrophages, which permit ongoing generation within the atherosclerotic plaque. In contrast, its activity has been proposed to promote the anti-oxidant and anti-inflammatory properties of HDL and in a Japanese cohort heterozygous deficiency of Lp-PLA$_2$ is associated with an increased rate of myocardial infarction, stroke and peripheral arterial disease. Regardless, it appears that Lp-PLA$_2$ plays an important role in orchestrating localized inflammatory events within the vessel wall *(57)*.

The ability of Lp-PLA$_2$ to reflect localized, rather than systemic, inflammation potentially provides greater specificity with regard to monitoring cardiovascular risk. Meta-analysis of a large number of cohorts has demonstrated that elevated Lp-PLA$_2$ levels are associated with greater prospective risk of cardiovascular events *(58)*. This association has been reported in studies that have employed assessment of either Lp-PLA$_2$ activity or mass. In a nested case-control analysis of the West of Scotland Coronary Prevention Study (WOSCOPS), baseline Lp-PLA$_2$ independently predicted the risk of a first vascular event, after controlling for traditional risk factors *(59)* (Fig. 3). This finding is supported by the Atherosclerosis Risk in the Community (ARIC) Study, although the ability to predict an adverse

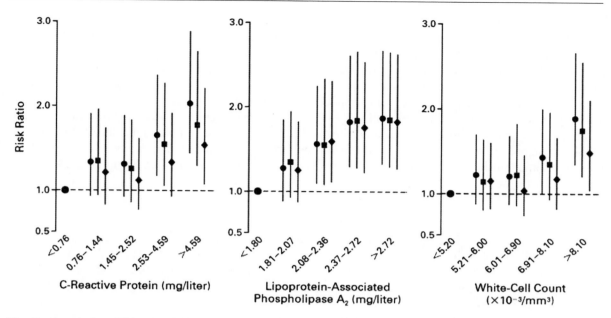

Fig. 3. Associations of levels of CRP, lipoprotein-associated phospholipase A_2 and white cell count with the risk of a coronary event in the WOSCOPS study. Copied with permission from *(59)*.

outcome was only observed in subjects with an LDL-C less than 130 mg/dL *(60)*. However, other investigators have reported that the ability of Lp-PLA_2 to predict cardiovascular risk does not persist after controlling for LDL-C levels *(61)*. The finding that Lp-PLA_2 predicts vascular events in patients presenting for coronary angiography, despite a lack of relationship with disease burden, supports its association with factors within the plaque that promote breakdown of the fibrous cap and progression to acute ischemia *(62)*.

Given the clear association with LDL-C, it is not surprising that Lp-PLA_2 levels decline in response to use of lipid-modifying therapies, and in contrast to CRP, this decline is largely predicted by reductions in LDL-C *(63, 64)*. The FDA has approved an assay for assessment of subjects deemed to be intermediate risk by traditional approaches, with recommendations that levels greater than 235 ng/mL identify an increase in prospective cardiovascular risk *(65)*. The development of new therapeutic agents that directly inhibit Lp-PLA_2 has been demonstrated to have a favorable impact on the size of the necrotic core in human atherosclerosis and is undergoing further evaluation in clinical trials *(66)*.

5.4.4. Additional Markers

Additional inflammatory mediators in atherosclerosis have been proposed as potential markers for use in risk prediction. Some, but not all, cohorts report an association between systemic levels of adhesion molecules *(67–69)*, chemokines *(70–72)* and cytokines *(73)* with the prevalence of coronary heart disease and prospective cardiovascular risk; it remains to be determined whether this persists after controlling for traditional risk factors.

5.4.5. Matrix Metalloproteinases

Pathology studies have established that matrix metalloproteinases (MMP) play an important role in vascular and ventricular remodeling and in the progression of atherosclerotic plaque to fibrous cap rupture and acute ischemic events *(74)*. Elevated systemic MMP levels have been reported in the setting of expansive arterial remodeling, a pattern of change in vascular dimension associated with acute coronary syndromes *(75)*. Several investigators have reported that MMP levels predict an increase risk of future cardiovascular events *(76)*. However, it remains to be determined whether the accuracy of risk prediction varies according to the specific form of MMP measured or if determination of activity rather than mass is more accurate. Furthermore, measurement of endogenous tissue inhibitors of metalloproteinases (TIMPs) may also provide important prognostic information *(77)*. Pregnancy associated plasma protein A (PAPP-A) is a specific metalloproteinase located within unstable, but not stable, plaques. The finding that circulating PAPP-A levels are elevated in patients with acute ischemic syndromes compared with stable angina or healthy controls suggests a potential role for this specific MMP in risk prediction *(78)*. Further evaluation is required to determine whether any measure of MMP provides clinical utility above and beyond that observed with assessment of traditional risk factors.

5.4.6. ADMA

Nitric oxide plays a pivotal role in the maintenance of vascular homeostasis. A reduction in nitric oxide bioavailability is the hallmark of changes in endothelial function that precede the formation of macroscopic changes within the artery wall. Given their short circulating half-life, no reliable and high throughput assay for the detection and quantitation of either nitric oxide or its metabolites has been developed. Increasing interest has focused on the role of methylated species of the nitric oxide precursor, L-arginine, in the pathogenesis of cardiovascular disease. The methylation product asymmetric dimethylarginine (ADMA) has been demonstrated to inhibit the activity of nitric oxide synthase (NOS) *(79)*. ADMA levels have been reported to be elevated in patients with cardiovascular risk factors and established atherosclerotic disease *(79)*. More recently elevated ADMA levels have been demonstrated to portend a poor prognosis in patients with acute myocardial infarction complicated by cardiogenic shock *(80)*.

5.5. EMERGING THROMBOTIC MARKERS

Given that thrombus formation is the major event leading to lumen occlusion and acute ischemia in the setting of plaque rupture, there is considerable interest in evaluating the propensity to thrombosis as a potential risk factor. Fibrinogen is an acute phase reactant that acts an important link between inflammation and thrombosis, via its pivotal role in promoting the coagulation cascade and plasma viscosity. Elevated fibrinogen levels are commonly observed in association with a number of risk factors including smoking, diabetes, obesity and increasing age *(81)*. Case-control studies have demonstrated that fibrinogen levels predict cardiovascular risk within all vascular territories persists following adjustment for conventional risk factors *(81)*. The lack of standardized assay, uniform cutoffs and evidence of benefit with a specific fibrinogen lowering intervention has limited its acceptance.

A number of additional factors involved in the regulation of thrombosis have been investigated with regard to a potential role in risk prediction. A range of platelet activation and aggregation assays has been used to characterize both the association between platelet activity and cardiovascular risk and the potential anti-platelet impact of medical therapies *(82)*. However, the lack of standardization of these assays has limited their use. The discovery that platelet-derived microparticles and CD40 both play a role in promoting both inflammatory and thrombotic pathways suggests that monitoring their systemic levels may predict cardiovascular risk. In studies of patients with acute coronary syndromes, systemic levels of soluble CD40 ligand predict prospective risk and correlate with the clinical benefit of early statin administration *(83)*. Monitoring systemic levels of factors involved in the control of thrombus dissolution, such as plasminogen activator inhibitor (PAI-1), has also been demonstrated to predict cardiovascular risk in case-control studies *(84)*.

5.6. ADDITIONAL MARKERS

5.6.1. Homocysteine

Homocysteine is a thiol-containing intermediate of methionine metabolism. Evidence supporting a potential role of homocysteine in cardiovascular disease is supported by the finding of atherosclerosis in young subjects with inborn errors of homocysteine metabolism and that laboratory experiments have demonstrated that homocysteine possesses inflammatory, oxidative, thrombotic and proliferative properties (85). A meta-analysis of case-control studies revealed that elevated homocysteine levels greater than 15 μmol/L are associated with a greater prevalence of atherosclerotic disease within coronary, cerebral and peripheral vascular territories (86). Subsequent meta-analyses also revealed that elevated homocysteine levels predict, albeit to a modest degree, the prospective risk of cardiovascular events (87).

The ability of homocysteine to predict cardiovascular risk appears to be enhanced in the setting of concomitant risk factors, such as diabetes mellitus, smoking and chronic renal impairment and in the setting of genetic variation in homocysteine metabolism (88–92). Meta-analyses have consistently demonstrated an association between a 677C→T polymorphism of methylene tetrahydrofolate reductase and a prospective cardiovascular risk (91, 92). Highlighting the distinction between the ability of a factor to predict risk and the ability of a factor to serve as a therapeutic target is consistent with the data from large prospective clinical trials that demonstrate that lowering of homocysteine levels with folic acid and vitamins is not associated with cardiovascular benefit (93).

5.6.2. Brain Natriuretic Peptide

A number of members of the natriuretic peptide family play an important role in the regulation of the cardiovascular system. Brain natriuretic peptide (BNP) is released from cardiac myocytes, predominantly in response to stretch. As a result, BNP levels have been consistently demonstrated to be elevated in the setting of heart failure (94). BNP has been subsequently incorporated into the diagnostic algorithm of patients evaluated for dyspnea and has been proposed to have a role in the titration of heart failure therapies. Similar findings have been demonstrated with use of the amino terminus proBNP (NT-proBNP) (95). Increasing evidence suggests that BNP may play a prognostic role as a biomarker in patients with atherosclerotic cardiovascular disease, without heart failure. BNP levels typically rise early in the setting of acute ST-elevation myocardial infarctions, followed by relatively rapid stabilization (96). Patients who demonstrate a biphasic pattern with an additional rise at day 5 are more likely to have large anterior wall infarcts with evidence of systolic dysfunction and clinical heart failure (96). Early observation that baseline BNP levels greater than 80 pg/mL at presentation with an acute coronary syndrome predict an elevated risk of cardiovascular events during the next 6 months (97) was confirmed by analysis of patients who participated in the Treat Angina with Aggrastat and Determine Cost of Therapy with an Invasive or Conservative Strategy-Thrombolysis in Myocardial Infarction (TACTICS-TIMI 18) Study (98) (Fig. 4).

The role of serial evaluation of BNP levels in patients presenting with an acute coronary syndrome was investigated in subjects participating in the A–Z trial. The subsequent presence of a BNP level greater than 80 pg/mL within the 12 months following presentation, despite having a lower level at baseline, was associated with an adverse outcome in terms of mortality and heart failure. In contrast, an initially high value, which decreased during follow-up, was accompanied by a relatively favorable prognosis. This highlights the potential importance of long-term serial measurements (99, 100). Similar findings for risk prediction in patients with acute coronary syndromes were found when levels of NT-proBNP were measured (101–103).

The underlying mechanistic link between BNP and subsequent incidence of ischemic cardiovascular events is supported by observations that BNP levels predict the extent of ischemic perfusion defects

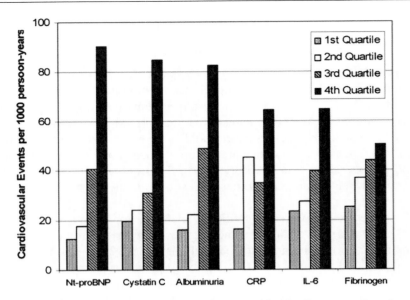

Fig. 4. Risk of death or myocardial infarction (MI) at 30 days stratified by B-type natriuretic peptide (BNP) and cardiac troponin I (cTnI) in the TACTICS-TIMI 18 study. Copied with permission from *(98)*.

on exercise myocardial scintigraphy *(104, 105)* and measures of atherosclerotic burden including the number of coronary arteries diseased on angiography *(106, 107)* and the degree of coronary calcification *(108)*. These observations support more recent findings that BNP levels can predict outcome in more stable patients with CAD at levels far below those used for the diagnostic threshold for heart failure. It remains to be determined whether BNP plays a direct pathologic role in the progression of atherosclerosis or reflects an increase in wall stress within the vascular system or some other aspect of the disease process.

5.6.3. Oxidative Stress

The pivotal role of oxidation in the pathology of atherosclerosis has also prompted the search to develop reliable markers of oxidative stress. The inability to monitor oxidant activity has been proposed as one of the limitations of clinical studies that have consistently demonstrated the lack of clinical efficacy of multivitamins. F_2-isoprostanes are stable peroxidation products of the arachidonic acid pathway, which can be reliably measured in a range of biological specimens. Increasing levels of F_2-isoprostanes have been reported in association with a range of cardiovascular risk factors *(109)* and within atherosclerotic lesions *(110)*. While F_2-isoprostane levels have been demonstrated to decrease in response to statin therapy *(111, 112)*, their use to predict prospective cardiovascular risk in case-control studies has not been elucidated.

Oxidative modification is an essential event required to convert LDL into an atherogenic species. Detection of oxidized LDL species reflects a broad spectrum of targets including both lipid and protein components of LDL particles. Support for the development of assays for quantitation of oxidized LDL (oxLDL) comes from findings of their localization within human atherosclerotic plaque *(113, 114)* and that immunization against a range of oxLDL epitopes is protective in animal models of atherosclerosis *(115)*. Three specific epitopes underlie the major oxLDL assays currently in use, targeting either phosphatidylcholine (E06 and DLH3) or apoB (4E6) *(61)*. A number of groups have reported that systemic oxLDL levels are elevated in the setting of the metabolic syndrome and endothelial dysfunction *(116, 117)*. Furthermore, elevated oxLDL levels predict the prospective risk of cardiovascular risk and progression of carotid intimal-medial thickness *(118, 119)*, but not coronary atherosclerosis *(120)*. Given the high correlation with LDL cholesterol and reduction in levels in response to statin therapy *(121)*, it remains to be determined what the incremental value of oxLDL measurement is in risk assessment. As a result, ongoing investigation and standardization are required to evaluate its potential clinical utility.

Endogenous anti-oxidant factors have also received attention with regard to development of therapeutic and diagnostic approaches. Paraoxonase (PON) is a lactase/esterase that is carried in the systemic circulation predominantly on the surface of high-density lipoprotein (HDL) particles. The demonstration that PON possesses anti-oxidant and anti-inflammatory activities in cellular studies and that genetic deletion of PON is associated with accelerated lesion formation in animal models of atherosclerosis suggests a potential role in vascular protection in humans *(122)*. However, considerable debate has continued on the role of PON in humans given that levels of PON mass and activity have been reported to be inversely associated with cardiovascular risk in some, but not all, patient cohorts and that it remains to be unequivocally demonstrated that PON actually acts as an anti-oxidant in humans *(123)*. A recent report appears to have provided some clarity in which increasing levels of PON activity were associated with low levels of measures of oxidative stress and relative protection from cardiovascular events *(123)*.

5.7. MEASURES OF RENAL IMPAIRMENT

Renal impairment is associated with an increase in cardiovascular disease, largely due to abnormalities of blood pressure and lipids. A number of reports have emerged that suggest an increase in cardiovascular risk in patients with biochemical evidence of impaired renal function that is independent of the presence of traditional risk factors. Cystatin C, calculated glomerular filtration rate (GFR) and the urinary albumin:creatinine ratio (UACR) are each markers of various degrees of renal impairment *(124)*. Each of these markers has been reported to predict incident cardiovascular events in cohorts of subjects with and without an established diagnosis of CAD. Neutrophil gelatinase-associated lipocalin (NGAL) is a marker of leukocyte elevation, which has emerged as a marker of early renal injury *(125)*. Pathology studies that localize NGAL within atherosclerotic plaque and the ventricular wall and its association with activation of matrix metalloproteinases implicate a potential role in the progression of atherosclerosis and remodeling *(126)*. While a number of reports suggest that an elevated NGAL level is associated with an increased risk of cardiovascular events *(127)*, this remains to be characterized in large cohorts.

5.8. PANELS OF MULTIPLE NOVEL BIOMARKERS

Pathological insights into the pathways that promote formation and subsequent clinical complications of atherosclerosis have stimulated the development of a large number of systemic biomarkers. The complexity of the disease process, involving the interaction of multiple pathological events, would imply that a panel of biomarkers that monitored a combination of these pathways might potentially be of greater clinical utility. In a review of 3,209 participants in the Framingham Heart Study, a panel of biomarkers including CRP, BNP, NT-pro-atrial natriuretic peptide, aldosterone, rennin, fibrinogen, D-dimer, PAI-1, homocysteine and the urinary albumin-to-creatinine ratio was evaluated. Subjects with a calculated multimarker score in the highest quartile were at a higher risk of a future cardiovascular event. However, the incremental increase in risk prediction when the multimarker score was combined with traditional risk factors was minimal *(128)*. In a cohort of elderly men in the Uppsala Longitudinal Study of Adult Men (ULSAM), the integration of a panel of markers reflecting myocardial necrosis (troponin I), ventricular dysfunction (NT-proBNP), renal impairment (cystatin C) and inflammation (CRP) improved the ability of traditional risk factors to predict the risk of cardio-vascular death *(129)*.

The approach of a biomarker panel was recently evaluated in patients with an established diagnosis of coronary heart disease in the Heart and Soul Study. When NT-proBNP, albuminuria and CRP were added to traditional risk factor assessment a significant increase in risk discrimination was observed *(130)* (Fig. 5). Accordingly, it would appear that there is a potential for multiple markers to be of clinical utility in both primary and secondary prevention settings. Further study is required to determine what combination of biomarkers improves risk stratification above and beyond that observed with assessment of traditional risk factors.

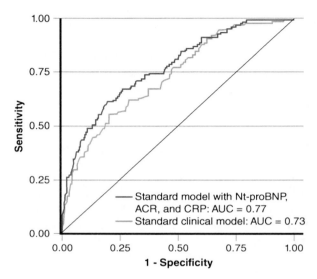

Fig. 5. Receiver operator characteristic curves for the standard clinical model and the standard clinical model plus NT-proBNP, albuminuria and CRP to predict major adverse cardiac events in the Heart and Soul Study. Copied with permission from *(130)*.

5.9. SUMMARY

The inability of traditional risk factor algorithms to accurately stratify cardiovascular risk in all subjects has stimulated the search to develop additional systemic biomarkers to enhance risk prediction. Systemic biomarkers that reflect the degree of inflammatory, oxidative and thrombotic activity within the coronary arteries provide an opportunity to identify patients who are more likely to progress to acute ischemic events. Emerging data suggest that a number of markers, particularly those that reflect systemic inflammatory activity, are independent predictors of clinical events.

REFERENCES

1. Murray CJ, Lopez AD. Alternative projections of mortality and disability by cause 1990–2020: Global Burden of Disease Study. *Lancet.* 1997;349:1498–1504.
2. Multiple Risk Factor Intervention Trial Research Group. Relationship between baseline risk factors and coronary heart disease and total mortality in the Multiple Risk Factor Intervention Trial. *Prev Med.* 1986;15:254–273.
3. D'Agostino RB Sr., Grundy S, Sullivan LM, Wilson P. Validation of the Framingham coronary heart disease prediction scores: results of a multiple ethnic groups investigation. *JAMA.* 2001;286:180–187.

4. Grundy SM, Cleeman JI, Merz CN, et al. Implications of recent clinical trials for the National Cholesterol Education Program Adult Treatment Panel III guidelines. *Circulation.* 2004;110:227–239.

5. Virani SS, Ballantyne CM. How to identify patients with vulnerable plaques. *Diabetes Obes Metab.* 2008;10:824–833.

6. Khot UN, Khot MB, Bajzer CT, et al. Prevalence of conventional risk factors in patients with coronary heart disease. *JAMA.* 2003;290:898–904.

7. Ross R. Atherosclerosis—an inflammatory disease. *N Engl J Med.* 1999;340:115–126.

8. Calabro P, Willerson JT, Yeh ET. Inflammatory cytokines stimulated C-reactive protein production by human coronary artery smooth muscle cells. *Circulation.* 2003;108:1930–1932.

9. Du Clos TW. Function of C-reactive protein. *Ann Med.* 2000;32:274–278.

10. Verma S, Wang CH, Li SH, et al. A self-fulfilling prophecy: C-reactive protein attenuates nitric oxide production and inhibits angiogenesis. *Circulation.* 2002;106:913–919.

11. Danenberg HD, Szalai AJ, Swaminathan RV, et al. Increased thrombosis after arterial injury in human C-reactive protein-transgenic mice. *Circulation.* 2003;108:512–515.

12. Pai JK, Pischon T, Ma J, et al. Inflammatory markers and the risk of coronary heart disease in men and women. *N Engl J Med.* 2004;351:2599–2610.

13. Pradhan AD, Manson JE, Rossouw JE, et al. Inflammatory biomarkers, hormone replacement therapy, and incident coronary heart disease: prospective analysis from the Women's Health Initiative Observational Study. *JAMA.* 2002;288:980–987.

14. Ridker PM, Buring JE, Shih J, Matias M, Hennekens CH. Prospective study of C-reactive protein and the risk of future cardiovascular events among apparently healthy women. *Circulation.* 1998;98:731–733.

15. Ridker PM, Cushman M, Stampfer MJ, Tracy RP, Hennekens CH. Inflammation, aspirin, and the risk of cardiovascular disease in apparently healthy men. *N Engl J Med.* 1997;336:973–979.

16. de Winter RJ, Koch KT, van Straalen JP, et al. C-reactive protein and coronary events following percutaneous coronary angioplasty. *Am J Med.* 2003;115:85–90.

17. Haverkate F, Thompson SG, Pyke SD, Gallimore JR, Pepys MB. Production of C-reactive protein and risk of coronary events in stable and unstable angina. European Concerted Action on Thrombosis and Disabilities Angina Pectoris Study Group. *Lancet.* 1997;349:462–466.

18. Lindahl B, Toss H, Siegbahn A, Venge P, Wallentin L. Markers of myocardial damage and inflammation in relation to long-term mortality in unstable coronary artery disease. FRISC Study Group. Fragmin during instability in coronary artery disease. *N Engl J Med.* 2000;343:1139–1147.

19. Liuzzo G, Biasucci LM, Gallimore JR, et al. The prognostic value of C-reactive protein and serum amyloid a protein in severe unstable angina. *N Engl J Med.* 1994;331:417–424.

20. Milazzo D, Biasucci LM, Luciani N, et al. Elevated levels of C-reactive protein before coronary artery bypass grafting predict recurrence of ischemic events. *Am J Cardiol.* 1999;84:459–461.

21. Morrow DA, Rifai N, Antman EM, et al. C-reactive protein is a potent predictor of mortality independently of and in combination with troponin T in acute coronary syndromes: a TIMI 11A substudy. Thrombolysis in myocardial infarction. *J Am Coll Cardiol.* 1998;31:1460–1465.

22. Retterstol L, Eikvar L, Bohn M, Bakken A, Eriks”sen J, Berg K. C-reactive protein predicts death in patients with previous premature myocardial infarction—a 10 year follow-up study. *Atherosclerosis.* 2002;160:433–440.

23. Ridker PM, Rifai N, Pfeffer MA, et al. Inflammation, pravastatin, and the risk of coronary events after myocardial infarction in patients with average cholesterol levels. Cholesterol and Recurrent Events (CARE) investigators. *Circulation.* 1998;98:839–844.

24. Miller M, Zhan M, Havas S. High attributable risk of elevated C-reactive protein level to conventional coronary heart disease risk factors: the Third National Health and Nutrition Examination Survey. *Arch Intern Med.* 2005;165:2063–2068.

25. Pepys MB, Hawkins PN, Kahan MC, et al. Proinflammatory effects of bacterial recombinant human C-reactive protein are caused by contamination with bacterial products, not by C-reactive protein itself. *Circ Res.* 2005;97:e97–e103.

26. Danesh J, Wheeler JG, Hirschfield GM, et al. C-reactive protein and other circulating markers of inflammation in the prediction of coronary heart disease. *N Engl J Med.* 2004;350:1387–1397.

27. Pearson TA, Mensah GA, Alexander RW, et al. Markers of inflammation and cardiovascular disease. Application to clinical and public health practice. A statement for healthcare professionals from the Centers for Disease Control and Prevention and the American Heart Association. *Circulation.* 2003;107:499–511.

28. Ridker PM, Buring JE, Rifai N, Cook NR. Development and validation of improved algorithms for the assessment of global cardiovascular risk in women: the Reynolds Risk Score. *JAMA.* 2007;297:611–619.

29. Albert MA, Danielson E, Rifai N, Ridker PM. Effect of statin therapy on C-reactive protein levels: the pravastatin inflammation/CRP evaluation (PRINCE): a randomized trial and cohort study. *JAMA.* 2001;286:64–70.

30. Jialal I, Stein D, Balis D, Grundy SM, Adams-Huet B, Devaraj S. Effect of hydroxymethyl glutaryl coenzyme a reductase inhibitor therapy on high sensitive C-reactive protein levels. *Circulation.* 2001;103:1933–1935.

31. Ridker PM, Rifai N, Pfeffer MA, Sacks F, Braunwald E. Long-term effects of pravastatin on plasma concentration of C-reactive protein. The Cholesterol and Recurrent Events (CARE) Investigators. *Circulation.* 1999;100:230–235.
32. Ridker PM, Rifai N, Clearfield M, et al. Measurement of C-reactive protein for the targeting of statin therapy in the primary prevention of acute coronary events. *N Engl J Med.* 2001;344:1959–1965.
33. Nissen SE, Tuzcu EM, Schoenhagen P, et al. Statin therapy, LDL cholesterol, C-reactive protein, and coronary artery disease. *N Engl J Med.* 2005;352:29–38.
34. Ridker PM, Cannon CP, Morrow D, et al. C-reactive protein levels and outcomes after statin therapy. *N Engl J Med.* 2005;352:20–28.
35. Ridker PM, Danielson E, Fonseca FA, et al. Rosuvastatin to prevent vascular events in men and women with elevated C-reactive protein. *N Engl J Med.* 2008;359:2195–2207.
36. Nicholls SJ, Hazen SL. Myeloperoxidase and cardiovascular disease. *Arterioscler Thromb Vasc Biol.* 2005;25: 1102–1111.
37. Daugherty A, Dunn JL, Rateri DL, Heinecke JW. Myeloperoxidase, a catalyst for lipoprotein oxidation, is expressed in human atherosclerotic lesions. *J Clin Invest.* 1994;94:437–444.
38. Hazen SL, Heinecke JW. 3-Chlorotyrosine, a specific marker of myeloperoxidase-catalyzed oxidation, is markedly elevated in low density lipoprotein isolated from human atherosclerotic intima. *J Clin Invest.* 1997;99:2075–2081.
39. Sugiyama S, Okada Y, Sukhova GK, Virmani R, Heinecke JW, Libby P. Macrophage myeloperoxidase regulation by granulocyte macrophage colony-stimulating factor in human atherosclerosis and implications in acute coronary syndromes. *Am J Pathol.* 2001;158:879–891.
40. Kutter D, Devaquet P, Vanderstocken G, Paulus JM, Marchal V, Gothot A. Consequences of total and subtotal myeloperoxidase deficiency: risk or benefit? *Acta Haematol.* 2000;104:10–15.
41. Nikpoor B, Turecki G, Fournier C, Theroux P, Rouleau GA. A functional myeloperoxidase polymorphic variant is associated with coronary artery disease in French-Canadians. *Am Heart J.* 2001;142:336–339.
42. Asselbergs FW, Reynolds WF, Cohen-Tervaert JW, Jessurun GA, Tio RA. Myeloperoxidase polymorphism related to cardiovascular events in coronary artery disease. *Am J Med.* 2004;116:429–430.
43. Exner M, Minar E, Mlekusch W, et al. Myeloperoxidase predicts progression of carotid stenosis in states of low high-density lipoprotein cholesterol. *J Am Coll Cardiol.* 2006;47:2212–2218.
44. Meuwese MC, Stroes ES, Hazen SL, et al. Serum myeloperoxidase levels are associated with the future risk of coronary artery disease in apparently healthy individuals: the EPIC-Norfolk Prospective Population Study. *J Am Coll Cardiol.* 2007;50:159–165.
45. Ndrepepa G, Braun S, Mehilli J, von Beckerath N, Schomig A, Kastrati A. Myeloperoxidase level in patients with stable coronary artery disease and acute coronary syndromes. *Eur J Clin Invest.* 2008;38:90–96.
46. Duzguncinar O, Yavuz B, Hazirolan T, et al. Plasma myeloperoxidase is related to the severity of coronary artery disease. *Acta Cardiol.* 2008;63:147–152.
47. Zhang R, Brennan ML, Fu X, et al. Association between myeloperoxidase levels and risk of coronary artery disease. *JAMA.* 2001;286:2136–2142.
48. Brennan ML, Penn MS, Van Lente F, et al. Prognostic value of myeloperoxidase in patients with chest pain. *N Engl J Med.* 2003;349:1595–1604.
49. Baldus S, Heeschen C, Meinertz T, et al. Myeloperoxidase serum levels predict risk in patients with acute coronary syndromes. *Circulation.* 2003;108:1440–1445.
50. Morrow DA, Sabatine MS, Brennan ML, et al. Concurrent evaluation of novel cardiac biomarkers in acute coronary syndrome: myeloperoxidase and soluble CD40 ligand and the risk of recurrent ischaemic events in TACTICS-TIMI 18. *Eur Heart J.* 2008;29:1096–1102.
51. Mocatta TJ, Pilbrow AP, Cameron VA, et al. Plasma concentrations of myeloperoxidase predict mortality after myocardial infarction. *J Am Coll Cardiol.* 2007;49:1993–2000.
52. Dominguez-Rodriguez A, Samimi-Fard S, Abreu-Gonzalez P, Garcia-Gonzalez MJ, Kaski JC. Prognostic value of admission myeloperoxidase levels in patients with ST-segment elevation myocardial infarction and cardiogenic shock. *Am J Cardiol.* 2008;101:1537–1540.
53. Ng LL, Pathik B, Loke IW, Squire IB, Davies JE. Myeloperoxidase and C-reactive protein augment the specificity of B-type natriuretic peptide in community screening for systolic heart failure. *Am Heart J.* 2006;152:94–101.
54. Tang WH, Tong W, Troughton RW, et al. Prognostic value and echocardiographic determinants of plasma myeloperoxidase levels in chronic heart failure. *J Am Coll Cardiol.* 2007;49:2364–2370.
55. Askari AT, Brennan ML, Zhou X, et al. Myeloperoxidase and plasminogen activator inhibitor 1 play a central role in ventricular remodeling after myocardial infarction. *J Exp Med.* 2003;197:615–624.
56. Vasilyev N, Williams T, Brennan ML, et al. Myeloperoxidase-generated oxidants modulate left ventricular remodeling but not infarct size after myocardial infarction. *Circulation.* 2005;112:2812–2820.
57. Lerman A, McConnell JP. Lipoprotein-associated phospholipase A_2: a risk marker or a risk factor? *Am J Cardiol.* 2008;101:11F–22F.

58. Garza CA, Montori VM, McConnell JP, Somers VK, Kullo IJ, Lopez-Jimenez F. Association between lipoprotein-associated phospholipase A$_2$ and cardiovascular disease: a systematic review. *Mayo Clin Proc.* 2007;82: 159–165.

59. Packard CJ, O'Reilly DS, Caslake MJ, et al. Lipoprotein-associated phospholipase A$_2$ as an independent predictor of coronary heart disease. West of Scotland Coronary Prevention Study Group. *N Engl J Med.* 2000;343:1148–1155.

60. Ballantyne CM, Hoogeveen RC, Bang H, et al. Lipoprotein-associated phospholipase A$_2$, high-sensitivity C-reactive protein, and risk for incident coronary heart disease in middle-aged men and women in the Atherosclerosis Risk in Communities (ARIC) study. *Circulation.* 2004;109:837–842.

61. Tsimikas S, Willerson JT, Ridker PM. C-reactive protein and other emerging blood biomarkers to optimize risk stratification of vulnerable patients. *J Am Coll Cardiol.* 2006;47:C19–C31.

62. Brilakis ES, McConnell JP, Lennon RJ, Elesber AA, Meyer JG, Berger PB. Association of lipoprotein-associated phospholipase A$_2$ levels with coronary artery disease risk factors, angiographic coronary artery disease, and major adverse events at follow-up. *Eur Heart J.* 2005;26:137–144.

63. Ballantyne CM, Nambi V. Markers of inflammation and their clinical significance. *Atheroscler Suppl.* 2005;6:21–29.

64. Davidson MH, Stein EA, Bays HE, et al. Efficacy and tolerability of adding prescription omega-3 fatty acids 4 g/d to simvastatin 40 mg/d in hypertriglyceridemic patients: an 8-week, randomized, double-blind, placebo-controlled study. *Clin Ther.* 2007;29:1354–1367.

65. Corson MA, Jones PH, Davidson MH. Review of the evidence for the clinical utility of lipoprotein-associated phospholipase A$_2$ as a cardiovascular risk marker. *Am J Cardiol.* 2008;101:41F–50F.

66. Serruys PW, Garcia-Garcia HM, Buszman P, et al. Effects of the direct lipoprotein-associated phospholipase A(2) inhibitor darapladib on human coronary atherosclerotic plaque. *Circulation.* 2008;118:1172–1182.

67. Hwang SJ, Ballantyne CM, Sharrett AR, et al. Circulating adhesion molecules VCAM-1, ICAM-1, and E-selectin in carotid atherosclerosis and incident coronary heart disease cases: the Atherosclerosis Risk in Communities (ARIC) Study. *Circulation.* 1997;96:4219–4225.

68. Luc G, Arveiler D, Evans A, et al. Circulating soluble adhesion molecules ICAM-1 and VCAM-1 and incident coronary heart disease: the PRIME Study. *Atherosclerosis.* 2003;170:169–176.

69. Malik I, Danesh J, Whincup P, et al. Soluble adhesion molecules and prediction of coronary heart disease: a prospective study and meta-analysis. *Lancet.* 2001;358:971–976.

70. Cipollone F, Marini M, Fazia M, Pini B, Iezzi A, Reale M, Paloscia L, Materazzo G, D'Annunzio E, Conti P, Chiarelli F, Cuccurullo F, Mezzetti A, et al. Elevated circulating levels of monocyte chemoattractant protein-1 in patients with restenosis after coronary angioplasty. *Arterioscler Thromb Vasc Biol.* 2001;21:327–334.

71. Deo R, Khera A, McGuire DK, et al. Association among plasma levels of monocyte chemoattractant protein-1, traditional cardiovascular risk factors, and subclinical atherosclerosis. *J Am Coll Cardiol.* 2004;44:1812–1818.

72. Hoogeveen RC, Morrison A, Boerwinkle E, et al. Plasma MCP-1 level and risk for peripheral arterial disease and incident coronary heart disease: Atherosclerosis Risk in Communities Study. *Atherosclerosis.* 2005;183:301–307.

73. Biasucci LM, Vitelli A, Liuzzo G, et al. Elevated levels of interleukin-6 in unstable angina. *Circulation.* 1996;94: 874–877.

74. Dollery CM, Libby P. Atherosclerosis and proteinase activation. *Cardiovasc Res.* 2006;69:625–635.

75. Schoenhagen P, Vince DG, Ziada KM, et al. Relation of matrix-metalloproteinase 3 found in coronary lesion samples retrieved by directional coronary atherectomy to intravascular ultrasound observations on coronary remodeling. *Am J Cardiol.* 2002;89:1354–1359.

76. Welsh P, Whincup PH, Papacosta O, et al. Serum matrix metalloproteinase-9 and coronary heart disease: a prospective study in middle-aged men. *QJM.* 2008;101:785–791.

77. Tayebjee MH, Lip GY, MacFadyen RJ. Matrix metalloproteinases in coronary artery disease: clinical and therapeutic implications and pathological significance. *Curr Med Chem.* 2005;12:917–925.

78. Bayes-Genis A, Conover CA, Overgaard MT, et al. Pregnancy-associated plasma protein A as a marker of acute coronary syndromes. *N Engl J Med.* 2001;345:1022–1029.

79. Cooke JP. ADMA, its role in vascular disease. *Vasc Med.* 2005;10(Suppl 1):S11–S17.

80. Nicholls SJ, Wang Z, Koeth R, et al. Metabolic profiling of arginine and nitric oxide pathways predicts hemodynamic abnormalities and mortality in patients with cardiogenic shock after acute myocardial infarction. *Circulation.* 2007;116:2315–2324.

81. Ernst E, Resch KL. Fibrinogen as a cardiovascular risk factor: a meta-analysis and review of the literature. *Ann Intern Med.* 1993;118:956–963.

82. Price MJ. Monitoring platelet function to reduce the risk of ischemic and bleeding complications. *Am J Cardiol.* 2009;103:35A–39A.

83. Kinlay S, Schwartz GG, Olsson AG, et al. Effect of atorvastatin on risk of recurrent cardiovascular events after an acute coronary syndrome associated with high soluble CD40 ligand in the Myocardial Ischemia Reduction with Aggressive Cholesterol Lowering (MIRACL) Study. *Circulation.* 2004;110:386–391.

84. Marcucci R, Brogi D, Sofi F, et al. PAI-1 and homocysteine, but not lipoprotein (a) and thrombophilic polymorphisms, are independently associated with the occurrence of major adverse cardiac events after successful coronary stenting. *Heart.* 2006;92:377–381.

85. Humphrey LL, Fu R, Rogers K, Freeman M, Helfand M. Homocysteine level and coronary heart disease incidence: a systematic review and meta-analysis. *Mayo Clin Proc.* 2008;83:1203–1212.

86. Boushey CJ, Beresford SA, Omenn GS, Motulsky AG. A quantitative assessment of plasma homocysteine as a risk factor for vascular disease. Probable benefits of increasing folic acid intakes. *JAMA.* 1995;274:1049–1057.

87. Homocysteine and risk of ischemic heart disease and stroke: a meta-analysis. *JAMA.* 2002;288:2015–2022.

88. Graham IM, Daly LE, Refsum HM, et al. Plasma homocysteine as a risk factor for vascular disease. The European Concerted Action Project. *JAMA.* 1997;277:1775–1781.

89. Klerk M, Verhoef P, Clarke R, Blom HJ, Kok FJ, Schouten EGMTHFR. 677C—>T polymorphism and risk of coronary heart disease: a meta-analysis. *JAMA.* 2002;288:2023–2031.

90. Moustapha A, Naso A, Nahlawi M, et al. Prospective study of hyperhomocysteinemia as an adverse cardiovascular risk factor in end-stage renal disease. *Circulation.* 1998;97:138–141.

91. Soinio M, Marniemi J, Laakso M, Lehto S, Ronnemaa T. Elevated plasma homocysteine level is an independent predictor of coronary heart disease events in patients with type 2 diabetes mellitus. *Ann Intern Med.* 2004;140: 94–100.

92. Wald DS, Law M, Morris JK. Homocysteine and cardiovascular disease: evidence on causality from a meta-analysis. *BMJ.* 2002;325:1202.

93. Antoniades C, Antonopoulos AS, Tousoulis D, Marinou K, Stefanadis C. Homocysteine and coronary atherosclerosis: from folate fortification to the recent clinical trials. *Eur Heart J.* 2009;30:6–15.

94. Maisel AS, Krishnaswamy P, Nowak RM, et al. Rapid measurement of B-type natriuretic peptide in the emergency diagnosis of heart failure. *N Engl J Med.* 2002;347:161–167.

95. Januzzi JL Jr., Camargo CA, Anwaruddin S, et al. The N-terminal Pro-BNP investigation of dyspnea in the emergency department (PRIDE) study. *Am J Cardiol.* 2005;95:948–954.

96. Morita E, Yasue H, Yoshimura M, et al. Increased plasma levels of brain natriuretic peptide in patients with acute myocardial infarction. *Circulation.* 1993;88:82–91.

97. de Lemos JA, Morrow DA, Bentley JH, et al. The prognostic value of B-type natriuretic peptide in patients with acute coronary syndromes. *N Engl J Med.* 2001;345:1014–1021.

98. Morrow DA, de Lemos JA, Sabatine MS, et al. Evaluation of B-type natriuretic peptide for risk assessment in unstable angina/non-ST-elevation myocardial infarction: B-type natriuretic peptide and prognosis in TACTICS-TIMI 18. *J Am Coll Cardiol.* 2003;41:1264–1272.

99. Morrow DA, de Lemos JA, Blazing MA, et al. Prognostic value of serial B-type natriuretic peptide testing during follow-up of patients with unstable coronary artery disease. *JAMA.* 2005;294:2866–2871.

100. Blazing MA, De Lemos JA, Dyke CK, Califf RM, Bilheimer D, Braunwald E. The A-to-Z Trial: methods and rationale for a single trial investigating combined use of low-molecular-weight heparin with the glycoprotein IIb/IIIa inhibitor tirofiban and defining the efficacy of early aggressive simvastatin therapy. *Am Heart J.* 2001;142:211–217.

101. Jernberg T, Stridsberg M, Venge P, Lindahl B. N-terminal pro brain natriuretic peptide on admission for early risk stratification of patients with chest pain and no ST-segment elevation. *J Am Coll Cardiol.* 2002;40:437–445.

102. Omland T, Persson A, Ng L, et al. N-terminal pro-B-type natriuretic peptide and long-term mortality in acute coronary syndromes. *Circulation.* 2002;106:2913–2918.

103. James SK, Lindahl B, Siegbahn A, et al. N-terminal pro-brain natriuretic peptide and other risk markers for the separate prediction of mortality and subsequent myocardial infarction in patients with unstable coronary artery disease: a Global Utilization of Strategies to Open occluded arteries (GUSTO)-IV substudy. *Circulation.* 2003;108:275–281.

104. Sabatine MS, Morrow DA, de Lemos JA, et al. Acute changes in circulating natriuretic peptide levels in relation to myocardial ischemia. *J Am Coll Cardiol.* 2004;44:1988–1995.

105. Weber M, Dill T, Arnold R, et al. N-terminal B-type natriuretic peptide predicts extent of coronary artery disease and ischemia in patients with stable angina pectoris. *Am Heart J.* 2004;148:612–620.

106. Sakai H, Tsutamoto T, Ishikawa C, et al. Direct comparison of brain natriuretic peptide (BNP) and N-terminal pro-BNP secretion and extent of coronary artery stenosis in patients with stable coronary artery disease. *Circ J.* 2007;71: 499–505.

107. Kim BS, Lee HJ, Shin HS, et al. Presence and severity of coronary artery disease and changes in B-type natriuretic peptide levels in patients with a normal systolic function. *Transl Res.* 2006;148:188–195.

108. Abdullah SM, Khera A, Das SR, et al. Relation of coronary atherosclerosis determined by electron beam computed tomography and plasma levels of n-terminal pro-brain natriuretic peptide in a multiethnic population-based sample (the Dallas Heart Study). *Am J Cardiol.* 2005;96:1284–1289.

109. Morrow JD. Quantification of isoprostanes as indices of oxidant stress and the risk of atherosclerosis in humans. *Arterioscler Thromb Vasc Biol.* 2005;25:279–286.

110. Pratico D, Iuliano L, Mauriello A, et al. Localization of distinct F2-isoprostanes in human atherosclerotic lesions. *J Clin Invest.* 1997;100:2028–2034.

111. De Caterina R, Cipollone F, Filardo FP, et al. Low-density lipoprotein level reduction by the 3-hydroxy-3-methylglutaryl coenzyme-A inhibitor simvastatin is accompanied by a related reduction of F2-isoprostane formation in hypercholesterolemic subjects: no further effect of vitamin E. *Circulation.* 2002;106:2543–2549.

112. Desideri G, Croce G, Tucci M, et al. Effects of bezafibrate and simvastatin on endothelial activation and lipid peroxidation in hypercholesterolemia: evidence of different vascular protection by different lipid-lowering treatments. *J Clin Endocrinol Metab.* 2003;88:5341–5347.

113. Ehara S, Ueda M, Naruko T, et al. Elevated levels of oxidized low density lipoprotein show a positive relationship with the severity of acute coronary syndromes. *Circulation.* 2001;103:1955–1960.

114. Nishi K, Itabe H, Uno M, et al. Oxidized LDL in carotid plaques and plasma associates with plaque instability. *Arterioscler Thromb Vasc Biol.* 2002;22:1649–1654.

115. Nilsson J, Nordin Fredrikson G, Schiopu A, Shah PK, Jansson B, Carlsson R. Oxidized LDL antibodies in treatment and risk assessment of atherosclerosis and associated cardiovascular disease. *Curr Pharm Des.* 2007;13:1021–1030.

116. Holvoet P, Kritchevsky SB, Tracy RP, et al. The metabolic syndrome, circulating oxidized LDL, and risk of myocardial infarction in well-functioning elderly people in the health, aging, and body composition cohort. *Diabetes.* 2004;53:1068–1073.

117. Matsumoto T, Takashima H, Ohira N, et al. Plasma level of oxidized low-density lipoprotein is an independent determinant of coronary macrovasomotor and microvasomotor responses induced by bradykinin. *J Am Coll Cardiol.* 2004;44:451–457.

118. Hulthe J, Fagerberg B. Circulating oxidized LDL is associated with subclinical atherosclerosis development and inflammatory cytokines (AIR Study). *Arterioscler Thromb Vasc Biol.* 2002;22:1162–1167.

119. Liu ML, Ylitalo K, Salonen R, Salonen JT, Taskinen MR. Circulating oxidized low-density lipoprotein and its association with carotid intima-media thickness in asymptomatic members of familial combined hyperlipidemia families. *Arterioscler Thromb Vasc Biol.* 2004;24:1492–1497.

120. Choi SH, Chae A, Miller E, et al. Relationship between biomarkers of oxidized low-density lipoprotein, statin therapy, quantitative coronary angiography, and atheroma: volume observations from the REVERSAL (Reversal of Atherosclerosis with Aggressive Lipid Lowering) study. *J Am Coll Cardiol.* 2008;52:24–32.

121. Crisby M, Nordin-Fredriksson G, Shah PK, Yano J, Zhu J, Nilsson J. Pravastatin treatment increases collagen content and decreases lipid content, inflammation, metalloproteinases, and cell death in human carotid plaques: implications for plaque stabilization. *Circulation.* 2001;103:926–933.

122. Mackness MI, Durrington PN, Mackness B. The role of paraoxonase 1 activity in cardiovascular disease: potential for therapeutic intervention. *Am J Cardiovasc Drugs.* 2004;4:211–217.

123. Bhattacharyya T, Nicholls SJ, Topol EJ, et al. Relationship of paraoxonase 1 (PON1) gene polymorphisms and functional activity with systemic oxidative stress and cardiovascular risk. *JAMA.* 2008;299:1265–1276.

124. Keller T, Messow CM, Lubos E, et al. Cystatin C and cardiovascular mortality in patients with coronary artery disease and normal or mildly reduced kidney function: results from the AtheroGene study. *Eur Heart J.* 2009;30:314–320.

125. Malyszko J, Bachorzewska-Gajewska H, Malyszko JS, Pawlak K, Dobrzycki S. Serum neutrophil gelatinase-associated lipocalin as a marker of renal function in hypertensive and normotensive patients with coronary artery disease. *Nephrology (Carlton).* 2008;13:153–156.

126. Hemdahl AL, Gabrielsen A, Zhu C, et al. Expression of neutrophil gelatinase-associated lipocalin in atherosclerosis and myocardial infarction. *Arterioscler Thromb Vasc Biol.* 2006;26:136–142.

127. Poniatowski B, Malyszko J, Bachorzewska-Gajewska H, Malyszko JS, Dobrzycki S. Serum neutrophil gelatinase-associated lipocalin as a marker of renal function in patients with chronic heart failure and coronary artery disease. *Kidney Blood Press Res.* 2009;32:77–80.

128. Wang TJ, Gona P, Larson MG, et al. Multiple biomarkers for the prediction of first major cardiovascular events and death. *N Engl J Med.* 2006;355:2631–2639.

129. Zethelius B, Berglund L, Sundstrom J, et al. Use of multiple biomarkers to improve the prediction of death from cardiovascular causes. *N Engl J Med.* 2008;358:2107–2116.

130. Shlipak MG, Ix JH, Bibbins-Domingo K, Lin F, Whooley MA. Biomarkers to predict recurrent cardiovascular disease: the Heart and Soul Study. *Am J Med.* 2008;121:50–57.

6 Deciphering Cardiovascular Genomics and How They Apply to Cardiovascular Disease Prevention

Kiran Musunuru

CONTENTS

Key Words: Genome-wide association; Genomics; Linkage dysequilibrium; Pharmacogenomics; Polymorphism.

KEY POINTS

- Genetic information is transmitted from DNA to RNA to proteins to metabolites.
- Genomics is the study of how DNA variants affect individuals' traits and diseases.
- The human genome has roughly 3 billion bases on 23 chromosome pairs and more than 11 million variants, or polymorphisms, that differ from person to person.
- The best-characterized polymorphisms are single nucleotide polymorphisms (SNPs), which differ at a single base.
- SNPs near a gene tend to remain together with that gene through many generations, a phenomenon called linkage disequilibrium.
- SNPs in linkage disequilibrium with genes can be used to "tag" the genes.
- Genome-wide association studies involve the genotyping of hundreds of thousands of SNPs and determining which are associated with a trait, a disease, or a response to medication.

From: *Contemporary Cardiology: Comprehensive Cardiovascular Medicine in the Primary Care Setting*
Edited by: Peter P. Toth, Christopher P. Cannon, DOI 10.1007/978-1-60327-963-5_6
© Springer Science+Business Media, LLC 2010

- Genome-wide association studies can identify SNPs to be used for disease risk prediction and pharmacogenomics, as well as identifying genes that are potential therapeutic targets.
- Genetic risk scores can be calculated but have not yet been demonstrated to be useful for disease risk prediction.
- Pharmacogenomics involves the use of SNP information to predict responses to therapy and may eventually allow the delivery of the "right drug for the right patient."
- Risks of genetic testing include the possibility of misinterpretation of the results, false reassurance or false worry, and ethical concerns.
- Discussions with patients about the genomics—particularly in regard to its current shortcomings—should be welcomed, keeping in mind that these discussions are opportunities to encourage traditional preventive health practices.

6.1. WHY IS GENOMICS IMPORTANT?

Genomics, or the study of genomes, is concerned with understanding how the deoxyribonucleic acid (DNA) of which genomes are constituted contributes to making an organism unique. Accordingly, human genomics focuses on how DNA sequences produce individuals' traits—e.g., skin color, cholesterol levels—and contribute to diseases—e.g., myocardial infarction, diabetes mellitus. The last few years have witnessed a remarkable leap forward in the use of genomics technology to understand human traits and diseases, to the point that new discoveries regarding what makes each person unique are being widely reported in the press and advertised by companies to the lay public. Although *no practical use of genomics yet exists*, there are high expectations that it will be clinically useful in the near future. Discussions with patients of the implications of genomics—whether it is in the form of genetic testing for disease risk, pharmacogenomics, or personalized medicine—will be unavoidable for primary care providers. This chapter seeks to: (1) explain the basic biology underlying genomics technology, (2) describe the potential future uses of genomics to improve patient care, particularly in cardiovascular medicine, and (3) set realistic expectations for the utility of genomics and explore the ethical implications of the technology.

6.2. A BRIEF INTRODUCTION TO MOLECULAR BIOLOGY

Deoxyribonucleic acid (DNA) is a molecule with two strands that are wrapped around each other in a helical formation, hence its description as a "double helix." The outer part of the helix contains the sugar and phosphate "backbone" of the DNA, and the inner part contains the "coding" portion of the molecule with four types of bases—adenine (A), cytosine (C), guanine (G), and thymine (T). An organism's genetic information is determined by the order of the sequence of the bases—with four bases available, the number of potential sequences is almost endless. The versatility of DNA results from the obligatory pairing of bases in the two strands. An adenine in one strand is always matched up with a thymine in the other strand, and cytosine is always paired with guanine. Thus, the two strands contain redundant information, and each can serve as a template on which a new complementary strand can be synthesized. This allows for easy duplication of the DNA so that when a cell divides into two, each descendant cell receives the same genetic information as the original cell.

An organism's DNA is organized into superlong strands that are packaged by a large complex of supporting proteins into chromosomes. Humans have 23 pairs of chromosomes, including the pair that determines gender, which in females comprises two X chromosomes, and in men, one X and one Y chromosome. For each chromosome pair, one was inherited from the mother and one from the father. The full set of chromosomes is collectively called the genome. The human genome is contained within the nucleus of each cell, where it is separated from the rest of the cell's functions.

In general, the genome is characterized by vast stretches of "non-coding" DNA sequence punctuated by small areas of "coding" DNA, also called genes, that represent the instructions needed by cells to perform their functions. Coding DNA is "transcribed" into a single-stranded molecule called ribonucleic acid (RNA) by a transcription enzyme complex. RNA is structurally similar to a DNA strand and also contains four types of bases, including adenine, cytosine, and guanine [in RNA, uracil (U) is substituted for DNA's thymine (T)]. The transcription enzymes have proofreading functions that ensure that the sequence of the RNA molecule perfectly matches the sequence of the DNA template from which it was synthesized. RNA is more flexible and mobile than DNA and is transported out of the nucleus of the cell into the outer compartment, the cytoplasm. Thus, RNA production is the mechanism by which genetic information is "expressed" and relayed from the central repository (DNA) to the rest of the cell, where it directs cellular functions.

While some RNAs have specialized functions—e.g., serving as structural components of certain parts of the cell—most RNAs take the form of "messenger" RNAs (mRNAs) that are "translated" by ribosomes into proteins. The ribosome reads from the beginning of the mRNA and uses it as a coding template with which to build proteins, with each non-overlapping set of three consecutive bases ("codons") serving to specify a particular amino acid. With four available types of bases, there are 64 possible codon combinations; with some redundancy, these codons are translated into any of 20 different amino acids or into a "stop" signal. In this way the RNA sequence is converted into an amino acid sequence until a stop signal is reached that prompts the ribosome to finish and release the protein. The protein is then processed by the cell and then deployed to serve its purpose (as an enzyme, as a secreted factor, etc.).

This highly organized progression from DNA, to transcribed RNA, to translated protein is known as the "central dogma" of molecular biology (Fig. 1), and while there are exceptions to this sequence of events, the central dogma explains the vast majority of cellular processes. By and large, in humans these processes combine with environmental influences to determine each person's individual characteristics, susceptibility to diseases, and responses to medications. The technology is now available to study the cellular processes at any step of the central dogma. When the investigation occurs at the level of DNA, it is termed "genomics;" when at the level of mRNAs, "transcriptomics;" when at the level of proteins, "proteomics." Processed proteins or other products of enzymatic reactions are called metabolites, the study of which is termed "metabolomics."

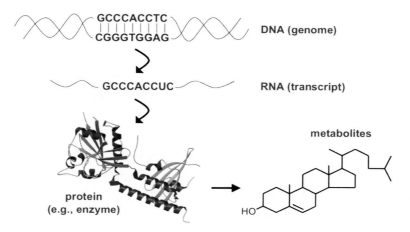

Fig. 1. Decoding and implementation of genetic information. Also known as the "central dogma," the cellular pathway begins with deoxyribonucleic acid (DNA) and proceeds with transcription of DNA into ribonucleic acid (RNA) transcripts, followed by translation of RNA into proteins (e.g., enzymes), which in turn produce metabolites.

6.3. THE PRINCIPLES OF HUMAN GENOMICS

The human genome is roughly 3 billion DNA bases in size, spanning the 23 chromosome pairs, and represents the complete list of coded instructions needed to make a person. There are an estimated 20,000–25,000 genes in the human genome, most of which encode proteins or components of proteins. What makes each person unique is a large number of DNA variations distributed throughout the genome. Some people have particular genetic variations that can predispose to heart disease; some of these variants require the presence of environmental factors (such as smoking and obesity) to trigger heart disease. Less commonly, certain variations have such a strong effect that they can cause heart disease outright. Other variations may determine how well patients respond to particular medications.

One reason some people are more susceptible to getting a disease than other people or respond differently to medications is that their DNA variants affect the function of genes. There are rare variants that have a large effect on a gene's function, either by significantly increasing or decreasing the gene's activity; these are the kind of variants that cause disease in many members of a single family and are also known as "mutations." There are common variants (>1% of the general population) that have a small effect on a gene's function. These variants do not change gene activity enough to cause disease by themselves, but, instead, need to be combined with other gene variants or with environmental factors in order for disease to occur. This is the case with most cardiovascular diseases where there are many contributing factors (e.g., hypercholesterolemia, myocardial infarction). Conversely, there are common variants that have the opposite effect—they offer modest protection against disease.

All of these differences at the DNA level are called "polymorphisms," of which there are several types (Fig. 2). The best characterized to date are single nucleotide polymorphisms (SNPs) in which a single base in the DNA differs from the usual base at that position. A copy number variant (CNV) is a polymorphism in which the number of repeats of a DNA sequence at a location varies from person to person. An "indel" (short for insertion–deletion) is a polymorphism in which a DNA sequence is either present or absent at a location, varying from person to person. SNPs are the most common and best understood of the polymorphisms, with an estimated 11 million SNPs across the human genome. Of these, more than 3 million have been identified, occurring on average once in every 1,000 bases.

"Locus" is one of the several terms used to describe a local area on a chromosome around an SNP. In most cases, each person has two copies of each locus because of the pairing of chromosomes;

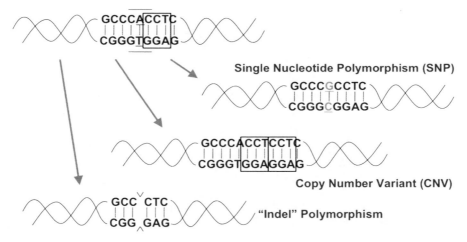

Fig. 2. Three types of polymorphisms. Variations in DNA sequence from person to person, or polymorphisms, can take the form of single nucleotide polymorphisms (SNPs), copy number variants (CNVs), and insertion–deletion variants ("indels").

the exceptions are loci on the X or Y chromosome in men, who have only one of each. A person's "genotype" at an SNP is the identity of the base position for each of the two copies—also called "alleles"—of the SNP on paired chromosomes; thus, a genotype is typically two letters. A "haplotype" is a combination of SNPs at multiple linked loci—often adjacent to each other—that are usually transmitted as a group from parent to child (Fig. 3).

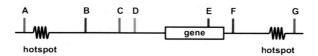

Fig. 3. Linkage disequilibrium. SNPs in proximity to a gene tend to stay together with that gene through many generations, a phenomenon known as linkage disequilibrium. In this example, only E is in the gene and directly affects its function. Genotypes at B, C, D, E, and F will stay together on a chromosome as it is passed from parents to offspring. In contrast, A and G are separated from the gene and the other SNPs by recombination hotspots, and thus they may not stay together on a chromosome through many generations—they will not be in linkage disequilibrium. Being linked, B through F make up a haplotype. Knowledge of any one of the five SNPs gives information on—acts as a "tag" for—the other four SNPs. Thus, genotyping B (or C or D or F) will indirectly yield information about the gene, even though the SNP is not in the gene.

Some SNPs lie in genes and affect the genes' function. Most SNPs lie outside genes, in the large stretches of non-coding DNA between genes, and do not directly affect the genes. Groups of SNPs near genes tend to stay together with the genes from generation to generation, over thousands of years, in what are called "linkage disequilibrium" blocks that are separated by chromosomal recombination hotspots (for a more detailed explanation of this phenomenon, please see *(1)*). Thus, even if it is not known which polymorphism in a gene causes a disease (which is usually the case), one can use an SNP that is not in the gene—but is in linkage disequilibrium with the gene—as a "tag" for that disease-causing variant of the gene (Fig. 3).

The technology is now available to decode hundreds of thousands of "tag" SNPs in a person's DNA all at once using "gene chips" or "gene arrays." By applying the gene chips to thousands of individuals, some with a disease and some without the disease, researchers are able to identify tag SNPs that are associated with disease (though the association is typically not perfect nor do associations imply causality). These studies are termed "genome-wide association studies" or "whole-genome studies."

As an example of how this technology might be used, consider a genome-wide association study performed for myocardial infarction. The study design would entail collecting DNA samples from several thousand patients who have suffered heart attacks and several thousand control individuals (who have not have had heart attacks but are otherwise similar to the patients). A gene chip is used to determine the genotype for more than 1 million SNPs in each of the study subjects. Despite having a massive amount of information (1 million genotypes for several thousand people, or billions of pieces of data), the statistical methods to analyze the information are relatively simple. The investigators set up computer software to analyze each SNP and ask: Does allele "A" versus allele "B" of this SNP occur in equal proportions in the myocardial infarction patients and the control individuals? In the vast majority of cases, there will be no difference in proportions; for a particular SNP, however, there may be a significant difference in the proportions (Fig. 4). Because the SNP "tags" any nearby genes, the implication is that there is a variant in one of the nearby genes that affects its function in such a way as to modify the risk of myocardial infarction (presumably through involvement in a pathophysiological process).

Several genome-wide association studies with precisely this design have been performed for myocardial infarction and coronary artery disease. These studies all found SNPs in a locus on chromosome 9p21 to be highly associated with coronary disease, with weaker associations seen for SNPs in other chromosomes *(2–4)*. (At the time of this writing, it remains unclear which gene near the 9p21

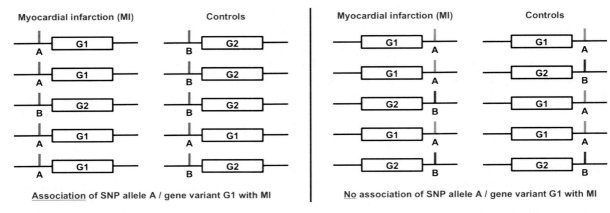

Association of SNP allele A / gene variant G1 with MI — No association of SNP allele A / gene variant G1 with MI

Fig. 4. General strategy for genome-wide association studies. For each of hundreds of thousands of SNPs distributed across the genome, the genotypes at the SNP are determined for both cases (myocardial infarction in this example) and controls. As shown on the *left*, an allele of the SNP may be seen in higher proportions in cases than controls. This SNP is therefore associated with the disease, and the strength of the association (*P* value) and exact increase in disease risk can be calculated using biostatistics. Even if this SNP is not in the causal gene (as in this example), it may be in linkage disequilibrium with a polymorphism in the gene, explaining the association with disease. On the *right*, the SNP alleles are present in the same proportions in cases and controls; this SNP is not associated with disease. Typically, out of hundreds of thousands of SNPs only a few (if any) show a statistically robust association with disease.

locus contributes to myocardial infarction.) Other studies have identified SNPs associated with atrial fibrillation *(5)*, lipid levels *(6–9)*, diabetes mellitus *(10–12)*, electrocardiographic QT interval *(13)*, abdominal aortic aneurysm *(14)*, and statin-induced myopathy *(15)*.

6.4. PRACTICAL USES OF GENOMICS STUDIES

Genome-wide association studies (GWAS) allow for the mapping of diseases (e.g., myocardial infarction) and clinical traits (e.g., cholesterol levels) to specific regions on chromosomes. They narrow the resolution from 3 billion bases (the entire human genome) to around 100,000 bases (chromosomal locus) surrounding a tag SNP. In principle, the tag SNP can then be used for disease risk prediction or for pharmacogenomics (see below). The tag SNP can also be used to pinpoint causal genes underlying the disease or trait or response to therapy. Subsequent studies on those genes can give important insights into basic biology as well as facilitate the development of new therapies that target the genes (Fig. 5).

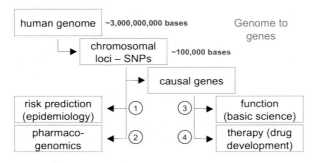

Fig. 5. Potential uses of information learned from genome-wide association studies.

6.5. GENETIC TESTING AND DISEASE RISK PREDICTION

After identifying a number of SNPs—in different chromosomal loci across the genome—that are associated with a disease of interest, one can use these SNPs to calculate a genetic risk score for the disease (Fig. 6). One simple example entails cataloging for each SNP: Does the patient have two copies of the lower-risk variant of the SNP, two copies of the higher-risk variant of the SNP, or one copy each of the lower-risk and the higher-risk variant? Risk "points" are assigned depending on the genotype at the SNP. These points are added up for all of the SNPs, yielding a total risk score. This risk score, especially when combined with a traditional risk score (e.g., Framingham risk estimate) that accounts for endogenous (blood pressure, serum lipids, age) and environmental factors (e.g., cigarette smoking), might be useful in predicting the likelihood of developing the disease. Eventually, clinicians would be able to order this panel of SNPs as a blood test and get back a risk score that would help guide patient management.

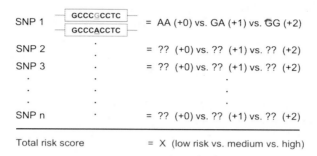

Fig. 6. Calculation of a genetic risk score.

One of the first published reports of a genetic risk score for cardiovascular disease, in early 2008, demonstrates the potential usefulness of a risk score *(16)*. The investigators calculated a lipid-based genetic risk score using nine SNPs associated with LDL cholesterol or HDL cholesterol (score from 0 to 18) and found that the score is associated with cardiovascular disease. The higher the risk score, the more likelihood the individual had of developing cardiovascular disease during the study period. However, when this particular genetic risk score was added to a traditional risk prediction model, it did not improve overall risk prediction. After adjustment for traditional risk factors, the relative risk between individuals with high genetic risk scores and those with low genetic risk scores was 1.63, a modest difference *(16)*. Although the degree of risk discrimination is likely to improve as additional SNPs discovered to be associated with cardiovascular disease are added to the genetic risk score, it remains to be seen whether it will be enough to significantly improve on current risk prediction strategies.

For a healthcare provider presented with this type of genetic information, it will be a challenge to meaningfully integrate it into clinical practice. This is especially true when the relative risks associated with SNP variants are in the 1.0–2.0 range—i.e., the at-risk genotype confers between 1 and 2 times the risk of developing the disease—as seems to be the case with most disease-associated genotypes. Providers must already ponder the utility of novel biomarkers, such as high-sensitivity C-reactive protein, that are only modestly predictive of cardiovascular disease and do not reclassify large proportions of patients into new risk categories *(17)*. To date, genetic risk scores do not appear to be any more predictive than these biomarkers. Indeed, it remains unclear in the absence of any clinical trials whether a genetic risk score will prove more useful than simply asking the question: "Do you have a family history of heart disease?"

Nevertheless, several companies see significant commercial potential in these types of risk scores and have already started marketing SNP panels to the general public, charging hundreds to thousands of US dollars. The implication of the advertising for these panels is that they will let patients know if they are at higher risk for particular diseases. None of these panels has yet been shown to add value to traditional risk factor algorithms, and they should not be recommended to patients at this time for that purpose.

There are other important limitations of these SNP panels. They do not include rare polymorphisms that cause disease (these include the mutations that are unique to one person, or to one family, and so are not going to be found on the SNP panels). So while the patient may learn from an SNP panel that she has a variant of a common SNP that modestly decreases the risk of a particular disease, e.g., breast cancer, she may unknowingly harbor a mutation—not found by the SNP panel—that dramatically increases her breast cancer risk. In this case, having only partial genetic information would give false reassurance and may even be harmful if the patient chooses to forego screening with mammography.

Furthermore, because the initial series of genome-wide studies were performed in Caucasian populations of European ancestry, the first generation of SNP panels may not be relevant to individuals of other ethnic or racial backgrounds. For now, non-Caucasian individuals will benefit less than Caucasians from the recent advances in genomics, although this situation should change as more genome-wide studies are performed in a wider variety of racial and ethnic groups.

When asked about SNP panels by patients, it is appropriate to say that the tests are experimental— they may eventually prove to be useful, but they may also prove to be a waste of money. It is also appropriate to point out that many old-fashioned preventative health practices—good diet, weight control, exercise, smoking cessation—can have a far larger impact on one's risk of getting a disease than any genetic influences that one may learn about from genetic testing.

6.6. PHARMACOGENOMICS

The field of pharmacogenomics—the use of human genomic variation to predict efficacy and toxicity of drug therapy—is a promising area for the clinical application of genomic information. Commonly used medications such as lipid-lowering therapy, antihypertensive drugs, antiarrhythmic drugs, and anticoagulants have differential effects depending on variation in certain genes. The ultimate objective of pharmacogenomics is to deliver the "right drug for the right patient" by accurately predicting both therapeutic response and safety before a drug is prescribed.

One scenario for the practical application for pharmacogenomics is the use of a screening test to identify patients who are at risk for adverse side effects from medications or who are unlikely to respond to a therapy (Fig. 7). A patient presenting to medical attention with a particular condition would undergo the screening test, which would identify the genotype of a relevant polymorphism or set of polymorphisms. The genotype information would be used to determine whether the patient's condition is likely to improve from the treatment, whether the treatment poses a risk and should be avoided altogether, or how much of the treatment should be given—i.e., tailoring the dose to the patient.

When associations between genotype and drug sensitivity have been identified, as in the case of INR response to warfarin therapy on the basis of *CYP2C9* genotypes and *VKORC1* haplotypes, trials

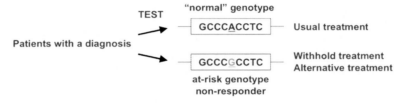

Fig. 7. The general strategy of pharmacogenomics.

must be conducted to evaluate the clinical efficacy of the gene-based prescribing strategy and determine whether the increment in efficacy or safety warrants the cost of genetic testing *(18)*. An initial trial reported in 2007 assessed an algorithm that used a patient's specific *CYP2C9* and *VKORC1* SNPs to calculate an ideal starting warfarin dose for anticoagulation (Fig. 8). When compared to the usual practice (i.e., providers picking a starting dose using best judgment), this specific algorithm did not improve the safety of warfarin initiation (out-of-range INR measurements were not reduced compared to traditional dosing), although it did reduce the number of dosing changes needed *(18)*. More research studies are underway to see whether genetic dosing of warfarin will be clinically useful.

Formula for dosing:

Estimated weekly coumadin dose = 1.64 + expe[3.984 + *1*1(0) + *1*2(-0.197) + *1*3(-0.360) + *2*3(-0.947) + *2*2(-0.265) + *3*3(-1.892) + Vk-CT(-0.304) + Vk-TT(-0.569) + Vk-CC(0) + age(-0.009) + male sex(0.094) + female sex(0) + weight in kg(0.003)]

where expe is the exponential to base e; *1, *2, *3 refer to CYP2C9 wild-type (*1) or variant (*2, *3) genotypes, respectively; and Vk refers to VKORC1 with variants CT, TT, or CC

Fig. 8. Genetic algorithm used to calculate starting warfarin dose in a recent clinical trial *(18)*.

Just as genome-wide association studies are being used to characterize disease risk, a similar strategy can be used to characterize appropriate or adverse responses to therapy. A genome-wide association study published in 2008 showed that individuals with one genotype at an SNP in the *SLCO1B1* gene have 17 times the risk of statin-induced myopathy than individuals with another genotype *(15)*. This dramatic difference in relative risk (though not absolute risk, given the overall rarity of statin-induced myopathy) suggests that a genetic test for this SNP could be helpful in predicting which patients are at risk of getting myopathy before they are started on statins. A *SLCO1B1* SNP test might be particularly useful for patients in whom there is already a clinical suspicion for risk of myopathy (e.g., family history, history of myalgias on statin therapy). As with all genetic findings to date, however, this strategy needs to be tested in a clinical trial before it can be recommended for general use.

Another potential application of genetics to predicting response to therapy involves the antiplatelet agent clopidogrel, which has become a mainstay of post-acute coronary syndrome (ACS) patient management, particularly after percutaneous coronary intervention. Clopidogrel is converted into its active metabolite in the liver by the cytochrome P-450 2C19 enzyme. In three large studies of post-ACS patients on clopidogrel therapy (TRITON-TIMI 38, FAST-MI, and AFIJI), the *CYP2C19* gene encoding this enzyme was genotyped, with identification of at least one reduced function allele in ~30% of individuals. In all of the three studies, carriers of reduced function *CYP2C19* alleles suffered significantly higher rates of cardiovascular death, myocardial infarction, and stroke *(19–21)*. This is consistent with the finding in TRITON-TIMI 38 that reduced function allele carriers had lower plasma levels of the active metabolite of clopidogrel *(19)*.

Thus, in principle, it should be possible to predict who will suffer worse cardiovascular outcomes while on clopidogrel therapy by determining patients' *CYP2C19* genotypes. Higher-risk individuals could be given higher doses of clopidogrel or preferentially receive alternative medications such as prasugrel. Further studies will be needed to determine if routine post-ACS genotyping of *CYP2C19* will be cost-effective and will improve patient outcomes.

6.7. RISKS OF GENETIC TESTING

Although some "early adopter" patients may take the initiative to avail themselves of commercial SNP genotyping services and then bring genetic information to providers for interpretation, others will approach their providers first and ask whether genetic testing is advisable. It may seem harmless for a patient to undergo SNP genotyping—typically involving only a swabbing of the inside of a cheek or a drawing of a blood sample—but there are important potential consequences to consider. As mentioned above, it is not yet clear how physicians should best interpret the results of genetic testing, since few clinical trials have been done. Furthermore, in the "Google era," there is the danger of patients overinterpreting the results of their tests based on misleading information available on the Internet.

One worrisome possibility is that a patient may be falsely reassured by hearing that his genetic risk score is low. He may not be vigorous about lifestyle changes that, if enacted, would reduce his risk of disease even more than the protection offered by his favorable genetic profile. Conversely, a high genetic risk score may cause undue worry and even strain family relations. For example, a person may learn that the spouse is more likely to develop a serious illness, and this may impact their relationship as well as relationships with parents and potential offspring. Arranging for a patient and family members to meet a genetic counselor is recommended if this type of situation should arise.

Finally, privacy issues should be seriously considered prior to the use of genetic tests. It remains to be seen what insurance companies will do if they obtain access to genetic data. The US Congress has acted to prohibit discrimination by employers and health insurers on the basis of genetic testing with the Genetic Information Nondiscrimination Act (GINA), but further ethical safeguards will undoubtedly be needed as the social implications of genomics become clearer.

6.8. CONCLUSION

Although genomics offers great promise for the improvement of cardiovascular medicine, it will be years before evidence-based applications of the technology are demonstrated and validated. Yet with the enormous publicity surrounding genomics discoveries, it will be natural for patients to seek advice about genetic testing from their providers. These inquiries should be welcomed, since they reflect patients taking an active interest in their own health, and they are opportunities for providers not only to educate patients about genomics—to highlight the present uncertainty of the clinical usefulness of the tests, as well as the potential hazards of obtaining the information—but also to reinforce old-fashioned preventive messages—good diet, weight control, exercise, smoking cessation—as well.

6.9. CASE STUDY 1

A 57-year-old Caucasian man presents to your clinic for the first time. He is eager to talk to you about the results of his "gene tests." Upon hearing about a commercial "personal genome service" that reads more than 500,000 locations in the genome and offers information on more than 100 diseases, he immediately signed up for the service. He has printed out all the results of the tests and brought them to you so you can read them and keep them in his medical record. He is particularly concerned because the tests reveal that he has an increased risk of having a heart attack. When you look at the specific information in the printouts, you see that on the basis of several SNP genotypes his relative risk of myocardial infarction is estimated to be 1.6 times that of the general population.

On physical examination, the patient is overweight and moderately hypertensive. He admits that he does not regularly exercise, smokes half a pack of cigarettes a day, and has not been taking the cholesterol medication prescribed to him by a physician 3 years ago. He asks how concerned he should be about the results of his genetic testing.

Answer: You can advise the patient that although his genetic testing may suggest a modestly increased risk of heart attack, the information is not useful at the present time because there has been no clinical trials testing whether this type of information is valid. You should point out that he has several traditional risk factors for myocardial infarction—high blood pressure, high cholesterol, tobacco use—all of which make it much more likely that he will get a heart attack in comparison to his putative 1.6-fold risk from his SNP genotypes. Importantly, he can do something about those risk factors—improve his diet, exercise regularly, take his prescribed medications, and stop smoking—while he cannot do anything about his genetics.

Given the potential privacy issues, keeping the results of nonclinical genetic testing in the medical record is not advisable at this time.

6.10. CASE STUDY 2

You are seeing in your clinic a 63-year-old woman whom you have been following for several years. She suffered a myocardial infarction 2 years ago, after which she was appropriately prescribed a statin drug for secondary prevention. She stopped taking the statin because she developed severe muscle aches, and she was switched to ezetimibe instead. On a fasting lipid profile taken several weeks ago in anticipation of today's visit, her LDL cholesterol remains quite elevated—135 mg/dL—far above the optimal goal of 70 mg/dL. You advise her that she really should be on a statin drug and you can prescribe her a different statin than the one she took before in the hope of avoiding her prior symptoms. She is hesitant to proceed; she has learned that her father developed bad "muscle disease" when he was taking a statin 10 years ago, requiring hospitalization, and both her brother and sister have experienced muscle aches when taking statins.

Is there a role for genetic testing in this patient's management?

Answer: At the time of this writing there is no genetic test for statin-induced myopathy; however, an SNP in the *SLCO1B1* gene has recently been reported to be strongly associated with myopathy *(15)*. Individuals with the at-risk genotype have 17 times the risk of developing myopathy compared to other individuals. It can be expected that a commercial test for this *SLCO1B1* variant will be available in the near future. Given this patient's prior symptoms and her strong family history, she appears to be at increased risk of statin-induced myopathy. Determining if she has the at-risk *SLCO1B1* genotype could be helpful in her management; if she does have the genotype, it would be prudent to avoid statin therapy altogether. If she does not have the genotype, one might be encouraged to cautiously start her on a different statin.

6.11. RECOMMENDED READING

1. Topol EJ, Murray SS, Frazer, KA. The genomics gold rush. *JAMA*. 2007;298:218–221.
2. Arnett DK, Baird AE, Barkley RA, et al. Relevance of genetics and genomics for prevention and treatment of cardiovascular disease: a scientific statement from the American Heart Association Council on epidemiology and prevention, the Stroke Council, and the Functional Genomics and Translational Biology Interdisciplinary Working Group. *Circulation*. 2007;115:2878–2901.
3. Musunuru K, Kathiresan S. HapMap and mapping genes for cardiovascular disease. *Circ Cardiovasc Genet*. 2008;1:66–71.

REFERENCES

1. Musunuru K, Kathiresan S. HapMap and mapping genes for cardiovascular disease. *Circ Cardiovasc Genet*. 2008;1: 66–71.
2. McPherson R, Pertsemlidis A, Kavaslar N, et al. A common allele on chromosome 9 associated with coronary heart disease. *Science*. 2007;316:1488–1491.

3. Helgadottir A, Thorleifsson G, Manolescu A, et al. A common variant on chromosome 9p21 affects the risk of myocardial infarction. *Science*. 2007;316:1491–1493.

4. Samani NJ, Erdmann J, Hall AS, et al. Genomewide association analysis of coronary artery disease. *N Engl J Med*. 2007;357:443–453.

5. Gudbjartsson DF, Arnar DO, Helgadottir A, et al. Variants conferring risk of atrial fibrillation on chromosome 4q25. *Nature*. 2007;448:353–357.

6. Willer CJ, Sanna S, Jackson AU, et al. Newly identified loci that influence lipid concentrations and risk of coronary artery disease. *Nat Genet*. 2008;40:161–169.

7. Kathiresan S, Melander O, Guiducci C, et al. Six new loci associated with blood low-density lipoprotein cholesterol, high-density lipoprotein cholesterol or triglycerides in humans. *Nat Genet*. 2008;40:189–197.

8. Wallace C, Newhouse SJ, Braund P, et al. Genome-wide association study identifies genes for biomarkers of cardiovascular disease: serum urate and dyslipidemia. *Am J Hum Genet*. 2008;82:139–149.

9. Sandhu MS, Waterworth DM, Debenham SL, et al. LDL-cholesterol concentrations: a genome-wide association study. *Lancet*. 2008;371:483–491.

10. Saxena R, Voight BF, Lyssenko V, et al. Diabetes genetics initiative of Broad Institute of Harvard and MIT, Lund University, and Novartis Institutes of BioMedical Research. Genome-wide association analysis identifies loci for type 2 diabetes and triglyceride levels. *Science*. 2007;316:1331–1336.

11. Zeggini E, Weedon MN, Lindgren CM, et al. Replication of genome-wide association signals in UK samples reveals risk loci for type 2 diabetes. *Science*. 2007;316:1336–1341.

12. Scott LJ, Mohlke KL, Bonnycastle LL, et al. A genome-wide association study of type 2 diabetes in Finns detects multiple susceptibility variants. *Science*. 2007;316:1341–1345.

13. Arking DE, Pfeufer A, Post W, et al. A common genetic variant in the NOS1 regulator NOS1AP modulates cardiac repolarization. *Nat Genet*. 2006;38:644–651.

14. Helgadottir A, Thorleifsson G, Magnusson KP, et al. The same sequence variant on 9p21 associates with myocardial infarction, abdominal aortic aneurysm and intracranial aneurysm. *Nat Genet*. 2008;40:217–224.

15. Link E, Parish S, Armitage J, et al. SEARCH Collaborative Group. SLCO1B1 variants and statin-induced myopathy—a genomewide study. *N Engl J Med*. 2008;359:789–799.

16. Kathiresan S, Melander O, Anevski D, et al. Polymorphisms associated with cholesterol and risk of cardiovascular events. *N Engl J Med*. 2008;358:1240–1249.

17. Musunuru K, Kral BG, Blumenthal RS, et al. The use of high-sensitivity assays for C-reactive protein in clinical practice. *Nat Clin Pract Cardiovasc Med*. 2008;5:621–635.

18. Anderson JL, Horne BD, Stevens SM, et al. Randomized trial of genotype-guided versus standard warfarin dosing in patients initiating oral anticoagulation. *Circulation*. 2007;116:2563–2570.

19. Mega JL, Close SL, Wiviott SD, et al. Cytochrome P-450 polymorphisms and response to clopidogrel. *N Engl J Med*. 2009;360:354–362.

20. Simon T, Verstuyft C, Mary-Krause M, et al. French registry of acute ST-elevation and non-ST-elevation myocardial infarction (FAST-MI) investigators. Genetic determinants of response to clopidogrel and cardiovascular events. *N Engl J Med*. 2009;360:363–375.

21. Collet JP, Hulot JS, Pena A, et al. Cytochrome P450 2C19 polymorphism in young patients treated with clopidogrel after myocardial infarction: a cohort study. *Lancet*. 2009;373:309–317.

7
The Metabolic Syndrome: 2009

Charles Reasner

CONTENTS

Key Words: Insulin resistance; Polycystic ovarian syndrome; Diabetes mellitus; Metformin; Fatty acids; Adipocytes.

KEY POINTS

- The metabolic syndrome describes a clustering of risk factors that increase an individual's likelihood of developing both type 2 diabetes mellitus and cardiovascular disease.
- In the United States, one-third of adults meet the criteria for the metabolic syndrome. In addition, each of the individual risk factors (central obesity, hypertriglyceridemia, low HDL-cholesterol, hypertension, and abnormal glucose metabolism) occurs in about one-third of adults.
- Obesity is increasing the fastest in children and adolescents. The prevalence of the metabolic syndrome in obese adolescents is 50%.
- An increase in intra-abdominal fat is the main driver of the metabolic syndrome. The amount of intra-abdominal fat is estimated by measuring the waist circumference.
- All patients with the metabolic syndrome should institute therapeutic lifestyle changes aimed at decreasing intra-abdominal obesity.
- Statins are first-line pharmacologic therapy for patients with atherogenic dyslipidemia. Niacin may be considered if the HDL-cholesterol is low after instituting statin therapy.
- Metformin is the first-line pharmacologic therapy for patients with hyperglycemia.
- Polycystic ovary syndrome (PCOS) is present in 10% of reproductive age females, making it the most common metabolic abnormality in young women.
- PCOS is often associated with insulin resistance, hyperinsulinemia, elevated androgen levels, and an increased risk of developing diabetes mellitus and cardiovascular disease.
- Lifestyle and pharmacologic interventions aimed at lowering insulin levels improve clinical outcomes in young women diagnosed with PCOS.

From: *Contemporary Cardiology: Comprehensive Cardiovascular Medicine in the Primary Care Setting*
Edited by: Peter P. Toth, Christopher P. Cannon, DOI 10.1007/978-1-60327-963-5_7
© Springer Science+Business Media, LLC 2010

7.1. DEFINITION

The association of insulin resistance with a clustering of risk factors that not only increased the risk of developing type 2 diabetes mellitus but also contributed to the development of cardiovascular disease was referred to as "syndrome X" by Reaven in 1988 *(1)*. Over the next several years the term "the insulin resistance syndrome" was used to describe these individuals with metabolic abnormalities including atherogenic dyslipidemia, hypertension, abdominal obesity, glucose intolerance, a prothrombotic profile, and a state of increased systemic inflammation. In 1998, the World Health Organization (WHO) task force on diabetes identified insulin resistance as the dominant cause of what we now term the metabolic syndrome and required indicators of insulin resistance to make the diagnosis *(2)*. Over time, the critical role played by abdominal obesity assumed a dominant position in the diagnostic criteria. The National Cholesterol Education Program (NCEP) Adult Treatment Panel III criteria for the metabolic syndrome replaced the requirement to demonstrate insulin resistance with a measure of waist circumference in the diagnostic criteria for the metabolic syndrome *(3)*. Since 2005 there has been general consensus regarding the clinical criteria needed to diagnose the metabolic syndrome. Thus, the American Heart Association/National Heart, Lung, and Blood Institute update of the NCEP criteria *(4)* and the International Diabetes Federation recommendations *(5)* are now largely in agreement. The core components for the WHO, NCEP, and the most recent International Diabetes Federation (IDF) criteria are outlined in Table 1.

Table 1
Criteria Proposed for Clinical Diagnosis of the Metabolic Syndrome

Clinical measure	WHO (1998)	NCEP (2001)	IDF (2005)
Insulin resistance	IGT, IFG, T2DM, or ↓ insulin sensitivity plus any two of the following	None Any 3 of the following	None
Body weight	M: waist-to-hip ratio >0.90 W: waist-to-hip ratio >0.85 and/or BMI >30 kg/m^2	M: waist circumference ≥102 cm W: waist circumference ≥88 cm	Increased waist circumference (population specific) plus any two of the following
Lipid	TG ≥150 mg/dL M: HDL-C <35 mg/dL W: HDL-C <39 mg/dL	TG ≥150 mg/dL M: HDL-C <40 mg/dL W: HDL-C <50 mg/dL	TG ≥150 mg/dL M: HDL-C <40 mg/dL W: HDL-C <50 mg/dL
Blood pressure	≥140/90 mmHg	≥130/85 mmHg	≥130 mmHg ≥85 mmHg diastolic
Glucose	IGT, IFG, or T2DM	≥110 mg/dL (includes diabetes)	≥100 mg/dL (includes diabetes)
Other	Microalbuminuria		

7.2. PREVALENCE OF THE METABOLIC SYNDROME

7.2.1. United States and Canada

The high prevalence of obesity in the United States (USA) is responsible for the alarming number of individuals affected in this country. About 30% of US adults are overweight (BMI: 25–29.9 kg/m^2) and another 32% are obese (BMI: >30 kg/m^2) *(6)*. By comparison, in Canada, 36% of adults are overweight and 23% are obese *(7)*. The National Health and Nutrition Examination Survey (NHANES) 1999–2002 is the most scientifically rigorous sample of the US population *(8)*. A total of 3,601 men and women aged >20 years were included in the survey. Using the NCEP definition, the prevalence of metabolic syndrome was 33.7% of men and 35.4% of women. Each of the individual risk factors—abdominal obesity, elevated triglycerides, low levels of HDL-cholesterol, hypertension, and elevated plasma glucose—occurred in about one-third of the population. As the population ages and becomes more obese, these numbers will undoubtedly increase.

There are important ethnic differences in the presentation of the metabolic syndrome. Black men have a relatively low prevalence of the metabolic syndrome compared with other ethnic groups due to a lower average waist circumference, lower triglycerides, and higher HDL-cholesterol levels *(9)*. On the other hand, Blacks are more likely to have hypertension and develop diabetes than Caucasians *(10, 11)*. The highest prevalence of the metabolic syndrome and type 2 diabetes in the United States is seen in the Hispanic population *(8, 12)*. Hispanics are more likely to have hypertriglyceridemia but less likely to have hypertension than either their Black or Caucasian counterparts. The highest prevalence of the metabolic syndrome in North America, almost 50% of the population, has been reported for the Oji–Cree population in Western Canada *(13)*. Functional polymorphisms in three candidate genes coding for plasma lipoproteins and blood pressure have been identified in this population *(14)*.

Results from a series of studies reporting the prevalence of the metabolic syndrome in Europe *(15–33)*, Asia *(34–50)*, and Latin America *(51–61)* have been published. Trials using the NCEP criteria for diagnosis are outlined in Tables 2, 3, and 4. In Europe and Latin America, approximately 25% of adults meet the criteria for the metabolic syndrome. In Asia, the prevalence is variable, with Japan and India having a relatively high prevalence compared with Central and Southeast Asia.

In the United States, the segment of the population that is growing fatter the fastest is children and teenagers. Data derived from the Third National Health and Nutrition Examination Survey III (NHANES III) showed between 1988–1994 and 1999–2000 the prevalence of overweight (≥95% of BMI for age) among adolescents aged 12–19 years increased from 11 to 16%. Among adolescent boys, prevalence increased from 12 to 13% in non-Hispanic whites, 11–21% in African-Americans, and from 14 to 28% in Mexican Americans. Among adolescent girls, overweight prevalence increased from 9 to 12% in non-Hispanic whites, 16–27% in African-Americans, and 15–19% in Mexican Americans *(62)*.

The role of obesity in childhood and the development of the metabolic syndrome were highlighted by a study done by Weiss and colleagues *(63)*. The effect of varying degrees of obesity on the prevalence of metabolic syndrome and its relation to insulin resistance in a large, multiethnic, multiracial cohort of children and adolescents was examined. A standard glucose tolerance test was administered

Table 2
Prevalence of Metabolic Syndrome in Europe

Country and reference	Population	Number	Criteria	Prevalence of MetS (% of population)		
				Men	Women	Total
France *(15)*	Men/women	3,359	NCEP	23.0	16.9	
France *(16)*	Men	10,592	NCEP	29.7		
Germany *(17)*	Men/women	4,816/2,315	NCEP	23.5	17.6	
Netherlands *(18)*	Adult men/women	1,364	NCEP	19.0	32.0	
Italy *(19)*	Men/women	1,877	NCEP	24.1	23.1	
Italy *(21)*	Men/women	2,100	NCEP	15	18	
Italy *(22)*	Men/women	5,632	NCEP	29.9	55.2	
Spain *(23)*	Men/women	2,540	NCEP	22.3	30.7	
Portugal *(24)*	Men/women	1,436	NCEP	19.1	27.0	
Croatia *(26)*	Men/women	996	NCEP			34.0
UK *(27)*	Women	3,589	NCEP		29.8	
Canary Islands *(29)*	Men/women	1,193	NCEP	20.3	21.1	

Table 3
Prevalence of Metabolic Syndrome in Asia

Country and reference	Population	Number	Criteria	Prevalence of MetS (% of population)	
				Men	Women
Central Asia					
India *(35)*	Men/women	1,123	NCEP	22.9	39.9
Southeast Asia					
Thailand *(38)*	Men/women	1,383	NCEP	15.7	11.7
Singapore *(39)*	Men/women	3,954	NCEP	14.1	12.3
	Men/women	4,816/2,315	NCEP	23.5	17.6
China					
(40)	Men/women	16,342	NCEP w/≥ 25 kg/m^2	15.7	10.2
(45)	Men/women type 2 DM	5,202	NCEP	23.9	12.8
Japan					
(47)	Men/women	8,144	NCEP	19.0	70.0
(48)	Men/women	3,264	Japanese criteria	12.1	1.7
(49)	Men/women	6,985	NCEP	30.2	10.3

Table 4
Prevalence of Metabolic Syndrome in Latin America

Country and reference	Population	Number	Criteria	Prevalence of MetS (% of population)		
				Men	Women	Total
Mexico *(51)*	Men/women	2,158	NCEP			26.6
Brazil *(52)*	Girls—overweight and non-overweight	388	3+ risk factors		Normal weight 14% Overweight 21.4%	
US Virgin Islands *(56)*	Caribbean-born adults No history of diabetes	893	NCEP			20.5
Brazil *(58)*	Japanese Brazilian men Women	151	NCEP	36.9	38.8	
Brazil *(60)*	Japanese Brazilians Men/women	877	NCEP modified for Asians	49.8	43.0	
Brazil *(61)*	Men/Women Spanish Migrants to Brazil	479	NCEP	29.6	22.6	

to 439 obese, 31 overweight, and 20 non-obese children and adolescents. Baseline measurements included blood pressure and plasma lipids, C-reactive protein (CRP), and adiponectin levels. Levels of TG, HDL-C, and blood pressure were adjusted for age and sex. Because the body mass index (BMI) varies according to age, the value for age and sex was standardized with the use of conversion to a Z-score. The prevalence of metabolic syndrome increased significantly with increasing insulin resistance and the degree of obesity. Fifty percent of severely obese children met the criteria for the metabolic syndrome. Compared to their normal weight siblings, obese children saw a doubling of their fasting triglyceride levels, an increase in systolic blood pressure of 20 mmHg, and a decrease of 20 mg/dL in their level of HDL-cholesterol. The fasting glucose was essentially unchanged because of a compensatory 3- to 4-fold rise in fasting plasma insulin levels. This study represents one of the clearest examples of the metabolic consequences of obesity as the 12- and 13-year-old children in this study had no medical problems other than obesity. It also should provide a clear signal that as the population develops greater degrees of obesity at younger ages, the prevalence of the metabolic syndrome will only increase.

7.3. PATHOGENESIS

7.3.1. Normal Insulin Action

In order to understand the insulin-resistant state associated with the metabolic syndrome we should first review physiologic insulin action. In the fasting state, approximately 85% of glucose production is derived from the liver, with the remainder produced by the kidney (64). Over half of this glucose production is essential to meet the needs of the brain and other neural tissues that metabolize glucose independent of insulin (65). In the fed state, carbohydrate ingestion leads to an increase in plasma glucose concentration and stimulates insulin release from the pancreatic beta cells. The resultant elevation in plasma insulin suppresses hepatic glucose production and stimulates glucose uptake by peripheral tissues, mainly skeletal muscle (66–69). Although fat tissue is responsible for only a small amount of total body glucose disposal, it plays a very important role in the maintenance of total body glucose homeostasis through the release of free fatty acids. Small increments in the plasma insulin exert a potent antilipolytic effect, leading to a marked reduction in the plasma-free fatty acid level (70). The decline in plasma FFA concentration results in increased glucose uptake in muscle and reduces hepatic glucose production (71, 72).

7.3.2. Central Obesity and Insulin Resistance

Imaging studies using measurements of central versus subcutaneous fat clearly demonstrate that excess intra-abdominal adipose tissue and not the subcutaneous adipose tissue correlates with insulin resistance and the metabolic syndrome (73–76). For example, individuals matched for central obesity with either high or low amounts of subcutaneous fat do not differ in their sensitivity to insulin (77, 78). Conversely, individuals matched for their amount of subcutaneous fat with either low or high levels of central fat are markedly different in their level of insulin resistance and glucose tolerance (77, 78). In fact, subcutaneous fat has been referred to as a "metabolic sink." As long as the subcutaneous fat cell has capacity to store fat, the body is protected. Once the storage capacity of the subcutaneous fat cell is exceeded, deposition of fat centrally leads to the development of the metabolic syndrome.

Increased amounts of visceral fat may lead to the metabolic syndrome in several ways. Visceral adipose tissue has a high lipolytic rate, which is especially refractory to insulin (75). Increased lipolysis of fat results in elevations of plasma FFAs and causes insulin resistance in muscle and liver (70–72) and impairs insulin secretion (79, 80). In addition to increased levels of circulating FFAs in plasma, type 2 diabetic and obese non-diabetic individuals have increased stores of triglycerides in muscle (81, 82) and liver (83), and the increased fat content correlates closely with the presence of insulin resistance in these tissues. Visceral fat cells are active endocrine cells producing many cytokines including leptin, tumor necrosis factor-alpha, and interleukin-6 (Fig. 1). These factors drain into the portal circulation and reduce insulin sensitivity in peripheral tissues (84). In a weight loss intervention trial carried out in obese, non-diabetic individuals, the best predictor of improvement in insulin sensitivity was a decrease in visceral adiposity (85).

Both the NCEP ATP III and IDF guidelines recognize central obesity as the driving force for the majority of individuals who are resistant to insulin. Both use waist circumference as a measure of central obesity. The measurement of waist circumference was felt to be superior to calculating the body mass index (BMI) because individuals with similar BMI values but different waistlines have different metabolic profiles (86, 87). In the landmark INTERHEART study, which compared risk factors in

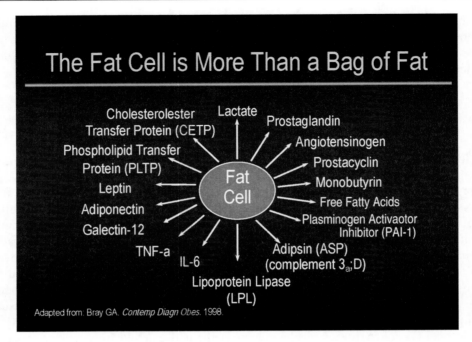

Fig. 1. This figure depicts the differential activity of the central versus peripheral fat cells. Increased intra-abdominal fat leads to production of cytokines which promote the development of the metabolic syndrome. Adapted from Bray GA. *(208).*

patients with myocardial infarctions with age-matched controls, the waist-to-hip ratio was associated with increased risk of cardiovascular disease *(88).* In the EPIC-Norfolk study which assessed the development of cardiovascular disease over a 9-year follow-up, an increased waist circumference was associated with an increased risk of an event, and a large hip girth was protective after adjusting for BMI *(87).* In spite of the appropriate importance given to waist circumference, it should be pointed out that an elevated BMI is associated with an increased metabolic risk. However, for any given BMI, a relative excess of intra-abdominal fat increases the risk even further. Finally, since there is a linear relationship between waist circumference and metabolic risk, any individual cut-off value will not be ideal at defining risk.

7.4. APPROACH TO THE PATIENT WITH THE METABOLIC SYNDROME: CASE STUDIES

Individuals with the metabolic syndrome are at increased risk for developing type 2 diabetes, cardiovascular disease, or both. While central obesity increases the risk of developing both disorders, low HDL and hypertension are strong predictors of heart disease, while hypertriglyceridemia and hyperglycemia are more strongly related to insulin resistance and the development of type 2 diabetes. In addition to therapeutic lifestyle changes, which should be recommended to all patients, some will benefit from strategies to reduce cardiovascular disease, while other individuals will need assistance in improving insulin resistance to reduce the risk of developing diabetes.

7.4.1. Case 1: A Patient with the Metabolic Syndrome and Atherogenic Dyslipidemia

A 56-year-old Mexican-American female presents for routine follow-up. Her past medical history is unremarkable. Her mother had a myocardial infarction at age 51 years, and one of her sisters has had a three-vessel coronary artery bypass graft. The patient is on no medications. The patient has no scheduled exercise program, but says she is "on her feet all day" at work.

Physical examination is remarkable for a well-developed woman with a blood pressure of 110/78 mmHg. Her BMI is 29 with a waist circumference of 88 cm. *Acanthosis nigricans* is present on the back of the neck. The remainder of the physical examination is unremarkable.

Lab findings include a fasting blood glucose of 92 mg/dL and a 2 h glucose value following a 75 g glucose load of 130 mg/dL. Fasting lipid profile revealed an LDL-C of 95 mg/dL, HDL-C of 41 mg/dL, and triglycerides of 190 mg/dL. A high sensitivity CRP level was elevated at 3.5. A CBC, UA, SMA-20, and thyroid function tests were normal. A baseline ECG was unremarkable.

7.4.1.1. CASE 1 DISCUSSION

This patient meets the IDF criteria for the metabolic syndrome based on her elevated waist circumference, low level of HDL-cholesterol, and elevated fasting triglyceride level. Her strong family history of cardiovascular disease underscores the importance of addressing her central obesity and "atherogenic dyslipidemia."

The lipoprotein profile characteristic of the metabolic syndrome is termed "atherogenic dyslipidemia." Atherogenic dyslipidemia is defined by the triad of high triglyceride levels (TG), low levels of high-density lipoprotein cholesterol (HDL-C), and the presence of small, dense low-density lipoprotein (LDL) particles. The atherogenic lipid profile is strongly associated with insulin resistance and typically precedes the diagnosis of type 2 diabetes *(89, 90)*. The pathogenesis of "atherogenic dyslipidemia" is outlined in Fig. 2.

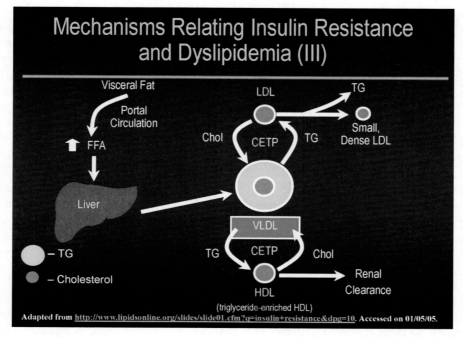

Fig. 2. Relationship between visceral fat and the development of "atherogenic dyslipidemia" characterized by (1) an increase in small, dense LDL particles, (2) elevated levels of VLDL triglycerides, and (3) low levels of HDL-cholesterol. Adapted from http://www.lipidsonline.org/slides/slide01.cfm?q=insulin+resistance&dpg=10. Accessed on 01/05/05.

7.4.1.1.1. Elevated Triglyceride Levels.   Insulin resistance or excessive visceral abdominal tissue (VAT) results in increased lipolysis and augmented fatty acid flux to the liver. In the liver, fatty acids are re-esterified into TGs and incorporated into very low-density lipoproteins (VLDL) *(90)*. The result is an increase in VLDL production and hypertriglyceridemia *(91, 92)*. VLDL particles are removed from the circulation by several high-affinity receptors that recognize its surface apoproteins (apo) B, C, and E. Glycosylation of these proteins may reduce their affinity for hepatic receptor-mediated clearance and increase their uptake by vascular macrophages *(93, 94)*. Therefore, central obesity and insulin resistance lead to elevated triglyceride as a result of both an overproduction and reduced catabolism of TG-rich VLDL.

7.4.1.1.2. Low Levels of HDL-Cholesterol.   HDL promotes the primary mechanism of lipid efflux from peripheral tissues ("reverse cholesterol transport"), has anti-inflammatory properties, and blocks LDL uptake by macrophages *(95, 96)*. HDL-cholesterol levels are lowered in patients with the metabolic syndrome as a result of elevated cholesterol ester transfer protein (CETP) activity, which enriches HDL particles with TG and apo E (Fig. 2). More apo E molecules per particle may promote greater HDL catabolism through receptor-mediated clearance. In addition, removal of cholesterol from the HDL particle results in an increase in small, lipid-poor HDL particles. Apo A-1, the primary apoprotein of HDL, appears to dissociate more easily from the smaller HDL species; free apo A-1 is then filtered in the kidney *(91)*. Apo A-1 deficiency subsequently leads to a decrease in new HDL production.

7.4.1.1.3. Small, Dense LDL Particles.   LDL particles are an end product of VLDL metabolism. While the LDL concentration is not elevated in individuals with the metabolic syndrome, there is a qualitative difference seen related to particle size and density. Elevated VLDL and TG levels stimulate CETP activity, transferring TG from VLDL to LDL particles (Fig. 2). Subsequent exposure to lipases further depletes LDL-TG, leaving a population of smaller, denser, and cholesterol-rich particles. This LDL subclass has a reduced affinity for the LDL receptor on the surface of hepatocytes, resulting in reduced clearance from plasma. If the patient develops diabetes, glycosylation of apo B in LDL particles may also diminish their affinity for the LDL receptor *(97)*. This leads to a greater opportunity for LDL oxidation by free radicals, preferential uptake by the scavenger receptors on tissue macrophages, and increased foam cell formation. The atherogenic potential of small, dense LDL particles may also derive from their greater ease of penetration into blood vessel walls.

The atherogenic triad has also been associated with a prothrombotic state *(98)*. The lipid abnormalities, together with hyperinsulinemia, are thought to induce plasminogen activator inhibitor expression, reduce endothelial cell tissue plasminogen activator production, promote platelet aggregation, elevate serum levels of factor VII, and increase blood and plasma viscosity *(99, 100)*. In a similar manner, a proinflammatory state, as identified by increased levels of the inflammatory marker C-reactive protein (CRP), has been linked with an increase in the number of CHD events in men and women *(101, 102)*. Patients with newly diagnosed diabetes have almost a 2-fold increased risk of having elevated CRP levels, compared with patients without diabetes *(103)*. The frequent concurrence of many suspected individual cardiovascular risk factors makes it difficult to identify any one of them as a truly independent predictor of CHD. However, it is clear that the presence of these features increases the risk for CHD at any level of LDL-C.

7.4.1.1.4. Lipid Goals for Patients with the Metabolic Syndrome.   Beginning in 1988, the National Cholesterol Education Program (NCEP) has issued several consensus reports addressing clinical management of high blood cholesterol levels based on the emergence of scientific information *(104–106)*. Each successive report has recommended progressively stricter lipid goals and indications for treatment that are directly related to an individual's degree of CHD risk. The highest risk is assigned to patients with clinically established CHD or other evidence of atherosclerosis. High LDL-C is the primary therapeutic target due to the significant cardiovascular benefits associated with LDL-C lowering demonstrated in primary and secondary prevention trials with statins. For patients in the high-risk category, the treatment goal for LDL-C lowering is <100 mg/dL *(106)*. The most recent guidelines state that the target for patients at *very high risk* may be lowered to 70 mg/dL. Patients considered to be at very high risk include patients with established cardiovascular disease *plus* other risk factors that include diabetes, the metabolic syndrome, or history of an acute coronary syndrome. The NCEP panel emphasized that the LDL target of <70 mg/dL does not apply to individuals who are not at very high risk. Once the LDL-C goal is achieved, however, many patients will still have persistent abnormalities of TGs and HDL-C.

Elevated TGs and low HDL-C levels are most often found together but may occur independently. Hypertriglyceridemia is a secondary target for lipid management. Serum TG values of >200 mg/dL may increase an individual's risk for CHD events substantially above that predicted by LDL-C values alone *(88)*. Some recommend lipid-lowering therapy targeted at correcting the serum level of non-HDL-C (total serum cholesterol minus HDL-C), representing the cholesterol carried by VLDL, intermediate-density lipoprotein (IDL), LDL, and Lp(a). All of these particles contain apo B lipoprotein and are atherogenic. Target non-HDL-C levels are 30 mg/dL above the LDL-C value goal *(104)*.

Low HDL-C is the most consistent predictor of CHD events in type 2 diabetics *(107)*. The most recent American Heart Association guidelines for cardiovascular disease prevention suggests a target HDL of >40 mg/dL in men and a level of >50 mg/dL in women *(108)*. NCEP ATP III states that there is insufficient clinical trial data to suggest a specific HDL target *(106)*.

The cornerstone of therapy for any patient with central obesity is therapeutic lifestyle changes (TLC). The ATP guidelines *(106)* make several dietary recommendations including

1. Reduced intakes of saturated fats (<7% of total calories) and cholesterol (<200 mg/day) Table 5. At all stages of dietary therapy, physicians are encouraged to refer patients to registered dietitians or other qualified nutritionists
2. Therapeutic options for enhancing LDL lowering such as plant sterols (2 g/day) and increased viscous (soluble) fiber (10–25 g/day)
3. Weight reduction, and
4. Increased physical activity

Finally, it should be stressed that the primary goal of TLC is to reduce abdominal obesity. In the centrally obese individual, weight loss alone may not reflect favorable changes in body composition. Figure 3 illustrates the response of a centrally obese man after a 1-year lifestyle modification program

Table 5
Nutrient Composition of the TLC Diet

Nutrient recommended intake
Saturated fat less than 7% of total calories
Polyunsaturated fat up to 10% of total calories
Monounsaturated fat up to 20% of total calories
Total fat 25–35% of total calories
Carbohydrate 50–60% of total calories
Fiber 20–30 g/day
Protein approximately 15% of total calories
Cholesterol less than 200 mg/day
Total calories (energy) Balance energy intake and expenditure to maintain desirable body weight/prevent weight gain

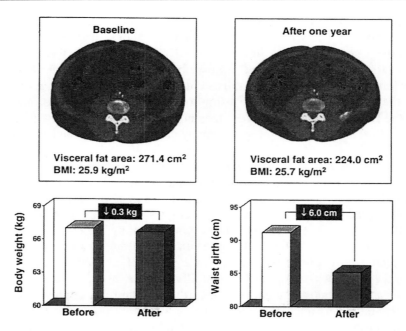

Fig. 3. Illustration of the response of a viscerally obese man involved in a 1-year lifestyle modification program at the Quebec Heart Institute. Despite the fact that this patient lost only 0.3 kg, he has reduced his waist girth by 6 cm as well as reduced his visceral adipose tissue by 17.5%. These findings emphasize the critical importance of assessing changes in waist circumference in addition to body weight.

at the Quebec Heart Institute *(109)*. The patient lost a modest 0.3 kg but reduced his waist girth by 6 cm. His documented 17.5% loss of visceral adipose tissue underscores the importance of following waist circumference along with weight loss in these individuals.

7.4.1.1.5. Pharmacologic Therapy.   The various classes of drugs used in the treatment of adult dyslipidemia provide a range of lipid alterations (Table 6) *(106)*. Clinical trials have established the value of these agents as monotherapy and in combination.

Table 6
Drugs for the Treatment of Adult Dyslipidemia *(106)*

Drug class	Lipid/lipoprotein	Effects
HMG CoA reductase	LDL-C	−18–55%
Inhibitors (statins)	HDL-C	+5–15%
	TG	−7–30%
Bile acid sequestrants	LDL-C	−15–30%
	HDL-C	+3–5%
	TG	No change or increase
Niacin	LDL-C	−5–25%
	HDH-C	+15–35%
	TG	−20–50%
Fibric acids	LDL-C	−5–20%[a]
	HDL-C	+10–20%
	TG	−20–50%

[a]Levels may rise in patients with hypertriglyceridemia.

STATINS. LDL-cholesterol is the initial target of therapy in a patient with the metabolic syndrome and atherogenic dyslipidemia. Statins (3-hydroxy-3-methylglutaryl co-enzyme A reductase inhibitors), the most powerful LDL-C-lowering class should be the initial treatment option. In both primary and secondary prevention trials, statin therapy has shown consistent reductions in cardiovascular events in patients with LDL-cholesterol levels between 100 and 200 mg/dL.

The Heart Protection Study randomized more than 20,000 patients considered to be at clinical risk of experiencing a new CHD event by virtue of prior CHD, other atherosclerotic disease, or diabetes *(110)*. This high-risk population included 5,963 men and women with diabetes, including 2,912 with no prior evidence of vascular disease *(111)*. After an average follow-up of 5 years, there was a 24% relative risk reduction in major vascular events (CHD death, myocardial infarction, stroke, or revascularization) with simvastatin treatment ($p < 0.0001$) in the total population. Notably, individuals with baseline LDL-cholesterol levels less than 100 mg/dL derived the same 24% reduction in major vascular events as patients with baseline LDL-cholesterol levels greater than 130 mg/dL. Based on the consistent reduction in CHD risk and the safety of statins demonstrated in these randomized clinical trials, it is recommended that all patients at high risk for cardiovascular disease be placed on statin therapy independent of LDL-C level.

Two large studies, the Treatment to New Targets Study (TNT) and the Incremental Decrease in End Points Through Aggressive Lipid Lowering (IDEAL) trial, assessed the possible benefit of further lowering LDL-C levels to 70 mg/dL or less in patients who are already at their LDL-C goal of less than 100 mg/dL on statin therapy. The TNT study *(112)* compared the effect of atorvastatin 80 mg daily to atorvastatin 10 mg daily in over 10,000 individuals with known cardiovascular disease. Baseline LDL-C in both groups was about 155 mg/dL. The mean on treatment LDL-C was 77 mg/dL in the atorvastatin 80 mg daily group compared to 101 mg/dL in the atorvastatin 10 mg daily group.

The reduction in LDL-cholesterol in this study had no impact on total mortality. The 22% reduction in cardiovascular events seen with the high-dose statin therapy was offset by a similar increase in noncardiovascular deaths. In addition, high-dose statin therapy was associated with more drug-related adverse events (8.1% versus 5.8%). Of most concern were the 60 cases of transaminase elevations above three times the upper limit of normal with atorvastatin 80 mg daily compared to the nine cases seen with atorvastatin 10 mg daily.

The IDEAL trial *(113)* compared therapy with simvastatin 20–40 mg daily to atorvastatin 80 mg daily in 8,882 patients with known coronary artery disease. As was the case in the TNT trial, there was no difference in total mortality between patients treated to an LDL-C target below 100 mg/dL. Surprisingly, there was no statistically significant reduction in the primary end point of cardiovascular events with more aggressive LDL lowering in this large, well-designed clinical trial.

Since our patient does not have documented cardiovascular disease and her baseline LDL-cholesterol is less than 100 mg/dL, the current NCEP ATP guidelines leave the decision to initiate statin therapy to discretion of the clinician *(106)*. However, these guidelines were made before the publication of the JUPITER trial *(114)*. The JUPITER trial randomly assigned 17,802 individuals without known cardiovascular disease with LDL-cholesterol levels less than 130 mg/dL and high-sensitivity C-reactive protein levels of 2.0 mg/dL or higher to rosuvastatin 20 mg daily or placebo. Rosuvastatin therapy was associated with a 50% reduction of LDL-cholesterol and a 37% reduction of C-reactive protein. After a median follow-up of 2 years there was a 46% reduction in major cardiovascular events and a 25% reduction in total mortality. Previous statin trials have reported a 20% reduction in cardiovascular risk over a 5-year period for each 40 mg/dL absolute reduction in LDL-cholesterol *(115, 116)*. This effect would have predicted only a 25% reduction in cardiovascular events. The observed reduction in cardiovascular events was almost twice the predicted benefit and was seen in half the time of the previous trials. The possible independent role played by lowering inflammation as reflected by the 37% reduction in CRP levels cannot be assessed by this study alone. However, the fact that the reduction in cardiovascular events was much greater than predicted and occurred sooner than seen in other statin trials suggests reducing inflammation may have played a significant role.

INTERVENTION. Our patient was placed on rosuvastatin 20 mg daily. At follow-up 3 months later, LDL-cholesterol was 52 mg/dL, HDL-cholesterol was 42 mg/dL, and triglyceride levels were 170 mg/dL.

7.4.1.1.6. Combination Therapy.

Statins primarily target LDL-C abnormalities. Because our patient presented with abnormal triglyceride and HDL-C levels, it may be beneficial to add an agent to address these lipid abnormalities. Fibric acid derivatives and niacin preparations address these abnormalities characteristic of "atherogenic dyslipidemia."

FIBRATES. The fibric acid derivatives include gemfibrozil, fenofibrate, and bezafibrate. Fibrates effectively reduce TG levels *(104, 105)* and have modest effects on LDL-C and HDL-C levels. The Helsinki Heart Study evaluated the effect of gemfibrozil in 4,081 hyperlipidemic men without prior evidence of CHD *(117)*. Treatment with gemfibrozil reduced TG levels by 26% and LDL-C levels by 10% and raised HDL-C levels by 6% from baseline. After 5 years, the rate of non-fatal myocardial infarction or CHD-related death was significantly reduced by gemfibrozil treatment.

The Veterans Administration HDL Intervention Trial (VA-HIT) enrolled 2,531 men with known CHD, low HDL-C levels, and normal LDL-C levels, including 1,092 with diabetes or impaired fasting glucose *(118)*. Treatment with gemfibrozil reduced TG levels by 31% and LDL-C levels by 2% and raised HDL-C levels by 6% from baseline. In the total population, major coronary events were reduced 22% more with gemfibrozil treatment than with placebo over a 5-year period *(119)*. The benefit tended to be greater in patients with diabetes than in those without diabetes (35% versus 18%; $p = 0.07$).

The Diabetes Atherosclerosis Intervention Study (DAIS) evaluated the coronary angiographic effects of fenofibrate treatment in 418 patients with type 2 diabetes and documented CHD *(120)*. Mean values for lipids at baseline were typical of diabetes, with LDL-C levels of 130 mg/dL, HDL-C levels of 39 mg/dL, and TG levels of 229 mg/dL. Treatment with fenofibrate reduced TG levels by 28% and LDL-C levels by 6% and raised HDL-C levels by 7% from baseline. After 3 years, the rate of atherosclerotic stenoses progression was less with fenofibrate than placebo (2.10% versus 3.65%; $p = 0.02$). Although the trial was not powered to assess clinical outcomes, there were fewer coronary events in the fenofibrate group than in the placebo group (38 versus 50) *(120)*.

The Fenofibrate Intervention and Event Lowering in Diabetes (FIELD) study *(121)* was designed to assess the effect of fenofibrate on cardiovascular disease in patients with diabetes both with and without known heart disease. Patients with type 2 diabetes between 50 and 75 years of age were randomized to treatment with fenofibrate 200 mg daily versus placebo. A total of 9,795 patients from 63 centers in Australia, New Zealand, and Finland were studied for 5 years making this by far the largest study ever completed in a diabetic population. The baseline lipid levels on no lipid altering medication included a mean LDL-cholesterol of 118 mg/dL (5.03 mmol/L), an HDL-cholesterol of 42.6 mg/dL (1.1 mmol/L), and a triglyceride level was 153.3 mg/dL (1.7 mmol/L) in both groups. The primary end point was the first occurrence of either a non-fatal myocardial infarction or death from coronary heart disease.

At the end of the trial a non-significant 11% reduction ($p = 0.16$) in the primary outcome of first myocardial infarction or coronary heart death was seen in the treatment group. This corresponded to a 24% reduction in non-fatal myocardial infarction in fenofibrate-treated patients ($p = 0.01$) and a 19% increase in coronary disease mortality ($p = 0.22$). A post hoc subgroup analysis showed a significant reduction in events in patients without previous cardiovascular events but no benefit in patients with known preexisting cardiovascular disease.

The non-significant 11% decrease in the primary end point of coronary events in diabetics treated with fenofibrate was surprising and the non-significant 11% increase in overall mortality is disturbing. Prior to the FIELD study, the Veterans Affairs High-Density Lipoprotein Intervention Trial (VA-HIT) provided the largest sample of diabetic patients treated with a fibric acid derivative *(118, 119)*. In

VA-HIT, 769 diabetics with known heart disease were randomized to either placebo or gemfibrozil 1,200 mg daily for 5 years. Baseline LDL-cholesterol and triglyceride levels were similar to those seen in the FIELD trial while HDL-cholesterol levels were significantly lower at 31 mg/dL. In the VA-HIT trial, diabetics treated with gemfibrozil had a 32% reduction in cardiovascular events ($p = 0.004$). The event reduction was due to a 22% reduction in myocardial infarction and a 41% reduction in cardiovascular death.

The reason(s) for the disappointing effect seen with fenofibrate in the FIELD study are unknown. The authors point out a greater use of statin therapy in patients allocated to the placebo group than in those on fenofibrate. While no patients were on statin therapy at the start of the study, statin therapy could be added during the study at the discretion of the patient's physician. In patients with known heart disease, 23% of placebo-allocated and 14% of fenofibrate-allocated patients received statins. In the primary prevention patients the corresponding numbers are 16% placebo treated and 7% fenofibrate treated. Since the vast majority of patients in this study did not receive statins, the "drop-in" statin effect can only be a partial explanation. If patients who were started on statin therapy in both groups were not included in the analysis, the benefit of fenofibrate was a non-significant 14% reduction in primary events ($p = 0.10$).

In my view, the most likely explanation for the disappointing effect of fenofibrate on cardiovascular event reduction in the FIELD trial was the lack of treatment effect on HDL-cholesterol levels. After 4 months of treatment HDL-cholesterol levels had increased 5% in patients randomized to therapy with fenofibrate. The initial increase in HDL-cholesterol seen in this study is similar to that seen in the VA-HIT trial *(118)*. In the VA-HIT study, diabetic patients' HDL-cholesterol levels increased 5% compared to the 8% increase in non-diabetic individuals and the 5% increase in HDL was maintained throughout the entire 5-year study. However, in the FIELD trial the initial increase in HDL-cholesterol was not sustained. By study close, the increase in HDL-cholesterol was only 1%. In the FIELD study the LDL-cholesterol level was reduced by 12% and triglyceride levels were 29% lower after 4 months of treatment. The reductions in LDL-cholesterol and triglycerides were maintained throughout the study. Thus the attenuation of effect on HDL-raising with fenofibrate is not likely due to a decrease in compliance with taking the medication as the lipid effects on LDL-cholesterol and triglycerides were maintained.

Analysis of the lipid values from the VA-HIT study demonstrated that baseline HDL and triglyceride levels were significant predictors of cardiovascular events; whereas, during the trial, only concentrations of HDL-cholesterol significantly predicted a reduction in cardiovascular end points *(122)*. Change in triglyceride levels was not predictive of a reduction in cardiovascular risk with gemfibrozil therapy. Similarly, the 29% reduction in triglyceride levels with fenofibrate therapy did not result in a significant reduction in the primary end point of non-fatal myocardial infarction or coronary death in the FIELD trial.

Although no clinical outcome trials of statin–fibrate treatment have been reported, combination therapy has been shown to be very effective in lowering TG and LDL-C levels in diabetic patients in small clinical studies. After 6 months, the combination of atorvastatin 20 mg and fenofibrate 200 mg/day reduced TG levels by 50% and LDL-C levels by 46% from baseline *(123)*. After 1 year, treatment with simvastatin 20 mg and bezafibrate 400 mg/day reduced TG levels by 42% and LDL-C levels by 29% *(124)*. HDL-C levels were increased by 21% with atorvastatin and fenofibrate and by 25% with simvastatin and bezafibrate *(123, 124)*.

Fibrate therapy is generally safe and well tolerated *(104, 105)*. Gastrointestinal symptoms are the most frequent adverse events reported. Fibrates are also associated with a small risk of myopathy (<0.1%) *(125)*. Use of statin–fibrate therapy has raised concern following reports in the literature of fatal rhabdomyolysis, especially with cerivastatin and gemfibrozil *(126, 127)*. More recent analyses show that statin–fibrate use is generally safe; in controlled clinical trials, including nearly 600 patients treated with this combination, only 1% of patients were withdrawn because of myalgias

(104, 105). Fenofibrate appears to be associated with a lower risk of myopathy than gemfibrozil, when used in combination with a statin. The Action to Control Cardiovascular Risk in Diabetes (ACCORD) trial will assess the potential additional benefit of adding fenofibrate to existing statin therapy *(128)*.

NIACIN. Niacin is the most effective pharmacologic agent currently available for increasing HDL-C levels *(105)*. In the Arbiter 3 trial *(129)*, 1,000 mg of Niaspan daily increased HDL by 25% after 24 months of therapy. The maximal effect of Niaspan to raise HDL-C may not be seen for 18 months.

Clinically, niacin's ability to decrease cardiovascular events was shown in the Coronary Drug Project, where CHD patients with hypercholesterolemia experienced a 27% relative reduction in non-fatal myocardial infarction rates and an 11% reduction in long-term mortality *(130, 131)*. Canner et al. published a post hoc analysis of these results based on the patient's baseline fasting and 1 h blood glucose levels *(132)*. Not surprisingly, niacin reduced non-fatal myocardial infarction and total mortality to a similar extent across all baseline glucose levels, even in patients with fasting blood glucose ≥ 126 mg/dL. Other trials of niacin in combination with LDL-C-lowering drugs have demonstrated significant regression of coronary stenoses and reductions in clinical events in patients with hypercholesterolemia *(133–135)*.

Statins and niacin have complementary actions on the atherogenic lipid profile. The HDL-Atherosclerosis Treatment Study (HATS), which enrolled 160 patients with CHD, included 34 patients with diabetes or impaired fasting glucose levels *(136)*. Substantial improvements were seen in this subgroup; simvastatin–niacin treatment was associated with a 31% decrease in LDL-C levels, a 40% decrease in TG levels, and a 30% increase in HDL-C levels, while placebo or antioxidant treatments alone had little effect *(136)*. After 3 years, average coronary stenosis progressed by 1.1% in patients taking simvastatin–niacin versus 4.8% in those not taking this combination ($p < 0.05$). The composite cardiovascular end point (CHD death, myocardial infarction, stroke, or revascularization) occurred in 11% of simvastatin–niacin-treated patients compared with 21% of those not taking simvastatin–niacin (RRR = 48%; P = NS), suggesting that substantial reductions in risk may be achieved with combination therapy. Smaller studies have shown that statin–niacin combinations also increase LDL particle size and the antiatherogenic HDL_2 subclass to a greater extent than statin monotherapy in patients with diabetes *(137, 138)*.

In the past, niacin has been considered to be relatively contraindicated in individuals with the metabolic syndrome due to concern that the modest hyperglycemic response to niacin may cause the individual to become diabetic. The hyperglycemic response to niacin is felt to be due to a secondary rebound in circulating oxidized-free fatty acids, leading to reduced insulin-stimulated glucose uptake and increased hepatic glucose output *(139)*. The Arterial Disease Multiple Interventions Trial (ADMIT) evaluated niacin therapy in 125 participants with diabetes and vascular disease for a period of 1 year. Niacin (average dose, 2.5 g/day) increased glucose levels by 8.1 mg/dL in the diabetic patients compared with an increase of 6.3 mg/dL in the non-diabetic patients, and A1C concentrations were not significantly changed from baseline *(140)*. Similarly, the Assessment of Diabetes Control and Evaluation of the Efficacy of Niaspan Trial (ADVENT) randomized 148 type 2 diabetic patients to placebo or extended-release niacin (niacin ER). Dose-dependent increases in HDL-C and decreases in TG occurred with niacin ER 1,000 and 1,500 mg, and these changes were accompanied by negligible increases in A1C *(141)*. In HATS, the combination of simvastatin and niacin was associated with small increases in fasting blood glucose during the first few months, which subsequently returned to baseline levels for the remainder of the study in the subgroup of patients with diabetes *(142)*.

Based on this accumulating evidence, the American Diabetes Association recommends that niacin ≤ 2 g/day can be used safely in diabetic patients with frequent glucose monitoring and adjustment of antidiabetic medication as necessary *(143)*.

INTERVENTION. Our patient was started on 500 mg of Niaspan daily. She was advised to take a 325 mg aspirin tablet with the Niaspan to reduce flushing. After 1 month at this dose, the Niaspan was increased to 1,000 mg daily. After 3 months of combined rosuvastatin and Niaspan therapy the patient's LDL-cholesterol was 54 mg/dL, her triglyceride levels were 118 mg/dL, and her HDL-C was 48 mg/dL.

7.4.2. Case 2: A Patient with the Metabolic Syndrome and Impaired Fasting Glucose

A 39-year-old African-American female presents for evaluation of abnormal glucose tolerance. She denies polyuria, polydipsia, or recent weight change. Her 41-year-old sister has been recently diagnosed with diabetes, which also afflicts her mother and maternal grandmother. Present medications include a diuretic, ACE-inhibitor, and beta blocker for hypertension. Physical exam is significant for central obesity and well-controlled hypertension. A fasting lipid panel is normal with an LDL-C of 85 mg/dL, HDL-C of 60 mg/dL, and TGs of 130 mg/dL. Her fasting glucose is 112 mg/dL. The patient requests therapy to prevent diabetes.

Our patient meets the criteria for metabolic syndrome based on the presence of central obesity, treated hypertension, and abnormal glucose. While my main concern for our first patient was to prevent cardiovascular disease, this patient's metabolic profile dramatically increases her risk of developing diabetes. The pattern of metabolic syndrome is quite common in the African-American population.

A mismatch between the patterns of nutrient intake and physical activity is responsible for the epidemic of obesity and diabetes seen in modern industrialized societies *(144)*. In addition to the diet changes outlined in our first case, this patient is free of cardiovascular disease and should be encouraged to begin a vigorous exercise program. The major component of physical fitness that has been related to the primary prevention of diabetes is aerobic exercise. A total of 5,990 male University of Pennsylvania alumni aged 39–68 years at baseline were followed an average of 14 years *(145)*. A total of 202 cases of diabetes occurred during 98,524 man-years of observation. After adjustment for age, body mass index (BMI), hypertension, and parental history of diabetes, the investigators observed a 6% lower risk of diabetes for each 50 kcal/week of self-reported leisure-time physical activity ($p - 0.01$).

As part of the Nurses' Health Study, 87,253 US female nurses aged 34–59 years were followed an average of 8 years, during which time 1,303 were diagnosed with diabetes *(146)*. Women who reported vigorous exercise at least once per week had a 33% lower age-adjusted risk of developing diabetes compared with women reporting no exercise ($p - 0.0001$). Similarly, an inverse relationship was seen between self-reported physical exercise and diabetes risk in 21,271 US male physicians aged 40–84 years were followed through 105,141 man-years, during which 285 developed diabetes *(147)*.

Significant graded inverse associations were consistently observed between levels of self-reported physical activity and incident diabetes over long follow-up periods in established cohorts of men in the British Regional Heart Study *(148)*; men and women in the Study of Eastern Finns *(149)*; and women in the Iowa Women's Health Study *(150)*, Nurses' Health Study *(151, 152)*, Women's Health Study *(153)*, and Women's Health Initiative Observational Study *(154)*. Each of the existing prospective studies of baseline fitness exposures and incident diabetes has shown that higher levels of fitness protect against the development of diabetes in women and men *(155–157)*.

Lynch et al. *(156)* followed 897 Finnish men aged 42–60 for 4 years during which time 46 cases of diabetes were identified with a 2-h postchallenge glucose level. Cardiorespiratory fitness was measured at baseline with ventilatory gas analysis during a maximal bicycle ergometry test. After adjusting for several confounders including age, BMI, and baseline glucose levels, odds ratios [95% confidence interval (CI)] for incident diabetes were 1.0 (referent), 0.77 (0.32–1.85), 0.26 (0.08–0.82), and 0.15 (0.03–0.79) in men in the first, second, third, and fourth quartile of fitness, respectively. Aerobics Center Longitudinal Study (ACLS) *(157)* followed 7,442 men aged 30–79 years with normal glucose metabolism who had two clinical examinations an average of 6 years apart. An inverse relationship between cardiovascular fitness and the development of both impaired fasting glucose and diabetes was demonstrated.

The rate of progression to diabetes over a 6-year period was assessed in four groups of Chinese patients with impaired glucose tolerance *(158)*. The interventions were control, diet, exercise, or diet plus exercise. Diet alone reduced risk by 31%. Exercise alone was even more effective, reducing risk 46%. The combination of diet plus exercise (42% reduction) was no better than exercise alone.

Two large randomized controlled studies conducted in Finland and the United States examined the effect of a comprehensive lifestyle intervention on the progression to diabetes in high-risk women and men with impaired glycemic control *(159, 160)*. In both studies, the lifestyle intervention included regular physical activity ($\geq$150 min/week of moderate to vigorous intensity activities), modest weight loss ($\geq$7% of baseline weight was targeted), reduction in fat intake, and increase in whole grains, fruits, and vegetables. Results of the studies were remarkably similar. During a mean follow-up of 3–4 years, the risk of developing diabetes was $\geq$60% lower for those in the lifestyle intervention compared with those in the control group. In the Finnish trial, study participants who met the intervention target of $\geq$4 h of moderate intensity activity/week, but who did not meet the weight loss goal, had a 70% lower risk of developing diabetes than those in the control arm ($p \geq 5$) *(160, 161)*. Therefore, regular exercise is able to prevent diabetes in the absence of weight loss.

INTERVENTION. Our patient was advised that she had impaired glucose tolerance and the metabolic syndrome. She was told that this information in addition to her strong family history of diabetes put her at great risk of developing diabetes in the future. She was given a heart healthy diet and asked to do a minimum of 30 min of aerobic exercise 5 days a week. She was also advised to do an additional 30 min of core training a minimum of 3 days each week.

7.4.2.1. PHARMACOLOGIC INTERVENTIONS FOR DIABETES PREVENTION

The STOP NIDDM trial evaluated the effect of the glucosidase inhibitor acarbose to prevent the development of diabetes in subjects with impaired glucose tolerance *(162)*. Individuals taking acarbose were 25% less likely to develop diabetes than placebo-treated subjects. The Diabetes Prevention Program compared the effect of metformin versus lifestyle changes in the prevention of diabetes *(163)*. After an average follow-up of 2.8 years, lifestyle changes were about twice as effective at preventing diabetes as metformin.

Several studies have examined the efficacy of thiazolidinediones to prevent diabetes. The TRIPOD study compared the effect of troglitazone 400 mg daily to placebo to prevent the development of diabetes in young women with a history of gestational diabetes *(164)*. Therapy with troglitazone reduced the risk of developing diabetes over a 4-year period about 60%. The DREAM study followed 5,269 people with impaired fasting glucose (IFG) and/or impaired glucose tolerance (IGT) from 191 clinical centers in 21 countries *(165)*. It was reported that 58% had isolated IGT, 14% had isolated IFG, and 28% had both. At study entry none of the patients had any prior evidence of cardiovascular disease (CVD). Patients were randomized to treatment with rosiglitazone or placebo and were followed for a median of 3 years (range 2.5–4.7 years) to determine the effect of drug intervention on the incidence of diabetes. There was a substantial reduction in the incidence of diabetes in the rosiglitazone-treated patients (HR 0.38, 95% CI 0.33–0.44, $p < 0.0001$). In addition, rosiglitazone treatment was associated with a 71% increase in the number of patients returning to normal glucose levels during the study: 1,330 (50.5%) individuals in the rosiglitazone-treated group became normoglycemic (FPG <6.1 mmol/L) compared with 798 (30.3%) of those given placebo (HR 1.71, 95% CI 1.57–1.87, $p < 0001$). Although the DREAM study was not statistically powered to detect a significant difference in cardiovascular (CV) event rates, more participants assigned to rosiglitazone than to placebo met the criteria for a composite CV end point (log HR 1.37, 95% CI 0.97–1.94, $p = 0.08$). In particular, more people treated with rosiglitazone developed congestive heart failure: 14 (0.5%) versus 2 (0.1%),

$p = 0.01$. ACTos NOW for the Prevention of Diabetes (ACT NOW) enrolled 602 individuals with impaired glucose tolerance, a prediabetic state, along with 102 healthy controls *(166)*. After randomization to pioglitazone 45 gm daily or placebo, patients were followed for 2 years. An 81% reduction in the incidence of diabetes was seen in individuals treated with pioglitazone.

INTERVENTION.   No pharmacologic intervention was recommended to our patient at this time.

7.4.3. Case 3: A Patient with Polycystic Ovary Syndrome

A 23-year-old female presents with a chief complaint of hirsutism and weight gain. She has noted excessive hair growth on her face, chest, and abdomen over the last 2 years. She has a documented weight gain of 20 kg between ages 17 and 18 years. She had pubarche at age 9 years but has never had regular menses. She has never had more than five periods in a year. She has had unprotected intercourse with her husband for the past 2 years and has not become pregnant.

Family history is significant for early onset of pubarche, irregular menses, and hirsutism in her mother and two older sisters. Her 50-year-old mother had diabetes since age 40 years. The patient denies breast discharge, change in ring or shoe size, use of steroids, or deepening of voice.

Physical exam is pertinent for the presence of A. *nigricans* and hyperpigmentation on the neck and groin. Terminal hair is present on the upper lip, chest, and abdomen. BP is 130/80 mmHg, BMI: 31, and waist circumference is 38 in.

Laboratory assessment shows free testosterone levels are 1.5 times the upper limit of normal. The LH:FSH ratio was greater than 2.0 on 2 determinations. Serum prolactin, DHEA-S, 17-OH progesterone, and a 24-h urine-free cortisol were normal. A fasting lipid profile showed an LDL-cholesterol of 110 mg/dL, triglycerides of 160 mg/dL and an HDL-cholesterol of 52 mg/dL. Fasting glucose is 106 mg/dL. Abdominal/pelvic ultrasound is significant for multiple cysts of the ovary.

A diagnosis of polycystic ovary syndrome is made based on the combination of oligomenorrhea, elevated levels of ovarian androgens, positive family history, multiple ovarian cysts, and exclusion of other hormonal disorders.

It is quite clear that PCOS has a variety of causes and may be inherited *(167–171)*. Disorders which affect the hypothalamic–pituitary–ovarian axis as well as genetic causes of insulin resistance may lead to a similar clinical picture. Dunaif and colleagues have shown defects in the insulin signaling pathways in both fat and skeletal muscle in patients with the polycystic ovarian syndrome *(172–174)*. Because insulin resistance and hyperinsulinemia play a central role in the development of the metabolic syndrome, the term "syndrome XX" has been suggested to describe this sex-specific metabolic syndrome *(105, 175)*. Obesity may cause or exacerbate PCOS. Up to 75% of women with PCOS in some series are obese *(176, 177)*. Polycystic ovary syndrome (PCOS) is present in 10% of reproductive age females making it the most common metabolic abnormality in young women *(178–180)*. A clinical diagnosis of PCOS can be made in a woman who has oligomenorrhea (fewer than nine menstrual cycles per year) or amenorrhea and elevated levels of ovarian androgens *(181)*. Patients will often present with cutaneous manifestations of androgen excess such as hirsutism, male pattern hair loss, or acne. Before a diagnosis of PCOS is made other causes of androgen excess such as congenital adrenal hyperplasia, adrenal or ovarian tumors producing androgens, hyperprolactinemia, or Cushing's syndrome should be ruled out.

The symptoms of PCOS usually begin around menarche *(182)* but may present several years after puberty, usually as a result of significant weight gain. Premature pubarche may predict future PCOS. About half of young girls with premature pubarche will develop ovarian hyperandrogenism *(183)*.

Women with PCOS are more efficient at making ovarian androgens than estrogen *(184, 185)*. Ovarian theca cells synthesize androstenedione which can be converted by 17 beta-hydroxysteroid dehydrogenase (17β-HSD) to testosterone in the theca cell or aromatized by the aromatase enzyme in the granulosa cell to form estrone (Fig. 4). Luteinizing hormone (LH) produced in pulsatile fashion by the anterior pituitary gland is responsible for theca cell androgen production while follicle stimulating

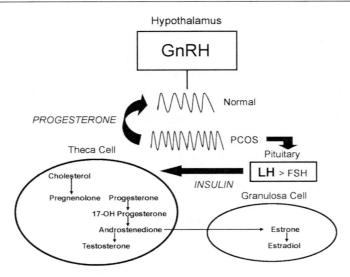

Fig. 4. Pathway of ovarian androgen and estrogen production. In PCOS an increase in the pulse frequency of GnRH increases LH production, which stimulates androgen production by the theca cells.

hormone (FSH) stimulates aromatase activity within the granulose cell and regulates the production of estrone. An increase in the production of LH in relation to FSH will result in preferential production of adrenal androgen.

The pulse frequency of the hypothalamic hormone gonadotropin-releasing hormone (GnRH) determines the relative proportion of LH and FSH release from the anterior pituitary. Increasing the pulse frequency of GnRH favors the production of LH while a slower frequency favors FSH production *(186)*. Since women with PCOS have an increased LH:FSH ratio, one of the causes of PCOS may be an increased pulse frequency of GnRH. This may be a primary defect or a result of low levels of progesterone in a woman with oligomenorrhea *(187)*.

Hyperinsulinemia, which results from insulin resistance, can cause or exacerbate PCOS. Insulin enhances the action of LH to stimulate the production of androgen by the theca cells. Insulin also inhibits the production of sex hormone binding globulin (SHBG), the main protein which binds testosterone. Since only unbound or "free" testosterone is active, a decrease in SHBG will increase the proportion of active testosterone.

Not surprisingly, the risk of cardiovascular disease and diabetes is increased in women with PCOS. A risk factor model analysis of 1,462 women in Sweden who underwent an assessment in a prospective population study estimated a 4- to 7-fold increase risk of myocardial infarction in women with PCOS compared with age-matched controls and 6-fold increased risk of developing diabetes *(188)*. In a study from the Czech Republic *(189)*, 28 women with PCOS were compared with 752 control women matched for BMI, waist–hip ratio, hypertension, dyslipidemia, and smoking. Women with PCOS were more likely to be diabetic (32% versus 8%) and have diagnosed coronary artery disease (21% versus 5%) than control subjects. In Holland, 346 lean (BMI:24.4 kg/m^2) women with PCOS had an increased prevalence of hypertension, diabetes mellitus, and cardiac symptoms *(190)*. The Nurses' Health Study is a prospective study of 101,000 female nurses. Oligomenorrhea was associated with a 2- to 2.5-fold increased risk of developing diabetes *(191)*. A 14-year prospective surveillance of 82,439 nurses aged 20–35 years in this study showed a history of oligomenorrhea was associated with a 100% increase in fatal and a 50% increase in non-fatal coronary artery disease *(192)*. While androgen status was not measured in this study, it is likely that the majority of women in this study with oligomenorrhea would have met the criteria for PCOS.

Obesity is associated with reduced fertility. In the Nurses Health Study, infertility increases above a BMI 26 mg/m^2 *(193)*. In addition, fat distribution is even more important than BMI in determining fertility. Comparing women with a waist:hip ratio <0.8 and >0.8 who had artificial insemination, women with central obesity were less likely to become pregnant *(194)*. Eighty-seven Australian women with PCOS who desired fertility were placed on a gradual weight loss program emphasizing sensible eating and exercise. Twenty of the women dropped out but 90% of those who stayed in the study ovulated and 78% became pregnant *(195)*.

INTERVENTION. Our patient was placed on a hypocaloric diet designed to lead to a weight loss of 1 lb/week. She was advised to do aerobic exercise for 30–45 min 5 days/week and participates in resistance training for 30–45 min twice weekly.

7.4.3.1. PHARMACOLOGIC TREATMENT OF PCOS

A reduction in insulin levels will lower the production of ovarian androgens. Both metformin and the thiazolidinediones (pioglitazone and rosiglitazone) have been used to treat PCOS. Metformin directly inhibits the production of ovarian androgens *(196, 197)* and decreases the amount of insulin necessary to control glucose by inhibiting hepatic glucose production. A meta-analysis of 13 studies in which metformin was administered to 543 women showed women treated with metformin were 3.9 times more likely to ovulate compared *(198)* with placebo-treated patients. Similarly, a woman treated with a combination of metformin and clomiphene was 4.4 times more likely to ovulate compared to a woman given clomiphene alone. Women who conceive while taking metformin have a lower rate of miscarriage and gestational diabetes *(199–202)*. Because metformin is a category B drug for pregnancy it is not contraindicated during pregnancy, although it cannot be stated to be safe. Most experts recommend it be discontinued when the patient becomes pregnant. Some have advocated using metformin during the first 12 week of pregnancy in women who have a history of early pregnancy loss *(202)*.

The thiazolidinediones (TZDs) directly reduce ovarian steroid synthesis *(203)* and indirectly lower ovarian androgen synthesis by reducing levels of insulin. The TZDs are the most potent insulin sensitizers available and have a major impact on fat and muscle and improve insulin sensitivity at the liver to a lesser degree. In a double-blind, randomized, placebo controlled trial ovulation was significantly more frequent in women given troglitazone *(176)*. Levels of free testosterone decreased, and sex hormone binding globulin increased in a dose-dependent manner. Similar findings were seen with rosiglitazone *(204, 205)* and pioglitazone *(206)*. Thiazolidinediones are category C drugs for pregnancy.

The combination of metformin and a thiazolidinedione has also been evaluated for the treatment of polycystic ovarian syndrome. In a study of normal weight women with PCOS (BMI: 24 kg/m^2) *(207)* treated for 6 months with 850 mg of metformin twice daily versus 4 mg of rosiglitazone twice daily, versus both or neither, ovulatory cycles were more frequent with metformin. Testosterone improved with both therapies and there was no evidence of synergist effect.

INTERVENTION. After 3 months of diet therapy, the patient expressed a desire to become pregnant. Metformin was given as an initial dose of 500 mg po daily and titrated to 1,000 mg twice daily over 1 month. After 4 months of combined diet and metformin treatment, the patient became pregnant.

REFERENCES

1. Reaven GM. Banting lecture 1988. Role of insulin resistance in human disease. *Diabetes.* 1988;37:1595–1607.
2. Alberti KG, Zimmet PZ. Definition, diagnosis and classification of diabetes mellitus and its complications. Part 1: diagnosis and classification of diabetes mellitus provisional report of a WHO consultation. *Diabet Med.* 1998;15:539–553.
3. Third Report of the National Cholesterol Education Program (NCEP). Expert Panel on detection, evaluation, and treatment of high blood cholesterol in adults (Adult Treatment Panel III). Final report. *Circulation.* 2002;106:3143–3421.

4. Grundy SM, Cleeman JI, Daniels SR, et al. American Heart Association; National Heart, Lung, and Blood Institute. Diagnosis and management of the metabolic syndrome: an America Heart Association/National Heart, Lung, and Blood Institute Scientific Statement. *Circulation.* 2005;112:2735–2752.

5. Alberti KGMM, Zimmet P, Shaw J, et al. IDF Epidemiology Task Force Consensus Group. The metabolic syndrome—a new worldwide definition. *Lancet.* 2005;366:1059–1062.

6. Ogden CL, Carroll MD, Curtin LR, McDowell MA, Tabak CJ, Flegal KM. Prevalence of overweight and obesity in the United States, 1999–2004. *JAMA.* 2006;295:1549–1555.

7. Shields M, Tjepkema M. Trends in adults obesity. *Health Rep.* 2006;17:53–59.

8. Ford ES, Giles WH, Dietz WH. Prevalence of the MetS among US adults: findings from the third National Health and Nutrition Examination Survey. *JAMA.* 2002;287:356–359.

9. Vega GL, Adams-Huet B, Peshock R, Willett D, Shah B, Grundy SM. Influence of body fat content and distribution on variation in metabolic risk. *J Clin Endocrinol Metab.* 2006;91:4459–4466.

10. Egede LE, Dagogo-Jack S. Epidemiology of type 2 diabetes: focus on ethnic minorities. *Med Clin North Am.* 2005;89:949–975.

11. Carter JS, Pugh JA, Monterrosa A. Non-insulin-dependent diabetes mellitus in minorities in the United States. *Ann Intern Med.* 1996;125:221–232.

12. Haffner SM, Hazuda HP, Mitchell BD, Patterson JK, Stern MP. Increased incidence of type II diabetes mellitus in Mexican Americans. *Diabetes Care.* 1991;14:102–108.

13. Kaler SN, Ralph-Campbell K, Pohar S, King M, Laboucan CR, Toth EL. High rates of the metabolic syndrome in a First Nations Community in Western Canada: prevalence and determinants in adults and children. *Int J Circumpolar Health.* 2006;65:389–402.

14. Pollex RL, Hanley AJ, Zinman B, Harris SB, Khan HM, Hegele RA. Metabolic syndrome in aboriginal Canadians: prevalence and genetic associations. *Atherosclerosis.* 2006;184:121–129.

15. Dallongeville J, Cottel D, Ferrieres J, et al. Household income is associated with the risk of metabolic syndrome in a sex-specific manner. *Diabetes Care.* 2005;28:409–415.

16. Bataille V, Perret B, Dallongeville J, et al. Metabolic syndrome and coronary heart disease risk in a population-based study of middle-aged men from France and Northern Ireland. A nested case-control study from the PRIME cohort. *Diabetes Metab.* 2006;32(5 Pt 1):475–479.

17. Assmann G, Guerra R, Fox G, et al. Harmonizing the definition of the metabolic syndrome: comparison of the criteria of the Adult Treatment Panel III and the International Diabetes Federation in United Statues American and European populations. *Am J Cardiol.* 2007;99:541–548.

18. Dekker JM, Girman C, Rhodes T, et al. Metabolic syndrome and 10-year cardiovascular disease risk in the Hoorn Study. *Circulation.* 2005;112:666–673.

19. Bo S, Gentile L, Ciccone G, et al. The metabolic syndrome and high C-reactive protein: prevalence and differences by sex in a southern-European population-based cohort. *Diabetes Metab Res Rev.* 2005;21:515–524.

20. Bonora E, Kiechl S, Willeit J, et al. Metabolic syndrome: epidemiology and more extensive phenotypic description. Cross-sectional data from the Bruneck Study. *Int J Obes Relat Metab Disord.* 2003;27:1283–1289.

21. Miccoli R, Bianchi C, Odoguardi L, et al. Prevalence of the metabolic syndrome among Italian adults according to ATP III definition. *Nutr Metab Cardiovasc Dis.* 2044;15:250–254.

22. Maggi S, Noale M, Gallina P, et al. ILSA Working Group. Metabolic syndrome, diabetes, and cardiovascular disease in an elderly Caucasian cohort: the Italian longitudinal study on aging. *J Gerontol A Biol Sci Med Sci.* 2006;61:505–510.

23. Lorenzo C, Serrano-Rios M, Martinez-Larrad MT, et al. Geographic variations of the International Diabetes Federation and the National Cholesterol Education Program-Adult Treatment Panel III definitions of the metabolic syndrome in nondiabetic subjects. *Diabetes Care.* 2006;29:685–691.

24. Santos AC, Barros H. Prevalence and determinants of obesity in an urban sample of Portuguese adults. *Public Health.* 2003;117:340–437.

25. Athyros VG, Ganotakis ES, Bathianaki M, et al. MetS-Greece Collaborative Group. Awareness, treatment and control of the metabolic syndrome and its components: a multicentre Greek study. *Hellenic J Cardiol.* 2005;46:380–386.

26. Kolcic I, Vorko-Jovic A, Salzer B, Smoljanovic M, Kern J, Vuletic S. Metabolic syndrome in a metapopulation of Croatian island isolates. *Croat Med J.* 2006;47:585–592.

27. Lawlor DA, Smith GD, Ebrahim S. Does the new International Diabetes Federation definition of the metabolic syndrome predict CHD any more strongly than older definitions? Findings from the British Women's Heart and Health Study. *Diabetologia.* 2006;49:41–48.

28. Tillin T, Forouhi N, Johnston DG, McKeigue PM, Chaturvedi N, Godsland IF. Metabolic syndrome and coronary heart disease in South Asians, African–Caribbeans and white Europeans: a UK population-based cross-sectional study. *Diabetologia.* 2005;48:649–656.

29. Boronat M, Chirino R, Varillas VF, et al. Prevalence of the metabolic syndrome in the island of Gran Canaria: comparison of three major diagnostic proposals. *Diabet Med.* 2005;22:1751–1756.

30. Gorter PM, Olijhoek JK, van der Graaf Y, Algra A, Rabelink TJ, Visseren FLSMART, Study G. Prevalence of the metabolic syndrome in patients with coronary heart disease, cerebrovascular disease, peripheral arterial disease or abdominal aortic aneurysm. *Atherosclerosis.* 2004;173:363–369.

31. Jerico C, Knobel H, Montero M, et al. Hypertens in HIV-infected patients: prevalence and related factors. *Am J Hypertens.* 2005;18:1396–1401.

32. Skoumas J, Papadimitriou L, Pitsavos C, et al. Metabolic syndrome prevalence and characteristics in Greek adults with familial combined hyperlipidemia. *Metabolism.* 2007;56:135–141.

33. Herva A, Rasanen P, Miettunen J. Timonen et al. Co-occurrence of metabolic syndrome with depression and anxiety in young adults: the Northern Finland 1955 Birth Cohort Study. *Psychosom Med.* 2006;68:213–216.

34. Deepa M, Farooq S, Datta M, Deepa R, Mohan V. Prevalence of metabolic syndrome using WHO, ATPIII and IDF definitions in Asian Indians: the Chennai Urban Rural Epidemiology Study (CURES-34). *Diabetes Metab Res Rev.* 2007;23:127–134.

35. Gupta R, Deedwania PC, Gupta A, Rastogi S, Panwar RB, Kothari K. Prevalence of metabolic syndrome in an Indian urban population. *Int J Cardiol.* 2004;97:257–261.

36. Ramachandran A, Snehalatha C, Satyavani K, Sivasankari S, Vijay V. Metabolic syndrome in urban Asian Indian adults—a population study using modified ATP III criteria. *Diabetes Res Clin Pract.* 2003;60:199–204.

37. Boonyavarakul A, Choosaeng C, Supasyndyh O, Panichkul S. Prevalence of the metabolic syndrome, and its association factors between percentage body fat and body mass index in rural Thai population aged 35 years and older. *J Med Assoc Thai.* 2005;88(Suppl 3):S121–S130.

38. Lohsoonthorn V, Dhanamun B, Williams MA. Prevalence of metabolic syndrome and its relationship to white blood cell count in a population of Thai men and women receiving routine health examinations. *Am J Hypertens.* 2006;19:339–345.

39. Heng D, Ma S, Lee JJ, et al. Modification of the NCEP ATP III definitions of the metabolic syndrome for use in Asians identifies individuals at risk of ischemic heart disease. *Atherosclerosis.* 2006;186:367–373.

40. Li ZY, Zu GB, Zia TA. Prevalence rate of metabolic syndrome and dyslipidemia in a large professional population in Beijing. *Atherosclerosis.* 2006;184:188–192.

41. Ko GT, Cockram CS, Chow CC, et al. High prevalence of metabolic syndrome in Hong Kong Chinese—comparison of three diagnostic criteria. *Diabetes Res Clin Pract.* 2005;69:160–168.

42. Feng Y, Hong X, Li Z, et al. Prevalence of metabolic syndrome and its relation of body composition in a Chinese rural population. *Obesity.* 2006;14:2089–2098.

43. Lao XQ, Thomas GN, Jiang CQ, et al. Association of the metabolic syndrome with vascular disease in an older Chinese populations: Guangzhou Biobank Cohort Study. *J Endocrinol Invest.* 2006;29:989–996.

44. Lu B, Yang Y, Song X, et al. An evaluation of the International Diabetes Federation definition of metabolic syndrome in Chinese patients older than 30 years and diagnosed with type 2 diabetes mellitus. *Metabolism.* 2006;55:1088–1096.

45. Fan JG, Zhu J, Li XJ, et al. Fatty liver and the metabolic syndrome among Shanghai adults. *J Gastroenterol Hepatol.* 2005;20:1825–1832.

46. Pei WD, Sun YH, Lu B, et al. Apolipoprotein B is associated with metabolic syndrome in Chinese families with familial combined hyperlipidemia, familial hypertriglyceridemia and familial hypercholesterolemia. *Int J Cardiol.* 2007;116:194–200.

47. Ishizaka N, Ishizaka Y, Toda E, Hashimoto H, Nagai R, Yamakado M. Hypertension is the most common component of metabolic syndrome and the greatest contributor to carotid arteriosclerosis in apparently healthy Japanese individuals. *Hypertens Res.* 2005;28:27–34.

48. Arai H, Yamamoto A, Matsuzawa Y, et al. Prevalence of metabolic syndrome in the general Japanese population in 2000. *J Atheroscler Thromb.* 2006;13:202–208.

49. Tanaka H, Shimabukuro T, Shimabukuro M. High prevalence of metabolic syndrome among men in Okinawa. *J Atheroscler Thromb.* 2005;12:284–288.

50. Aizawa Y, Kamimura N, Watanabe H, et al. Cardiovascular risk factors are really linked in the metabolic syndrome: this phenomenon suggests clustering rather than coincidence. *Int J Cardiol.* 2006;109:213–218.

51. Aguilar-Salinas CA, Rojas R, Gomez-Perez FJ, et al. The metabolic syndrome: a concept hard to define. *Arch Med Res.* 2005;36:223–231.

52. Alvarez MM, Vieira AC, Moura AS, da Veiga GV. Insulin resistance in Brazilian adolescent girls: association with overweight and metabolic disorders. *Diabetes Res Clin Pract.* 2006;74:183–188.

53. Florez H, Silva E, Fernandez V, et al. Prevalence and risk factors associated with the metabolic syndrome and dyslipidemia in White, Black, American and Mixed Hispanics in Zulia State, Venezuela. *Diabetes Res Clin Pract.* 2005;69:63–77.

54. Hidalgo LA, Chedraui PA, Morocho N, Alvarado M, Chavez D, Huc A. The metabolic syndrome among postmenopausal women in Ecuador. *Gynecol Endocrinol.* 2006;22:447–454.

55. Sherry N, Hassoun A, Oberfield SE, et al. Clinical and metabolic characteristics of an obese, Dominican, pediatric population. *J Pediatr Endocrinol Metab.* 2006;18:1063–1071.

56. Tull ES, Thurland A, LaPorte RE. Metabolic syndrome among Caribbean-born persons living in the U.S. Virgin Islands. *Rev Panam Salud Publica.* 2005;186:418–426.

57. Hashimoto SM, Gimeno SG, Matsumura L, Franco LJ, Miranda WL, Ferreira SR. Autoimmunity does not contribute to the highly prevalent glucose metabolism disturbances in a Japanese Brazilian population. *Ethn Dis.* 2007 Winter;17(1):78–87 (Japanese Brazilian Diabetes Study Group. Summary for patients in: *Ethn Dis.* 2007; 17:169).

58. Damiao R, Castro TG, Cardoso MA, Gimeno SG, Ferreira SR. Japanese–Brazilian Diabetes Study Group. Dietary intakes associated with metabolic syndrome in a cohort of Japanese ancestry. *Br J Nutr.* 2006;96:532–538.

59. Lanz JR, Pereira AC, Martinez E, Kriegr JE. Metabolic syndrome and coronary artery disease: is there a gender specific effect? *Int J Cardio.* 2006;107:317–321.

60. Freire RD, Cardoso MA, Gimeno SG, Ferreira SR. Japanese–Brazilian Diabetes Study Group. Dietary fat is associated with metabolic syndrome in Japanese Brazilians. *Diabetes Care.* 2005;28:1779–1785.

61. Pousada JM, Britto MM, Cruz T, et al. The metabolic syndrome in Spanish migrants to Brazil: unexpected results. *Diabetes Res Clin Pract.* 2006;72:75–80.

62. Ogden CL, Flegal KM, Carroll MD, Johnson CL. Prevalence and trends in overweight among US children and adolescents, 1999–2000. *JAMA.* 2002;288:1728–1732.

63. Weiss R, Dziura J, Burgert TS, et al. Obesity and the metabolic syndrome in children and adolescents. *N Engl J Med.* 2004;350:2362–2374.

64. Ekberg K, Landau BR, Wajngot A, et al. Contributions by kidney and liver to glucose production in the postabsorptive state and after 60 h of fasting. *Diabetes.* 1999;48:292–298.

65. Huang SC, Phelps ME, Hoffman EJ, Sideris K, Selin CJ, Kuhl DE. Non-invasive determination of local cerebral metabolic rate of glucose in man. *Am J Physiol.* 1980;238:E69–E82.

66. DeFronzo RA, Jacot E, Jequier E, Maeder E, Wahren J, Felber JP. The effect of insulin on the disposal of intravenous glucose: results from indirect calorimetry. *Diabetes.* 1981;30:1000–1007.

67. Katz LD, Glickman MG, Rapoport S, Ferrannini E, DeFronzo RA. Splanchnic and peripheral disposal of oral glucose in man. *Diabetes.* 1983;32:675–679.

68. Ferrannini E, Bjorkman O, Reichard GA Jr, et al. The disposal of an oral glucose load in healthy subjects. *Diabetes.* 1985;34:580–588.

69. Mandarino L, Bonadonna R, McGuinness O, Wasserman D. Regulation of muscle glucose uptake in vivo. In: Jefferson LS, Cherrington AD, eds. *Handbook of Physiology.* Vol. II. Oxford: Oxford University Press; 2001:803–848.

70. Bergman RN. Non-esterified fatty acids and the liver: why is insulin secreted into the portal vein? *Diabetologia.* 2000;43:946–952.

71. Boden G. Role of fatty acids in the pathogenesis of insulin resistance and NIDDM. *Diabetes.* 1997;46:3–10.

72. McGarry JD. Banting lecture 2001: dysregulation of fatty acid metabolism in the etiology of type 2 diabetes. *Diabetes.* 2002;51:7–18.

73. Lebovitz HE, Banerji MA. Point: visceral adiposity is causally related to insulin resistance. *Diabetes Care.* 2005;28:2322–2325.

74. Björntorp P. Visceral obesity: a "civilization syndrome". *Obes Res.* 1993;1:206–222.

75. Björntorp P. Metabolic implications of body fat distribution. *Diabetes Care.* 1991;14:1132–1143.

76. Goodpaster BH, Krishnaswami S, Resnick H, et al. Association between regional adipose tissue distribution and both type 2 diabetes and impaired glucose tolerance in elderly men and women. *Diabetes Care.* 2003;26:372–379.

77. Ross R, Aru J, Freeman J, Hudson R, Janssen I. Abdominal adiposity and insulin resistance in obese men. *Am J Physiol Endocrinol Metab.* 2002;282:E657–E663.

78. Ross R, Aru J, Freeman J, Hudson R, Janssen I. Abdominal obesity, muscle composition, and insulin resistance in premenopausal women. *J Clin Endocrinol Metab.* 2002;87:5044–5051.

79. Kashyap S, Belfort R, Pratipanawatr T, et al. Chronic elevation in plasma free fatty acids impairs insulin secretion in non-diabetic offspring with a strong family history of T2DM. *Diabetes.* 2002;51(Suppl 2):A12.

80. Carpentier A, Mittelman SD, Bergman RN, Giacca A, Lewis GF. Prolonged elevation of plasma free fatty acids impairs pancreatic beta-cell function in obese nondiabetic humans but not in individuals with type 2 diabetes. *Diabetes.* 2000;49:399–408.

81. Goodpaster BH, Thaete FL, Kelley BE. Thigh adipose tissue distribution is associated with insulin resistance in obesity and in type 2 diabetes mellitus. *Am J Clin Nutr.* 2000;71:885–892.

82. Greco AV, Mingrone G, Giancaterini A, et al. Insulin resistance in morbid obesity. Reversal with intramyocellular fat depletion. *Diabetes.* 2002;51:144–151.

83. Ryysy L, Hakkinen AM, Goto T, et al. Hepatic fat content and insulin action on free fatty acids and glucose metabolism rather than insulin absorption are associated with insulin requirements during insulin therapy in type 2 diabetic patients. *Diabetes.* 2000;49:749–758.

84. Kelley DE. The Impact of Obesity, Regional Adiposity and Ectopic Fat on the Pathophysiology of Type 2 Diabetes. Council on Obesity Diabetes Education. 2003;12–20.

85. Goodpaster BH, Kelley DE, Wing RR, Meier A, Thaete FL. Effects of weight loss on insulin sensitivity in obesity: influence of regional adiposity. *Diabetes.* 1999;48:839–847.

86. Balkau B, Deanfield JE, Després JP, et al. International day for the evaluation of abdominal obesity (IDEA): a study of waist circumference, cardiovascular disease, and diabetes mellitus in 168,000 primary care patients in 63 countries. *Circulation.* 2007;116:1942–1951.

87. Canoy D, Boekholdt SM, Wareham N, et al. Body fat distribution and risk of coronary heart disease in men and women in the European Prospective Investigation Into Cancer and Nutrition in Norfolk cohort: a population-based prospective study. *Circulation.* 2007;116:2933–2943.

88. Yusuf S, Hawken S, Ounpuu S, et al. Obesity and the risk of myocardial infarction in 27,000 participants from 52 countries: a case-control study. *Lancet.* 2005;366:1640–1649.

89. Haffner SM. Management of dyslipidemia in adults with diabetes. *Diabetes Care.* 1998;21:160–178.

90. Austin MA, King MC, Vranizan KM, Krauss RM. Atherogenic lipoprotein phenotype. A proposed genetic marker for coronary heart disease risk. *Circulation.* 1990;82:495–506.

91. Ginsberg HN. Diabetic dyslipidemia: basic mechanisms underlying the common hypertriglyceridemia and low HDL cholesterol levels. *Diabetes.* 1996;45(Suppl 3):S27–S30.

92. Brown MS, Kovanen PT, Goldstein JL. Regulation of plasma cholesterol by lipoprotein receptors. *Science.* 1981;212:628–635.

93. Bucala R, Makita Z, Vega G, et al. Modification of low density lipoprotein by advanced glycation end products contributes to the dyslipidemia of diabetes and renal insufficiency. *Proc Natl Acad Sci USA.* 1994;91:9441–9445.

94. Verges BL. Dyslipidaemia in diabetes mellitus. Review of the main lipoprotein abnormalities and their consequences on the development of atherogenesis. *Diabetes Metab.* 1999;25(Suppl 3):32–40.

95. Tall AR. An overview of reverse cholesterol transport. *Eur Heart J.* 1998;19(Suppl A):A31–A35.

96. Rohrer L, Hersberger M, von Eckardstein A. High density lipoproteins in the intersection of diabetes mellitus, inflammation and cardiovascular disease. *Curr Opin Lipidol.* 2004;15:269–278.

97. Howard BV. Insulin resistance and lipid metabolism. *Am J Cardiol.* 1999;84(Suppl 1):28–32.

98. Calles-Escandon J, Garcia-Rubi E, Mirza S, Mortensen A. Type 2 diabetes: one disease, multiple cardiovascular risk factors. *Coron Artery Dis.* 1999;10:23–30.

99. Rosenson RS, Lowe GDO. Effects of lipids and lipoproteins on thrombosis and rheology. *Atherosclerosis.* 1998;140:271–280.

100. Reaven GM. Multiple CHD risk factors in type 2 diabetes: beyond hyperglycaemia. *Diabetes Obes Metab.* 2002;4(Suppl 1):S13–S18.

101. Ridker PM, Hennekens CH, Buring JE, Rifai N. C-reactive protein and other markers of inflammation in the prediction of cardiovascular disease in women. *N Engl J Med.* 2000;342:836–843.

102. Koenig W, Sund M, Fröhlich M, et al. C-Reactive protein, a sensitive marker of inflammation, predicts future risk of coronary heart disease in initially healthy middle-aged men: results from the MONICA (Monitoring Trends and Determinants in Cardiovascular Disease) Augsburg Cohort Study, 1984 to 1992. *Circulation.* 1999;99:237–242.

103. Ford ES. Body mass index, diabetes, and C-reactive protein among U.S. adults. *Diabetes Care.* 1999;22:1971–1977.

104. Expert Panel on Detection, Evaluation, and Treatment of High Blood Cholesterol in Adults. Report of the National Cholesterol Education Program Expert Panel on Detection, Evaluation, and Treatment of High Blood Cholesterol in Adults. *Arch Intern Med.* 1988;148:36–69.

105. Expert Panel on Detection, Evaluation, and Treatment of High Blood Cholesterol in Adults. National Cholesterol Education Program (Adult Treatment Panel III): Full report. NIH Publication No. 02-5215. September 2002. Bethesda, MD: NIH National Heart, Lung, and Blood Institute; 2002.

106. Grundy SM, Cleeman JI, Merz CN, et al. Coordinating Committee of the National Cholesterol Education Program. Implications of recent clinical trials for the National Cholesterol Education Program Adult Treatment Panel III guidelines. *Circulation.* 2004;110:227–239.

107. American Diabetes Association. Management of dyslipidemia in adults with diabetes. *Diabetes Care.* 2002;25(Suppl 1):S74–S77.

108. Mosca L, Appel LJ, Benjamin EJ, et al. Evidence-based guidelines for cardiovascular disease prevention in women. *Circulation.* 2004;109:672–693.

109. Després J-P, Lemieux I, Bergeron J, et al. Abdominal obesity and the metabolic syndrome: contribution to global cardiometabolic risk. *Arterioscler Thromb Vasc Biol.* 2008;28:1039–1049.

110. Heart Protection Study Collaborative Group. MRC/BHF Heart Protection Study of cholesterol lowering with simvastatin in 20 536 high-risk individuals: a randomised placebo-controlled trial. *Lancet.* 2002;360:7–22.

111. Heart Protection Study Collaborative Group. MRC/BHF Heart Protection Study of cholesterol-lowering with simvastatin in 5963 people with diabetes: a randomised placebo-controlled trial. *Lancet.* 2003;361:2005–2016.

112. LaRosa JC, Grundy SM, Waters DD, et al. Treating to New Targets (TNT) Investigators. Intensive lipid lowering with atorvastatin in patients with stable coronary disease. *N Engl J Med.* 2005;352:1425–1435.

113. Pederson TR, Faergeman O, Kastelein JJP, et al. Incremental Decrease in End Points Through Aggressive Lipid Lowering (IDEAL) Study Group. High-dose atorvastatin vs. usual-dose simvastatin for secondary prevention after myocardial infarction. The IDEAL Study: a randomized controlled trial. *JAMA*. 2005;294:2437–2445.

114. Ridker PM, Danielson E, Fonseca FAH, et al. JUPITER Study Group. Rosuvastatin to prevent vascular events in men and women with elevated C-reactive protein. *N Engl J Med*. 2008;359:2195–2207.

115. Baigent C, Keech A, Kearney PM, et al. Efficacy and safety of cholesterol-lowering treatment: prospective meta-analysis of data from 90,056 participants in 14 randomised trials of stains. *Lancet*. 2005;366:1267–1278.

116. Cannon CP, Steinberg BA, Murphy SA, Mega JL, Braunwald E. Meta-analysis of cardiovascular outcomes trials comparing intensive versus moderate statin therapy. *J Am Coll Cardiol*. 2006;48:438–445.

117. Koskinen P, Mänttäri M, Manninen V, Huttunen JK, Heinonen OP, Frick MH. Coronary heart disease incidence in NIDDM patients in the Helsinki Heart Study. *Diabetes Care*. 1992;15:820–825.

118. Rubins HB, Robins SJ, Collins D, et al. Diabetes, plasma insulin, and cardiovascular disease: subgroup analysis from the Department of Veterans Affairs high-density lipoprotein intervention trial (VA-HIT). *Arch Intern Med*. 2002;162:2597–2604.

119. Rubins HB, Robins SJ, Collins D, et al. Veterans Affairs High-Density Lipoprotein Cholesterol Intervention Trial Study Group. Gemfibrozil for the secondary prevention of coronary heart disease in men with low levels of high-density lipoprotein cholesterol. *N Engl J Med*. 1999;341:410–418.

120. Diabetes Atherosclerosis Intervention Study Investigators. Effect of fenofibrate on progression of coronary-artery disease in type 2 diabetes: the Diabetes Atherosclerosis Intervention Study, a randomised study. *Lancet*. 2001;357:905–910.

121. The FIELD Study Investigators. Effects of long-term fenofibrate therapy on cardiovascular events in 9795 people with type 2 diabetes mellitus (The FIELD Study): randomized, controlled trial. *Lancet*. 2005;366:1849–1861.

122. Robins SJ, Collins D, Wittes JT, et al. VA-HIT Study Group. Relation of gemfibrozil treatment and lipid levels with major coronary events: VA-HIT: a randomized controlled trial. *JAMA*. 2001;285:1585–1591.

123. Athyros VG, Papageorgiou AA, Athyrou VV, Demitriadis DS, Kontopoulos AG. Atorvastatin and micronized fenofibrate alone and in combination in type 2 diabetes with combined hyperlipidemia. *Diabetes Care*. 2002;25:1198–1202.

124. Gavish D, Leibovitz E, Shapira I, Rubinstein A. Bezafibrate and simvastatin combination therapy for diabetic dyslipidaemia: efficacy and safety. *J Intern Med*. 2000;247:563–569.

125. Pasternak RC, Smith SC Jr., Bairey-Merz CN, Grundy SM, Cleeman JI, Lenfant C. ACC/AHA/NHLBI clinical advisory on the use and safety of statins. *J Am Coll Cardiol*. 2002;40:567–572.

126. Omar MA, Wilson JP. FDA adverse event reports on statin-associated rhabdomyolysis. *Ann Pharmacother*. 2002;36:288–295.

127. Ballantyne CM, Corsini A, Davidson MH, et al. Risk for myopathy with statin therapy in high-risk patients. *Arch Intern Med*. 2003;163:553–564.

128. Study Group. Effects of intensive glucose lowering in type 2 diabetes. The action to control cardiovascular risk in diabetes study group. *N Engl J Med*. 2008;258(24):2545–2559.

129. Taylor AS, Lee HS, Sullenberger LE. The effect of 24 months of combination satin and extended-release niacin on carotid intima-media thickness: ARBITER 3. *Curr Med Res Opin*. 2006;22:2243–2250.

130. The Coronary Drug Project Research Group. Clofibrate and niacin in coronary heart disease. *JAMA*. 1975;231:360–381.

131. Canner PL, Berge KG, Wenger NK, et al. Coronary Drug Project Research Group. Fifteen year mortality in Coronary Drug Project patients: long-term benefit with niacin. *J Am Coll Cardiol*. 1986;8:1245–1255.

132. Canner PL, Furberg CD, McGovern ME. Niacin decreases myocardial infarction and total mortality in patients with impaired fasting glucose or glucose intolerance: results from the Coronary Drug Project [abstract 3138]. *Circulation*. 2002;106(Suppl II):636.

133. Kane JP, Malloy MJ, Ports TA, Phillips NR, Diehl JC, Havel RJ. Regression of coronary atherosclerosis during treatment of familial hypercholesterolemia with combined drug regimens. *JAMA*. 1990;264:3007–3012.

134. Blankenhorn DH, Nessim SA, Johnson RL, Sanmarco ME, Azen SP, Cashin-Hemphill L. Beneficial effects of combined colestipol-niacin therapy on coronary atherosclerosis and coronary venous bypass grafts. *JAMA*. 1987;257:3233–3240.

135. Brown G, Albers JJ, Fisher LD, et al. Regression of coronary artery disease as a result of intensive lipid-lowering therapy in men with high levels of apolipoprotein B. *N Engl J Med*. 1990;323:1289–1298.

136. Brown BG, Zhao XQ, Chait A, et al. Simvastatin and niacin, antioxidant vitamins, or the combination for the prevention of coronary disease. *N Engl J Med*. 2001;345:1583–1592.

137. Van JT, Pan J, Wasty T, Chan E, Wu X, Charles MA. Comparison of extended-release niacin and atorvastatin monotherapies and combination treatment of the atherogenic lipid profile in diabetes mellitus. *Am J Cardiol*. 2002;89:1306–1308.

138. Pan J, Lin M, Kesala R, Van J, Charles M. Niacin treatment of the atherogenic lipid profile and Lp(a) in diabetes. *Diabetes Obes Metab.* 2002;4:255–261.

139. Boden G, Chen X, Ruiz J, White JV, Rossetti L. Mechanisms of fatty acid-induced inhibition of glucose uptake. *J Clin Invest.* 1994;93:2438–2446.

140. Elam MB, Hunninghake DB, Davis KB, et al. . ADMIT Investigators. Effect of niacin on lipid and lipoprotein levels and glycemic control in patients with diabetes and peripheral arterial disease. The ADMIT study: a randomized trial. *JAMA.* 2000;284:1263–1270.

141. Grundy SM, Vega GL, McGovern ME, et al. Diabetes Multicenter Research Group. Efficacy, safety, and tolerability of once-daily niacin for the treatment of dyslipidemia associated with type 2 diabetes: results of the Assessment of Diabetes Control and Evaluation of the Efficacy of Niaspan Trial. *Arch Intern Med.* 2002;162:1568–1576.

142. Zhao X-Q, Morse JS, Dowdy AA, et al. Safety and tolerability of simvastatin plus niacin in patients with coronary artery disease and low high-density lipoprotein cholesterol (The HDL Atherosclerosis Treatment Study). *Am J Cardiol.* 2004;93:307–312.

143. American Diabetes Association. Dyslipidemia management in adults with diabetes. *Diabetes Care.* 2004;27(Suppl 1):S68–S71.

144. Eaton SB, Konner M, Shostak M. Stone agers in the fast lane: chronic degenerative diseases in evolutionary perspective. *Am J Med.* 1988;84:739–749.

145. Helmrich SP, Ragland DR, Leung RW, Paffenbarger RS Jr.. Physical activity and reduced occurrence of non-insulin-dependent diabetes mellitus. *N Engl J Med.* 1991;325:147–152.

146. Manson JE, Rimm EB, Stampfer MJ, et al. Physical activity and incidence of non-insulin-dependent diabetes mellitus in women. *Lancet.* 1991;338:774–778.

147. Manson JE, Nathan DM, Krolewski AS, Stampfer MJ, Willett WC, Hennekens CH. A prospective study of exercise and incidence of diabetes among US male physicians. *JAMA.* 1992;268:63–67.

148. Wannamethee SG, Shaper AG, Alberti KG. Physical activity, metabolic factors, and the incidence of coronary heart disease and type 2 diabetes. *Arch Intern Med.* 2000;160:2108–2116.

149. Hu G, Lindstrom J, Valle TT, et al. Physical activity, body mass index, and risk of type 2 diabetes in patients with normal or impaired glucose regulation. *Arch Intern Med.* 2004;164:892–896.

150. Folsom AR, Kushi LH, Hong CP. Physical activity and incident diabetes mellitus in postmenopausal women. *Am J Public Health.* 2000;90:134–138.

151. Hu FB, Manson JE, Stampfer MJ, et al. Diet, lifestyle, and the risk of type 2 diabetes mellitus in women. *N Engl J Med.* 2001;345:790–797.

152. Hu FB, Sigal RJ, Rich-Edwards JW, et al. Walking compared with vigorous physical activity and risk of type 2 diabetes in women: a prospective study. *JAMA.* 1999;282:1433–1439.

153. Weinstein AR, Sesso HD, Lee IM, et al. Relationship of physical activity vs. body mass index with type 2 diabetes in women. *JAMA.* 2004;292:1188–1194.

154. Hsia J, Wu L, Allen C, et al. Physical activity and diabetes risk in postmenopausal women. *Am J Prev Med.* 2005;28:19–25.

155. Carnethon MR, Gidding SS, Nehgme R, Sidney S, Jacobs DR Jr, Liu K. Cardiorespiratory fitness in young adulthood and the development of cardiovascular disease risk factors. *JAMA.* 2003;290:3092–3100.

156. Lynch J, Helmrich SP, Lakka TA, et al. Moderately intense physical activities and high levels of cardiorespiratory fitness reduce the risk of non-insulin-dependent diabetes mellitus in middle-aged men. *Arch Intern Med.* 1996;156:1307–1314.

157. Wei M, Gibbons LW, Mitchell TL, Kampert JB, Lee CD, Blair SN. The association between cardiorespiratory fitness and impaired fasting glucose and type 2 diabetes mellitus in men. *Ann Intern Med.* 1999;130:89–96.

158. Pan XR, Li GW, Hu YH, et al. Effects of diet and exercise in preventing NIDDM in people with impaired glucose tolerance. The Da Qing IGT and Diabetes Study. *Diabetes Care.* 1997;20:537–544.

159. Knowler WC, Barrett-Connor E, Fowler SE, et al. Reduction in the incidence of type 2 diabetes with lifestyle intervention or metformin. *N Engl J Med.* 2002;346:393–403.

160. Tuomilehto J, Lindstrom J, Eriksson JG, et al. Prevention of type 2 diabetes mellitus by changes in lifestyle among subjects with impaired glucose tolerance. *N Engl J Med.* 2001;344:1343–1350.

161. Laaksonen DE, Lindstrom J, Lakka TA, et al. Physical activity in the prevention of type 2 diabetes: the Finnish Diabetes Prevention Study. *Diabetes.* 2005;54:158–165.

162. Chiasson JL, Josse RG, Gomis R, Hanefeld M, Karasik A, Laakso M. STOP-NIDDM Trial Research Group. Acarbose for prevention of type 2 diabetes mellitus: the STOP-NIDDM randomized trial. *Lancet.* 2002;359:2072–2077.

163. Knowler WC, Barrett-Connor E, Fowler SE, et al. Diabetes Prevention Program Research Group. Reduction in the incidence of type 2 diabetes with lifestyle intervention or metformin. *N Engl J Med.* 2002;346:393–403.

164. Buchannan T, Xiang AH, Peters RK, et al. Preservation of pancreatic [beta]-cell function and prevention of type 2 diabetes by pharmacological treatment of insulin resistance in high-risk Hispanic women. *Diabetes.* 2002;51:2796–2803.

165. The DREAM (Diabetes Reduction Assessment with Ramipril and Rosiglitazone Medication) Trial Investigators. Effect of rosiglitazone on the frequency of diabetes in patients with impaired glucose tolerance or impaired fasting glucose: a randomized controlled trial. *Lancet.* 2006;368:1096–1105.

166. ACT NOW results. Presented at the American Diabetes Association Annual Meeting, June 2008.

167. Azziz R, Kashar-Miller MD. Family history as a risk factor for the polycystic ovary syndrome. *J Pediatr Endocrinol Metab.* 2000;13:1303–1306.

168. Urbanek M, Legro R, Driscoll DA, et al. Thirty-seven candidate genes for polycystic ovary syndrome: strongest evidence for linkage is with follistatin. *Proc Natl Acad Sci USA.* 1999;86:8573–8578.

169. Ehrmann DA, Sturis J, Byrne MM, Karrison T, Rosenfield RL, Polonsky KS. Insulin secretory defects in polycystic ovary syndrome: relationship to insulin sensitivity and family history of non-insulin-dependent diabetes mellitus. *J Clin Invest.* 1995;96:520–527.

170. Legro RS, Driscoll D, Strauss JFIII, Fox J, Dunaif A. Evidence for a genetic basis for hyperandrogenemia in polycystic ovary syndrome. *Proc Natl Acad Sci USA.* 1998;95:14956–14960.

171. Kahsar-Miller MD, Nixon C, Boots LR, Go RC, Azziz R. Prevalence of polycystic ovary syndrome (PCOS) in first-degree relatives of patients with PCOS. *Fertil Seril.* 2001;75:53–58.

172. Dunaif A, Segal KR, Futterweit W, Dobrjansky A. Profound peripheral insulin resistance, independent of obesity, in polycystic ovary syndrome. *Diabetes.* 1989;38:1165–1174.

173. Dunaif A. Insulin resistance and the polycystic ovary syndrome: mechanism and implications for pathogenesis. *Endocr Rev.* 1997;18:774–800.

174. Dunaif A, Wu X, Lee A, Diamanti-Kandarakis E. Defects in insulin receptor signaling in vivo in the polycystic ovary syndrome (PCOS). *Am J Physiol Endocrinol Metab.* 2001;281:E392–E399.

175. Sam S, Dunaif A. Polycystic ovary syndrome: syndrome XX? *Trends Endocrinol Metab.* 2003;14:365–370.

176. Azziz R, Ehrmann D, Legro RS, et al. Troglitazone improves ovulation and hirsutism in the polycystic ovary syndrome: a multicenter, double blind, placebo-controlled trial. *J Clin Endocrinol Metab.* 2001;86:1626–1632.

177. Franks S. Polycystic ovary syndrome: a changing perspective. *Clin Endocrinol.* 1989;31:87–120.

178. Knochenhauer E, Key TJ, Kahsar-Miller M, Waggoner W, Boots LR, Assiz R. Prevalence of the polycystic ovary syndrome in unselected black and white women of the southeastern United States: a Prospective study. *J Clin Endocrinol Metab.* 1998;83:3078–3082.

179. Diamanti-Kandarakis E, Kouli CR, Bergiele AT, et al. A survey of the polycystic ovary syndrome in the Greek island of Lesbos: hormonal and metabolic profile. *J Clin Endocrinol Metab.* 1999;84:4006–4011.

180. Asuncion M, Calvo RM, San Millan JL, Sancho J, Avila S, Escobar-Morreale HE. A prospective study of the prevalence of the polycystic ovary syndrome in unselected Caucasian women from Spain. *J Clin Endocrinol Metab.* 2000;85:2434–2438.

181. Ayala C, Steinberger E, Smith KD, Rodriguez-Rigau L, Petak SM. Serum testosterone levels and reference ranges in reproductive-age women. *Endocr Pract.* 1999;5:322–329.

182. Franks S. Adult polycystic ovary syndrome begins in childhood. *Best Pract Res Clin Endocrinol Metab.* 2002;16:263–272.

183. Ibanez L, Valls C, Marcos MV, Ong K, Dunger DB, De Zegher F. Insulin sensitization for girls with precocious pubarche and with risk for polycystic ovary syndrome: effects of prepubertal initiation and postpubertal discontinuation of metformin treatment. *J Clin Endocrinol Metab.* 2004;89:4331–4337.

184. Nelson VL, Legro RS, Strauss JF III, McAllister JM. Augmented androgen production is a stable steroidogenic phenotype of propagated theca cells from polycystic ovaries. *Mol Endocrinol.* 1999;13:946–947.

185. Nelson VL, Qin KN, Rosenfield RL, et al. The biochemical basis for increased testosterone production in theca cells propagated from patients with polycystic ovary syndrome. *J Clin Endocrinol Metab.* 2001;85:5925–5933.

186. Haisenleder DJ, Dalkin AC, Ortolano GA, Marshall JC, Shupnik MA. A pulsatile gonadotropin-releasing hormone stimulus is required to increase transcription of the gonadotropin subunit genes: evidence for differential regulation of transcription by pulse frequency in vivo. *Endocrinology.* 1991;128:509–517.

187. Eagleson CA, Gingrich MB, Pastor CL, et al. Polycystic ovarian syndrome: evidence that flutamide restores sensitivity of the gonadotropin-releasing hormone pulse generator to inhibition by estradiol and progesterone. *J Clin Endocrinol Metab.* 2000;85:4047–4052.

188. Dahlgren E, Janson PO, Johansson S, Lapidus L, Oden A. Polycystic ovary syndrome and risk for myocardial infarction: evaluated from a risk factor model based on a prospective population study of women. *Acta Obstet Gynecol Scand.* 1992;71:599–604.

189. Cibula D, Cifkova R, Fanta M, Poledne R, Zivny J, Skibova J. Increased risk of non-insulin dependent diabetes mellitus, arterial hypertension and coronary heart disease in perimenopausal women with a history of the polycystic ovary syndrome. *Hum Reprod.* 2000;15:785–789.

190. Elting MW, Korsen TJ, Bezemer PD, Schoemaker J. Prevalence of diabetes mellitus, hypertension and cardiac complaints in a follow-up study of a Dutch PCOS population. *Hum Reprod.* 2001;16:556–560.

191. Solomon CG, Hu FB, Dunaif A, et al. Long or highly irregular menstrual cycles as a marker for risk of type 2 diabetes mellitus. *JAMA.* 2001;286:2421–2426.

192. Solomon CG, Hu FB, Dunaif A, et al. Menstural cycle irregularity and risk for future cardiovascular disease. *J Clin Endocrinol Metab.* 2002;87:2013–2017.

193. Rich-Edwards JW, Goldman MB, Willett WC, et al. Adolescent body mass index and infertility caused by ovulatory disorder. *Am J Obstet Gynecol.* 1994;171:171–177.

194. Zaadstra BM, Seidell JC, Van Noord PA, et al. Fat and female fecundity: prospective study of effect of body fat distribution on conception rates. *BMJ.* 1993;306:484–487.

195. Clark AM, Thornley B, Tomlinson L, Galletley C, Norman RJ. Weight loss in obese infertile women results in improvement in reproductive outcome for all forms of fertility treatment. *Hum Reprod.* 1998;13:1502–1505.

196. Mansfield R, Galea R, Brincat M, Hole D, Mason H. Metformin has direct effects on human ovarian steroidogenesis. *Fertil Steril.* 2003;79:956–962.

197. Attia GR, Rainey WE, Carr BR. Metformin directly inhibits androgen production in human thecal cells. *Fertil Steril.* 2001;76:517–524.

198. Lord JM, Flight IHK, Nroman RJ. Insulin-sensitising drugs (metformin, troglitazone, rosiglitazone, pioglitazone, D-chi-ro-inositol) for polycystic ovary syndrome. *Cochrane Database Syst Rev.* 2003;3:CD003053.

199. Glueck CJ, Goldenberg N, Pranikoff J, Loftspring M, Sieve L, Wang P. Height, weight, and motor-social development during the first 18 months of life in 126 infants born to 109 mothers with polycystic ovary syndrome who conceived on and continued metformin through pregnancy. *Hum Reprod.* 2004;19:1323–1330.

200. Glueck CJ, Wang P, Kobayashi S, Phillips H, Sieve-Smith L. Metformin therapy throughout pregnancy reduces the development of gestational diabetes in women with polycystic ovary syndrome. *Fertil Steril.* 2002;77:520–525.

201. Glueck CJ, Wang P, Goldenberg N, Sieve-Smith L. Pregnancy outcomes among women with polycystic ovary syndrome treated with metformin. *Hum Reprod.* 2002;17:2858–2864.

202. Gluck CJ, Phillips H, Cameron D, Sieve-Smith L, Wang P. Continuing metformin throughout pregnancy in women with polycystic ovary syndrome appears to safely reduce first-trimester spontaneous abortion: a pilot study. *Fertil Steril.* 2001;75:46–52.

203. Mitwally MF, Witchel SF, Casper RF. Troglitazone: a possible modulator of ovarian steroidogenesis. *J Soc Gynecol Investig.* 2002;9:163–167.

204. Ghazeeri G, Kutteh WH, Bryer-Ash M, Haas D, Ke RW. Effect of rosiglitazone on spontaneous and clomiphene citrate-induced ovulation in women with polycystic ovary syndrome. *Fertil Steril.* 2003;79:562–566.

205. Belli SH, Graffigna MN, Oneto A, Otero P, Schurman L, Levalle OA. Effect of rosiglitazone on insulin resistance, growth factors, and reproductive disturbances in women with polycystic ovary syndrome. *Fertil Steril.* 2004;81:624–629.

206. Romualdi D, Guido M, Ciampelli M, et al. Selective effects of pioglitazone on insulin and androgen abnormalities in normo- and hyperinsulinaemic obese patients with polycystic ovary syndrome. *Hum Reprod.* 2003;18:1210–1218.

207. Baillargeon JP, Jakubowicz DJ, Iuorno MJ, Jakubowicz S, Nestler JE. Effects of metformin and rosiglitazone, alone and in combination, in nonobese women with polycystic ovary syndrome and normal indices of insulin sensitivity. *Fertil Steril.* 2004;82:893–902.

208. Bray GA. How do we get fat? An epidemiologic and metabolic approach. *Clin Dermatol.* 2004;22(4):281–288.

8

Chronic Kidney Disease in the Primary Care Setting: Importance for Estimating Cardiovascular Disease Risk and Use of Appropriate Therapies

Matthew R. Weir and Miguel Portocarrero

CONTENTS

Key Words: Chronic kidney disease; Cardiovascular disease; Microalbuminuria; Estimated glomerular filtration rate; Creatinine clearance; Nephropathy; Proteinuria; Albuminuria; End-stage renal disease.

KEY POINTS

- Chronic kidney disease is unequivocally associated with more CVD. This relationship persists whether or not patients have albuminuria. Whether the definition of CKD should be based on estimated GFR or albuminuria, or both, is not yet agreed upon.
- The much greater frequency of CVD in patients with CKD can be explained by traditional CVD risk factors such as hypertension, diabetes, and dyslipidemia. However, a large number of other nontraditional risk factors could explain the independent association of CKD and CVD.

From: *Contemporary Cardiology: Comprehensive Cardiovascular Medicine in the Primary Care Setting*
Edited by: Peter P. Toth, Christopher P. Cannon, DOI 10.1007/978-1-60327-963-5_8
© Springer Science+Business Media, LLC 2010

- Future clinical research is necessary to establish optimal goals and treatment strategies for blood pressure, cholesterol, and glucose in patients with CKD. The available epidemiological data indicate that a threshold-based algorithm is not appropriate. Certainly, the data for blood pressure and LDL cholesterol indicate a continuous relationship between levels and CVD events. There may be more controversy as to the safety of achieving lower levels of hemoglobin A1C in patients with diabetes.
- Also important are the nontraditional risk factors. Whether they will also require treatment to reduce CV events is an important area of future study. Vitamin D deficiency may be the most important of the new nontraditional risk fractions that require screening and treatment.
- Perhaps the most important consideration is that earlier recognition of CKD, whether by using estimated GFR determination, or an albumin:creatinine ratio, is an important and a valuable way to recognize patients who need global cardiovascular risk-reducing strategies.

8.1. BACKGROUND

This chapter provides a clinical perspective on how the kidney can be used as a sentinel for cardiovascular disease (CVD) burden and, perhaps, as a means of measuring therapeutic success for the treatment of cardiovascular disease. To accomplish these goals, we will first provide some background about the relationship between chronic kidney disease and CVD. Next, we will discuss the value of estimating glomerular filtration rate (GFR) as a better measure of overall kidney function as opposed to simply using a serum creatinine. In addition, we will also focus on the importance of residual albuminuria or proteinuria and its implications for predicting CVD. These observations will set the stage for assessing appropriate blood pressure, cholesterol and glucose goals for patients, and the pharmacologic means of attaining these goals.

Chronic kidney disease (CKD) is a worldwide public health problem that is increasing in frequency and cost. Clinicians usually recognize the need for dialysis or transplantation as a result of CKD; however, much more important is the cardiovascular disease (CVD) burden, which remains unrecognized until the patient has a fatal CVD event. In fact, patients with CKD are much more likely to die of CVD than they are to reach kidney failure. As shown in Fig. 1, regardless of gender or ethnicity, the cardiovascular mortality in the general population is substantially less at all ages compared to patients

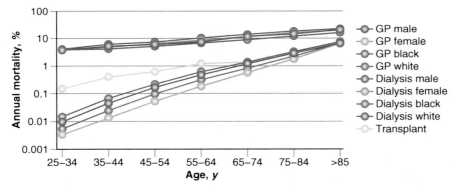

Fig. 1. Cardiovascular mortality in the general population (GP; National Center for Health Statistics [NCHS] multiple cause mortality data files, International Classification of Diseases, 9th Revision [ICD 9] codes 402, 404, 410–414, and 425–429, 1993) compared with the same events in patients with kidney failure treated by dialysis or kidney transplant (United States Renal Data System [USRDS] special data request Health Care Financing Administration form 2746 Nos. 23, 26–29, and 31, 1994–1996). Data are stratified by age, race, and sex. CVD mortality is underestimated in kidney transplant recipients owing to incomplete ascertainment of cause of death. Reproduced and modified with permission from Foley et al. *(66).*

with end-stage renal failure being treated with either dialysis or transplantation. This difference is most remarkable in younger age groups and remains statistically different even in older age groups. Consequently, it is important to develop strategies to better define CKD and discuss the relationship between CKD and CVD in the general population.

Table 1
Stages of CKD

Stage	Description	GFR (mL/min/173 m²)	US prevalence 1,000 s	US prevalence percent
1	Kidney damage with normal or increased GFR	≥90	5,900	3.3
2	Kidney damage with mildly decreased GFR	60–89	5,300	3.0
3	Moderately decreased GFR	30–59	7,600	4.3
4	Severely decreased GFR	15–29	400	0.2
5	Kidney failure	<15 or dialysis	300	0.1

Data for Stages 1–4 from NHANES III (1988–1994) based on population of 177 million with age ≥20 years. Data for Stage 5 from United States Renal Data System (1998) include 230,000 patients treated by dialysis and assumes 70,000 additional patients not on dialysis. GFR estimated from serum creatinine by abbreviated Modification of Diet in Renal Disease Study equation based on age, sex, race, and calibration for serum creatinine. For Stages 1 and 2, kidney damage was assessed by spot albumin-to-creatinine ratio >17 mg/g (men) or >25 mg/g (women) on two measurements.

Reproduced and modified with permission from the National Kidney Foundation.

In 2002, the National Kidney Foundation published clinical guidelines that provide definitions and risk stratification for CKD (1). These guidelines are based on estimated GFR and are staged from 1 to 5 (Table 1). This table depicts the US prevalence of kidney disease based on these staging criteria. A GFR less than 60 mL/min/1.73 m² was selected as the cutoff for definition of CKD because it represents an approximate 50% reduction of what is assumed to be a normal GFR in young men and women. As will be examined later, when the GFR drops below 60 mL/min/1.73 m², there is a clear increase in the risk for cardiovascular events. End-stage kidney failure is defined as a GFR less than 15 mL/min/1.73 m², or treatment by dialysis or transplantation. Most patients beginning dialysis have an estimated GFR below 15 mL/min/1.73 m².

Although this classification system is based on GFR, it should be appreciated that another measure of kidney disease is evidence of albumin or protein in the urine. This measure also has important implications for CVD, to be addressed later in this chapter. However, an important issue is how this classification system needs to be adjusted based on the presence or absence of proteinuria at each CKD stage of GFR. For example, might a patient with Stage 2 CKD with proteinuria have more CVD risk than a patient with Stage 3 CKD but without proteinuria? These are interesting issues that need to be clarified in future clinical studies evaluating the CVD outcome of patients with CKD both with and without varying degrees of proteinuria.

8.2. WHY IS THERE A RELATIONSHIP BETWEEN CKD AND CVD?

Are CKD and CVD just epiphenomena, or are they causally related? Many CVD risk factors also explain the risk for CKD, largely because they explain an increased risk for vascular disease throughout the circulatory system. They can be considered traditional risk factors. However, there are also nontraditional risk factors that must be more carefully explored (2, 3).

Most of the traditional CVD risk factors—such as older age, diabetes mellitus, systolic hypertension, left ventricular hypertrophy (LVH), and dyslipidemia—are prevalent in patients with CKD *(2, 3)* (Table 2). However, a large number of nontraditional risk factors occur in patients with CKD, which may also relate to the development of CVD *(2)*. Perhaps the most important nontraditional risk factors are inflammation, oxidant stress, and vitamin D deficiency. The interplay of hyperhomocysteinemia,

Table 2
Traditional and Nontraditional Cardiovascular Risk Factors in CKD

Traditional risk factors	*Nontraditional risk factors*
Older age	Albuminuria
Male gender	Homocysteine
Hypertension	Lipoprotein(a) and apolipoprotein(a) isoforms
Higher LDL cholesterol	Lipoprotein remnants
Lower HDL cholesterol	Anemia
Diabetes	Abnormal calcium/phosphate metabolism
Smoking	Extracellular fluid volume overload
Physical inactivity	Electrolyte imbalance
Menopause	Oxidative stress
Family history of CVD	Inflammation (C-reactive protein)
LVH	Malnutrition
	Thrombogenic factors
	Sleep disturbances
	Altered nitric oxide/endothelin balance

LDL = low-density lipoprotein, HDL = high-density lipoprotein.
Reproduced and modified with permission from *(3)*.

Table 3
Approximate Prevalence of CVD in the General Population and CKD

	Ischemic heart disease (clinical)	*LVH (echo)*	*Heart failure (clinical)*
General population	8–13[a]	20[b]	3–6[c]
CKD Stages 3–4 (diabetic and nondiabetic kidney disease)	NA	25–50 (varies with level of kidney function)[d]	NA
CKD Stages 1–4 (kidney transplant recipients)	15[e]	50–70[f]	NA
CKD Stage 5 (hemodialysis)	40[g]	75[h]	40[g]
CKD Stage 5 (peritoneal dialysis)	40[g]	75[h]	40[g]

NA = not available.

Values are percentages.

[a]Age 55–64 years. The higher percentage is for men. Data are from NHANES III, American Heart Association Statistical Web *(7)*.

[b]Data from *(8)*.

[c]Age 55–64 years. The higher percentage is for men. Data are from NHANES III, American Heart Association Statistical Web *(7)*.

[d]Data from *(9)*.

[e]Data from *(10)*.

[f]Data from *(11–15)*.

[g]Data from *(16, 17)*.

[h]Data from *(5)*.

lipoprotein abnormalities, abnormal calcium and phosphorus metabolism, malnutrition, sleep disturbances, prothrombotic factors, etc. may also be involved.

The most important point is that classic CVD risk factors do not entirely explain the heightened CVD risk seen in patients with CKD. Thus, there must be interplay between these two elements to explain the increased risk. In fact, if one looks at the types of vascular disease seen in patients with CKD versus the general population, there is a higher prevalence of large vessel atherosclerotic disease, which is frequently calcified, as opposed to fibroatheromatous *(4)*. In addition, there is also a high prevalence of arteriolosclerosis and remodeling of large arteries associated with a loss of arterial compliance and increased systolic blood pressure. Cardiac dysfunction frequently occurs, with impaired pumping capability due to pressure or volume overload *(5)*. As depicted in Table 3, there is a greater prevalence of heart disease, including ischemic disease, hypertrophic disease, and heart failure, in patients with CKD compared to the general population.

8.3. REDUCED GFR AS A CVD EQUIVALENT

Figure 2 shows the smoothed 3-year predicted probability of developing CVD based on level of GFR in the Cardiovascular Health Study (CHS) *(6)*. The figure contrasts unadjusted with adjusted data for known CVD risk factors. These results show that much CKD risk arises from its association with CVD risk factors, but there is still evidence that the presence of CKD, in and of itself, is an important independent risk factor for cardiovascular events. For example, a GFR of 30 mL/min is associated with a 22% CVD risk compared to a 15% risk associated with a GFR of 130 mL/min even after one adjusts for other CVD risk factors.

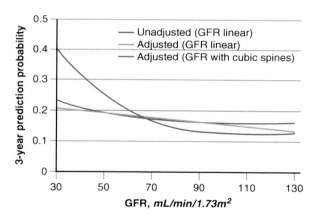

Fig. 2. Smoothed 3-year probability of developing CVD by level of GFR in the Cardiovascular Health Study. Unadjusted curve shows risk incorporating each individual's value for other individual's value for each other covarites. Adjusted curve shows average risk in population if everyone had GFR value shown on *x*-axis. Tick marks along the *x*-axis indicate GFR values for individual participants with events (marks from solid bar in GFR regions with many events). Reproduced and modified with permission from Manjunath et al. *(6)*.

These observations from the CHS study are not unique. In fact, decreased GFR has been consistently observed to be an important risk factor for CVD outcomes and all cause mortality in a variety of different populations with varying degrees of vascular disease, diabetes, or other cardiovascular risk factors *(6–9)*. Although in low-risk populations the relationship between the level of kidney function and outcomes is not as clear as it is in patients with more CVD burden *(10, 11)*, some of these studies have not used adequate measures of kidney function nor have they noted whether the patients had proteinuria. Duration of follow-up also may not have been sufficient to evaluate the long-term impact of reduced kidney function on outcome.

Many clinicians and investigators have discussed possible explanations for the independent association of impaired kidney function and increased risk for cardiovascular events. Some have hypothesized that reduced GFR may be just a surrogate measure of diffuse vascular disease. Others have suggested that reduced GFR may be a measure of residual confounding from traditional CVD risk factors (3). There is also concern that people with reduced GFR also have more of the nontraditional CVD risk factors, which, coupled with traditional risk factors, could increase the risk for cardiovascular events (12). Another, perhaps even more important, concern is that patients with reduced GFR may not always receive the appropriate medications to reduce cardiovascular event risk (drugs that block the renin–angiotensin system, aspirin, statins, etc.). Many patients with CKD, who may be malnourished or have a lot of inflammation, may have reduced low-density lipoprotein (LDL) cholesterol levels, which may not be indicative of a healthy lipoprotein profile. Reduced GFR may be a risk factor for progressive cardiac remodeling and dysfunction in addition to blood vessel disease.

Because of their increased CVD risk, patients with CKD benefit as much as, if not more than, non-CKD patients from appropriate medications and therapies. The higher the serum creatinine level, the greater the CVD risk and greater the advantage of directed cardiovascular risk-reduction strategies. From an epidemiologic standpoint, kidney dysfunction predicts increased cardiovascular event rate risk in the general population as well as increased mortality after acute myocardial infarction and stroke.

8.4. WHAT MUST WE DO DIFFERENTLY TO SCREEN PATIENTS FOR CKD?

The two most important considerations are to estimate GFR and to quantitate albumin or protein in the urine. It is important to appreciate that the serum creatinine level is not a good measure of GFR. As shown in Fig. 3, there is not a linear relationship between serum creatinine and GFR, particularly with a serum creatinine 0.8–1.2 mg/dL. A doubling of serum creatinine level, for example, from 2 to 4 mg/dL, is associated with a reduction in creatinine clearance. However, the relationship is much

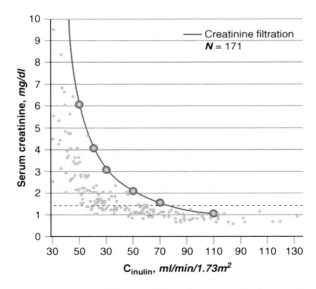

Fig. 3. The relationship between serum creatinine mg/dL and measured glomerular filtration rate. Reproduced with permission from Kidney International (67).

steeper with serum creatinines in the 1–2 mg/dL range. Note that changes in the serum creatinine level of only 1–1.5 mg/dL are associated with a substantial reduction in creatinine clearance that may not otherwise be clinically apparent. Simple formulae such as the Cockcroft–Gault equation *(13)* and abbreviated MDRD study equation *(14)* shown in Table 4 can be used to predict GFR based on serum creatinine. Many of these formulae can be preprogrammed into the laboratory or computer to provide quick estimation of GFR in older patients of smaller body habitus.

Table 4
Equations to Predict GFR Based on Serum Creatinine

Cockcroft–Gault equation	$$C_{Cr} \text{ (mL/min)} = \frac{(140 - \text{age}) \times \text{weight}}{72 \times S_{Cr}} \times (0.85 \text{ if female})$$
Abbreviated MDRD study equation	$GFR \text{ (mL/min/1.73 m}^2) = 186 \times (S_{Cr})^{-1.154} \times (\text{age})^{-0.203} \times (0.742 \text{ if female}) \times (1.210 \text{ if black})$

C_{Cr} = creatinine clearance, MDRD = Modification of Diet in Renal Disease, S_{Cr} = serum creatinine in mg/dL.

Age in years, weight in kilograms.

Objective measurement of albumin or protein in the urine is important. The traditional urine dipstick is not an objective measure of protein in the urine, but a concentration-dependent means of measuring albumin. The higher the specific gravity, the more likely albumin will be detectable. The lower the specific gravity, the less likely albumin will be detectable. A microalbumin dipstick, which is much more sensitive for small amounts of albumin, or a laboratory measurement of a spot urine albumin:creatinine ratio is much more objective at quantifying albumin or protein in the urine. Table 5 shows urine col-

Table 5
Definitions of Proteinuria

Urine collection method	Normal	Microalbuminuria	Albuminuria or clinical proteinuria
Total protein			
24-h excretion (varies with method)	<300 mg/day	NA	≥300 mg/day
Spot urine dipstick	<30 mg/dL	NA	≥30 mg/dL
Spot urine protein-to-creatinine ratio (varies with method)	<200 mg/g	NA	≥200 mg/g
Albumin			
24-h excretion	<300 mg/day	30–30 mg/day	>300 mg/day
Spot urine albumin-specific dipstick	<3 mg/dL	>3 mg/dL	NA
Spot urine albumin-to-creatinine ratio (varies by sex[a])	<17–250 mg/g (men) <25–355 mg/g (women)	17–250 mg/g (men) 25–355 mg/g (women)	>250 mg/g (men) > 355 mg/g (women)

NA = not applicable.

[a]Sex-specific cutoff values are from a single study. Use of the same cutoff value for men and women leads to higher values of prevalence for women than men. Current recommendations from the American Diabetes Association define cutoff values for spot urine albumin-to-creatinine ratio for microalbuminuria and albuminuria as 30 and 300 mg/g, respectively, without regard to sex.

Reproduced and modified with permission from the National Kidney Foundation.

lection methods and their associated definitions of normal, microalbuminuria, or clinical proteinuria. Although it is customary to obtain a 24-h urine sample, these samples are as easily overcollected as they are undercollected. Consequently, the ratio of the albumin or protein to creatinine is a more valid measure because it eliminates the variability of timed collections. A spot urine protein:creatinine ratio can be used because urine creatinine production remains constant as a measure of muscle breakdown from day to day. Thus, the only variable is the urine albumin or protein concentration. Although albuminuria or proteinuria can vary from day to day based on blood pressure, salt intake, posture, exercise, illness, etc., one can use repetitive measurements over time, just like the blood pressure, to screen for albumin or protein in the urine, as well as response to therapy.

8.5. WHY IS MICROALBUMINURIA SUCH A POWERFUL PREDICTOR OF CVD OUTCOMES?

Microalbuminuria is a predictor of CVD whether a patient has diabetes mellitus or not *(15–17)*. The relationship between microalbuminuria or proteinuria and clinical CVD has been confirmed in multiple different racial and ethnic groups and is strongest in patients with type 2 diabetes mellitus, largely because of their older age. In addition, there is also a strong association between albuminuria and subclinical measures of CVD such as carotid intimal media thickness, LVH, coronary artery disease, and even peripheral vascular disease *(18–20)*. Longitudinal studies also demonstrate the relationship between the amount of albumin in the urine and cardiovascular events. In the Heart Outcomes Prevention Evaluation (HOPE) study, as depicted in Fig. 4, a spot urine albumin:creatinine ratio at the start of this study was predictive of cardiovascular events in all participants, whether diabetic or not *(17)*. The albumin:creatinine ratio decile predicted events even below the traditional microalbuminuria threshold of 30 mg albumin/g creatinine. This indicates that the presence of albumin in the urine may be an important biomeasure of CVD burden and risk for events. In fact, this proved to be the most important predictor of cardiovascular events in the HOPE study.

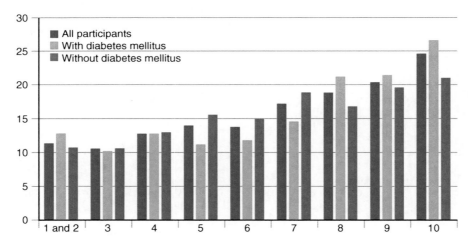

Fig. 4. All participants in the HOPE study had a spot urine microalbumin:creatinine ratio performed at the beginning of the trial. Note the continuous relationship between the albumin:creatinine ratio and cardiovascular events. Reproduced with permission from Gerstein et al. *(17) JAMA.*

Like reduced GFR, microalbuminuria could indicate a higher prevalence of traditional risk factors such as hypertension, dyslipidemia, and diabetes. However, there is still an independent adverse prognostic risk for cardiovascular events even after one adjusts for these factors. Some have suggested that the presence of microalbuminuria may be reflective of generalized endothelial dysfunction with increased vascular permeability coupled with abnormalities of the coagulation and fibrinolytic systems *(21–23)*. However, albumin in the urine could be nothing more than evidence of diffuse vascular and target organ disease throughout the body. Therapeutic strategies that result in a reduction in microalbuminuria or proteinuria result in better long-term kidney and CVD outcomes.

8.6. TREATMENT STRATEGIES OF TRADITIONAL RISK FACTORS

Routine lifestyle modifications should include increased physical activity, moderation of salt and alcohol intake, weight loss, and, most importantly, smoking cessation. Cigarette smoking is the most important preventable cause of early mortality in the United States *(24)*. In patients with CKD, there is evidence that cigarette smoking may increase the risk of incident kidney disease *(24)*. In addition, since many patients with CKD also have diabetes, it is important to note that studies have found a 2–11-fold increase in early death in smokers with diabetes compared with others who did not smoke *(15)*. Similarly, smoking potentiates the microvascular complications of diabetes and can substantially worsen renal and peripheral vascular disease *(25, 26)*.

Cigarette smoking appears to interfere with vascular health in multiple ways. The smoke itself acts as a direct source of the glycosylation end products that destroy vascular integrity *(27)*. Smoking increases the oxidation of LDL cholesterol, as well as its uptake by monocytes and vascular smooth muscle cells, thereby promoting atherogenesis. Smoking also appears to interfere with the benefits of modifying other cardiovascular risk factors. Consequently, smoking cessation needs to be a top priority in diabetes management.

Dietary salt intake may also be a concern in the patient with CKD *(28)*. There is abundant evidence that it raises blood pressure, and experimental evidence linking increased salt exposure with kidney tissue injury *(26)*. Proper diet, exercise, and weight control are likely also important for CKD patients, not just because they have increased risk for kidney disease but also because obesity has been linked to glomerular kidney disease and may be associated with increased risk for renal disease progression *(29)*.

8.7. DIABETES CONTROL

Diabetes mellitus is the leading cause of ESRD in the United States and contributes to nearly 50% of the total number of patients on dialysis. More patients would develop ESRD secondary to diabetes were it not for the competing hazard of cardiovascular events. Consequently, earlier diagnosis and management of diabetes in the CKD patient is essential. Unfortunately, most of the data on treatment benefits are in the general population, and often patients with CKD are excluded from the studies. It was not until the last decade that the importance of vigorous glucose control was proven in patients with type 2 diabetes. The United Kingdom Prospective Diabetes Study (UKPDS) demonstrated that in non-CKD patients, tighter glucose control (HbA1c 0.9% lower than the control group) is linked to reductions in combined endpoints for diabetes-related events of sudden death, hypoglycemia and hyperglycemia, myocardial infarction (MI), angina, heart failure, stroke, renal failure, amputations, and blindness *(30)*. Importantly, the risk of fatal and nonfatal MI was reduced by 16% with tighter control. These results, although modest, in no way minimize the importance of better glucose control, but they emphasize the impact that the other cardiovascular risk factors can have on these endpoints. The Diabetes Complications and Control Trial (DCCT) unequivocally demonstrated a significant reduction in the microvascular complications of retinopathy, neuropathy, and nephropathy in non-CKD patients with type 1 diabetes with more intensive glycemic control *(31, 32)*. Thus, both these trials showed that any reduction in HbA1c reduced the risk of complications, with the lowest risk being in those patients with HbA1c in the normal range (less than 6%).

In a recent large-pooled analysis *(33)*, there was a continuous and significant relationship between the risks for macrovascular disease and HbA1c level in non-CKD patients. In this analysis, a 1% increase in HbA1c represented a 20% increase in the risk for CVD. Interestingly, this relationship was also seen in among normoglycemic (nondiabetic) adults along the continuum of HbA1C between 5 and 6.9%.

Some controversy about optimal achieved levels of the HbA1c exists in the literature. The more intensive glycemic control arm of the Action to Control Cardiovascular Risk in Diabetes (ACCORD) study was terminated early due to increased evidence of cardiovascular events *(34)*. In this study, non-CKD patients with type 2 diabetes were randomized to two treatment levels of HbA1c (7.0–7.9%, or less than 6.0) and systolic blood pressure (less than 130 mmHg or less than 120 mmHg). The median HbA1c in the standard group was 7.5%, and in the intensive group 6.4%. The study was stopped after 3.5 years because of increased mortality (HR 1.22, $p = 0.04$) in the intensive group *(34)*.

It is beyond the scope of this chapter to make specific recommendations about hypoglycemic therapy. Many effective strategies exist using insulin and oral antidiabetic medications. Unfortunately, one of the most effective oral medications, metformin, is not indicated in patients with CKD (estimated GFR below 50 mL/min/1.73 m^2) due to increased risk of life-threatening lactic acidosis.

8.8. HYPERTENSION CONTROL

Epidemiological evidence indicates that there is a continuous relationship between blood pressure and cardiovascular events *(35, 36)*. Needless to say, the patient with CKD is at increased risk for cardiovascular events, and the choice of a blood pressure goal is of great importance. Current guidelines indicate that a goal systolic blood pressure below 130 mmHg is indicated for patients with CKD, whether or not they have diabetes *(37)*. Previous guidelines have suggested that if there is evidence of proteinuria, a lower goal of 125/75 mmHg may be preferable *(38)*. However, there are no prospective studies evaluating the benefit of lower blood pressure goals on the incidence of either cardiovascular events or the rate of progression of kidney disease.

One might infer from epidemiological data that patients treated to lower blood pressure goals would have the same CV risk as people with lower blood pressure who do not require treatment. Yet, prospective studies have not been done to test this consideration. What is clear, however, from secondary analyses from numerous trials of patients with CKD, is that lower levels of systolic blood pressure (preferably into the 120–130 mmHg range) are associated with less likelihood for progression of kidney disease. This benefit is seen sooner in those patients with more protein in the urine. For example, in the Modification of Diet in Renal Disease (MDRD) study, patients with more than 3 g/day of protein in their urine demonstrated the benefit of a blood pressure goal of 125/75 mmHg versus the traditional goal of 140/90 mmHg within 8 months of randomization *(39)*. For patients with 1–3 g/day of protein in their urine, it took 2 years to demonstrate the advantage of the lower blood pressure treatment goal. Whereas, in patients with less than 1 g/day of protein in the urine, there did not appear to be a difference in favor of lower blood pressure on the rate of progression of kidney disease after 3 years of follow-up.

So, whether a patient has diabetic or nondiabetic kidney disease, it is evident in the literature from secondary analyses of clinical trials that achieved levels of systolic blood pressure, between 120 and 130 mmHg, appear optimal for slowing progression of kidney disease *(40, 41)*. Unfortunately, these studies were not powered to evaluate the advantage of lower systolic blood pressure and the risk for cardiovascular events. In a sense, one must take it on faith that those lower levels of blood pressure associated with stabilization of kidney disease progression, likely will also provide benefits with regard to cardiovascular events. This was certainly the case when Berl and his colleagues evaluated levels of achieved systolic blood pressure on cardiovascular events in the Irbesartan Diabetic Nephropathy

Trial *(42)*. It was evident from their analysis that achieved levels of systolic blood pressure in the 120–130 mmHg range also appeared to be beneficial with regard to the relative risk for cardiovascular events.

Often patients with kidney disease will need multiple drugs to control blood pressure. This requirement is in large part related to the multiple factors that contribute to blood pressure elevation in the patient with CKD such as volume overload, sympathetic nervous system activation, and perhaps excess activity of the renin–angiotensin system within the kidneys. Another factor that contributes to the requirement of multiple medications in the patient with CKD is the need for lower systolic blood pressure goals. As a result, it is not uncommon for patients with CKD to require three to five medications for achieving blood pressure control *(43, 44)*.

Often patients with CKD will require some form of diuretic support. For patients with estimated glomerular filtration rate (GFR) below 50 mL/min, loop diuretics may be preferred, as thiazide diuretics lose their natriuretic efficacy at lower levels of GFR. On the other hand, not well tested is whether the vasodilatory effects of thiazide diuretics are of importance in patients with lower GFR. Beta-blockers may be useful in patients with CKD to assist in blood pressure reduction, and cardioprotection. The negative chronotropic effects of beta-blockers may be of value in limiting the risk for ischemia, particularly in patients with CKD who are at higher risk for CVD. Beta-blockers may also be helpful if the patient has had a previous MI, known coronary ischemia, systolic heart failure, or hypertrophic cardiomyopathy.

Drugs that modify the activity of the renin–angiotensin system are routinely indicated in patients with CKD by all of the major guidelines (American Diabetes Association, National Kidney Foundation, Joint National Commission). In large part, this recommendation stems from the evidence from multiple clinical trials in patients with diabetic and nondiabetic kidney disease indicating that lower blood pressure in conjunction with renin–angiotensin system blockade is associated with delayed progression of kidney disease and fewer patients reaching end-stage renal disease *(40, 41, 45, 46)*. Many of the clinical trials of CKD have used composite endpoints of doubling of serum creatinine, end-stage renal disease, or all cause death. Consistently, lower achieved levels of blood pressure coupled with renin–angiotensin system blockade are associated with reduction in the composite endpoint *(40, 41, 45, 46)*.

The data indicating renal protection with ACE inhibitors and angiotensin receptor blockers in clinical trials of patients with CKD are very similar. More clinical trials have been done with ACE inhibitors in patients with nondiabetic kidney disease and in patients with type 1 diabetes, whereas the majority of data in patients with CKD due to type 2 diabetes have been performed with angiotensin receptor blockers. The only head-to-head clinical trial comparing an ACE inhibitor and angiotensin receptor blocker in diabetics did not show a difference in renoprotective benefits *(47)*. It is for these reasons that current guidelines endorse the use of drugs that block the renin–angiotensin system in patients with all forms of kidney disease, particularly, if there is evidence of proteinuria. Another interesting finding in the clinical trials of patients with CKD is that the higher the serum creatinine, the greater the risk-reduction benefits of drugs that block the renin–angiotensin system *(48)*. Although these drugs do require greater vigilance and patient monitoring when used in patients with higher serum creatinine levels, it is quite apparent, probably due to the patient's increased risk for kidney and CVD progression, that renin–angiotensin system blockade coupled with lower blood pressure goals provides important cardiovascular and kidney risk-reduction benefits. A recent paper by Hou et al. demonstrated that even patients with nondiabetic kidney disease with a creatinine as high as 5.0 mg/dL can be safely and effectively treated with renin–angiotensin system blockade *(49)*. Likewise, in diabetic nephropathy, there is ample safety and efficacy data in patients with estimated glomerular filtration rates in the 20–40 mL/min/1.73 m^2 range to demonstrate the advantage of renin–angiotensin system inhibition *(43, 44)*. Although the frequency of hyperkalemia defined as a serum potassium of 5.5 mEq/L or greater is more common in patients receiving renin–angiotensin system blocking drugs, one has to remember that only 1–2% of patients have to stop these drugs due to problems with serum potassium. Often elevated potassium levels are related to hemolysis. As many as two thirds of these readings normalize when repeated *(44)*. Thus, the important take-home message is that lower blood pressure and blocking the renin–angiotensin system are the key aspects of all therapeutic approaches for the treatment of hypertension in patients with CKD.

Measuring a urine albumin:creatinine ratio is also an important opportunity to identify patients at greater cardiovascular risk. This is true not only in patients with CKD, but also in the general population *(28)*. Epidemiological data indicate that there is a continuous relationship between the amount of albumin in the urine and risk for cardiovascular events *(50, 51)*. Moreover, secondary analyses of clinical trials indicate that net levels of achieved proteinuria reduction are also predictive of modification of risk for progression of kidney disease or the development of cardiovascular events *(45, 52)*. Thus, residual albuminuria may serve as an important biomeasure, not only of risk for CVD, but also, perhaps, for adequacy of response to the treatment strategy (blood pressure level achieved and medications used). Although there are no prospective studies showing that purposeful reduction of proteinuria with medication reduces the risk of cardiovascular events or progression of kidney disease, many clinicians would agree that given the consistency of the data from many clinical studies, monitoring change in urinary albumin excretion may be a worthwhile endeavor to gauge the adequacy of the antihypertensive treatment regimen.

It is important to note that albumin or protein in the urine should be objectively measured. This is preferably done with urine albumin or protein:creatinine ratio *(28)*. Either a spot specimen or an overnight collection will suffice. Since muscle mass can be assumed to be constant, the urine creatinine should not vary. Thus, the albumin or protein:creatinine ratio can provide an approximate assessment of daily urine albumin or protein excretion without the problems of an under- or overcollection of a 24-h urine specimen. Due to the simplicity of this test, it can be repeated longitudinally as one would also measure blood pressure. In Table 2, the traditional definitions in ways of measuring urine protein and albumin are listed.

8.9. HYPERLIPIDEMIA CONTROL

As with blood pressure and serum glucose levels, there is some debate as to what are optimal treatment goals, particularly with regard to LDL cholesterol in patients with CKD. Although the risk for CVD is abnormally high in patients with CKD, there is limited data to guide the use of lipid-lowering drugs in these populations because the majority of trials in the general population have often excluded patients with CKD *(51)*. Also, since there are both pathophysiologic and epidemiological differences in the patterns of CVD in the patients with CKD compared to the general population, perhaps the study findings derived from the observations in the general population may not be directly applicable to patients with CKD. The National Kidney Foundation Disease Outcomes Quality Initiative Workgroup provided some guidelines several years ago for managing dyslipidemia in individuals with CKD *(1)*. However, since these guidelines were published, additional data may refine some of these recommendations.

Two major studies in the general population provide important consideration. The Heart Protection Study was a randomized clinical trial in more than 20,000 individuals, which demonstrated clear benefits of a statin in patients with and without diabetes for primary and secondary prevention for cardiovascular events, regardless of initial untreated LDL cholesterol *(53)*. The Cholesterol Treatment Trial Collaboration analyzed the data of more than 90,000 people *(54)*. Statin therapy significantly reduced the incidence of the primary outcome in the patients with impaired kidney function. The hazard ratio was 0.77 (95% confidence interval 0.68–0.86). This effect was very similar to the primary outcome in patients with normal kidney function. In general, the current literature supports the recommendations of the guidelines with regard to patients with CKD, indicating that an LDL cholesterol goal below

100 mg/dL is desirable and that fasting triglycerides should also be corrected with therapeutic lifestyle changes and triglyceride-lowering agents (1). These guidelines have also suggested that non-HDL cholesterol should also be targeted to below 130 mg/dL (55).

Despite the scarcity of literature on statin use and cardiovascular outcomes in patients with CKD, it is reasonable to apply currently accepted NCEP ATP III guidelines to the treatment of LDL cholesterol levels in patients with CKD (55). However, it is also important to note that given the results of the Heart Protection Study and the Cholesterol Treatment Trial Collaboration (54), there is a strong argument to abandon a threshold-based algorithm for treating dyslipidemia. It may be more appropriate to consider that lower achieved levels of LDL cholesterol in patients with increased cardiovascular risks is advisable, regardless of initial LDL level. Rather, it may be more appropriate to achieve at least a 30–40% reduction in LDL cholesterol from baseline, and to reduce LDL cholesterol at least to below NCEP ATP III LDL goal levels. Given the results of the Pravastatin Pooling Project (56), it is advisable to aggressively treat patients with CKD who have an estimated GFR in the 30–60 mL/min/1.73 m^2 range with known coronary heart disease and probably also those without known coronary heart disease. As mentioned previously, all the major guidelines now indicate that estimated GFR below 60 mL/min/1.73 m^2, proteinuria, or microalbuminuria are coronary artery disease equivalents, and should be treated to LDL-C and non-HDL-C goals of <100 mg/dL and <130 mg/dL.

8.10. NONTRADITIONAL RISK FACTORS FOR CVD

There are numerous non-traditional cardiovascular risk factors for CVD in patients with CKD (3). Whether specific treatment of these risk factors will result in cardiovascular risk reduction or possibly even slowing progression of kidney disease is unknown. The importance of microalbuminuria as a predictive factor for CVD and residual albuminuria as a potential biomeasure of therapeutic success has already been discussed. The treatment of homocysteine with folic acid and vitamin B$_6$ does not appear to be beneficial in the general population (57). There is a large ongoing study in kidney transplant recipients, which may provide insight as to whether homocysteine lowering is beneficial for CVD event reduction or not (57). The treatment of lipoprotein(a) and its various isoforms is an active area of ongoing research. No definitive studies are available at the current time.

The treatment of anemia was once thought to be important in the patient for CKD, not only to restore vitality, but perhaps also to reduce likelihood of CVD progression. Two large studies in patients with CKD have not demonstrated the benefit of hemoglobin correction above 12 mg/dL (58, 59). If anything, there was a paradoxical increase in risk for kidney disease progression and cardiovascular events if hemoglobin was treated above 13 mg/dL. Although these studies were flawed because of the large number of dropouts, and the short duration of follow-up, they both indicated trends that higher hemoglobin correction is not advantageous for patients. Consequently, current recommendations are to use erythrocyte-stimulating agents to correct hemoglobin into the 11–12 mg/dL range, and no higher. One important consideration about anemia correction with erythrocyte-stimulating agents is the associated increase in blood pressure (60). This may be related to the dose of the erythropoietic drugs rather than the net level of hemoglobin correction. Consequently, when using these agents, blood pressure needs to be monitored carefully and aggressively treated.

Oxidative stress, inflammation, malnutrition, and thrombogenic factors are all suspected to be important factors that may contribute to cardiovascular risk in patients with CKD (3). Unfortunately, there are no available data to suggest that the correction of these abnormalities results in fewer cardiovascular events. Sleep disturbances are also more common in patients with CKD. Although positive pressure oxygen therapy at night improves sleep, and may even lower blood pressure, there are no data to show that it improves longevity.

Perhaps the one area that is of greatest interest of all the nontraditional risk factors is the use of activated vitamin D supplementation in patients with CKD. Recent reports suggest that activated vitamin D supplementation in patients with CKD is associated with improved survival *(60)*. In addition, there is evidence to suggest potential health benefits of vitamin D beyond reducing serum parathyroid hormone levels in both the general population and in patients with CKD(s). Lower 25-hydroxyvitamin D and 1,25-dihydroxyvitamin D levels have been associated with cardiovascular risk factors including inflammation, glucose intolerance, and albuminuria *(61)*. In contrast, investigators have noted lower risk for death or dialysis with activated vitamin D use in patients with Stage 3 and Stage 4 CKD *(62)*. Moreover, there is experimental evidence indicating unique cellular benefits of activated vitamin D, as well as evidence that inadequate vitamin D receptor activation worsens diabetic nephropathy *(63)*. In clinical studies of activated vitamin D supplementation, investigators have noted reduced proteinuria in patients with chronic kidney disease *(64)*. Others have demonstrated that activated vitamin D has antiproteinuric effects in patients with nephropathy *(65)*, despite concomitant use of renal angiotensin system blockers.

Unfortunately, there are no prospective clinical trials that have been completed to test the hypothesis that activated vitamin D supplementation will reduce the likelihood of cardiovascular events in patients with CKD. Fortunately, there is one ongoing trial to answer this intriguing question. In the meantime, it is fair to say that patients with CKD should have vitamin D and parathyroid hormone levels measured, and activated vitamin D supplementation should be provided in deficient patients as part of good general clinical care. Whether it will prove to be a strategy of the future for reducing the risk for CVD is unknown.

8.11. SUMMARY

Chronic kidney disease is unequivocally associated with more CVD. This relationship persists whether or not patients have albuminuria. Whether the definition of CKD should be based on estimated GFR or albuminuria, or both, is not yet agreed upon.

The much greater frequency of CVD in patients with CKD can be explained by traditional CVD risk factors such as hypertension, diabetes, and dyslipidemia. However, a large number of other nontraditional risk factors could explain the independent association of CKD and CVD.

Future clinical research is necessary to establish optimal goals and treatment strategies for blood pressure, cholesterol, and glucose in patients with CKD. The available epidemiological data indicate that a threshold-based algorithm is not appropriate. Certainly, the data for blood pressure and LDL cholesterol indicate a continuous relationship between levels and CVD events. There may be more controversy as to the safety of achieving lower levels of hemoglobin A1C in patients with diabetes.

Also important are the nontraditional risk factors. Whether they will also require treatment to reduce CV events is an important area of future study. Vitamin D deficiency may be the most important of the new nontraditional risk fractions that require screening and treatment.

Perhaps the most important consideration is that earlier recognition of CKD, whether by using estimated GFR determination, or an albumin:creatinine ratio, is an important and a valuable way to recognize patients who need global cardiovascular risk-reducing strategies.

8.12. CASE STUDIES

8.12.1. Case 1

A 58-year-old black female with type 2 diabetes mellitus, hypertension, and CKD. She admits to dietary indiscretion and noncompliance with her medication regimen and is asymptomatic except for minor fatigue. She has evidence of retinopathy and 2+ pitting edema. BP is 148/104 mmHg, $P = 78$ BPM. Current medications include insulin 15 units NPH q 12H, amlodipine 5 mg daily, HCTZ 25 mg daily, and simvastatin 40 mg daily.

8.12.1.1. LABORATORY DATA

BUN: 40 mg/dL
Creatinine: 2.0 mg/dL
24-h urine protein: 1 g
K: 4.5 mEq/L
LDL cholesterol: 150 mg/dL
HDL cholesterol: 35 mg/dL
TG: 300 mg/dL
Glucose: 220 mg/dL
HbA1C: 7.8%

8.12.1.2. ISSUES

1. Discuss use of diuretics in patients with CKD and poorly controlled diabetes.
2. How would you manage this patient's hypertension?
3. What impact does edema have on your treatment decision?
4. Is edema related to use of amlodipine and/or decreased renal function?

8.12.1.3. DISCUSSION POINTS

- Both ACEIs and ARBs have proven to be beneficial for the treatment of diabetic nephropathy (independent of BP effects).
- ACEIs have been studied primarily in Type 1 DM and ARBs in T2DM.
- Loop diuretics may be required rather than thiazides if creatinine >1.8 mg/dL to restore euvolemia and water retention.
- Beta-blockers would be indicated with CHF or a history of myocardial infarction.
- Edema likely will require diuretics. Some edema may be due to amlodipine, which could be alleviated by renin–angiotensin system blockade.
- More aggressive management of this patient's lipids and glucose should be considered as well.

8.12.2. Case 2

A 65-year-old white obese male with a history of stroke, diabetes mellitus, PAD, hyperlipidemia, and hypertension. He does not smoke. Current medications include metformin 1.5 g, HCTZ 12.5 mg, and atenolol 50 mg daily.

8.12.2.1. PHYSICAL EXAMINATION

BMI: 35 kg/m^2
Waist circumference: 46 in.
BP: 154/108
PL: 60 BPM
Peripheral pulses diminished
Bilateral carotid bruits
ECG: First-degree AV block, old IWMI

8.12.2.2. LABORATORY RESULTS

Total cholesterol: 225 mg/dL
LDL cholesterol: 145 mg/dL
HDL cholesterol: 33 mg/dL
TG: 160 mg/dL
FBG: 140 mg/dL

Creatinine: 1.5 mg/dL
HbA1C: 7.2%
Microalbuminuria: 250 mg/g creatinine

8.12.2.3. ISSUES

1. What are the glucose, lipid, and BP treatment goals in this patient?
2. How would you treat this patient?
3. Which antiplatelet therapy would you institute?
4. How low should you treat blood pressure?

8.12.2.4. DISCUSSION POINTS

- Lifestyle modification should be attempted, but will likely not be entirely helpful.
- Framingham 10-year risk is 27%, hence need to institute aggressive lipid management. Begin with a statin.
- Selection of an agent other than metformin (contraindicated with creatinine >1.5 mg/dL) to improve blood glucose control should be considered to achieve HbA1C <6.5% or 7.0%. Can transition to sulfonylurea plus a dipeptidyl peptidase inhibitor, or to insulin.
- Beta-blockers in the setting of PAD no longer contraindicated. Moreover, he has evidence of an old inferior wall MI on EKG. Continue the beta-blocker.
- ACEI or ARB would be indicated in view of albuminuria and history of stroke.
- Goal blood pressure should be less than 130 mmHg.
- Substitution of loop diuretic for thiazide may be worthwhile.
- Antiplatelet agent is also warranted (aspirin 81 mg daily).
- ABI determination would be useful to determine severity of PAD.
- Carotid ultrasound should be performed given history of stroke.
- LDL cholesterol below 100 mg/dL, or preferably below 70 mg/dL, is optimal. In addition, given his high-risk status, non-HDL-C should be reduced to <130 mg/dL or preferably <100 mg/dL and effort should be made to raise his HDL-C, per NCEP recommendations for a high-risk patient.

REFERENCES

1. K/DOQI NKF. Clinical practice guidelines for management of dyslipidemias in patients with kidney disease: evaluation, classification, and stratification. *Am J Kidney Dis.* 2003;41:I–91.
2. Sarnak MJ, Levey AS. Cardiovascular disease and chronic renal disease: a new paradigm. *Am J Kidney Dis.* 2000;35:S117–S131.
3. Sarnak MJ, Levey AS, Schoolwerth AC, et al. Kidney disease as a risk factor for development of cardiovascular disease: a statement from the American Heart Association Councils on Kidney in Cardiovascular Disease, High Blood Pressure Research, Clinical Cardiology, and Epidemiology and Prevention. *Circulation.* 2003;108:2154–21569.
4. London GM, Marchais SJ, Guerin AP, Metivier F, Adda H. Arterial structure and function in end-stage renal disease. *Nephrol Dial Transplant.* 2002;17:1713–1724.
5. Foley RN, Parfrey PS, Harnett JD, et al. Clinical and echocardiographic disease in patients starting end-stage renal disease therapy. *Kidney Int.* 1995;47:186–192.
6. Manjunath G, Tighiouart H, Coresh J, et al. Level of kidney function as a risk factor for cardiovascular outcomes in the elderly. *Kidney Int.* 2003;63:1121–1129.
7. Henry RM, Kostense PJ, Bos G, et al. Mild renal insufficiency is associated with increased cardiovascular mortality: the Hoorn Study. *Kidney Int.* 2002;62:1402–1407.
8. Schillaci G, Reboldi G, Verdecchia P. High-normal serum creatinine concentration is a predictor of cardiovascular risk in essential hypertension. *Arch Intern Med.* 2001;161:886–891.
9. Shulman NB, Ford CE, Hall WD, et al. Prognostic value of serum creatinine and effect of treatment of hypertension on renal function. Results from the hypertension detection and follow-up program. The Hypertension Detection and Follow-up Program Cooperative Group. *Hypertension.* 1989;13:I80–I93.

10. Culleton BF, Larson MG, Wilson PW, Evans JC, Parfrey PS, Levy D. Cardiovascular disease and mortality in a community-based cohort with mild renal insufficiency. *Kidney Int.* 1999;56:2214–2219.

11. Garg AX, Clark WF, Haynes RB, House AA. Moderate renal insufficiency and the risk of cardiovascular mortality: results from the NHANES I. *Kidney Int.* 2002;61:1486–1494.

12. Shlipak MG, Fried LF, Crump C, et al. Elevations of inflammatory and procoagulant biomarkers in elderly persons with renal insufficiency. *Circulation.* 2003;107:87–92.

13. Cockcroft DW, Gault MH. Prediction of creatinine clearance from serum creatinine. *Nephron.* 1976;16:31–41.

14. Levey AS, Bosch JP, Lewis JB, Greene T, Rogers N, Roth D. A more accurate method to estimate glomerular filtration rate from serum creatinine: a new prediction equation. Modification of Diet in Renal Disease Study Group. *Ann Intern Med.* 1999;130:461–470.

15. Agewall S, Wikstrand J, Ljungman S, Fagerberg B. Usefulness of microalbuminuria in predicting cardiovascular mortality in treated hypertensive men with and without diabetes mellitus. Risk Factor Intervention Study Group. *Am J Cardiol.* 1997;80:164–169.

16. Dinneen SF, Gerstein HC. The association of microalbuminuria and mortality in non-insulin-dependent diabetes mellitus. A systematic overview of the literature. *Arch Intern Med.* 1997;157:1413–1418.

17. Gerstein HC, Mann JFE, Yi Q, et al. Albuminuria and risk of cardiovascular events, death, and heart failure in diabetic and nondiabetic individuals. *JAMA.* 2001;286:421–426.

18. Mykkanen L, Zaccaro DJ, O'Leary DH, Howard G, Robbins DC, Haffner SM. Microalbuminuria and carotid artery intima-media thickness in nondiabetic and NIDDM subjects. The Insulin Resistance Atherosclerosis Study (IRAS). *Stroke.* 1997;28:1710–1716.

19. Stephenson JM, Kenny S, Stevens LK, Fuller JH, Lee E. Proteinuria and mortality in diabetes: the WHO Multinational Study of Vascular Disease in Diabetes. *Diabet Med.* 1995;12:149–155.

20. Suzuki K, Kato K, Hanyu O, Nakagawa O, Aizawa Y. Left ventricular mass index increases in proportion to the progression of diabetic nephropathy in type 2 diabetic patients. *Diabetes Res Clin Pract.* 2001;54:173–180.

21. Festa A, D'Agostino R, Howard G, Mykkanen L, Tracy RP, Haffner SM. Inflammation and microalbuminuria in nondiabetic and type 2 diabetic subjects: The Insulin Resistance Atherosclerosis Study. *Kidney Int.* 2000;58:1703–1710.

22. Stehouwer CD, Nauta JJ, Zeldenrust GC, Hackeng WH, Donker AJ, den Ottolander GJ. Urinary albumin excretion, cardiovascular disease, and endothelial dysfunction in non-insulin-dependent diabetes mellitus. *Lancet.* 1992;340:319–323.

23. Stehouwer CD, Lambert J, Donker AJ, van H V. Endothelial dysfunction and pathogenesis of diabetic angiopathy. *Cardiovasc Res.* 1997;34:55–68.

24. Jones-Burton C, Seliger SL, Scherer RW, et al. Cigarette smoking and incident chronic kidney disease: a systematic review. *Am J Nephrol.* 2007;27:342–351.

25. Chuahirun T, Khanna A, Kimball K, Wesson DE. Cigarette smoking and increased urine albumin excretion are interrelated predictors of nephropathy progression in type 2 diabetes. *Am J Kidney Dis.* 2003;41:13–21.

26. Messerli FH, Weir MR, Neutel JM. Combination therapy of amlodipine/benazepril versus monotherapy of amlodipine in a practice-based setting. *Am J Hypertens.* 2002;15:550–556.

27. Tracy RE, Malcom GT, Oalmann MC, Newman WP III, Guzman MA. Nephrosclerosis, glycohemoglobin, cholesterol, and smoking in subjects dying of coronary heart disease. *Mod Pathol.* 1994;7:301–309.

28. Weir MR, Dworkin LD. Antihypertensive drugs, dietary salt, and renal protection: how low should you go and with which therapy? *Am J Kidney Dis.* 1998;32:1–22.

29. Young JA, Hwang SJ, Sarnak MJ, et al. Association of visceral and subcutaneous adiposity with kidney function. *Clin J Am Soc Nephrol.* 2008;3:1786–1791.

30. Intensive blood-glucose control with sulphonylureas or insulin compared with conventional treatment and risk of complications in patients with type 2 diabetes (UKPDS 33). *Lancet.* 1998;352:837–853.

31. Nathan DM, Cleary PA, Backlund JY, et al. Retinopathy and nephropathy in patients with type 1 diabetes four years after a trial of intensive therapy. *N Engl J Med.* 2000;342:381–389.

32. Nathan DM, Cleary PA, Backlund JY, et al. Intensive diabetes treatment and cardiovascular disease in patients with type 1 diabetes. *N Engl J Med.* 2005;353:2643–2653.

33. Khaw KT, Wareham N, Luben R, et al. Glycated haemoglobin, diabetes, and mortality in men in Norfolk cohort of European prospective investigation of cancer and nutrition (EPIC-Norfolk). *BMJ.* 2001;322:15–18.

34. The Action to Control Cardiovascular Risk in Diabetes Study Group. Effects of intensive glucose lowering in type 2 diabetes. *N Engl J Med.* 2008;358:2545–2559.

35. Lewington S, Clarke R, Qizilbash N, Peto R, Collins R. Age-specific relevance of usual blood pressure to vascular mortality: a meta-analysis of individual data for one million adults in 61 prospective studies. *Lancet.* 2002;360:1903–1913.

36. Vasan RS, Larson MG, Leip EP, et al. Impact of high-normal blood pressure on the risk of cardiovascular disease. *N Engl J Med.* 2001;345:1291–1297.

37. Chobanian AV, Bakris GL, Black HR, et al. The seventh report of the Joint National Committee on Prevention, Detection, Evaluation, and Treatment of High Blood Pressure: the JNC 7 report. *JAMA*. 2003;289:2560–2571.

38. Joint National Committee on Detection, Evaluation and Treatment of High Blood Pressure. The sixth report of the Joint National Committee on Detection, Evaluation, and Treatment of High Blood Pressure (JNC VI). NIH Publications, Bethesda, MD. 1997:98–4080.

39. Klahr S, Levey AS, Beck GJ, et al. The effects of dietary protein restriction and blood-pressure control on the progression of chronic renal disease. Modification of Diet in Renal Disease Study Group. *N Engl J Med*. 1994;330:877–884.

40. Jafar TH, Stark PC, Schmid CH, et al. Progression of chronic kidney disease: the role of blood pressure control, proteinuria, and angiotensin-converting enzyme inhibition: a patient-level meta-analysis. *Ann Intern Med*. 2003;139:244–252.

41. Pohl MA, Blumenthal S, Cordonnier DJ, et al. Independent and additive impact of blood pressure control and angiotensin ii receptor blockade on renal outcomes in the Irbesartan Diabetic Nephropathy Trial: clinical implications and limitations. *J Am Soc Nephrol*. 2005;16(10):3027–3037.

42. Berl T, Hunsicker LG, Lewis JB, et al. Impact of achieved blood pressure on cardiovascular outcomes in the Irbesartan Diabetic Nephropathy Trial. *J Am Soc Nephrol*. 2005;16:2170–2179.

43. Brenner BM, Cooper ME, de Zeeuw D, et al. Effects of losartan on renal and cardiovascular outcomes in patients with type 2 diabetes and nephropathy. *Engl J Med*. 2001;345:861–869.

44. Lewis EJ, Hunsicker LG, Clarke WR, Berl T, Pohl MA, Lewis JB, et al. Renoprotective effect of the angiotensin-receptor antagonist irbesartan in patients with nephropathy due to type 2 diabetes. *N Engl J Med*. 2001;345:851–860.

45. Dezeeuw D, Remuzzi G, Parving HH, et al. Proteinuria, a target for renoprotection in patients with type 2 diabetic nephropathy: lessons from RENAAL. *Kidney Int*. 2004;65:2309–2320.

46. Wright JT Jr, Bakris G, Greene T, et al. Effect of blood pressure lowering and antihypertensive drug class on progression of hypertensive kidney disease: results from the AASK Trial. *JAMA*. 2002;288:2421–2431.

47. Barnett AH, Bain SC, Bouter P, et al. Angiotensin-receptor blockade versus converting-enzyme inhibition in type 2 diabetes and nephropathy. *N Engl J Med*. 2004;351:1952–1961.

48. Lewis EJ, Hunsicker LG, Bain RP, Rohde RD. The Collaborative Study Group. The effect of angiotensin-converting-enzyme inhibition on diabetic nephropathy. *N Engl J Med*. 1993;329:1456–1462.

49. Hou FF, Zhang X, Zhang GH, et al. Efficacy and Safety of benazepril for advanced chronic renal insufficiency. *N Engl J Med*. 2006;354:131–140.

50. Mann JF, Gerstein HC, Pogue J, Bosch J, Yusuf S. Renal insufficiency as a predictor of cardiovascular outcomes and the impact of ramipril: the HOPE Randomized Trial. *Ann Intern Med*. 2001;134:629–636.

51. Nogueira J, Weir M. The unique character of cardiovascular disease in chronic kidney disease and its implications for treatment with lipid-lowering drugs. *Clin J Am Soc Nephrol*. 2007;2:766–785.

52. Atkins RC, Briganti EM, Lewis JB, et al. Proteinuria reduction and progression to renal failure in patients with type 2 diabetes mellitus and overt nephropathy. *Am J Kidney Dis*. 2005;45:281–287.

53. Collins R, Armitage J, Parish S, Sleigh P, Peto R. MRC/BHF Heart Protection Study of cholesterol-lowering with simvastatin in 5963 people with diabetes: a randomised placebo-controlled trial. *Lancet*. 2003;361:2005–2016.

54. Baigent C, Keech A, Kearney PM. Efficacy and safety of cholesterol-lowering treatment: prospective meta-analysis of data from 90,056 participants in 14 randomised trials of statins. *Lancet*. 2005;366:1267–1278.

55. Expert Panel on Detection EaToHBCiA. Executive summary of the third report of the National Cholesterol Education Program (NCEP) Expert Panel on Detection, Evaluation, and Treatment of High Blood Cholesterol in Adults (Adult Treatment Panel III). *JAMA*. 2001;285:2486–2497.

56. Tonelli M, Isles C, Curhan GC, et al. Effect of pravastatin on cardiovascular events in people with chronic kidney disease. *Circulation*. 2004;110:1557–1563.

57. Jamison RL, Hartigan P, Kaufman JS, et al. Effect of homocysteine lowering on mortality and vascular disease in advanced chronic kidney disease and end-stage renal disease: a randomized controlled trial. *JAMA*. 2007;298:1163–1170.

58. Singh AK, Szczech L, Tang KL, et al. Correction of anemia with epoetin alfa in chronic kidney disease. *N Engl J Med*. 2006;355:2085–2098.

59. The CREATE, Trial G. Effects of Reviparin, a low-molecular-weight heparin, on mortality, reinfarction, and strokes in patients with acute myocardial infarction presenting with st-segment elevation. *JAMA*. 2005;293:427–435.

60. Fishbane S, Besarab A. Mechanism of increased mortality risk with erythropoietin treatment to higher hemoglobin targets. *Clin J Am Soc Nephrol*. 2007;2:1274–1282.

61. de Boer I, Ioannou GN, Kestenbaum B, Brunzell JD, Weiss NS. 25-Hydroxyvitamin D levels and albuminuria in the Third National Health and Nutrition Examination Survey (NHANES III). *Am J Kidney Dis*. 2007;50:69–77.

62. Kovesdy CP, Ahmadzadeh S, Anderson JE, Kalantar-Zadeh K. Association of activated vitamin D treatment and mortality in chronic kidney disease. *Arch Int Med*. 2008;168:397–403.

63. Zhang Z, Sun L, Wang Y, et al. Renoprotective role of the vitamin D receptor in diabetic nephropathy. *Kidney Int*. 2008;73:163–171.

64. Szeto CC, Chow KM, Kwan BC, Chung KY, Leung CB, Li PK. Oral calcitriol for the treatment of persistent proteinuria in immunoglobulin A nephropathy: an uncontrolled trial. *Am J Kidney Dis*. 2008;51:724–731.

65. Alborzi P, Patel N, Agarwal R. Home blood pressures are of greater prognostic value than hemodialysis unit recordings. *Clin J Am Soc Nephrol*. 2007;2:1228–1234.

66. Foley RN, Parfrey PS, Sarnak MJ. Clinical epidemiology of cardiovascular disease in chronic renal disease. *Am J Kidney Dis* 1998;32:S112–S119.

67. Shemesh O, Golbetz H, Kriss JP, and Myers BD. Limitations of creatinine as a filtration marker in glomerulopathic patients. *Kidney Int*. 1985;28:830–838.

II

CORONARY ARTERY DISEASE

9 Evaluation of Chest Pain and Myocardial Ischemia

Joshua M. Kosowsky and Calvin Huang

CONTENTS

Key Words: Chest pain; Electrocardiogram; Helical chest CT; Ischemia; Respiratory distress; Shock.

9.1. INTRODUCTION

Chest pain is one of the most common presentations that clinicians are called upon to evaluate on an urgent basis in the office, clinic, or emergency department (ED). The CDC recorded 6.4 million visits to the ED for chest pain in 2006 *(1)*. Some of the challenges in the evaluation of chest pain include the broad spectrum of potential etiologies for chest pain, limited availability of definitive diagnostic modalities, and the potentially lethal consequences of serious conditions when not recognized early. Even when armed with all the tools of a full-service ED, often a definitive diagnosis cannot be arrived at. Instead, clinicians are forced to rely on the power of exclusion to discern if there is a threat to life and to decide how best to manage uncertain risks.

The initial evaluation of chest pain revolves around the theme of early recognition of the life-threatening problem. It is important to approach each patient with a differential diagnosis in mind and to evaluate and treat in a systematic fashion (Table 1). Although there are several potentially life-threatening causes of chest pain, the focus of this chapter is on the exclusion of cardiac ischemia. In the United States, myocardial infarction (MI) is the number one cause of mortality *(2)*. Furthermore, from a risk management standpoint, cases of missed MI are very commonly litigated on the basis of "failure to diagnose" *(3)*. Missed and delayed diagnoses of cardiac ischemia are associated with increased mortality. On the other hand, 75% or more of the greater than 5 million patients who present to EDs in the United States annually with chest pain have no objective evidence of an acute coronary syndrome, and "rapid rule-out" protocols for these patients in short-stay observation units have been shown to be safe and cost effective by reducing the need for hospitalization.

From: *Contemporary Cardiology: Comprehensive Cardiovascular Medicine in the Primary Care Setting*
Edited by: Peter P. Toth, Christopher P. Cannon, DOI 10.1007/978-1-60327-963-5_9
© Springer Science+Business Media, LLC 2010

Table 1
Differential Diagnosis of Chest Pain

Thoracic aortic dissection
Abrupt onset of maximal pain
Pain radiating to back/shoulder
Neurologic deficits
Chest X-ray may be suggestive, but not sensitive or specific
High-resolution helical CT with contrast is diagnostic

Pericarditis
Recent viral illness
Positional/pleuritic component
Friction rub
Effusion may be evident on echocardiogram

Pulmonary embolus
Visceral pain and shortness of breath with acute PE
Pleuritic pain with pulmonary infarct
Sinus tachycardia is the most common EKG finding
D-dimer may be helpful in ruling out PE in low to moderate probability patients
High-resolution helical CT with contrast is diagnostic

Pneumothorax
Unilateral decreased breath sounds
Hypotension/tachycardia with tension pneumothorax
Chest X-ray diagnostic for significant pneumothorax

Pneumonia
Fever and other constitutional symptoms
Cough, shortness of breath
Chest X-ray findings

Gastrointestinal pain
Relation to meals
Abdominal tenderness

Musculoskeletal pain
Worse with movement
Symptoms reproducible with palpation

Herpes zoster
History of varicella
Pain/tenderness does not cross midline
Rash may be a delayed finding

9.2. INITIAL PRESENTATION

Upon initial presentation, it is essential to quickly form a mental impression of the patient's clinical status. This evaluation may be formed by quickly assessing the patient's general appearance, vital signs, and chief complaint. For any patient presenting in extremis, it is advisable to begin with the ABCs, starting with airway and breathing, and moving next to circulation. At each stage, as a problem is encountered, a working differential diagnosis is generated with empiric treatment provided as needed.

For the patient presenting to an outpatient setting with chief complaint of chest pain, the threshold to transfer the patient to an ED by ambulance should be appropriately low. Any patient with abnormal vitals or active chest pain of potentially ischemic origin should be transferred without delay, along with any relevant records, imaging, and prior cardiac testing, and EKGs should be sent with the patient if doing so does not delay transfer.

9.3. CHEST PAIN AND RESPIRATORY DISTRESS

Chest pain and respiratory distress should guide the physician to a short but emergent list of differential diagnoses. Although many conditions can present this way, there are some that present with some frequency and typically require immediate diagnosis and treatment. These would include massive pulmonary embolus, tension pneumothorax, and myocardial infarction with acute heart failure.

The initial management of the patient with chest pain or respiratory distress is the same, regardless of etiology. The awake patient with adequate respiratory effort should be started on 100% oxygen delivered by nonrebreather face mask. If there is inadequate respiratory effort, ventilations should be assisted with a bag–valve mask device. Pulse oximetry and continuous cardiac monitoring should begin as soon as possible.

The decision of whether or not to intubate the trachea is an important one. Considerations include the ability to deliver higher levels of positive pressure, the need to protect the airway from soft tissue collapse or aspiration in the setting of decreased mental status, and the ability to ensure secure ventilation and oxygenation during patient transport. However, intubation is not an end in and of itself and should not delay definitive evaluation and treatment. Noninvasive positive pressure ventilation via face mask can be used as a temporizing measure, either to support the patient until intubation can occur, or until treatment of the underlying disease is able to take effect.

Once these initial measures are begun, the clinician must quickly obtain a basic history from the patient, EMS personnel, family members, and whatever medical records are available. The physical examination should focus on the cardiovascular and pulmonary systems. Obviously, an electrocardiogram should be obtained without delay. Depending upon the degree of extremis, the patient may require decisive treatment before a definitive diagnosis can be made.

9.4. CHEST PAIN AND SHOCK

The presentation of chest pain and shock should trigger an automatic series of coordinated actions from the evaluating team. Large bore intravenous access should be obtained, pulse oximetry and cardiac monitoring initiated, and a 12-lead electrocardiogram performed as soon as possible. In cases of actual or impending cardiac arrest, cardiac resuscitation should occur following ACLS guidelines with attention to early defibrillation.

Life-threatening etiologies of chest pain with shock include massive MI, tension pneumothorax, cardiac tamponade, and aortic dissection with rupture. Although an initial bolus of intravenous fluid is almost always reasonable, one must recognize that life-threatening causes of chest pain may not be fluid responsive and that additional fluid boluses may further complicate a patient's physiological status. Resuscitation, whether with fluids or vasopressor agents, should be seen as a temporizing measure until definitive diagnosis and treatment can be attained. Additional diagnoses to consider would include massive pulmonary embolus, pneumonia with sepsis, and perforated peptic ulcer.

9.5. EVALUATION OF THE STABLE PATIENT WITH CHEST PAIN

After the vital signs are screened for any immediate life-threatening abnormalities, an EKG should be obtained and reviewed by an attending physician within 10 min of the patient's arrival (Fig. 1). In settings where chest pain is evaluated with frequency, such as the emergency department or urgent care clinic, a protocol to ensure this 10-min door to EKG time should be in place. This goal is listed as Class I by the ACC/AHA *(4)*.

The EKG should be immediately reviewed for evidence of ST-elevation myocardial infarction, which, if present, should prompt immediate plans for revascularization. In the appropriate setting, hyper-acute T waves, a new left bundle-branch-block, or findings consistent with an acute posterior MI

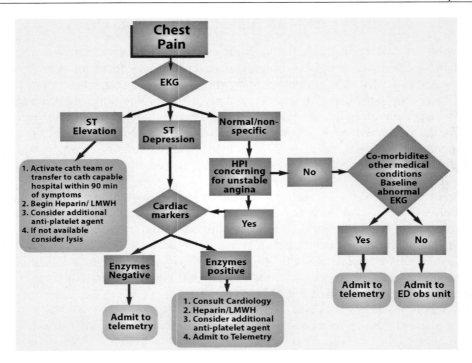

Fig. 1. Evaluation of the stable patient with chest pain.

should be considered ST-elevation equivalents. The standards established by the ACC/AHA include a "door-to-needle" time of 30 min and a "door-to-balloon" time of 90 min.

For most other patients, a directed history and physical examination, together with review of the initial ECG, will lead to a diagnosis of possible (or probable) ischemic chest pain. The classic presentation of cardiac ischemia is visceral chest pain with radiation to the shoulder, arms, neck, back, and/or jaw. The pain may be exertional but is typically not pleuritic or reproducible with palpation. A patient with only brief twinges of pain is unlikely having cardiac ischemia. Likewise, in the absence of abnormal vital signs or electrocardiographic changes, the patient with constant pain for days on end is unlikely to be having myocardial ischemia. A sizable proportion of patients will present with a history of chest pain that has now resolved, making diagnosis all the more difficult. The resolution of pain with nitroglycerin, however, should not be viewed as a diagnostic tool. Several other diagnoses under consideration may also respond to nitrates including esophageal spasm.

For any patient in whom the diagnosis of myocardial ischemia is being entertained, cardiac biomarkers should be measured. For patients with ongoing symptoms, the ECG should be repeated at regular intervals (at least once within 30 min) and with any change in clinical status to assess for ST segment or T-wave changes. New or dynamic ECG changes in the appropriate clinical context should be taken as evidence of ischemia. By the time the ECG is repeated and initial cardiac markers have returned (and frequently much sooner), the clinician (having also had time to review medical records and potentially discuss the case with the patient's cardiologist) should be able to assess whether the patient is considered to have unstable angina (UA) or a non-ST-elevation myocardial infarction (NSTEMI). It should be emphasized that UA remains essentially a clinical diagnosis that in some cases requires a great deal of judgment (e.g., in the absence of obvious ST segment depression or positive cardiac markers). Patients with UA/NSTEMI generally require hospital admission.

For patients who are not felt to have UA/NSTEMI, but whose chest pain is not clearly nonischemic, a rapid "rule-out MI" protocol can be initiated in an observation unit setting (Fig. 2). The common

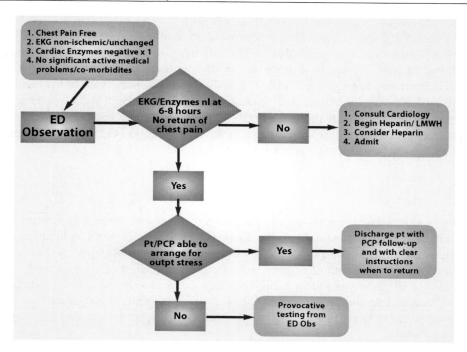

Fig. 2. Observation protocol for chest pain.

practice is to obtain two sets of cardiac markers separated by either 6 or 8 h, although one set of negative biomarkers may be adequate if there is more than 8–12 h from onset of symptoms to time of testing *(4)*. During the observation period, a comprehensive assessment of cardiac risk factors should be made, including an assessment of lipid profile and C-reactive protein (CRP) if indicated. Patients who develop recurrent pain must have a prompt repeat ECG and clinical reassessment. New ECG changes or positive cardiac markers should prompt hospital admission.

Having successfully completed the "rule-out" portion (i.e., no recurrent ischemic pain, no ECG changes, negative markers) of the evaluation, the decision as to when and how to further risk-stratify patients will vary from clinician to clinician. In general, most patients are sent for a standard Bruce Protocol exercise tolerance test (ETT), which has been shown to be a good prognostic indicator of adverse cardiac events in low- to moderate-risk chest pain patients. In studies evaluating the treadmill stress, patients with a low risk assignment had 1 year cardiac mortality in the range of less than 0.5% *(5)*. However, depending on the baseline ECG, capacity for exercise, and prior history of provocative testing, an individual patient may be considered for alternative testing or, in some cases, no testing at all. As per ACC/AHA guidelines, it is acceptable for a stress test to occur as an outpatient within 72 h of presentation of symptoms in an individual who is "low risk" after negative serial enzymes and serial EKGs *(6)*.

Functional testing with imaging (e.g., SPECT-MIBI, echocardiography) should be considered whenever a standard ETT is not felt to be diagnostic, such as when the patient's baseline EKG has ST segment abnormalities or left bundle-branch-block. Additionally, for patients with a very high pretest likelihood of CAD, perfusion imaging may be favored. For patients who are unable to exercise, a pharmacologic stress test (e.g., dobutamine, adenosine) can be arranged. All results (whether negative, positive, or nondiagnostic) must be considered in the context of the individual patient's presentation. Although a negative stress test is generally reassuring enough to allow for discharge, no patient should go home without arranging for follow-up, specifically if there are outstanding issues of risk-factor modification or a need for additional testing. Patients with nondiagnostic or positive results do not necessarily require admission, but will almost always warrant at least consultation with a cardiologist.

Helical chest CT is a powerful technology with an emerging role in the evaluation of chest pain and myocardial ischemia. Current-generation CT with contrast can exclude the diagnosis of aortic dissection with a sensitivity approaching 100% *(7)*, and exclude pulmonary embolism with a sensitivity of over 90% *(8)*. More recently, multidetector helical chest CT has been used to image the coronary arteries. Coronary artery CT can evaluate for both cutoff of flow to the myocardium as well as for the presence of plaque, which correlates with the extent of CAD. A single CT can thus be used for "triple rule-out," evaluating for CAD, aortic dissection, and segmental PE.

9.6. CONCLUSION

Chest pain is a symptom that almost any type of physician will frequently encounter in clinical practice. Quickly obtaining a sense of the patient's severity of illness as well as focusing on the timely diagnosis of life-threatening conditions is a key skill to develop. Following this, close attention to the natural history and progression of disease will often reveal the underlying pathology. In the cases where an immediate diagnosis is not at hand, life-threatening disease should be excluded by either observation or diagnostic testing. Close follow-up is always essential. The approach to evaluation and treatment of chest pain, when performed in a systematic but efficient manner, can safely and positively impact patient outcomes.

9.7. CASE STUDIES

9.7.1. Case 1

A 54-year-old woman presents to your office for her annual physical. She has a history of hypertension and hypercholesterolemia, but no known coronary artery disease. She mentions that she has been having intermittent chest pain. These episodes last several minutes and are not brought on by exertion. They have been ongoing for about 1 month with two to three episodes a week. The frequency and severity have not changed.

The patient has a pulse of 70 and a blood pressure of 154/86. Her lungs are clear to auscultation bilaterally; her heart sounds include a regular S1 and S2 with no murmurs or rub. Her EKG shows a normal sinus rhythm with an incomplete right bundle-branch-block. There are no ST or T-wave changes. She is not currently having symptoms; she reports that the last time she had pain was 4 days ago. What is the next appropriate step in the management of this patient?

Although the symptoms are somewhat atypical, angina cannot be excluded. Reassuringly, her symptoms are mild and not progressive. She is currently asymptomatic and her EKG shows no evidence of ischemia; therefore, she can be safely managed in the outpatient setting. The next step in assessing this patient's chest pain should be to arrange for an outpatient stress test to assess for inducible ischemia. In the meantime, management of the patient's coronary risk factors (hypertension, hypercholesterolemia) should be initiated, and the patient should be given clear instructions about symptoms that should prompt immediate medical attention.

9.7.2. Case 2

A 62-year-old man presents to your office for an unscheduled visit. He has a history of hypertension but often does not take his medications. He reports that he was shoveling snow earlier in the day, when he developed a dull chest pain, which improved with rest but has not entirely subsided. He reports no other symptoms.

The patient has a pulse of 92 and a blood pressure of 164/94. His lungs are clear to auscultation bilaterally; his heart sounds include a regular S1 and S2 with no murmurs or rub. An EKG performed in your office shows 2 mm depressions in leads I, V5, and V6. What is the appropriate management for this patient?

This patient is having symptoms that are concerning for a non-ST-elevation myocardial infarction (NSTEMI) in a lateral distribution. Even though the patient is feeling better, he should be transported to the nearest hospital as soon as possible by EMS. If available, aspirin should be given to the patient to chew and swallow. He should not be allowed to drive himself. Any relevant medical records should be sent with the patient.

REFERENCES

1. Pitts SR, Niska RW, Xu J, Burt CW. *National Hospital Ambulatory Medical Care Survey: 2006 Emergency Department Summary*. National Health Statistics Reports, No 7. Hyattsville, MD: National Center for Health Statistics; 2008.

2. Heron MP, Hoyert DL, Xu J, Scott C, Tejada-Vera B. *Deaths: Preliminary Data for 2006*. National Vital Statistics Reports, Vol 56, No 16. Hyattsville, MD: National Center for Health Statistics; 2008.

3. General and Family Practice Claim Summary. Rockville, MD: Physician Insurers Association of America; 2002.

4. Anderson JL, Adams CD, Antman EM, et al. ACC/AHA 2007 guidelines for the management of patients with unstable angina/non–ST-elevation myocardial infarction: executive summary: a report of the American College of Cardiology/American Heart Association Task Force on Practice Guidelines (Writing Committee to Revise the 2002 Guidelines for the Management of Patients with Unstable Angina/Non-ST-Elevation Myocardial Infarction). *Circulation*. 2007;116:803–877.

5. Hochman JS, McCabe CH, Becker RC, Stone PH, et al. Outcome and profile of women and men presenting with acute coronary syndromes: a report from TIMI IIIB. TIMI Investigators. Thrombolysis in Myocardial Infarction. *J Am Coll Cardiol*. 1997;30:141–148.

6. Gibbons RJ, Balady GJ, Bricker JT, et al. ACC/AHA 2002 guideline update for exercise testing: a report of the American College of Cardiology/American Heart Association Task Force on Practice Guidelines (Committee on Exercise Testing). *Circulation*. 2002;106:1883–1892.

7. Shiga T, Wajima Z, Apfel CC. Diagnostic accuracy of transesophageal echocardiography, helical computed tomography, and magnetic resonance imaging for suspected thoracic aortic dissection: systematic review and meta-analysis. *Arch Int Med*. 2006;166:1350–1356.

8. Stein PD, Fowler SE, Goodman LR, et al. Contrast enhanced multidetector spiral CT of the chest and lower extremities in suspected acute pulmonary embolism: results of the Prospective Investigation of Pulmonary Embolism Diagnosis II (PIOPED II). *N Engl J Med*. 2006;345:2317–2327.

10 Unstable Angina and Non-ST Elevation Myocardial Infarction

Ali Mahajerin and Eli V. Gelfand

CONTENTS

Key Words: Atherosclerotic plaque; Unstable angina; Heparin; Myocardial infarction; Troponin.

KEY POINTS

- Acute coronary syndromes represent a major public health concern, with 1.4 million hospitalizations occurring annually in the United States; NSTEACS account for 71–83% of these.
- NSTEACS is characterized by anginal chest discomfort accompanied by ischemic electrocardiographic ST-segment abnormalities and/or elevation of cardiac biomarkers.
- The differential diagnosis of NSTEACS includes other life-threatening diagnoses, such as pulmonary embolism, aortic dissection, tension pneumothorax, esophageal rupture, and pericardial tamponade.
- Rupture of a vulnerable atherosclerotic plaque and subsequent thrombus formation are central to the pathophysiology of acute coronary syndromes.
- Risk stratification for recurrent MI, death, or heart failure is central to decision making in NSTEACS.
- The management of NSTEACS includes application of anti-ischemic therapies, antiplatelet therapies, and anticoagulation, as well as selective use of coronary revascularization.
- Secondary prevention includes agents such as aspirin, beta-blockers, lipid-lowering agents, and ACE inhibitors, as well as weight control, smoking cessation, and management of hyperglycemia if present.

From: *Contemporary Cardiology: Comprehensive Cardiovascular Medicine in the Primary Care Setting*
Edited by: Peter P. Toth, Christopher P. Cannon, DOI 10.1007/978-1-60327-963-5_10
© Springer Science+Business Media, LLC 2010

10.1. INTRODUCTION

Unstable angina (UA) and non-ST elevation myocardial infarction (NSTEMI) represent part of the acute coronary syndrome (ACS) spectrum that also includes ST elevation myocardial infarction (STEMI). Combined, UA and NSTEMI are known as non-ST elevation acute coronary syndrome (NSTEACS). Recent estimates suggest that 1.4 million hospitalizations occur annually for ACS events in the United States, with 558,000 for UA alone (1). Of those patients with elevated cardiac biomarkers suggestive of myocardial infarction (MI), at least one-half may be classified as NSTEMI (1, 2).

10.2. DEFINITIONS AND CLASSIFICATION

Myocardial infarction can be broadly defined as a pathologic process of myocardial necrosis resulting from sustained ischemia. Recently, the European Society of Cardiology (ESC), American College of Cardiology (ACC), American Heart Association (AHA), and World Heart Federation (WHF) developed an updated classification scheme for MI that considers the underlying mechanism of myocardial ischemia and clinical circumstances that have led to infarction (3), seen in Table 1. NSTEACS are characterized by a syndrome of anginal chest discomfort, accompanied by ischemic electrocardiographic (ECG) ST-segment abnormalities and/or elevation in cardiac biomarkers (4). The presence of elevated cardiac biomarkers distinguishes NSTEMI from UA (1). The recommendations set forth by the ACC and AHA are classified by the strength of supporting evidence. This classification scheme is outlined in Table 2 (4).

Table 1
Joint ESC/ACC/AHA/WHF Task Force Classification Scheme for Myocardial Infarction (3)

Type 1	Spontaneous myocardial infarction related to ischemia due to a primary coronary event such as plaque erosion and/or rupture, fissuring, or dissection
Type 2	Myocardial infarction secondary to ischemia due to either increased oxygen demand or decreased supply, e.g., coronary artery spasm, coronary embolism, anemia, arrhythmias, hypertension, or hypotension
Type 3	Sudden unexpected cardiac death, including cardiac arrest, often with symptoms suggestive of myocardial ischemia, accompanied by presumably new ST elevation, or new left bundle-branch-block, or evidence of fresh thrombus in a coronary artery by angiography and/or at autopsy, but death occurring before blood samples could be obtained, or at a time before the appearance of cardiac biomarkers in the blood
Type 4a	Myocardial infarction associated with percutaneous coronary intervention
Type 4b	Myocardial infarction associated with stent thrombosis as documented by angiography or at autopsy
Type 5	Myocardial infarction associated with coronary artery bypass grafting

Reproduced from *Circulation* © 2007 with permission from LWW.

10.3. PATHOPHYSIOLOGY

ACS is the culmination of an atheroinflammatory process originating at the site of a cholesterol-laden plaque within a coronary artery. Braunwald proposed a pentad of pathophysiologic processes that contribute to the development of an acute atherothrombotic event (5) including: (a) rupture of a vulnerable atherosclerotic plaque that disrupts the local balance of thrombosis and endogenous fibrinolysis, leading to formation of a superimposed nonocclusive thrombus; (b) dynamic obstruction of the vessel such as spasm of a major epicardial coronary vessel in Prinzmetal's angina or constriction of small

Table 2
ACC and AHA Classification Scheme for Recommendations *(4)*

Class	Risk–benefit profile	Recommendation
I	Benefit >>> Risk	Procedure/treatment *should* be performed/administered
IIa	Benefit >> Risk Additional studies with focused objectives needed	*It is reasonable* to perform procedure/administer treatment
IIb	Benefit ≥ Risk Additional studies with broad objectives needed; additional registry data would be helpful	Procedure/treatment *may be considered*
III	Risk ≥ Benefit No additional studies needed	Procedure/treatment should *not* be performed/administered *since it is not helpful and may be harmful*

Reproduced from the *Journal of the American College of Cardiology* © 2007 with permission from Elsevier.

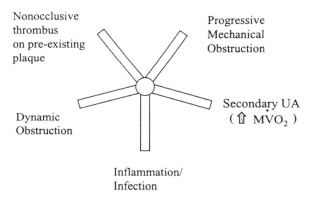

Fig. 1. Framework for considering five major causes of unstable angina *(5)*. Reproduced from *Circulation* © 1998 with permission from LWW.

muscular coronary arteries; (c) progressive mechanical obstruction of the vessel; (d) inflammation; and (e) secondary unstable angina, related to oxygen supply–demand mismatch *(5, 6)* (Fig. 1). These processes are not mutually exclusive, and ACS can arise as a combination of some or all of these factors. STEMI typically results from transmural ischemia, when the coronary thrombus is occlusive, while the thrombus is nonocclusive in UA or NSTEMI.

10.3.1. Thrombosis

The central role of thrombosis in the pathogenesis of ACS is supported by the presence of thrombi at the site of a ruptured atherosclerotic coronary plaque at autopsy in atherectomy specimens from patients with UA and on angioscopy and angiography of patients with UA. Marked improvement in clinical outcomes of patients with ACS is achieved with specific antithrombotic therapy including aspirin *(7)*, heparin (unfractionated or low-molecular weight) *(8–10)*, platelet glycoprotein (GP) IIb/IIIa inhibitors *(11–13)*, and clopidogrel *(14)* (Fig. 2).

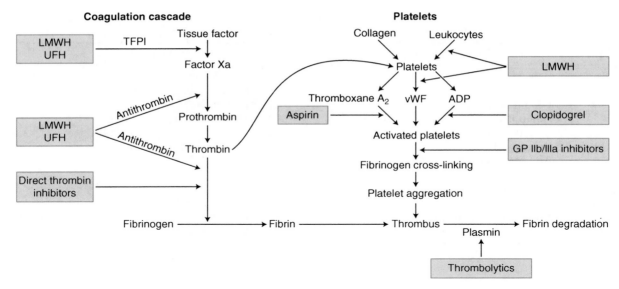

Fig. 2. Main sites of action of antithrombotic therapies. ADP = Adenosine Diphosphate GP = Glycoprotein, LMWH = Low-Molecular Weight Heparin, TFPI = Tissue Factor Pathway Inhibitor, UFH = Unfractionated Heparin, vWF = von Willebrand Factor *(118)*. Reproduced from *American Journal of Cardiology* © 2003 with permission from Elsevier.

10.3.2. Role of Platelets

When an atherosclerotic plaque ruptures, collagen and tissue factor are exposed to blood. Platelet adhesion occurs through the interaction of the GP Ib receptor with von Willebrand factor. Platelet activation involves a conformational change of platelet shape, degranulation with release of several proaggregatory and chemoattractant mediators, and expression of GP IIb/IIIa receptors on the platelet surface, which binds fibrinogen in their activated conformation. Platelet aggregation is mediated through this interaction. Because of this central role, antiplatelet therapy is a cornerstone of therapy and includes decreasing formation of thromboxane A2 (aspirin), inhibiting the adenosine diphosphate receptor pathway of platelet activation (clopidogrel and prasugrel) *(15)*, and directly inhibiting platelet aggregation (GP IIb/IIIa inhibitors). The precise sites of antiplatelet therapy activity on the platelet activation cascade are highlighted in Fig. 2.

10.3.3. Plasma Coagulation System in Acute Coronary Syndrome

Concurrently, with formation of the platelet aggregate, the plasma coagulation system is activated. Rupture of the atherosclerotic plaque and release of tissue factor activate factor X, converting it to factor Xa, which in turn generates thrombin (factor IIa). Thrombin converts fibrinogen to fibrin in the final common pathway for clot formation. Thrombin stimulates platelet aggregation and activates factor XIII, thereby cross-linking and stabilizing the fibrin clot. Concurrently, endogenous fibrinolytic mechanisms are activated including plasmin, which functions to cleave fibrin-specific peptide bonds and break apart the clot. Pharmacological inhibition of thrombin and factor Xa plays an important role in the primary treatment of ACS, and specific anticoagulation targets are highlighted in Fig. 2.

10.3.4. Dynamic Coronary Obstruction

Coronary vasoconstriction commonly occurs in the region of atherosclerotic plaques and may result from local vasoconstrictors released by platelets (serotonin and thromboxane A_2), as well as from mediators present within the thrombus, such as thrombin. *Prinzmetal's angina* is caused by focal constriction of a coronary artery segment that occurs even in the absence of significant atherosclerotic narrowing. *Microcirculatory angina* occurs as a consequence of vasoconstriction in small intramural arteries where coronary flow is slow despite the lack of epicardial stenoses. Adrenergic stimuli, exposure to cold, cocaine *(16)*, and profound mental stress *(17)* can also lead to coronary vasoconstriction.

10.3.5. Progressive Mechanical Obstruction

Progressive narrowing of the coronary lumen has been observed most commonly in the setting of restenosis after percutaneous coronary intervention (PCI) prior to the widespread use of drug-eluting stents. Angiographic and atherectomy studies have demonstrated that many patients without previous intracoronary procedures have also shown progressive luminal narrowing of the culprit vessel preceding the onset of NSTEACS that is related to rapid cellular proliferation *(18)*.

10.3.6. Secondary Unstable Angina

This form of UA is caused by profound imbalances in myocardial oxygen supply and demand, sometimes on a background of underlying coronary stenoses. Examples are given in Table 3. Infarction in this setting would be classified as Type II MI by the updated ESC/ACC/AHA/WHF classification scheme *(3)* (Table 1).

Table 3
Causes of Myocardial Oxygen Supply–Demand Mismatch that May Lead
to Secondary Unstable Angina

Conditions that cause *increased oxygen demand*
 Tachycardia
 Systemic infection/fever
 Thyrotoxicosis
 Hyperadrenergic states
 Elevations of left ventricular afterload (hypertension, severe aortic stenosis)

Conditions that cause *impaired oxygen delivery*
 Anemia
 Hypoxemia
 Hypotension

10.4. CLINICAL PRESENTATION

Patients with NSTEACS typically present with anginal chest pain occurring at rest or with minimal exertion, though as many as half of all MIs may be clinically silent and unrecognized by the patient *(19)*. Angina is characterized by a poorly localized chest or arm discomfort (only infrequently described as "pain"), often associated with physical exertion or emotional stress, relieved within 5–15 min by rest and/or nitroglycerin. A grading system for angina, developed by the Canadian Cardiovascular Society, is outlined in Table 4 *(20)*. *Unstable angina* has one or more of the following features: (a) occurs at rest (or with light exertion), usually lasting at least 20 min; (b) is severe and

Table 4
Canadian Cardiovascular Society Grading of Angina Pectoris *(20)*

Class	Description
I	Ordinary physical activity does not cause angina, such as walking and climbing stairs. Angina with strenuous or rapid or prolonged exertion at work or recreation
II	Slight limitation of ordinary activity. Walking or climbing stairs rapidly, walking uphill, walking or stair climbing after meals, or in cold, or in wind, or under emotional distress, or only during the few hours after awakening. Walking more than two blocks on the level and climbing more than one flight of ordinary stairs at a normal pace and in normal conditions
III	Marked limitation of ordinary physical activity. Walking one or two blocks on the level and climbing one flight of stairs in normal conditions and at normal pace
IV	Inability to carry on any physical activity without discomfort, anginal syndrome may be present at rest

Reproduced from *Circulation* © 1976 with permission from LWW.

described as frank pain, and of recent onset (i.e., within 1 month); or (c) occurs with an accelerating pattern (i.e., more severe, prolonged, or frequent than previous occurrences, and with a lower threshold for occurrence with exertion). Anginal equivalents may include arm pain, lower jaw pain, diaphoresis, shortness of breath, or extreme fatigue.

Physical examination can be unremarkable, though signs of a large infarct are highlighted in Table 5. A sufficiently large infarction will cause end-organ hypoperfusion and cardiogenic shock, which developed in 2.5% of patients without ST elevation on presentation and carried a mortality rate greater than 70% in the GUSTO-IIb Trial *(21)*. Right ventricular (RV) infarction is a distinct entity, usually caused by occlusion of the proximal right coronary artery and commonly occurs in association with inferior left ventricular (LV) infarction. Physical signs of RV infarction include hypotension and elevation of jugular venous pressure in the setting of few signs of LV failure.

Table 5
Signs of a Large Myocardial Infarction

Evidence of low cardiac output
  Diaphoresis
  Pale cool skin
  Sinus tachycardia
  Confusion

Evidence of elevated filling pressures
  Audible S3 or S4 on cardiac auscultation
  Rales on lung auscultation
  Jugular venous distention

Symptoms of ACS must be differentiated from other causes of chest pain, many of which can be life threatening (Table 6). Acute aortic dissection should be considered given the potential ramifications of treating patients for suspected ACS with antithrombotic and antiplatelet agents. In cases of suspected RV infarction, care must be exercised in differentiating this scenario from the overlapping presentations of acute pulmonary embolism or cardiac tamponade. Acute pericarditis may be misdiagnosed as acute MI since presentation commonly involves chest discomfort with ST-segment ECG changes. One study suggests that the following features of chest pain identify a subgroup of patients who are at "low" risk for having ongoing MI (<3%): (i) sharp or stabbing pain, (ii) no history of angina or MI

Table 6
Differential Diagnosis of Chest Discomfort

Conditions with immediate life-threatening potential
    Acute coronary syndrome
    Acute aortic dissection
    Pulmonary embolism/infarction
    Esophageal rupture
    Tension pneumothorax
    Cardiac tamponade

Other conditions
    Acute pericarditis
    Gastroesophageal reflux disease
    Costochondritis and related musculoskeletal conditions
    Acute myocarditis
    Transient apical ballooning syndrome ("takotsubo-type" cardiomyopathy)
    Esophageal spasm
    Pleurisy
    Herpes zoster
    Pancreatitis
    Gallbladder disease

and (iii) pain with pleuritic or positional components, or (iv) pain that was reproduced by palpation of the chest wall *(22)*.

10.5. INITIAL EVALUATION AND RISK STRATIFICATION

Prompt evaluation of patients with suspected ACS is essential. Patients who contact primary care providers by phone with symptoms suggestive of accelerating angina or angina at rest should be advised that a full evaluation cannot be performed solely via the telephone and prompt evaluation in an emergency room should be strongly encouraged. Use of emergency medical services rather than private transportation is advised.

An initial-focused history should concentrate on the nature of the anginal symptoms, any prior history of coronary artery disease (CAD), and traditional cardiovascular risk factors. Cocaine use should be addressed and urine toxicology should be performed when substance abuse is suspected as a cause of, or contributor to, ACS.

Physical examination should be directed toward the assessment of possible precipitants of NSTEACS, such as severe hypertension, thyroid disease, gastrointestinal bleeding, or other causes of severe anemia. Evidence for extracardiac vascular disease, such as carotid bruits or diminished distal pulses, should be sought. Alternate life-threatening diagnoses should be considered (see Table 6), and hemodynamic ramifications of a large MI should also be evaluated as highlighted in Table 5.

10.5.1. ECG

A 12-lead ECG should be interpreted within 10 min of the patient's arrival to the emergency department. A recording made during active chest pain is of particular value. The presence of ST deviation and/or T-wave inversions in contiguous leads indicating active ischemia (Fig. 3), or pathologic Q-waves suggesting prior myocardial infarction (Fig. 4), should be evaluated. If the initial ECG is not diagnostic of ACS, follow-up ECG should be performed every 15–30 min, or with episodes of recurrent chest pain, to evaluate for evolving ST changes. Posterior leads V_7–V_9 should be utilized to

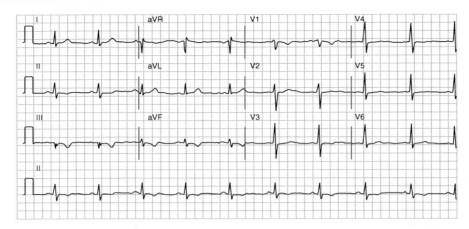

Fig. 3. ECG evidence of myocardial ischemia, with T-wave inversions in the inferior leads II, III, and aVF. Subtle ST depression is suggested in lead aVF, though ST deviation is not noted elsewhere on this ECG.

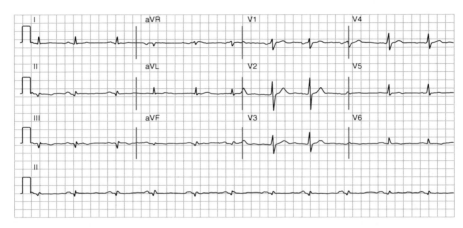

Fig. 4. ECG evidence of prior myocardial infarction, with Q-waves in the inferior leads II, III, and aVF. Minimal Q-waves in leads I, aVL, and V6 are also noted.

enhance the detection of posterior MI, since acute MI due to left circumflex coronary artery occlusion can often present with a non-diagnostic 12-lead ECG and 4% of acute MI patients have ST elevation solely in the posterior leads *(23)*. When RV infarction is suspected based on the clinical presentation, right-sided precordial leads should be obtained to assess for ST elevation in lead V_4R *(24)*.

10.5.2. Cardiac Biomarkers

Cardiac-specific troponin is highly sensitive and specific in detecting myocardial cell necrosis *(3)*. Troponin elevation can be detected in blood as early as 2–4 h after symptom onset, for 5–14 days following an acute event *(25)* (Fig. 5). Creatine kinase-MB (CK-MB), though less sensitive and less specific for MI, is typically used as an adjunctive assay. For patients presenting less than 6 h from symptom onset, repeat troponin levels should be drawn in 6–8 h, or as guided by symptom onset.

B-type natriuretic peptide (BNP) is a cardiac neurohormone released in response to ventricular stretch. While BNP has been used as a diagnostic and prognostic marker in congestive heart failure, it also serves as a strong predictor of short- and long-term mortality in patients with ACS independent of previous heart failure or clinical signs of LV dysfunction *(26)*. In a 2001 study, plasma BNP levels

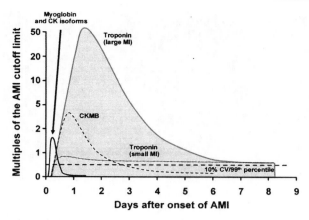

Fig. 5. Time course of the appearance biomarkers in the blood after acute MI. Shown are the time concentrations/activity curves for myoglobin and creatine kinase (CK) isoforms, troponin after large and small infarctions, and CK-MB. Note that with the cardiac troponin some patients have a second peak in addition. CV = coefficient of variation *(25)*. Reproduced from the *Journal of the American College of Cardiology* © 2006 with permission from Elsevier.

were measured at a mean of 40 h after the onset of symptoms in patients presenting with NSTEACS. Patients with BNP levels above a threshold of 80 pg/mL had an increased incidence of death, new or progressive heart failure, and new or recurrent MI at 30 days and 10 months from the index event *(27)*. It is reasonable to measure BNP in the first few days after an ACS event for the purpose of risk stratification.

CD40 ligand (CD40L) is an investigational inflammatory marker expressed on the platelet surface during platelet activation. A soluble fragment is cleaved and measurable by lab assay. CD40L is prothrombotic and proinflammatory, along with having a role in atherosclerosis progression *(28, 29)*. CD40L is a marker of platelet activation, with increased levels of CD40L being associated with increased risk of death, MI, and recurrent ischemic events independent of troponin and C-reactive protein, both in clinically stable patients *(30)* and those with ACS *(31)*.

Other biomarkers of ischemia are being developed to assess for myocardial ischemia before necrosis occurs, such as ischemia-modified albumin (IMA). The metal-binding site on the amino terminus of albumin is damaged in ischemic tissue, perhaps due to free radical formation within this acidotic environment *(32)*. The sensitivity and specificity of the test have been variable, though IMA has a consistently high negative predictive value *(33)* and therefore may be clinically useful for "ruling out" patients presenting with chest pain when cardiac ischemia is suspected.

10.5.3. Cardiac-Computed Tomography

Cardiac-computed tomography (CCT) is being investigated for its use in diagnosing suspected NSTEACS. CCT has short examination times of approximately 5 min and excellent image quality, along with observed high negative predictive values in selected patient groups (ranging 91–100% in various studies) *(34–36)*, thereby making it an attractive tool for "ruling out" CAD and facilitating more rapid triage from the emergency department. The primary use of CCT in acute chest pain is, therefore, for patients with an intermediate pre-test probability of CAD, it can provide diagnostic information and also facilitate more rapid triage decisions. Cardiac CT is inappropriate in patients with a high pre-test probability of CAD presenting with suspected NSTEACS, because post-test probability of CAD will remain unacceptably high despite a negative CCT scan *(37)*. Patients with a very low pre-test probability of CAD presenting with chest pain may be subjected to an unnecessary study

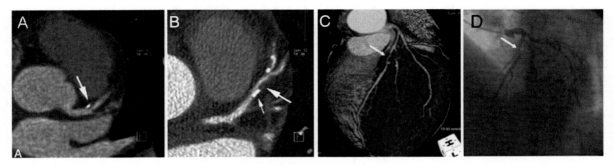

Fig. 6. Cardiac CT imaging. (**a**) Small, partly calcified coronary atherosclerotic plaque in the very proximal segment of the left anterior descending artery (*arrow*). (**b**) In a patient with severe coronary atherosclerosis, calcified (*smaller arrow*) and non-calcified plaque (*larger arrow*) are visible in the mid-section of the left anterior descending coronary artery *(119)*. Volume-rendered three-dimensional imaging (**c**) in a different patient shows severe discrete stenosis located in the proximal left anterior descending artery (*arrow*). Conventional angiography (**d**) reveals significant stenosis at the corresponding area of the left anterior descending coronary artery (*arrow*) *(120)*. Reproduced from the *Journal of the American College of Cardiology* © 2006 and © 2008 with permission from Elsevier.

if sent for CCT. Cardiac CT permits the visualization of non-stenotic coronary plaque, both calcified and non-calcified, as seen in Fig. 6.

10.5.4. Cardiovascular Magnetic Resonance

Cardiovascular magnetic resonance (CMR) is being investigated for its use in early triage of patients presenting with chest pain. CMR can provide a wide range of information including global and regional cardiac function, myocardial perfusion, myocardial viability, and proximal coronary anatomy. CMR has been shown to add diagnostic value over the usual clinical parameters such as ECG, troponin, and thrombolysis in myocardial infarction (TIMI) score in suspected NSTEACS *(38, 39)*. The inability to differentiate non-viable myocardium as acute versus chronic MI previously limited the value of CMR in the triage of patients with chest pain. A more recent study evaluated an expanded CMR protocol including T2-weighted imaging and assessment of LV wall thickness, finding increased specificity (84–96%), positive predictive value (55–85%), and overall accuracy (84–93%) versus the conventional CMR protocol for determining if myocardial abnormalities on late gadolinium enhancement (LGE) CMR are acute versus chronic in nature *(40)*. CMR may facilitate the triage of acute chest pain while also identifying specific myocardial territories at risk, leading to a more prompt and targeted revascularization strategy. Disadvantages of CMR include long scan times, a steep learning curve, high set-up cost, and the inability to scan patients with implanted pacemakers/defibrillators. An example of myocardial infarction detected by LGE CMR is provided in Fig. 7.

10.5.5. Risk Stratification in NSTEACS

NSTEACS is a spectrum of diseases with variable clinical course and prognoses (Fig. 8). Optimal management strategies in NSTEACS are, therefore, dependent on an individual patient's risk of major adverse cardiac events. High-risk features of NSTEMI are highlighted in Table 7. Rapid bedside evaluation of individual risk profile can be accomplished using the TIMI risk score *(41)*, which was derived and validated through the TIMI-11B *(9, 42)* and the ESSENCE *(10)* trials. Seven variables were iden-

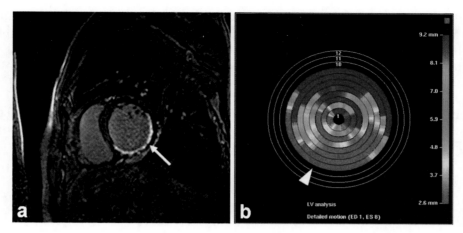

Fig. 7. (a) LGE CMR image, taken from a sagittal view. Normal myocardium is dark, while infarcted myocardium appears bright in this protocol. This patient has had a prior infarct in the basal and mid-inferior and inferolateral walls (*arrow*). **(b)** Wall motion analysis from a bull's eye depiction of the left ventricle. Normal segments are *blue*, while abnormal or hypokinetic/akinetic segments are *red*. Decreased excursion of the inferior wall is suggested (*arrowhead*) and correlates with the infarct identified with LGE CMR.

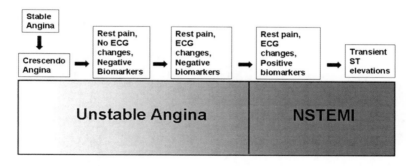

Fig. 8. Spectrum of severity in unstable angina and non-ST elevation myocardial infarction.

Table 7
Indicators of Increased Risk in Patients with NSTEACS (6)

1. Recurrent ischemia at rest or with minimal activity, despite intensive anti-ischemic therapy
2. Elevated serum troponin level
3. New ST-segment depression
4. Recurrent ischemia with heart failure symptoms, an S_3 gallop, pulmonary edema, rales or new mitral regurgitation
5. High-risk findings on noninvasive stress testing
6. LV ejection fraction <40%
7. Hemodynamic instability or angina at rest accompanied by hypotension
8. Sustained ventricular tachycardia
9. Percutaneous intervention within 6 months
10. Prior coronary artery bypass graft surgery

tified that, when present, contributed to increased risk of end points such as all-cause mortality, new or recurrent MI, or severe recurrent ischemia prompting urgent revascularization within 14 days *(41)* (Table 8). The risk of adverse events increases as the TIMI risk score increases, as demonstrated in Fig. 9. Patients with a high TIMI risk score (≥ 3) benefit from GP IIb/IIIa inhibitors (versus placebo) *(13, 43, 44)*, low-molecular weight heparin (versus unfractionated heparin) *(9, 41)*, and invasive (versus conservative) strategy *(45)*.

The Global Registry of Acute Coronary Events (GRACE) risk score is another powerful risk prediction model, validated by the GRACE and GUSTO-IIb cohorts, which can predict all-cause mortality from hospital discharge to 6 month after any form of ACS. The GRACE risk score is based on

Table 8
TIMI Risk Score for NSTEACS *(41)*

Components	Points
Age ≥ 65 years	1
Documented prior coronary artery stenosis >50%	1
At least three conventional cardiac risk factors	1
Use of aspirin in the preceding 24 h	1
At least two anginal episodes in the preceding 24 h	1
ST-segment deviation	1
Elevated cardiac biomarkers	1
Total possible score	0–7

0–2: low risk, 3–4: intermediate risk, 5–7: high risk.

Copyright © 2000 American Medical Association. All Rights Reserved.

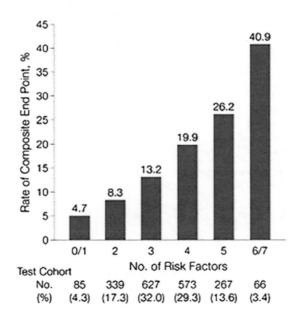

Fig. 9. Rates of all-cause mortality, myocardial infarction, and severe recurrent ischemia prompting urgent revascularization through 14 days after randomization based on the number of risk factors present. Event rates increased significantly as the TIMI risk score increased ($p < 0.001$ by χ^2 for trend) *(41)*. Copyright © 2000 American Medical Association. All Rights Reserved.

eight variables including older age, Killip class, systolic blood pressure, ST-segment deviation, cardiac arrest during presentation, serum creatinine level, positive initial cardiac biomarkers, and heart rate *(46)*.

10.6. MANAGEMENT OF NSTEACS

10.6.1. Routine Initial Measures in NSTEACS

Patients who are hemodynamically stable should be admitted to an inpatient telemetry unit for continuous ECG monitoring. Reliable intravenous access, rapid availability of bedside cardioverters–defibrillators, and frequent monitoring of vital signs are essential. Hemodynamic instability, sustained arrhythmia, or progressive ischemic discomfort may necessitate placement in a coronary care unit if a higher level of care is necessary. Bed rest should be implemented during active ischemia, and physical activity should initially be permitted only to the extent that it does not provoke symptom recurrence. Oxygen should be administered to patients with arterial saturation of <90%, patients in respiratory distress, or those with other high-risk features for hypoxemia.

10.6.2. Anti-ischemic and Analgesic Therapies

10.6.2.1. NITRATES

Nitroglycerin increases myocardial oxygen supply through endothelium-dependent coronary vasodilation while also reducing myocardial oxygen demand through venodilation and reduction of LV preload and wall stress. Nitroglycerin can be given sublingually as a tablet or buccal spray; for persistent angina, a continuous intravenous infusion of nitroglycerin may be initiated. Contraindications to nitrates include hypotension (initial systolic BP <90 mmHg or 30 mmHg below baseline) and use of phosphodiesterase-5 inhibitors within the preceding 24 h (sildenafil or vardenafil) to 48 h (tadalafil) *(47)*. *Nitrates should be avoided in patients with RV infarction, where the decrease in preload that results from nitrate-mediated venodilation may provoke hypotension.* Nitrates appear to have a neutral effect on mortality in MI *(48, 49)*; therefore, the goal of nitrate therapy is the relief of anginal discomfort.

10.6.2.2. MORPHINE

Judicious use of morphine is reasonable for patients with persistent anginal discomfort despite nitroglycerin therapy. A dose of morphine sulfate (1–5 mg IV) may be considered in such cases with careful blood pressure monitoring, with repeat doses every 5–30 min as needed. No randomized controlled clinical trials have been performed to determine the impact on mortality with morphine administration during ACS.

10.6.2.3. BETA-ADRENERGIC BLOCKERS

Beta-adrenergic blockers (BBs) competitively block the effects of catecholamines on beta-adrenergic receptors. In NSTEACS, the primary benefits of BBs are due to inhibition of beta-1 adrenergic receptors, which results in decreased myocardial contractility and heart rate and, therefore, reduced cardiac work and myocardial oxygen demand. Trials in the prethrombolytic era, when STEMI and NSTEMI were included, showed a reduction in infarct size, reinfarction, and mortality with BBs *(50, 51)*. Several placebo-controlled trials in NSTEACS have shown benefit of BBs in reducing progression to MI and/or recurrent ischemia *(52, 53)*.

The COMMIT trial, which evaluated 45,852 patients with acute MI (93% with STEMI, 7% with NSTEMI), suggested a modest reduction in reinfarction and ventricular fibrillation with metoprolol after day 1 but was counterbalanced by an increase in cardiogenic shock mainly during days 0–1 and primarily occurring in patients who were initially hemodynamically unstable or in acute heart failure

(54). Therefore, BBs are recommended for patients with ACS who do not have contraindications to beta-adrenergic blockade, as outlined in Table 9. A focused update to the *ACC/AHA Guidelines for STEMI Management* suggests that intravenous BBs should be avoided in the setting of severe acute heart failure or cardiogenic shock *(55)*.

Table 9
Contraindications to Beta-Adrenergic Blockers

History of severe bronchospasm
Bradycardia
Second- or third-degree atrioventricular (AV) block
Persistent hypotension
Previously known systolic dysfunction with *acute* pulmonary edema
Cardiogenic shock

10.6.2.4. CALCIUM CHANNEL BLOCKERS

Calcium channel blockers (CCBs) have been shown to relieve or prevent ischemic symptoms to a degree similar to BBs *(56–58)*, though meta-analyses have not found any beneficial effect of CCBs reducing mortality or subsequent reinfarction *(50, 59)*. Diltiazem and verapamil have been shown to be harmful to patients with acute MI with LV dysfunction or CHF *(57, 60, 61)*. Likewise, short-acting nifedipine, which does not lower heart rate (and instead causes a reflex *tachycardia*), has been shown to be harmful in patients when administered without a BB *(62)*. CCBs should be used in patients with ACS only if needed for recurrent ischemia despite beta-adrenergic blockade or in patients in whom BBs are contraindicated, with diltiazem and verapamil being avoided in patients with LV dysfunction and/or CHF and nifedipine being avoided altogether. When atrial fibrillation with rapid ventricular response complicates NSTEACS, BBs may be considered for rate-control strategies if CCBs are being avoided.

10.6.2.5. ANGIOTENSIN-CONVERTING ENZYME INHIBITORS

The benefits of angiotensin-converting enzyme (ACE) inhibition in STEMI have been considerable, but routine ACE inhibition in NSTEACS is less established. Three large trials showed a 0.5% absolute reduction in mortality with early ACE inhibition in patients with acute MI *(48, 49, 63)*, but no benefit was observed in patients without ST elevations in the ISIS-4 study *(49)*. Therefore, ACE inhibition in the short term does not appear to confer any benefit for patients with NSTEACS. Long-term ACE inhibition, on the other hand, has been beneficial in preventing recurrent ischemic events and mortality in patients with *stable* CAD *(64, 65)*. Recurrent MI and need for revascularization were reduced with captopril and enalapril in the SAVE and SOLVD trials *(66, 67)*, and these results have been confirmed in the HOPE and EUROPA trials *(64, 65)*. Extrapolation of these results in patients with *stable* CAD leads many clinicians to prescribe ACE inhibitors to all patients after NSTEACS. ACE inhibitors are often used within the first 24 h of NSTEACS when systemic hypertension persists despite the use of BBs and nitrates and in patients with LV dysfunction or congestive heart failure.

10.6.2.6. LIPID-LOWERING THERAPY

Long-term lipid-lowering therapy, especially with 3-hydroxy-3-methyl-glutaryl coenzyme A (HMG-CoA) reductase inhibitors (statins), has been shown to be beneficial in patients following ACS *(68–70)*. In the landmark 4S trial, simvastatin reduced mortality by 30% and coronary deaths by 42% in patients with hypercholesterolemia with a history of angina or prior MI *(68)*. Recurrent MI and the need for coronary revascularization were likewise decreased by 37% *(68, 71)*.

The benefit of early statin initiation in the setting of NSTEMI has been investigated in several studies *(72–75)*. The MIRACL trial found that a 4-month course of atorvastatin 80 mg/day, initiated between 24 and 96 h after hospital admission for NSTEMI, reduced the incidence of cardiovascular death, nonfatal MI, resuscitated sudden cardiac death, or urgent rehospitalization for recurrent ischemia by 16% *(76)*, with similar findings in the longer-term A-to-Z TIMI 21 trial of early aggressive simvastatin treatment *(77)*.

The role of intensive lipid-lowering therapy (atorvastatin 80 mg/day) was compared to standard lipid-lowering therapy (pravastatin 40 mg/day) in patients with ACS in the PROVE-IT-TIMI 22 study *(78)*. Standard therapy led to a low-density lipoprotein cholesterol (LDL-C) value of 95 mg/dL, while intensive therapy lowered LDL to a median value of 62 mg/dL. The risk of death, MI, UA, revascularization, or stroke was reduced by 16% with intensive therapy, with rates at 2 year (mean time of follow-up) falling from 26.3 to 22.4% in the standard versus intensive therapy groups. Benefits were emerged within 30 days of randomization and continued throughout 2.5 year of follow-up. Patients with ACS should be initiated on high-dose statin therapy and continued to achieve target LDL-C levels.

The latest update to the National Cholesterol Education Panel (NCEP) guidelines considers those with a history of ACS as very high risk and recommends an optional goal LDL-C of <70 mg/dL for these patients *(79)*.

10.6.3. Antiplatelet Therapies

10.6.3.1. ASPIRIN

Aspirin decreases platelet aggregation by irreversibly modifying the enzyme cyclooxygenase (COX)-1 and attenuating thromboxane release. The Antithrombotic Trialists' Collaboration included over 5,000 patients with NSTEACS enrolled in 12 trials treated with antiplatelet therapy (mostly with aspirin) and demonstrated that the combined end point of MI, stroke, or death from cardiovascular disease was reduced by 46% with antiplatelet therapy *(80)*. The optimal dosage of aspirin during the acute phase of ACS appears to be at least 160 mg/day, based on the mortality benefit seen among STEMI patients enrolled in the ISIS-2 trial *(81)*. For long-term treatment, a dose of 75–100 mg/day is equally effective compared to the higher dosage and appears to have lower bleeding complications *(82)*. Aspirin resistance has been reported in 5–8% of patients during chronic therapy and is not dose dependent *(83–85)*, though this phenomenon may simply reflect inadequate blockade of the thromboxane pathway.

Contraindications to aspirin are rare, but include documented aspirin allergy (e.g., bronchoconstriction), active life-threatening bleeding, or a known platelet disorder. For patients with mild gastrointestinal symptoms such as non-ulcer dyspepsia, it is usually safe to continue such therapy, at least in the short term, clopidogrel therapy (see subsequent discussion) *(4)*, or strong consideration of performing aspirin desensitization in an intensive care unit setting.

10.6.3.2. CLOPIDOGREL

Clopidogrel blocks platelet adenosine diphosphate (ADP) receptors, thereby interfering with platelet aggregation and increasing bleeding time. The CAPRIE trial compared clopidogrel to aspirin for secondary prevention in a broad range of patients with atherosclerotic disease, finding that clopidogrel resulted in an 8.7% relative reduction in the long-term combined end point of stroke, MI, or cardiovascular death *(86)*. Dual antiplatelet therapy with clopidogrel and aspirin in NSTEACS was addressed in the CURE trial, where patients were randomized to receive aspirin alone or with clopidogrel. Cardiovascular death, MI, or stroke at 9th month was reduced by 20%, and the benefit persisted for 1 year *(14)*. Similar findings were observed in the PCI-CURE trial, which evaluated a subset of CURE patients who underwent percutaneous coronary intervention (PCI) *(87)*. In CURE, dual antiplatelet therapy was associated with a 35% increase in major bleeding, but the absolute increase was only small at 1%: from 2.7 to 3.7%, and there was no increase in intracranial hemorrhage rate *(14)*.

Clopidogrel at a loading dose of 300 mg orally, and a maintenance dose of 75 mg daily, should be administered to all eligible patients with NSTEACS *(4)*. Higher loading doses, such as 600 mg or 900 mg orally, also appear to be safe and more rapidly acting. To reduce the risk of acute stent thrombosis, a potentially catastrophic complication, clopidogrel should be continued for a minimum of 1 month for bare-metal stents (and ideally for up to 1 year) and a minimum 12 month uninterrupted therapy for drug-eluting stents. It is also ideal to continue clopidogrel for 12 month in patients treated with medical therapy alone.

Perioperative bleeding is increased in patients undergoing coronary artery bypass graft (CABG) surgery within 5 days of clopidogrel treatment versus patients treated with aspirin. In this subset of CURE patients, 9.6% of patients treated with clopidogrel had significant bleeding (defined as receipt of ≥ 2 units of blood) compared to 6.3% of patients treated with aspirin. If surgery was delayed beyond 5 days of clopidogrel treatment, no excess bleeding was observed *(14)*.

A newer ADP-receptor antagonist, prasugrel, has been shown to have a more rapid onset of action along with a higher dose of platelet inhibition than clopidogrel *(88)*. The TRITON-TIMI 38 trial directly compared prasugrel to clopidogrel in 13,608 moderate- to high-risk patients with ACS undergoing PCI, including 10,074 with NSTEACS *(89)*. At 15-month follow-up, the rate of definite or probable stent thrombosis was significantly reduced in the prasugrel group (1.1% versus 2.4%). The rates of cardiovascular death, nonfatal MI, or stroke were also significantly less with prasugrel versus clopidogrel (9.9% versus 12.1%), though major bleeding events were slightly higher in the prasugrel group (2.4% versus 1.8%). Though FDA approval is still pending, prasugrel may be more beneficial than clopidogrel for reducing stent thrombosis events in selected patients for whom this slightly higher bleeding risk would still be acceptable.

10.6.3.3. Glycoprotein IIb/IIIa Inhibitors

GP IIb/IIIa inhibitors are useful in selected patients with NSTEACS, primarily where an early invasive strategy is employed. The benefit is seen in high-risk patients: those with elevated cardiac biomarkers, TIMI risk score ≥ 3, or continued ischemic discomfort. Current ACC/AHA guidelines recommend using an IV GP IIb/IIIa inhibitor, along with aspirin, clopidogrel, and unfractionated heparin (UFH) or low-molecular weight heparin (LMWH), in patients with NSTEMI in whom catheterization with PCI is planned *(4)*. The GP IIb/IIIa inhibitors eptifibatide or tirofiban are also encouraged in patients treated conservatively, whereas abciximab is not approved for this indication. Several moderate-sized clinical trials have evaluated the role of GP IIb/IIIa inhibitors, with many demonstrating a reduction in death, recurrent MI, and urgent revascularization *(11–13, 90)*. A meta-analysis of six trials of 31,000 patients with NSTEACS who were not scheduled to undergo early revascularization demonstrated significant reduction in death and MI at 5 days (5.7% versus 6.9%) and 30 days (10.8% versus 11.8%) *(91)*. The benefit was limited to patients who underwent PCI or CABG within 30 days and only to those patients in whom the troponin was elevated.

As powerful inhibitors of platelet aggregation, GP IIb/IIIa inhibitors are associated with higher rates of major bleeding (2.4% versus 1.4% for placebo in a meta-analysis) *(91)*. Dose reductions are necessary for renal insufficiency when administering tirofiban and eptifibatide, and their use is discouraged in patients with a creatinine >4.0 mg/dL. Abciximab may be used in patients with renal insufficiency, including those on hemodialysis. An important side effect of GP IIb/IIIa inhibitors is thrombocytopenia (incidence ranging 0.2–2% in clinical trials), and routine measurement of platelet count is indicated prior to initiation, 6–8 h later, and daily thereafter until infusion is terminated. If the platelet count drops below 50,000 per μL, the GP IIb/IIIa inhibitor should be discontinued. Platelet transfusion should be considered if the platelet count is <10,000 per μL, if there is severe bleeding, or if an emergency invasive procedure is needed.

10.6.3.4. ANTICOAGULATION

Addition of subcutaneous LMWH, intravenous UFH, or fondaparinux to therapy with aspirin and/or clopidogrel is a Class I recommendation for all patients with NSTEACS *(4)*, with an alternative option of bivalirudin for patients treated with an invasive strategy.

10.6.3.5. UNFRACTIONATED OR LOW-MOLECULAR WEIGHT HEPARIN

Several trials demonstrated superiority of combined therapy with intravenous UFH and aspirin versus aspirin alone for preventing death or MI in ACS. A meta-analysis by Oler et al. demonstrated that addition of IV heparin to aspirin reduced the death or MI rate by one-third *(8)*. The dosing regimen of IV heparin that results in the best aPTT control and the highest safety is 60 units/kg IV bolus, followed by 12 units/kg IV infusion with subsequent drip rate adjustments based on aPTT; measurement of aPTT is done 6 h after starting the IV infusion of heparin, and then every 12–24 h during the infusion, with goal aPTT 50–70 s.

Enoxaparin has several potential advantages over UFH in ACS. It has a higher anti-Xa to anti-IIa activity ratio (which results in less thrombin generation), higher bioavailability, and more predictable and potent antithrombin activity. Administration is simplified, and frequent laboratory monitoring is not necessary. In several trials of enoxaparin versus either placebo or UFH, enoxaparin was more effective in preventing death or MI, while bleeding rates were overall equivalent between LMWH and UFH *(92)*; similar findings have been observed in more recent studies employing GP IIb/IIIa inhibitors and an early invasive approach *(93, 94)*. In a meta-analysis of contemporary trials of enoxaparin versus UFH in NSTEACS, enoxaparin resulted in a statistically significant 9% reduction in the odds of death or MI at 30 days *(92)*. Current guidelines give a Class IIa indication to enoxaparin as the preferred antithrombin versus UFH in NSTEACS, unless the patient has renal failure or is scheduled to undergo CABG within 24 h *(4)*.

10.6.3.6. DIRECT THROMBIN INHIBITORS

Direct thrombin inhibitors (DTIs) such as bivalirudin have undergone extensive evaluation in NSTEACS. The ACUITY trial tested bivalirudin alone or with a GP IIb/IIIa inhibitor, versus UFH or LMWH with a GP IIb/IIIa inhibitor in patients undergoing PCI for NSTEACS *(95)*. Bivalirudin with or without GP IIb/IIIa inhibitor was found to be noninferior to UFH/LMWH and GP IIb/IIIa inhibitor, and bivalirudin monotherapy had a superior net clinical benefit driven primarily by a reduction in bleeding *(95)*. Patients needed to be pretreated with clopidogrel to have the clinical benefit. Until further data are available, the primary niche for DTIs in ACS may be antithrombin therapy for patients with heparin-induced thrombocytopenia thrombosis syndrome (HITTS) or for use during PCI, especially in patients with an increased risk of bleeding.

10.6.3.7. FONDAPARINUX

Fondaparinux is a synthetic polysaccharide that directly inhibits factor Xa activity. Potential advantages over UFH include decreased binding to plasma proteins, dose-independent clearance, and a longer half-life with more predictable and sustained anticoagulation with fixed once-daily subcutaneous dosing. Fondaparinux, like enoxaparin, does not require laboratory monitoring. Fondaparinux and enoxaparin had similar rates of death, MI, or refractory ischemia at 9 days in the OASIS-5 trial *(96)*, but fondaparinux had a significantly lower rate of bleeding which was also observed in a subgroup analysis of patients who underwent PCI *(97)*. Current ACC/AHA guidelines give a Class I recommendation to the use of fondaparinux in patients undergoing an early invasive strategy for NSTEACS, with a Class IIa recommendation for its use rather than UFH in patients managed with an initial conservative strategy *(4)*. Because of a higher risk of catheter-associated thrombus in OASIS-5 patients who underwent PCI after pretreatment with fondaparinux (0.9% versus 0.3%) *(96)*, current guidelines recommend that patients receiving fondaparinux pre-PCI should receive an additional anticoagulant with anti-IIa activity to support PCI and specifically recommend UFH for this purpose *(4)*. Fondaparinux is preferable in patients with an increased risk of bleeding. If CABG is planned within 24 h, UFH is preferred since its anticoagulant effect can be more rapidly reversed *(4)*.

10.6.3.8. WARFARIN

The combination of aspirin plus warfarin in MI appears to be more effective than aspirin alone for long-term secondary prevention, but results in a significant increase in the risk of major bleeding *(98)*. Given the similar benefit seen with dual antiplatelet therapy of aspirin plus clopidogrel with the added convenience of less frequent laboratory monitoring, as well as the common use of PCI in the patient population (where clopidogrel use is firmly established), the clinical use of aspirin plus warfarin is limited. Currently, such an approach should be taken in patients with a separate clinical indication for warfarin, such as chronic atrial fibrillation or severe LV dysfunction with high risk of systemic embolization. A 3–6-month course of warfarin should be strongly considered following the diagnosis of new LV aneurysm, especially if intracardiac thrombus is present. Data on long-term anticoagulation of such patients are limited.

10.6.3.9. FIBRINOLYSIS

Fibrinolytic therapy is *contraindicated* in patients with NSTEACS. Several trials, including TIMI-IIIB, showed conclusively that such therapy in NSTEACS was associated with *more* fatal and nonfatal MI and a higher rate of intracranial hemorrhage than heparin alone *(99)*. Coronary arteriography during NSTEACS demonstrates that the culprit artery is not occluded in 60–85% of cases *(100)*, and the nonocclusive thrombus is often platelet rich and therefore less likely to respond to fibrinolytic therapy *(101)*. In contrast, patients with STEMI often have an occlusive thrombus that is fibrin rich *(102)* and therefore more likely to respond to fibrinolytic therapy.

10.6.4. Invasive versus Conservative Strategy

Early invasive strategy generally refers to coronary angiography and, when indicated, percutaneous intervention within the first 48 h after NSTEACS presentation. A suggested algorithm for this strategy from the *ACC/AHA Guidelines* is shown in Fig. 10. *Conservative strategy* encompasses full medical management, followed by functional coronary evaluation such as treadmill or pharmacologic stress testing or echocardiography. Angiography is then performed for recurrent ischemia, hemodynamic instability, malignant arrhythmia, or high-risk findings on noninvasive testing. A suggested algorithm for this strategy from the *ACC/AHA Guidelines* is shown in Fig. 11.

Nine large randomized trials have compared invasive to conservative strategies in NSTEACS, and all trials except for the VANQWISH trial have demonstrated an advantage to early invasive strategy in patients with moderate-to-high risk for nonfatal MI, heart failure, or death *(45, 99, 103, 104)*. Markers of increased risk differed between the trials and included age in TIMI-IIIB, elevated serum troponin in FRISC II and TACTICS-TIMI 18, and ST depression in TIMI-IIIB, FRISC II, and TACTICS-TIMI 18. Early invasive strategy currently receives a Class I recommendation in NSTEACS patients with high-risk indicators *(4)*.

Per current *ACC/AHA Guidelines* for antiplatelet therapy, aspirin should be administered to UA/NSTEMI patients as soon as possible after hospital presentation *(4)*. If an initial invasive strategy is selected, additional antiplatelet therapy should be administered before diagnostic angiography as a Class I recommendation and can consist of either clopidogrel (loading dose followed by daily maintenance dose) or an intravenous GP IIb/IIIa inhibitor; the combination of these three antiplatelet agents prior to diagnostic angiography is also recommended as a Class IIa recommendation for patients managed with an initial invasive strategy *(4)*. If an early conservative strategy is selected, clopidogrel should be added to aspirin as a Class I recommendation and administered for at least 1 month and

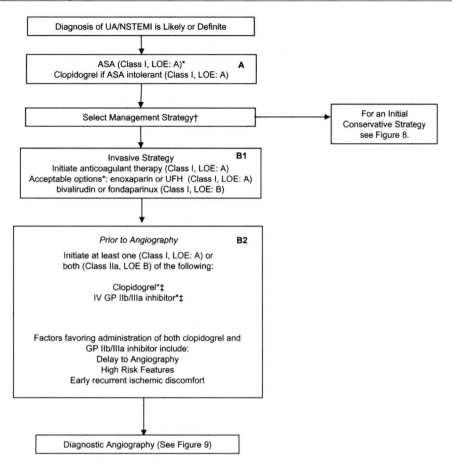

Fig. 10. Algorithm for patients with NSTEACS managed by an initial invasive strategy. When multiple drugs are listed, they are in alphabetical order and not in order of preference (e.g., Boxes B1 and B2) *(4)*. ASA = Aspirin, GP = Glycoprotein, I = Intravenous, LOE = Level of Evidence, UA/NSTEM = Unstable Angina/Non-ST-Elevation Myocardial Infarction, UFH = Unfractionated Heparin. Reproduced from the *Journal of the American College of Cardiology* © 2007 with permission from Elsevier.

ideally up to 1 year *(4)*. If recurrent symptoms, ischemia, heart failure, or serious arrhythmias occur in patients being managed with an initial early conservative strategy, diagnostic angiography should be performed and either GP IIb/IIIa inhibitor or clopidogrel should be added to aspirin and anticoagulation therapy before diagnostic angiography as Class I recommendations *(4)*. An intravenous GP IIb/IIIa inhibitor can also be given to patients receiving aspirin, clopidogrel, and anticoagulant therapy as part of an initial conservative strategy if recurrent ischemic discomfort occurs as a Class IIa recommendation *(4)*.

Anticoagulant therapy should be given in addition to antiplatelet therapy in UA/NSTEMI patients as soon as possible after presentation per current ACC/AHA guidelines *(4)*. If an invasive strategy is selected, regimens can include either enoxaparin or UFH (Class I, level of evidence [LOE] A), or either bivalirudin or fondaparinux (Class I, LOE B). For a conservative strategy, enoxaparin and UFH have established efficacy (Class I, LOE A) along with fondaparinux (Class I, LOE B), with fondaparinux being preferred if bleeding risk is increased *(4)*; enoxaparin or fondaparinux is preferred over UFH as a Class IIa recommendation, unless CABG is planned within 24 h *(4)*.

If PCI is performed as a post-angiography management strategy, aspirin and clopidogrel should be continued along with intravenous GP IIb/IIIa inhibitor (if not started before diagnostic angiography),

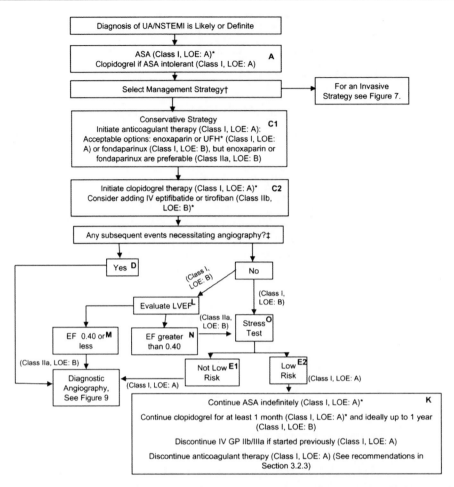

Fig. 11. Algorithm for patients with NSTEACS managed by an initial conservative strategy. When multiple drugs are listed, they are in alphabetical order and not in order of preference (e.g., Boxes C, C1, and C2). ‡Recurrent symptoms/ischemia, heart failure, serious arrhythmia *(4)*. ASA = Aspirin; EF = ejection fraction; GP = glycoprotein; IV = Intravenous; LOE = Level of Evidence; LVEF = Left Ventricular Ejection Fraction, UA/NSTEMI = Unstable Angina/Non-ST Elevation Myocardial Infarction, UFH = Unfractionated Heparin. Reproduced from the *Journal of the American College of Cardiology* © 2007 with permission from Elsevier.

while anticoagulant therapy should be discontinued post-PCI for uncomplicated cases as Class I recommendations *(4)*. If angiography identified CAD but no PCI was performed, aspirin and clopidogrel should be continued post-angiography, while GP IIb/IIIa inhibitor should be discontinued and UFH should be continued for at least 48 h or until discharge. If either enoxaparin or fondaparinux were selected for anticoagulation pre-angiography, they should be continued for the duration of hospitalization (up to 8 days) as a Class I recommendation. These guidelines for appropriate cessation of therapy are also applicable to patients managed with a conservative strategy who did not undergo angiography *(4)*.

10.6.5. Predischarge Non-invasive Risk Stratification After UA/NSTEMI

Several situations may arise where non-invasive risk stratification would be helpful in patients with suspected or definite NSTEACS prior to discharge from the hospital

1. To diagnose or rule out ACS in patients with an intermediate probability for this diagnosis.
2. To diagnose exercise-induced ischemia in patients, in whom early conservative strategy has been employed, and to assess ischemia extent and severity.
3. To diagnose and localize residual ischemia in patients, where complete percutaneous or surgical revascularization has not been fully accomplished (e.g., patient with multivessel coronary disease, who underwent PCI of a culprit vessel).
4. To assess myocardium for viability and thus determine utility of future revascularization.

Treadmill exercise tolerance testing (ETT) with echocardiography or myocardial perfusion imaging is most commonly employed. Pharmacologic stress testing with a vasodilator (e.g., adenosine or dipyridamole) may be performed if patients cannot exercise and is safe as early as 48 h after presentation with a definite ACS if the ECG is stable for 24 h prior to the test, biomarkers are downtrending, and the patient is free of anginal discomfort at rest.

If an early invasive strategy has been employed, and revascularization has been complete, there is generally no need for functional testing prior to hospital discharge. Such testing may be undertaken later, primarily to determine the patient's functional exercise capacity, provide a new "baseline" study, and prescribe an appropriate exercise program for cardiac rehabilitation.

10.7. SECONDARY PREVENTION MEASURES AFTER NSTEACS

Diagnosis of ACS is commonly perceived as a "life-changing" event, and risk factor modification and secondary prevention measures become central to long-term management. Table 10 provides a comprehensive checklist of issues to be addressed at the first outpatient appointment following a hospital discharge for NSTEACS.

10.7.1. Pharmacologic Measures

10.7.1.1. ASPIRIN

Following ACS, aspirin reduces the risk of recurrent MI, stroke, or cardiovascular death by approximately 25% (80). A dose of 75–162 mg/day should be continued in all patients unless contraindicated, with a higher initial dose of 162–325 mg/day given for a prespecified duration as outlined in Table 11 (4).

10.7.1.2. CLOPIDOGREL

Clopidogrel therapy following ACS is outlined in Table 11 (4). Given the potentially catastrophic consequences of stent thrombosis, the importance of adhering to these post-PCI dual antiplatelet therapy guidelines must be reinforced.

10.7.1.3. BETA-ADRENERGIC BLOCKERS

BBs reduce mortality after ACS by as much as 23%, mainly by reducing the incidence of fatal ventricular tachyarrhythmias and blocking the effects of adverse cardiac remodeling in patients with LV systolic dysfunction (105). Unless contraindicated, BBs should be administered indefinitely to all patients recovering from NSTEACS.

10.7.1.4. ACE INHIBITORS

Multiple studies have demonstrated the efficacy of ACE inhibitors for secondary prevention of CAD (64–67). The greatest benefit is derived from patients at higher risk, such as those with depressed LV ejection fraction (LVEF) or large anterior MI. Because of their beneficial effects in hypertension, diabetes mellitus, or chronic renal insufficiency, ACE inhibitors are strongly recommended in patients with these conditions. The 2007 ACC/AHA guidelines give a Class I recommendation to

Table 10
Outpatient Visit Checklist for Patients Discharged with Diagnosis of NSTEACS

Demographics
Name:_____
DOB:_____   Age:_____
PCP:_____
Cardiologist:_____
Cardiologist Phone #:_____
Date of ACS:_____

Coronary Anatomy at Discharge
Date:_____
LMCA:_____
LAD:_____
LCx:_____
RCA:_____
LIMA:_____
SVG:_____
SVG:_____
SVG:_____
LVEF:_____ by Echo Cath Nuclear CMR

Risk Factor Modification
Diabetic: Yes/No
Smoker: Yes/No
Hypertension: Yes/No
Hyperlipidemia: Yes/No
Overweight: Yes/No
Chronic renal insufficiency: Yes/No
Congestive heart failure: Yes/No
Depression: Yes/No

Stents Used (circle all that apply)
Bare-metal   Heparin-coated
Drug-eluting
Type_____
Date implanted:_____

Follow-Up Issues to Be Addressed
☐ Reinforce dual antiplatelet therapy
☐ Aspirin for life
☐ Plavix per guidelines
☐ Beta-blocker indefinitely
☐ ACE inhibitor if CHF/LVEF <40%, diabetic,
    hypertensive, renal insufficiency
☐ Statin therapy post-ACS
☐ Check HbA1c, goal <7.0
☐ Goal LDL <70, HDL >40, trig <150
☐ Goal BP <130/80
☐ Check weight, BMI, waist circumference goal
    BMI 18.5–24.9, goal waist circumference
    <40 in. (men) or <35 in. (women)
☐ Smoking cessation
☐ NTG Rx as needed; refill regularly
☐ Stop HRT
☐ Avoid COX-2 inhibitors
☐ Dietary changes – ADA, DASH diets
☐ Cardiac rehabilitation program

Labs
☐ Hemoglobin:_____
☐ Platelets:_____
☐ Creatinine:_____
☐ Fasting glucose:_____
☐ HbA1c:_____
☐ Total cholesterol:_____
☐ LDL:_____
☐ HDL:_____
☐ Triglycerides:_____
☐ CRP:_____

Antiplatelet Therapy Dosing Guidelines
☐ Aspirin: 325 mg/day for _____ months
    then 81 mg/day **indefinitely**
☐ Plavix: 75 mg/day for _____ months
    mandatory uninterrupted therapy

ACE inhibitors being prescribed indefinitely for patients recovering from NSTEACS with heart failure, LV systolic dysfunction (LVEF <40%), hypertension, or diabetes mellitus, unless contraindicated *(4)*. Angiotensin-receptor blockers may be prescribed in cases of ACE inhibitor intolerance (e.g., persistent cough, history of angioedema).

10.7.1.5. STATINS AND LIPID-LOWERING THERAPY

Multiple studies have demonstrated that statins reduce CAD death and recurrent MI post-ACS through a wide range of pretreatment levels *(68–76, 78)*. The PROVE-IT and MIRACL studies suggest

Table 11
Suggested Antiplatelet Therapy Duration Post-NSTEACS

Type of stent	Duration of high-dose aspirin therapy (month)	Duration of clopidogrel therapy (mandatory for prevention of stent thrombosis if stent placed) (month)
None	1	1
Bare-metal stent	1	1
Cypher DES	3	12
Taxus DES	6	12

that early high-dose statin therapy appears to confer additional benefits after MI *(76, 78)*. Updated NCEP guidelines recommend an optional LDL-C goal of less than 70 mg/dL for very high-risk patients, including those with a recent NSTEACS *(79)*. If the LDL goal is not achieved with diet and statin therapy, options include adding a bile acid binding resin, ezetimibe, niacin, or fibrate therapy, depending upon the specific derangements in the lipid profile. Post-ACS patients with near-goal LDL but low HDL (<40 mg/dL) benefit from treatment to raise HDL, and both gemfibrozil and niacin have been demonstrated to reduce cardiac events when used for this purpose.

10.7.2. Medications of No Benefit or Harm Following ACS

10.7.2.1. VITAMINS/ANTIOXIDANTS

Although there is an association between elevated homocysteine (HCY) levels and CAD, reduction of HCY levels by folic acid supplementation does not seem to reduce the risk of ACS events *(106, 107)* Additionally, clinical trials have failed to demonstrate a benefit of antioxidant vitamins for primary or secondary prevention of CAD *(108)*. Neither of these strategies should be used for secondary prevention following NSTEACS.

10.7.2.2. HORMONE REPLACEMENT THERAPY

The heart and estrogen/progestin replacement study (HERS) trial of estrogen/progestin therapy for secondary prevention of CAD in post-menopausal women failed to demonstrate benefit *(109)*, with a pattern of early increased risk of CAD events. The Women's Health Initiative (WHI) also identified an increased risk of coronary events associated with hormone replacement therapy (HRT), especially within the first year after beginning HRT *(110, 111)*. These studies were stopped early in light of these observed risks. Post-menopausal women receiving HRT at the time of NSTEACS should discontinue its use, and HRT should not be initiated for secondary prevention of coronary events *(4)*.

10.7.2.3. NON-STEROIDAL ANTI-INFLAMMATORY DRUGS

Selective COX-2 inhibitors and other non-selective, non-steroidal, anti-inflammatory drugs (NSAIDs) have been associated with increased cardiovascular risk, particularly in patients with established CAD *(112)*. Alternative agents, such as acetaminophen, tramadol, or short-term narcotic analgesics, should be considered for musculoskeletal pain management. Non-selective NSAIDs such as naproxen should only be used very sparingly for refractory pain.

10.7.3. Therapy for Co-morbidities Following NSTEACS

10.7.3.1. DIABETES MELLITUS

Diabetes mellitus confers a significant additional risk of mortality during ACS, and meticulous control of serum glucose becomes paramount following discharge. A target hemoglobin A1c of <7%

is recommended by the ACC/AHA for diabetics post-MI *(113)* through diet, physical activity, oral hypoglycemics, and insulin. Thiazolidinedione drugs should be used with caution, however, since they may cause substantial sodium and fluid retention and are therefore contraindicated in patients with decompensated (NYHA Class III–IV) heart failure after ACS.

10.7.3.2. HYPERTENSION

The *2007 AHA Statement on the Treatment of Hypertension in CAD* and the 2007 European Society of Hypertension–European Society of Cardiology (ESH-ESC) recommend a goal BP below 130/80 mmHg in patients with established CAD or a coronary risk equivalent such as carotid artery disease, peripheral arterial disease, abdominal aortic aneurysm, or diabetes mellitus *(114, 115)*. Home blood pressure monitoring should be emphasized.

10.7.3.3. DEPRESSION

Major depression is common among patients hospitalized for CAD, and depression after MI is associated with a 5.7-fold increase in cardiac mortality within 6 months *(116)*. A combination of short-term individual cognitive behavioral therapy and selective serotonin re-uptake inhibitors (SSRIs), when needed, may reduce depressive symptoms over the 6-month post-MI period in depressed or socially isolated patients.

10.7.4. Lifestyle Modifications

10.7.4.1. SMOKING CESSATION

Patients should be advised to quit smoking at every visit. Assistance through counseling and developing a plan for quitting is essential and can be done by arranging follow-up, referral to special programs, and/or pharmacotherapy (including nicotine replacement therapy, bupropion, or varenicline). Patients should be encouraged to reduce their exposure to second-hand smoke.

10.7.4.2. DIET/NUTRITION AND WEIGHT LOSS

Diabetics should consider the American Diabetes Association (ADA) diet, and patients with hypertension may consider the JNC-7 DASH diet recommendations. Following ACS, intake of saturated fats, trans-fatty acids, and cholesterol should be reduced to less than 200 mg/day. Patients should be encouraged to increase consumption of omega-3 fatty acids in the form of fish or capsule form (1 g/day) for risk reduction. Salt intake should be minimized.

Body mass index (BMI) and waist circumference should be assessed at each visit. Weight maintenance should be encouraged through a combination of physical activity, caloric intake modification, and dietary changes. A BMI of 18.5–24.9 kg/m^2 and a waist circumference (measured horizontally at the iliac crest) of <40 in. for men and <35 in. for women is recommended *(4)*. When weight loss is necessary, the initial goal should be a 10% reduction from baseline with further goals determined by response to initial weight loss strategies.

10.7.4.3. ALCOHOL

Dietary studies have consistently demonstrated a J-shaped relationship between the amount of routinely consumed alcohol and cardiovascular events including ACS and stroke. Moderate consumption (0.5–1 drink daily for women, 1–2 drinks daily for men) increases HDL levels and has a positive effect on post-prandial glucose and insulin levels, while also reducing the risk of recurrent events after MI. However, the AHA reinforces that alcohol consumption cannot be recommended solely for cardiovascular disease risk reduction and recommends that "if alcoholic beverages are consumed, they should be limited to no more than 2 drinks/day for men and 1 drink/day for women, and ideally should be consumed with meals" *(117)*.

10.7.4.4. Physical Activity

For all NSTEACS patients, daily walking for 30–60 min should be encouraged immediately after discharge. Participating in a comprehensive cardiac rehabilitation program is a Class I recommendation from the ACC/AHA guidelines, and exercise training can generally begin within 1–2 wk after NSTEACS treated with PCI or CABG *(4)*. Decisions regarding returning to work will likely be influenced not only by a patient's cardiac functional status but also by factors such as job satisfaction, financial stability, and company policies and may need to be addressed with each patient on an individual basis depending on their functional status, the nature of their employment, and the circumstances surrounding their ACS event.

In stable patients without complications, sexual activity with the usual partner can be resumed within 7–10 days. Driving can begin 1 week after discharge, though this may also depend on individual state laws. Patients whose MI was complicated by cardiac arrest or other complications, such as high-degree heart block or serious arrhythmias, should delay driving for 2–3 week after symptoms have resolved. Air travel within the first 2 weeks after MI should be undertaken only if there is no angina, dyspnea, or hypoxemia at rest, and the patient should have a companion with them at all times *(4)*. Patients who had UA but no infarction can return to these activities sooner (often within a few days) than those who experienced NSTEMI.

10.8. CASE STUDIES

10.8.1. Case 1

A 54-year-old male with type 2 diabetes mellitus, hypertension, hyperlipidemia, and a 30 pack/year smoking history presents to the emergency room with central non-radiating chest pressure while watching television. He has had this intermittently in the past 3 months, but usually after exertion or walking fast. He takes aspirin chronically, including on the day of symptom onset. Physical examination reveals blood pressure 160/85, heart rate 85, O_2 saturation 95% on room air; he has no murmurs, normal S1, S2, and his lungs are clear. Peripheral pulses are intact and equal, and exam is otherwise unremarkable. His initial ECG suggests T-wave inversions in the inferior leads (Fig. 3), but no ST elevation. Chest x-ray is unremarkable. Cardiac biomarkers return elevated with a CPK 400, CK-MB 85, troponin-T 1.36. He is given aspirin 325 mg by mouth. His pain is initially responsive to sublingual nitroglycerin, but later becomes recurrent requiring intravenous nitroglycerin drip.

10.8.1.1. Management Strategies

This patient's clinical presentation is consistent with an NSTEMI. Initial risk stratification is important in this setting to guide further decision-making. In this case, his TIMI risk score (Table 8) would be 3 (1 point for having at least three conventional cardiac risk factors, 1 point for using aspirin in the preceding 24 h, and 1 point for elevated cardiac biomarkers), classifying him as at least intermediate risk for major adverse events.

Appropriate anti-ischemic therapy for this patient would include continuing the intravenous nitroglycerin drip as necessary for symptomatic relief. Beta-adrenergic blockade would be appropriate as well. Given his higher TIMI risk score, he should receive anticoagulation with either unfractionated heparin or low-molecular weight heparin. Additionally, with a TIMI risk score of 3, cardiac catheterization should be performed within 48 h of initial presentation as part of an initial invasive strategy. His antiplatelet regimen should include aspirin, and it would be reasonable to add clopidogrel with a loading dose being given prior to cardiac catheterization. Given the possibility of PCI being performed during cardiac catheterization, and in light of his TIMI risk score, an IV GP IIb/IIIa inhibitor should be administered as adjunctive antiplatelet therapy. If his symptoms are refractory to anti-ischemic therapies, performing cardiac catheterization more expeditiously may need to be considered.

10.8.2. Case 2

A 75-year-old female with obesity, hypertension, hyperlipidemia, and a 40 pack/year smoking history presents to the office for follow-up. She had recently been admitted to the hospital for an inferior non-ST elevation myocardial infarction and was taken for cardiac catheterization during which a sirolimus-eluting stent was placed in her mid-RCA. A transthoracic echocardiogram prior to discharge revealed preserved biventricular systolic function (LVEF 55%) and mild left ventricular hypertrophy, with no significant valvular disease seen. Her current ECG demonstrates inferior Q-waves consistent with her myocardial infarction (Fig. 4). She is currently on aspirin 325 mg/day, clopidogrel 7 mg/day, atorvastatin 80 mg/day, and metoprolol succinate 25 mg/day. Her blood pressure remains elevated at 155/90, correlating with her home readings. She continues to smoke 10 cigarettes/day.

10.8.2.1. MANAGEMENT DECISIONS

This patient has had a recent NSTEMI in the setting of several cardiac risk factors. Since she had a sirolimus-eluting stent placed, she should remain on high-dose aspirin for 3 months and then be transitioned to 81 mg daily dose indefinitely. She should remain on clopidogrel for 12 months mandatory uninterrupted therapy to reduce the risk of stent thrombosis (Table 11).

She remains hypertensive, and left ventricular hypertrophy on her echocardiogram suggests this has been a chronic process. An ACE inhibitor would be a reasonable therapy for this patient, not only for management of her hypertension but also for long-term reduction of recurrent ischemic events in patients with stable CAD. Her beta-adrenergic blocker could be advanced as tolerated as well. An appropriate target blood pressure would be less than 130/80 mmHg.

She should remain on a statin, and given her recent NSTEACS event, a target LDL-C of less than 70 mg/dL should be considered. Her HDL target should be greater than 40 mg/dL, and gemfibrozil or niacin may be added to her regimen if necessary to help achieve this target HDL.

Table 12
Suggested Online Resources for Further Information

Name	Web address	Features
CardioSource	http://www.cardiosource.com/	American College of Cardiology site with extensive library of images, reviews of current literature, and references to ACC/AHA guidelines
TheHeart.org	http://www.theheart.org/	An independent website with news updates from current clinical trials as well as streaming discussions, educational programs, and slide downloads
Clinical trial results	http://www.clinicaltrialresults.org/	Current clinical trials, with streaming interviews with clinical investigators, slide downloads
ACC guidelines database	http://www.acc.org/qualityand science/clinical/topic/topic.htm	Index of ACC clinical guidelines
AHA statistics	http://www.americanheart.org/ presenter.jhtml?identifier=3055922	Latest cardiovascular disease statistics from the American Heart Association
ECG wave maven	http://ecg.bidmc.harvard.edu/maven/ mavenmain.asp	A leading free online ECG education tool, with many ECGs pertaining to acute coronary syndrome diagnosis and complications

Further risk factor modification should also be addressed at this visit. Weight maintenance should be encouraged to achieve a goal BMI of 18.5–24.9 and a waist circumference of >35 in. for a female patient. Smoking cessation is imperative, and all available options should be reviewed in order to develop a plan for quitting. Physical activity should be encouraged immediately after discharge, and it would be reasonable to refer this patient to a comprehensive cardiac rehabilitation program.

10.9. FURTHER READING

Several online resources are available for further detailed information regarding management of patients with NSTEACS. These resources can be found in Table 12.

REFERENCES

1. Rosamond W, Flegal K, Furie K, et al. Heart disease and stroke statistics—2008 update: a report from the American Heart Association Statistics Committee and Stroke Statistics Subcommittee. *Circulation*. 2008;117(4):e25–e146.
2. Fox KA, Steg PG, Eagle KA, et al. Decline in rates of death and heart failure in acute coronary syndromes, 1999–2006. *JAMA*. 2007;297(17):1892–1900.
3. Thygesen K, Alpert JS, White HD, et al. Universal definition of myocardial infarction. *Circulation*. 2007;116(22):2634–2653.
4. Anderson JL, Adams CD, Antman EM, et al. ACC/AHA 2007 guidelines for the management of patients with unstable angina/non-ST-elevation myocardial infarction: a report of the American College of Cardiology/American Heart Association Task Force on Practice Guidelines (Writing Committee to Revise the 2002 Guidelines for the Management of Patients with Unstable Angina/Non-ST-Elevation Myocardial Infarction) developed in collaboration with the American College of Emergency Physicians, the Society for Cardiovascular Angiography and Interventions, and the Society of Thoracic Surgeons endorsed by the American Association of Cardiovascular and Pulmonary Rehabilitation and the Society for Academic Emergency Medicine. *J Am Coll Cardiol*. 2007;50(7):e1–e157.
5. Braunwald E. Unstable angina: an etiologic approach to management. *Circulation*. 1998;98(21):2219–2222.
6. Gelfand EV, Cannon CP. Myocardial infarction: contemporary management strategies. *J Intern Med*. 2007;262(1):59–77.
7. Theroux P, Ouimet H, McCans J, et al. Aspirin, heparin or both to treat unstable angina. *N Engl J Med*. 1988;319:1105–1111.
8. Oler A, Whooley MA, Oler J, Grady D. Adding heparin to aspirin reduces the incidence of myocardial infarction and death in patients with unstable angina. A meta-analysis. *JAMA*. 1996;276:811–815.
9. Antman EM, McCabe CH, Gurfinkel EP, et al. Enoxaparin prevents death and cardiac ischemic events in unstable Angina/Non-Q-wave myocardial infarction: results of the Thrombolysis In Myocardial Infarction (TIMI) 11B trial. *Circulation*. 1999;100(15):1593–1601.
10. Cohen M, Demers C, Gurfinkel EP, et al. A comparison of low-molecular-weight heparin with unfractionated heparin for unstable coronary artery disease. *N Engl J Med*. 1997;337:447–452.
11. The PURSUIT Trial Investigators. Inhibition of Platelet Glycoprotein IIb/IIIa with eptifibatide in patients with acute coronary syndromes. *N Engl J Med*. 1998;339:436–443.
12. The Platelet Receptor Inhibition for Ischemic Syndrome Management (PRISM) Study Investigators. A comparison of aspirin plus tirofiban with aspirin plus heparin for unstable angina. *N Engl J Med*. 1998;338:1498–1505.
13. The Platelet Receptor Inhibition for Ischemic Syndrome Management in Patients Limited by Unstable Signs and Symptoms (PRISM-PLUS) Trial Investigators. Inhibition of the platelet glycoprotein IIb/IIIa receptor with tirofiban in unstable angina and non-Q-wave myocardial infarction. *N Engl J Med*. 1998;338:1488–1497.
14. Clopidogrel in Unstable Angina to Prevent Recurrent Events Trial Investigators. Effects of clopidogrel in addition to aspirin in patients with acute coronary syndromes without ST-segment elevation. *N Engl J Med*. 2001;345:494–502.
15. Storey RF, Newby LJ, Heptinstall S. Effects of P2Y(1) and P2Y(12) receptor antagonists on platelet aggregation induced by different agonists in human whole blood. *Platelets*. 2001;12(7):443–447.
16. Pitts WR, Lange RA, Cigarroa JE, Hillis LD. Cocaine-induced myocardial ischemia and infarction: pathophysiology, recognition, and management. *Prog Cardiovasc Dis*. 1997;40(1):65–76.
17. Strike PC, Steptoe A. Systematic review of mental stress-induced myocardial ischaemia. *Eur Heart J*. 2003;24(8):690–703.
18. Kaski JC. Rapid coronary artery disease progression and angiographic stenosis morphology. *Ital Heart J*. 2000;1(1):21–25.

19. Kannel WB. Silent myocardial ischemia and infarction: insights from the Framingham Study. *Cardiol Clin.* 1986;4(4):583–591.
20. Campeau L. Letter: grading of angina pectoris. *Circulation.* 1976;54(3):522–523.
21. Holmes DR Jr., Berger PB, Hochman JS, et al. Cardiogenic shock in patients with acute ischemic syndromes with and without ST-segment elevation. *Circulation.* 1999;100(20):2067–2073.
22. Lee TH, Cook EF, Weisberg M, Sargent RK, Wilson C, Goldman L. Acute chest pain in the emergency room. Identification and examination of low-risk patients. *Arch Intern Med.* 1985;145(1):65–69.
23. Matetzky S, Freimark D, Feinberg MS, et al. Acute myocardial infarction with isolated ST-segment elevation in posterior chest leads V7-9: "hidden" ST-segment elevations revealing acute posterior infarction. *J Am Coll Cardiol.* 1999;34(3):748–753.
24. Robalino BD, Whitlow PL, Underwood DA, Salcedo EE. Electrocardiographic manifestations of right ventricular infarction. *Am Heart J.* 1989;118(1):138–144.
25. Jaffe AS, Babuin L, Apple FS. Biomarkers in acute cardiac disease: the present and the future. *J Am Coll Cardiol.* 2006;48(1):1–11.
26. Galvani M, Ottani F, Oltrona L, et al. N-terminal pro-brain natriuretic peptide on admission has prognostic value across the whole spectrum of acute coronary syndromes. *Circulation.* 2004;110(2):128–134.
27. de Lemos JA, Morrow DA, Bentley JH, et al. The prognostic value of B-type natriuretic peptide in patients with acute coronary syndromes. *N Engl J Med.* 2001;345:1014–1021.
28. Andre P, Prasad KS, Denis CV, et al. CD40L stabilizes arterial thrombi by a beta3 integrin-dependent mechanism. *Nat Med.* 2002;8(3):247–252.
29. Schonbeck U, Sukhova GK, Shimizu K, Mach F, Libby P. Inhibition of CD40 signaling limits evolution of established atherosclerosis in mice. *Proc Natl Acad Sci USA.* 2000;97(13):7458–7463.
30. Schonbeck U, Varo N, Libby P, Buring J, Ridker PM. Soluble CD40L and cardiovascular risk in women. *Circulation.* 2001;104(19):2266–2268.
31. Heeschen C, Dimmeler S, Hamm CW, et al. Soluble CD40 ligand in acute coronary syndromes. *N Engl J Med.* 2003;348(12):1104–1111.
32. Collinson PO, Gaze DC. Ischaemia-modified albumin: clinical utility and pitfalls in measurement. *J Clin Pathol.* 2008;61(9):1025–1028.
33. Peacock F, Morris DL, Anwaruddin S, et al. Meta-analysis of ischemia-modified albumin to rule out acute coronary syndromes in the emergency department. *Am Heart J.* 2006;152(2):253–262.
34. Leber AW, Johnson T, Becker A, et al. Diagnostic accuracy of dual-source multi-slice CT-coronary angiography in patients with an intermediate pretest likelihood for coronary artery disease. *Eur Heart J.* 2007;28(19):2354–2360.
35. Weustink AC, Meijboom WB, Mollet NR, et al. Reliable high-speed coronary computed tomography in symptomatic patients. *J Am Coll Cardiol.* 2007;50(8):786–794.
36. Ropers U, Ropers D, Pflederer T, et al. Influence of heart rate on the diagnostic accuracy of dual-source computed tomography coronary angiography. *J Am Coll Cardiol.* 2007;50(25):2393–2398.
37. Dewey M, Teige F, Schnapauff D, et al. Noninvasive detection of coronary artery stenoses with multislice computed tomography or magnetic resonance imaging. *Ann Intern Med.* 2006;145(6):407–415.
38. Kwong RY, Schussheim AE, Rekhraj S, et al. Detecting acute coronary syndrome in the emergency department with cardiac magnetic resonance imaging. *Circulation.* 2003;107(4):531–537.
39. Plein S, Greenwood JP, Ridgway JP, Cranny G, Ball SG, Sivananthan MU. Assessment of non-ST-segment elevation acute coronary syndromes with cardiac magnetic resonance imaging. *J Am Coll Cardiol.* 2004;44(11):2173–2181.
40. Cury RC, Shash K, Nagurney JT, et al. Cardiac magnetic resonance with T2-weighted imaging improves detection of patients with acute coronary syndrome in the emergency department. *Circulation.* 2008;118(8):837–844.
41. Antman EM, Cohen M, Bernink PJ, et al. The TIMI risk score for unstable angina/non-ST elevation MI: a method for prognostication and therapeutic decision making. *JAMA.* 2000;284:835–842.
42. Antman EM, Cohen M, Radley D, et al. Assessment of the treatment effect of enoxaparin for unstable Angina/Non-Q-wave myocardial infarction: TIMI 11B-ESSENCE meta- analysis. *Circulation.* 1999;100:1602–1608.
43. Roffi M, Chew DP, Mukherjee D, et al. Platelet glycoprotein IIb/IIIa inhibitors reduce mortality in diabetic patients with non-ST-segment-elevation acute coronary syndromes. *Circulation.* 2001;104(23):2767–2771.
44. Morrow DA, Antman EM, Snapinn SM, McCabe CH, Theroux P, Braunwald E. An integrated clinical approach to predicting the benefit of tirofiban in non-st elevation acute coronary syndromes: application of the TIMI risk score for UA/NSTEMI in PRISM-PLUS. *Eur Heart J.* 2002;23:223–229.
45. Cannon CP, Weintraub WS, Demopoulos LA, et al. Comparison of early invasive and conservative strategies in patients with unstable coronary syndromes treated with the glycoprotein IIb/IIIa inhibitor tirofiban. *N Engl J Med.* 2001;344(25):1879–1887.
46. Eagle KA, Lim MJ, Dabbous OH, et al. A validated prediction model for all forms of acute coronary syndrome: estimating the risk of 6-month postdischarge death in an international registry. *JAMA.* 2004;291(22):2727–2733.

47. Cheitlin MD, Hutter AM Jr., Brindis RG, et al. ACC/AHA Expert Consensus Document. Use of sildenafil (Viagra) in patients with cardiovascular disease. American College of Cardiology/American Heart Association. *J Am Coll Cardiol.* 1999;33(1):273–282.

48. Gruppo Italiano per lo Studio della Sopravvivenza nell'Infarto Miocardico. GISSI-3: effect of lisinopril and trasdermal glyceryl trinitrate singly and together on 6-week mortality and ventricular function after acute myocardial infarction. *Lancet.* 1994;343:1115–1122.

49. ISIS-4 Collaborative Group. ISIS-4: randomized factorial trial assessing early oral captopril, oral mononitrate, and intravenous magnesium sulphate in 58,050 patients with suspected acute myocardial infarction. *Lancet.* 1995;345:669–685.

50. Yusuf S, Wittes J, Friedman L. Overview of results of randomized clinical trials in heart disease. II. Unstable angina, heart failure, primary prevention with aspirin and risk factor reduction. *JAMA.* 1988;260:2259–2263.

51. Yusuf S, Peto R, Lewis J, Collins R, Sleight P. Beta-blockade during and after myocadial infarction: an overview of the randomized trials. *Prog Cardiovasc Dis.* 1985;27:335–371.

52. Gottlieb SO, Weisfeldt ML, Ouyang P, et al. Effect of the addition of propranolol to therapy with nifedipine for unstable angina pectoris: a randomized, double-blind, placebo- controlled trial. *Circulation.* 1986;73(2):331–337.

53. The Holland Interuniversity Nifedipine/Metoprolol Trial (HINT) Research Group. Early treatment of unstable angina in the coronary care unit: a randomised, double blind, placebo controlled comparison of recurrent ischaemia in patients treated with nifedipine or metoprolol or both. *Br Heart J.* 1986;56(5):400–413.

54. Chen ZM, Pan HC, Chen YP, et al. Early intravenous then oral metoprolol in 45,852 patients with acute myocardial infarction: randomised placebo-controlled trial. *Lancet.* 2005;366(9497):1622–1632.

55. Antman EM, Hand M, Armstrong PW, et al. 2007 focused update of the ACC/AHA 2004 guidelines for the management of patients with ST-elevation myocardial infarction: a report of the American College of Cardiology/American Heart Association Task Force on Practice Guidelines. *J Am Coll Cardiol.* 2008;51(2):210–247.

56. Pepine CJ, Faich G, Makuch R. Verapamil use in patients with cardiovascular disease: an overview of randomized trials. *Clin Cardiol.* 1998;21(9):633–641.

57. Gibson RS, Boden WE, Theroux P, et al. Diltiazem and reinfarction in patients with non-Q-wave myocardial infarction. Results of a double-blind, randomized, multicenter trial. *N Engl J Med.* 1986;315(7):423–429.

58. Lubsen J, Tijssen JG. Efficacy of nifedipine and metoprolol in the early treatment of unstable angina in the coronary care unit: findings from the Holland Interuniversity Nifedipine/metoprolol Trial (HINT). *Am J Cardiol.* 1987;60(2):18A–25A.

59. Hennekens CH, Albert CM, Godfried SL, Gaziano JM, Buring JE. Adjunctive drug therapy of acute myocardial infarction—evidence from clinical trials. *N Engl J Med.* 1996;335:1660–1667.

60. The Multicenter Diltiazem Postinfarction Trial Research Group. The effect of diltiazem on mortality and reinfarction after myocardial infarction. *N Engl J Med.* 1988;319:385–392.

61. Hansen JF, Hagerup L, Sigurd B, et al. Cardiac event rates after acute myocardial infarction in patients treated with verapamil and trandolapril versus trandolapril alone. *Am J Cardiol.* 1997;79(6):738–741.

62. Wilcox RG, Hampton JR, Banks DC, et al. Trial of early nifedepine in acute myocardial infarction: the TRENT study. *BMJ.* 1986;293:1204–1208.

63. Chinese Cardiac Study Collaborative Group. Oral captopril versus placebo among 13,634 patients with suspected myocardial infarction: interim report from the Chinese Cardiac Study (CCS-1). *Lancet.* 1995;345:686–687.

64. Yusuf S, Sleight P, Pogue J, et al. Effects of an angiotensin-converting-enzyme inhibitor, ramipril, on cardiovascular events in high-risk patients. *N Engl J Med.* 2000;342(3):145–153 [published erratum appears in *N Engl J Med.* 2000 Mar 9;342(10):748].

65. Fox KM. Efficacy of perindopril in reduction of cardiovascular events among patients with stable coronary artery disease: randomised, double-blind, placebo-controlled, multicentre trial (The EUROPA Study). *Lancet.* 2003;362(9386):782–788.

66. Rutherford JD, Pfeffer MA, Moye LA, et al. Effects of captopril on ischemic events after myocardial infarction. Results of the Survival and Ventricular Enlargement Trial. *Circulation.* 1994;90:1731–1738.

67. The SOLVD Investigators. Effect of enalapril on survival in patients with reduced left ventricular ejection fractions and congestive heart failure. *N Engl J Med.* 1991;325(5):293–302.

68. Scandinavian Simvastatin Survival Study Group. Randomised trial of cholesterol lowering in 4444 patients with coronary heart disease: the Scandinavian Simvastatin Survival Study (4S). *Lancet.* 1994;344:1383–1389.

69. The Long-Term Intervention with Pravastatin in Ischaemic Disease (LIPID) Study Group. Prevention of cardiovascular events and death with pravastatin in patients with coronary heart disease and a broad range of initial cholesterol levels. *N Engl J Med.* 1998;339(19):1349–1357.

70. Heart Protection Study Collaborative Group. MRC/BHF Heart Protection Study of cholesterol lowering with simvastatin in 20,536 high-risk individuals: a randomised placebo controlled trial. *Lancet.* 2002;360:7–22.

71. Pedersen TR, Kjekshus J, Berg K, et al. Cholesterol lowering and the use of healthcare resources. Results of the Scandinavian Simvastatin Survival Study. *Circulation.* 1996;93:1796–1802.

72. Arntz HR, Agrawal R, Wunderlich W, et al. Beneficial effects of pravastatin (+/-colestyramine/niacin) initiated immediately after a coronary event (the randomized lipid-coronary artery disease [L-CAD] study). *Am J Cardiol.* 2000;86(12):1293–1298.

73. Liem AH, van Boven AJ, Veeger NJ, et al. Effect of fluvastatin on ischaemia following acute myocardial infarction: a randomized trial. *Eur Heart J.* 2002;23(24):1931–1937.

74. Aronow HD, Topol EJ, Roe MT, et al. Effect of lipid-lowering therapy on early mortality after acute coronary syndromes: an observational study. *Lancet.* 2001;357(9262):1063–1068.

75. Stenestrand U, Wallentin L. Early statin treatment following acute myocardial infarction and 1-year survival. *JAMA.* 2001;285(4):430–436.

76. Schwartz GG, Olsson AG, Ezekowitz MD, et al. Effects of atorvastatin on early recurrent ischemic events in acute coronary syndromes: the MIRACL study: a randomized controlled trial. *JAMA.* 2001;285(13):1711–1718.

77. De Lemos JA, Blazing MA, Wiviott SD, et al. Early intensive vs a delayed conservative simvastatin strategy in patients with acute coronary syndromes: phase z of the A to Z trial. *JAMA.* 2004;292:1307–1316.

78. Cannon CP, Braunwald E, McCabe CH, et al. Intensive versus moderate lipid lowering with statins after acute coronary syndromes. *N Engl J Med.* 2004;350(15):1495–1504.

79. Grundy SM, Cleeman JI, Merz CN, et al. Implications of recent clinical trials for the National Cholesterol Education Program Adult Treatment Panel III guidelines. *Circulation.* 2004;110(2):227–239.

80. Antithrombotic Trialists' Collaboration. Collaborative meta-analysis of randomised trials of antiplatelet therapy for prevention of death, myocardial infarction, and stroke in high risk patients. *BMJ.* 2002;324(7329):71–86.

81. ISIS-2 (Second International Study of Infarct Survival) Collaborative Group. Randomised trial of intravenous streptokinase, oral aspirin, both, or neither among 17,187 cases of suspected acute myocardial infarction: ISIS-2. *Lancet.* 1988;2:349–360.

82. Topol EJ, Easton D, Harrington RA, et al. Randomized, double-blind, placebo-controlled, international trial of the oral IIb/IIIa antagonist lotrafiban in coronary and cerebrovascular disease. *Circulation.* 2003;108(4):399–406.

83. Eikelboom JW, Hirsh J, Weitz JI, Johnston M, Yi Q, Yusuf S. Aspirin-resistant thromboxane biosynthesis and the risk of myocardial infarction, stroke, or cardiovascular death in patients at high risk for cardiovascular events. *Circulation.* 2002;105(14):1650–1655.

84. Gum PA, Kottke-Marchant K, Poggio ED, et al. Profile and prevalence of aspirin resistance in patients with cardiovascular disease. *Am J Cardiol.* 2001;88(3):230–235.

85. Gum PA, Kottke-Marchant K, Welsh PA, White J, Topol EJ. A prospective, blinded determination of the natural history of aspirin resistance among stable patients with cardiovascular disease. *J Am Coll Cardiol.* 2003;41(6):961–965.

86. CAPRIE Steering Committee. A randomised, blinded, trial of clopidogrel versus aspirin in patients at risk of ischaemic events (CAPRIE). *Lancet.* 1996;348:1329–1339.

87. Mehta SR, Yusuf S, Peters RJ, et al. Effects of pretreatment with clopidogrel and aspirin followed by long-term therapy in patients undergoing percutaneous coronary intervention: the PCI-CURE study. *Lancet.* 2001;358(9281): 527–533.

88. Wiviott SD, Antman EM, Winters KJ, et al. Randomized comparison of prasugrel (CS-747, LY640315), a novel thienopyridine P2Y12 antagonist, with clopidogrel in percutaneous coronary intervention: results of the Joint Utilization of Medications to Block Platelets Optimally (JUMBO)-TIMI 26 Trial. *Circulation.* 2005;111(25):3366–3373.

89. Wiviott SD, Braunwald E, McCabe CH, et al. Prasugrel versus clopidogrel in patients with acute coronary syndromes. *N Engl J Med.* 2007;357(20):2001–2015.

90. The EPIC Investigators. Use of a monoclonal antibody directed against the platelet glycoprotein IIb/IIIa receptor in high risk angioplasty. *N Engl J Med.* 1994;330:956–961.

91. Boersma E, Harrington RA, Moliterno DJ, et al. Platelet glycoprotein IIb/IIIa inhibitors in acute coronary syndromes: a meta-analysis of all major randomised clinical trials. *Lancet.* 2002;359:189–198.

92. Petersen JL, Mahaffey KW, Hasselblad V, et al. Efficacy and bleeding complications among patients randomized to enoxaparin or unfractionated heparin for antithrombin therapy in non-ST-segment elevation acute coronary syndromes: a systematic overview. *JAMA.* 2004;292(1):89–96.

93. Blazing MA, de Lemos JA, White HD, et al. Safety and efficacy of enoxaparin vs unfractionated heparin in patients with non-ST-segment elevation acute coronary syndromes who receive tirofiban and aspirin: a randomized controlled trial. *JAMA.* 2004;292(1):55–64.

94. Ferguson JJ, Califf RM, Antman EM, et al. Enoxaparin vs unfractionated heparin in high-risk patients with non-ST-segment elevation acute coronary syndromes managed with an intended early invasive strategy: primary results of the SYNERGY Randomized Trial. *JAMA.* 2004;292(1):45–54.

95. Stone GW, McLaurin BT, Cox DA, et al. Bivalirudin for patients with acute coronary syndromes. *N Engl J Med.* 2006;355(21):2203–2216.

96. Yusuf S, Mehta SR, Chrolavicius S, et al. Comparison of fondaparinux and enoxaparin in acute coronary syndromes. *N Engl J Med.* 2006;354(14):1464–1476.

97. Mehta SR, Granger CB, Eikelboom JW, et al. Efficacy and safety of fondaparinux versus enoxaparin in patients with acute coronary syndromes undergoing percutaneous coronary intervention: results from the OASIS-5 Trial. *J Am Coll Cardiol.* 2007;50(18):1742–1751.

98. Rothberg MB, Celestin C, Fiore LD, Lawler E, Cook JR. Warfarin plus aspirin after myocardial infarction or the acute coronary syndrome: meta-analysis with estimates of risk and benefit. *Ann Intern Med.* 2005;143(4):241–250.

99. The TIMI IIIB Investigators. Effects of tissue plasminogen activator and a comparison of early invasive and conservative strategies in unstable angina and non-Q-wave myocardial infarction: results of the TIMI IIIB trial. *Circulation.* 1994;89:1545–1556.

100. Kerensky RA, Wade M, Deedwania P, Boden WE, Pepine CJ. Revisiting the culprit lesion in non-Q-wave myocardial infarction. Results from the VANQWISH Trial Angiographic Core Laboratory. *J Am Coll Cardiol.* 2002;39(9):1456–1463.

101. Jang IK, Gold HK, Ziskind AA, et al. Differential sensitivity of erythrocyte-rich and platelet-rich arterial thrombi to lysis with recombinant tissue-type plasminogen activator. A possible explanation for resistance to coronary thrombolysis. *Circulation.* 1989;79(4):920–928.

102. Mizuno K, Satumo K, Miyamoto A, et al. Angioscopic evaluation of coronary artery thrombi in acute coronary syndromes. *N Engl J Med.* 1992;326:287–291.

103. Boden WE, O'Rourke RA, Crawford MH, et al. Outcomes in patients with acute non-Q-wave myocardial infarction randomly assigned to an invasive as compared with a conservative strategy. *N Engl J Med.* 1998;338:1785–1792.

104. FRagmin and Fast Revascularisation during Instability in Coronary Artery Disease Investigators. Invasive compared with non-invasive treatment in unstable coronary-artery disease: FRISC II prospective randomised multicentre study. *Lancet.* 1999;354(9180):708–715.

105. Freemantle N, Cleland J, Young P, Mason J, Harrison J. Beta blockade after myocardial infarction: systematic review and meta regression analysis. *BMJ.* 1999;318(7200):1730–1737.

106. Lonn E, Yusuf S, Arnold MJ, et al. Homocysteine lowering with folic acid and B vitamins in vascular disease. *N Engl J Med.* 2006;354(15):1567–1577.

107. Bonaa KH, Njolstad I, Ueland PM, et al. Homocysteine lowering and cardiovascular events after acute myocardial infarction. *N Engl J Med.* 2006;354(15):1578–1588.

108. Bjelakovic G, Nikolova D, Gluud LL, Simonetti RG, Gluud C. Mortality in randomized trials of antioxidant supplements for primary and secondary prevention: systematic review and meta-analysis. *JAMA.* 2007;297(8):842–857.

109. Hulley S, Grady D, Bush T, et al. Heart and Estrogen/progestin Replacement Study (HERS) Research Group. Randomized trial of estrogen plus progestin for secondary prevention of coronary heart disease in postmenopausal women. *JAMA.* 1998;280(7):605–613.

110. Manson JE, Hsia J, Johnson KC, et al. Estrogen plus progestin and the risk of coronary heart disease. *N Engl J Med.* 2003;349(6):523–534.

111. Rossouw JE, Anderson GL, Prentice RL, et al. Risks and benefits of estrogen plus progestin in healthy postmenopausal women: principal results from the Women's Health Initiative Randomized Controlled Trial. *JAMA.* 2002;288(3):321–333.

112. Kearney PM, Baigent C, Godwin J, Halls H, Emberson JR, Patrono C. Do selective cyclo-oxygenase-2 inhibitors and traditional non-steroidal anti-inflammatory drugs increase the risk of atherothrombosis? Meta-analysis of randomised trials. *BMJ.* 2006;332(7553):1302–1308.

113. Smith SC Jr., Allen J, Blair SN, et al. AHA/ACC guidelines for secondary prevention for patients with coronary and other atherosclerotic vascular disease: 2006 update endorsed by the National Heart, Lung, and Blood Institute. *J Am Coll Cardiol.* 2006;47(10):2130–2139.

114. Mancia G, De Backer G, Dominiczak A, et al. 2007 guidelines for the management of arterial hypertension: the Task Force for the Management of Arterial Hypertension of the European Society of Hypertension (ESH) and of the European Society of Cardiology (ESC). *Eur Heart J.* 2007;28(12):1462–1536.

115. Rosendorff C, Black HR, Cannon CP, et al. Treatment of hypertension in the prevention and management of ischemic heart disease: a scientific statement from the American Heart Association Council for High Blood Pressure Research and the Councils on clinical cardiology and epidemiology and prevention. *Circulation.* 2007;115(21):2761–2788.

116. Frasure-Smith N, Lesperance F, Talajic M. Depression following myocardial infarction. Impact on 6-month survival. *JAMA.* 1993;270(15):1819–1825.

117. Lichtenstein AH, Appel LJ, Brands M, et al. Diet and lifestyle recommendations revision 2006: a scientific statement from the American Heart Association Nutrition Committee. *Circulation.* 2006;114(1):82–96.

118. Selwyn AP. Prothrombotic and antithrombotic pathways in acute coronary syndromes. *Am J Cardiol.* 2003;91(12A):3H–11H.

119. Achenbach S. Computed tomography coronary angiography. *J Am Coll Cardiol.* 2006;48(10):1919–1928.

120. Choi EK, Choi SI, Rivera JJ, et al. Coronary computed tomography angiography as a screening tool for the detection of occult coronary artery disease in asymptomatic individuals. *J Am Coll Cardiol.* 2008;52(5):357–365.

11 ST Elevation Myocardial Infarction

Eric R. Bates and Brahmajee K. Nallamothu

CONTENTS

Key Words: Atheroslcerotic plaque; Electrocardiogram; Myocardial infarction; Thrombosis; Troponin.

KEY POINTS

- Age, blood pressure, heart rate, congestive heart failure, and ECG findings allow early risk stratification for patients presenting with acute ST-segment elevating myocardial infarction (STEMI).
- Expeditious reperfusion therapy should be the goal for all patients with STEMI.
- Primary PCI is superior to fibrinolytic therapy if performed in a timely manner (less than 90 min) in an excellent interventional cardiology laboratory.
- Echocardiography should be performed in hemodynamically unstable patients to exclude mechanical complications.
- All patients should receive dual antiplatelet therapy with aspirin for life and clopidogrel for 1 year.
- Patients should receive anticoagulation therapy with either unfractionated heparin, enoxaparin, fonda- parinux, or bivalirudin.
- Patients should receive an oral beta-blocker within 24 h unless contraindications exist.
- Aspirin, beta-blockers, statins, and ACE inhibitors have each been shown to reduce long-term mortality.
- Aldosterone blockade is indicated in patients with LVEF ≤40% and either symptomatic heart failure or diabetes mellitus, unless they have renal dysfunction or hyperkalemia.
- Risk stratification should be performed to select high-risk patients for elective coronary artery revascu- larization and ICD therapy.
- Patients should be referred to a cardiac rehabilitation program subsequent to discharge from hospital.

From: *Contemporary Cardiology: Comprehensive Cardiovascular Medicine in the Primary Care Setting*
Edited by: Peter P. Toth, Christopher P. Cannon, DOI 10.1007/978-1-60327-963-5_11
© Springer Science+Business Media, LLC 2010

- Long-term adoption of American Heart Association Step II diet, exercise, and smoking cessation are indicated. Control of hypertension, hyperlipidemia, diabetes mellitus, and weight to target values should be aggressively pursued.

11.1. INTRODUCTION

Acute ST elevation myocardial infarction (STEMI) is the leading cause of death in the United States. The American Heart Association estimated that there were 920,000 Americans with acute myocardial infarction (MI) in 2005 *(1)*. Approximately 30–45% of these were STEMI. Excellent societal guideline recommendations exist for STEMI care *(2–4)*.

Atherosclerotic coronary artery disease and plaque rupture with resultant thrombosis remains the most common cause of MI. Other, less common, causes include arteritis, trauma, embolization, congenital anomalies, hypercoagulable states, and substance abuse.

11.2. PATIENT EVALUATION

11.2.1. History

The risk for STEMI increases with age. Patients often have a family history of coronary artery disease or risk factors including smoking, hypertension, diabetes mellitus, dyslipidemia, or obesity. The classic symptom is crushing retrosternal chest discomfort with radiation to the left arm. Some individuals may present with epigastric pain, which can lead to the misdiagnosis of heartburn or another abdominal disorder. Elderly individuals may not have any chest discomfort, but may present with symptoms of left ventricular failure, marked weakness, or syncope. Postoperative patients and diabetic patients are other subgroups that may not experience classic symptoms. Patients may also present with neck, jaw, back, shoulder, or right arm pain as the sole manifestation. Other associated symptoms can include diaphoresis, dyspnea, fatigue, weakness, dizziness, palpitations, acute confusion, nausea, or emesis.

11.2.2. Physical Examination

The physical examination is more important in excluding other diagnoses and in risk-stratifying patients than in establishing the diagnosis of MI. Patients presenting with STEMI often appear anxious and distressed. All patients should have a thorough cardiovascular examination as a baseline to monitor for complications that may develop, such as ventricular septal rupture or acute mitral regurgitation. A fourth heart sound is almost universally present in patients who are in sinus rhythm. Systolic blood pressure, heart rate, rales, and a third heart sound are important prognostic determinants. A baseline neurologic examination is important, particularly before fibrinolytic therapy is initiated.

11.2.3. Electrocardiogram

The electrocardiographic diagnosis of STEMI requires at least 1 mm of acute ST-segment elevation in two or more contiguous leads. The presence of prior left bundle branch block may confound the diagnosis, but striking ST-segment deviation that cannot be explained merely by conduction abnormality is suggestive of STEMI. The electrocardiogram (ECG) also is a valuable clinical tool for determining infarct location and estimating potential infarct size.

11.2.4. Cardiac Biomarkers

The serum cardiac markers used in the diagnosis of MI include creatine kinase (CK), creatine kinase–myocardial band (CK–MB) isoenzyme, and cardiac-specific troponins. The diagnosis of MI has recently been expanded to include any elevation of serum cardiac biomarkers (preferably troponin) combined with symptoms, ECG signs, or cardiac imaging evidence consistent with myocardial ischemia *(5)*.

11.2.5. Echocardiography

The portability of echocardiography makes it a valuable clinical tool. This technique can be useful to confirm or exclude the diagnosis and to help with risk stratification. The echocardiogram is very helpful in diagnosing the mechanical complications of STEMI.

11.3. DIFFERENTIAL DIAGNOSIS

Pulmonary embolism can present with chest pain associated with severe shortness of breath without clinical or radiographic evidence of pulmonary edema. Echocardiography may be useful by demonstrating normal left ventricular wall motion and right ventricular dilatation and strain, although spiral computed tomography has more recently routinely been used. Patients with pneumothorax and pleuritis may also present with substernal chest discomfort, but the character of the pain is different, and the pain is often worse with inspiration.

Acute aortic dissection pain is typically central, severe, and often described by the patient as a tearing sensation. The pain is maximal at onset and persists for many hours. It is extremely important to diagnose this condition because fibrinolytic therapy usually results in death. Chest radiography often shows a widened mediastinum. The diagnosis is usually confirmed with transesophageal echocardiography, computed tomography, or magnetic resonance imaging.

Pericardial pain is usually aggravated by inspiration and lying supine. It is important to distinguish pericarditis from STEMI because inadvertent fibrinolysis in patients with pericarditis may lead to hemopericardium. The ST-segment changes in pericarditis are diffuse, with a concave upward slope. Other important diagnostic features include PR-segment depression and absence of reciprocal ST-segment depression.

Myocarditis typically presents with more gradual onset of symptoms and prior upper respiratory tract symptoms in a relatively young patient. Serum cardiac markers usually remain elevated rather than peaking and returning to baseline levels.

Patients with hypertrophic cardiomyopathy may present with chest discomfort similar to angina, related to increased myocardial oxygen demand. Transthoracic echocardiography is a useful test for diagnosing this condition. Use of nitroglycerin or dobutamine may precipitate hypotension and syncope in affected patients.

Patients with acute cholecystitis may present with symptoms and occasionally ECG findings suggestive of inferior MI. The presence of fever, marked leukocytosis, and right upper quadrant tenderness favor the diagnosis of cholecystitis. Esophageal and other upper gastrointestinal symptoms may also mimic ischemic chest discomfort.

Costochondritis pain is usually associated with localized swelling and redness, and the character of the pain is usually sharp with marked focal tenderness.

Patients with a hyperventilation or panic attack present with chest discomfort, panic/acute anxiety, lightheadedness, air hunger, and paresthesias.

11.4. THERAPY

11.4.1. Pre-hospital Care

There is increasing emphasis on establishing a regional pre-hospital system of care network of hospitals connected with efficient ambulance services *(6)*. Early activation of the emergency medical system, public education in cardiopulmonary resuscitation, and a well-trained ambulance service are important components. Shared written protocols, pre-hospital diagnosis and treatment, and rapid transport to the most appropriate hospital facility by ambulance or helicopter are crucial for optimal management. The ability to treat out-of-hospital cardiac arrest with prompt cardiopulmonary resuscitation, early defibrillation, and advanced cardiac life support is the greatest opportunity for increasing survival with STEMI. Rapid diagnosis and early risk stratification of patients with acute chest pain more quickly identify patients who are candidates for reperfusion therapy.

11.4.2. General Treatment Measures

Several interventions should quickly be undertaken while patients are being evaluated for reperfusion therapy (Table 1). First, patients with overt pulmonary congestion and arterial oxygen desaturation (saturation less than 90%) should be given supplemental oxygen, as should all patients with MI during the first 2–3 h. Second, sublingual nitroglycerin every 5 min for a total of three doses should be given,

Table 1
Diagnostic and Treatment Measures in Patients with ST Elevation Myocardial Infarction

Initial diagnostic measures
1. Use continuous ECG; automated BP, HR monitoring
2. Take targeted history (for MI inclusions, fibrinolysis exclusions). Check vital signs, perform-focused examination
3. Start IV(s); draw blood for serum cardiac markers, hematology, chemistry, lipid profile
4. Obtain 12-lead ECG
5. Obtain chest X-ray

General treatment measures
1. Oxygen 2–4 L/min by nasal cannula
2. Nitroglycerin 0.4 mg sublingual every 2–5 min 3 times
3. Morphine (2–4 mg) as needed

Specific treatment measures
1. Reperfusion therapy
   Primary PCI: door-to-balloon time <90 min
   Fibrinolytic therapy: door-to-needle time <30 min
   Alteplase: 15 mg IV bolus, infusion 0.75 mg/kg over 30 min (max 50 mg), then 0.5 mg/kg over 60 min (max 35 mg)
   Reteplase: 10 U IV over 2 min, repeated in 30 min
   Tenecteplase: 0.5 mg/kg IV bolus
2. Antiplatelet therapy:
   Aspirin: 160–325 mg, chew and swallow
   Clopidogrel: 75 mg (600 mg load with primary PCI, 300 mg load if age ≤75 year)
   Abciximab: 0.25 mg/kg bolus, 0.125 mcg/kg/min (maximum 10 mcg/min) over 12 h IV
   Eptifibatide: 180 mcg/kg bolus repeated at 10 min, 2.0 mcg/kg/min for 18–24 h IV
   Tirofiban: 25 mcg/kg bolus, 0.15 mcg/kg/min for 18–24 h IV
3. Antithrombotic therapy:
   Unfractionated heparin: 60 U/kg (max, 4,000 U), 12 U/kg/h (max, 1,000/h) adjusted to keep aPTT
      50–70 s × 48 h
   Enoxaparin: 30 mg IV load, 1 mg/kg SC twice daily if age ≤75 year; no bolus, 0.75 mg/kg SC twice daily
      if age >75 year
   Fondaparinux: 2.5 mg IV bolus, 2.5 mg SC once daily
   Bivalirudin: 0.75 mg/kg bolus, 1.75 mg/kg/h infusion

ECG = electrocardiogram, BP = blood pressure, HR = heart rate, MI = myocardial infarction, IV = intravenous administrations, PCI = percutaneous coronary intervention, S = subcutaneous.

with intravenous therapy considered for ongoing ischemic discomfort, control of hypertension, and management of congestive heart failure. Patients should first be asked about recent use of sildenafil because administration of nitroglycerin within 24 h of sildenafil ingestion, or a similar agent, may cause severe hypotension. Third, morphine sulfate is the analgesic of choice to manage pain.

11.4.3. Reperfusion Therapy

Patients within 12 h of symptom onset are candidates for reperfusion therapy for survival benefit, although little myocardial salvage occurs after 3–4 h of myocardial ischemia. Therefore, the overarching goal in STEMI is to initiate reperfusion therapy within 2 h (ideally within 60 min) of symptom onset (Fig. 1). An underutilized strategy for improving systems of care for STEMI patients is to expand the use of pre-hospital 12-lead electrocardiography programs by emergency medical systems *(2)*.

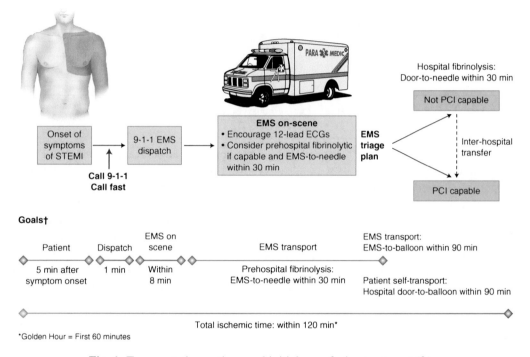

Fig. 1. Transportation options and initial reperfusion treatment *(2)*.

It is increasingly clear that two types of hospital systems provide reperfusion therapy: those with PCI capability and those without PCI capability. STEMI patients presenting to a hospital with PCI capability should be treated with primary PCI within 90 min of first medical contact as a systems goal. The best outcomes are achieved by offering this strategy 24 h/day, 7 days/week.

Because of the critical importance of time-to-treatment, fibrinolytic therapy is generally preferred, if there are no contraindications (Table 2), in hospital systems that do not have the capability of meeting the time goal for primary PCI. There need to be transfer protocols in place for arranging rescue PCI when clinically indicated. For fibrinolytic therapy, the systems goal is to deliver drug within 30 min of hospital presentation.

11.4.4. Primary PCI

In unstable patients, such as those with cardiogenic shock (especially those less than 75 years of age), severe congestive heart failure/pulmonary edema, or hemodynamically compromising ventricular

Table 2
Absolute and Relative Contraindications for Fibrinolytic Therapy (2)

Contraindications
Previous hemorrhagic stroke at any time; other strokes or cerebrovascular events with 1 year
Known intracranial neoplasm
Active internal bleeding (does not include menses)
Suspected aortic dissection

Cautions/relative contraindications
Severe uncontrolled hypertension on presentation (blood pressure >180/110 mmHg)
History of prior cerebrovascular accident or known intracerebral pathology not covered in contraindications
Current use of anticoagulants in therapeutic doses (INR 2.0–3.0); known bleeding diathesis
Recent trauma (within 2–4 week), including head trauma or traumatic or prolonged (>10 min) CPR or major
    surgery (<3 week)
Non-compressible vascular punctures
Recent (within 2–4 week) internal bleeding
For streptokinase/antistreplase: prior exposure (especially within 5 days–2 years) or prior allergic reaction
Pregnancy
Active peptic ulcer
History of chronic severe hypertension

INR = international normalized ratio, CPR = cardiopulmonary resuscitation.

arrhythmias (regardless of age), a strategy of immediate coronary angiography with intent to perform PCI is a useful approach regardless of symptom duration or prior therapy. In stable patients, primary PCI has been associated with better outcomes than fibrinolytic therapy, when performed quickly in an excellent interventional cardiology laboratory (7). Routine coronary stent implantation decreases the need for subsequent target vessel revascularization but does not reduce death or reinfarction rates. Drug-eluting stents further reduce the risk of reintervention, compared with bare metal stents, without changing the risk for stent thrombosis, reinfarction, or death. However, they should generally be avoided in patients who need oral anticoagulation (atrial fibrillation, left ventricular thrombus, mechanical valves) because of the bleeding risk associated with long-term triple antithrombotic therapy. PCI may be considered in stable patients from 12 to 24 h after symptom onset, but is contraindicated after 24 h if the artery is totally occluded and there are no signs of ischemia (4). PCI of a hemodynamically significant stenosis in a patent infarct artery greater than 24 h after STEMI may be considered as part of an invasive strategy to maintain long-term patency.

11.4.5. Rescue PCI

Failed fibrinolysis can be assumed when there is <50% ST-segment resolution 90 min following initiation of therapy in the lead showing the greatest degree of ST-segment elevation at presentation. Rescue PCI should be considered if there is clinical or ECG evidence of a moderate or large infarct and the procedure can be performed within 12 h of symptom onset (8). Facilitated PCI, defined as a pharmacological reperfusion treatment delivered prior to planned PCI in order to improve coronary patency, has not been shown to reduce infarct size or improve outcomes (9).

11.4.6. Coronary Angiography

When it is likely that fibrinolysis was successful (ST-segment resolution >50% at 90 min, typical reperfusion arrhythmia, resolution of chest pain), coronary angiography within 3–24 h is recommended if there are no contraindications (4). Early PCI decreases the risk and complications of infarct artery re-occlusion. In patients who did not receive reperfusion therapy, angiography is recommended before hospital discharge *(4)*.

11.4.7. Antiplatelet Therapy

Clopidogrel should be added to aspirin as dual antiplatelet therapy in all STEMI patients. With fibrinolytic therapy, a 300-mg oral loading dose should be administered if age is ≤75 year, but not if age is >75 year *(10)*. The loading dose with primary PCI should be 600 mg. Intravenous glycoprotein IIb/IIIa inhibitors are often used during primary PCI. Non-steroidal anti-inflammatory drugs (NSAIDs) and selective cyclo-oxygenase (COX-2) inhibitors increase the risk of death, reinfarction, cardiac rupture, and other complications and should be discontinued.

11.4.8. Antithrombin Therapy

Bivalirudin *(11)* is an alternative to unfractionated heparin with primary PCI, but fondaparinux *(12)* should be avoided as the sole anticoagulant because of the risk of catheter thrombosis. Enoxaparin *(13)* and fondaparinux are alternatives to unfractionated heparin *(14)* with fibrinolytic therapy or in patients not receiving reperfusion therapy. For age >75 year, enoxaparin should be started at a reduced dose (0.75 mg/kg) without an intravenous bolus. If PCI is not performed, enoxaparin and fondaparinux should be administered for the duration of the hospital stay, but unfractionated heparin should only be administered for 48 h because of the risk of heparin-induced thrombocytopenia.

11.4.9. Routine Prophylactic Therapies in the Acute Phase

There is no mortality benefit for the early routine use of intravenous beta-blocker therapy, although it can be useful in treating hypertension *(15)*. Oral beta-blockers, statins (irrespective of baseline total cholesterol or low-density lipoprotein cholesterol), and ACE inhibitors should be started in stable patients within 24 h, if no contraindications are present. No benefit has been demonstrated with routine use of calcium channel blockers, magnesium, lidocaine, or glucose–insulin–potassium infusions.

11.5. COMPLICATIONS

Sudden cardiac death before hospital admission is the most common cause of mortality in STEMI. In-hospital mortality is primarily due to circulatory failure resulting from either severe left ventricular dysfunction or one of the mechanical complications. The complications of STEMI may be broadly classified as hemodynamic, mechanical, electrical, ischemic, embolic, and pericardial.

11.5.1. Hemodynamic Complications

11.5.1.1. Hypotension

Hypotension (systolic pressure <90 mmHg or 30 mm below previous pressure) can result from hypovolemia, hemorrhage, arrhythmia, heart failure, mechanical complications, or other complications such as sepsis or pulmonary embolism (Fig. 2). Rapid volume loading and correction of underlying etiologies are recommended. Persistent hypotension should be evaluated with echocardiography to define cardiac anatomy. Vasopressor and inotropic agents may be required for inotropic failure.

11.5.1.2. Left Ventricular Failure

The degree of left ventricular failure can be categorized by the Killip classification: class 1, no rales or third heart sound; class 2, pulmonary congestion with rales over <50% of the lung fields or third heart sound; class 3, pulmonary edema with rales over 50% of the lung fields; and class 4,

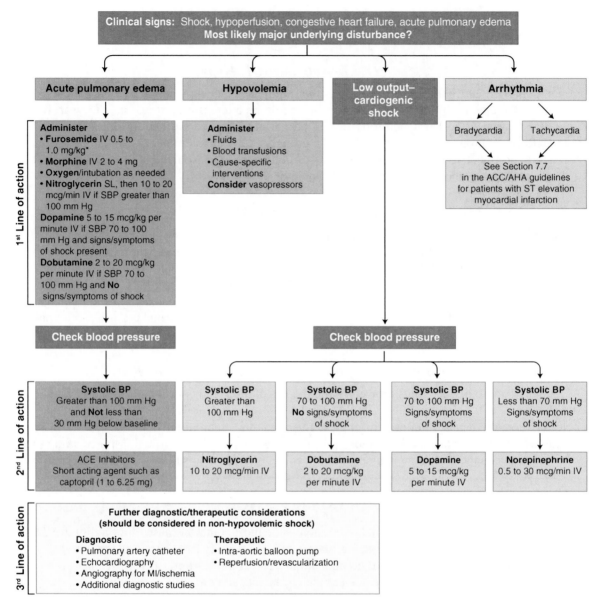

Fig. 2. Emergency management of complicated ST elevation myocardial infarction *(2)*.

shock. Therapeutic measures for Killip class 2 and 3 heart failure include oxygen, nitrates, morphine, diuretics, vasodilator therapy, and correction of arrhythmia and electrolyte abnormalities.

11.5.1.3. RIGHT VENTRICULAR FAILURE

Mild right ventricular dysfunction is common after inferior MI, but hemodynamically significant right ventricular impairment is seen in only 10% of patients. The triad of hypotension, jugular venous distention, and clear lungs is very specific but has poor sensitivity for right ventricular infarction. Patients with severe right ventricular failure have symptoms of low cardiac output, including diaphoresis, clammy extremities, and altered mental status. Patients are often oliguric and hypotensive. The ECG usually shows an inferior injury current. ST elevation in V4R in the setting of suspected right ventricular infarction has a positive predictive value of 80%. Hemodynamic monitoring with a pulmonary artery catheter usually reveals high right atrial (RA) pressures relative to the pulmonary artery wedge pressure (PCWP). Acute right ventricular failure results in underfilling of the left ventricle and the low cardiac output state. An RA pressure higher than 10 mmHg and an RA/PCWP ratio of 0.8 or higher are strongly suggestive of right ventricular infarction. Treatment of right ventricular infarction involves volume loading, inotropic support with dobutamine, and maintenance of atrioventricular synchrony. Patients who undergo successful reperfusion of the right coronary artery and the right ventricular branches have improved right ventricular function and decreased 30-day mortality rates.

11.5.1.4. CARDIOGENIC SHOCK

Cardiogenic shock is a clinical state of hypoperfusion, hypotension, and low cardiac output due to extensive loss of viable myocardium. Urgent echocardiography and placement of a pulmonary artery catheter can confirm the diagnosis and exclude other conditions. Mechanical ventilation and intra-aortic balloon counterpulsation (IABP) assist in stabilizing the patient. Vasopressor agents and dobutamine are required to improve perfusion. Emergency revascularization of viable myocardium with PCI or surgery can be lifesaving.

11.5.2. Mechanical Complications

11.5.2.1. FREE WALL RUPTURE

Left ventricular free wall rupture occurs in 3% of patients and accounts for about 10% of deaths from STEMI. Advanced age, female gender, hypertension, first MI, and poor coronary collateral vessels are risk factors for free wall rupture. Emergency thoracotomy with surgical repair is the definitive therapy, but most patients die within minutes. Pseudoaneurysm results from a contained rupture of the left ventricular free wall by the pericardium and mural thrombus. Spontaneous rupture occurs without warning in approximately one-third of patients; therefore, surgical resection is recommended for both symptomatic and asymptomatic patients, irrespective of the aneurysm size.

11.5.2.2. VENTRICULAR SEPTAL RUPTURE

Ventricular septal rupture occurs in 0.5–2% of patients. The diagnosis should be suspected with sudden hemodynamic deterioration and a new loud pansystolic murmur. Echocardiography with color flow imaging or an increase in oxygen saturation in the right ventricle can confirm the diagnosis. An IABP should be inserted as early as possible, unless there is significant aortic regurgitation. Nitroprusside can be used with close hemodynamic monitoring. Early surgical repair is the treatment of choice.

11.5.2.3. MITRAL REGURGITATION

Mitral regurgitation is common and is usually caused by mitral valve annulus dilatation due to left ventricular dysfunction or to papillary muscle dysfunction. However, rupture of the papillary muscle trunk or tip occurs in 1% of patients and contributes to 5% of the deaths. It is more common with inferior MI. Sudden hemodynamic deterioration and a new soft pansystolic murmur at the cardiac apex is the usual clinical presentation. Two-dimensional echocardiography with Doppler and color flow imaging is the diagnostic modality of choice. Hemodynamic monitoring with a pulmonary artery catheter may reveal large V waves in the PCWP tracing. Vasodilator and IABP therapy should be initiated and immediate surgery should be performed.

11.5.2.4. LEFT VENTRICULAR ANEURYSM

An acute aneurysmal segment expands in systole, wasting contractile energy generated by the normal myocardium. Chronic aneurysms develop in 10% of patients without reperfusion therapy and are more commonly seen after anterior MI. Heart failure, ventricular arrhythmias, and systemic embolism of mural thrombus are possible sequelae. Heart failure with acute aneurysm is treated with intravenous vasodilators and IABP. Anticoagulation with warfarin is indicated for patients with mural thrombus. In patients with refractory heart failure or ventricular arrhythmias, surgical resection of the aneurysm should be considered. Revascularization may be beneficial in patients with a large amount of viable myocardium in the aneurysmal segment.

11.5.3. Electrical Complications

Arrhythmias are the most common complications after STEMI, affecting approximately 90% of patients. Conduction abnormalities causing hypotension may necessitate temporary or permanent pacemaker therapy. These are briefly summarized in Table 3. An implantable cardioverter defibrillator is indicated in patients with sustained ventricular fibrillation or ventricular tachycardia more than 2 days after the MI if recurrent ischemia or transient causes have been excluded and may be implanted for primary prevention if left ventricular function is significantly reduced 1 month after STEMI.

11.5.4. Ischemic Complications

Infarct extension is a progressive increase in the amount of myocardial necrosis within the same arterial territory as the original MI. Recurrent angina within a few hours to 30 days after MI is defined as postinfarction angina. The frequency of postinfarction angina is higher after fibrinolytic therapy than after primary PCI. Patients with postinfarction angina have an increased incidence of sudden death, reinfarction, and acute cardiac events. Either PCI or surgical revascularization improves prognosis in these patients. It may be difficult to differentiate ECG changes of reinfarction from the evolving ECG changes of the index MI. Recurrent elevations in CK–MB after normalization or to more than 50% of the prior value are diagnostic of reinfarction.

11.5.5. Embolic Complications

The incidence of systemic embolism after MI is approximately 2%; the incidence is higher in patients with anterior MI. Patients with large anterior MI or mural thrombi should be treated with intravenous heparin for 3–4 days with a target partial thromboplastin time of 50–70 s. Oral therapy with warfarin should be continued for at least 3 months in patients with mural thrombus and in those with large akinetic areas detected by echocardiography.

11.5.6. Pericardial Complications

Early pericarditis usually develops within 24–96 h. The pain is constant, worse with lying supine, alleviated by sitting up and leaning forward, usually pleuritic in nature, and worsened with deep inspiration, coughing, and swallowing. Postinfarction pericarditis is treated with aspirin in doses of 650 mg every 4–6 h. Non-steroidal anti-inflammatory agents and corticosteroids should not be administered to these patients because they may interfere with myocardial healing and contribute to infarct expansion. Colchicine may be beneficial in patients with recurrent pericarditis. Dressler's syndrome (post-MI syndrome) occurs in 1–3% of patients and is seen 1–8 weeks after MI. Patients present with chest discomfort suggestive of pericarditis, fever, arthralgia, malaise, elevated leukocyte count, and elevated erythrocyte sedimentation rate. Treatment is similar to that for early postinfarction pericarditis.

Table 3
Electrical Complications of Acute Myocardial Infarction and Their Management

Category	Arrhythmia	Objective	Treatment
1. Electrical instability	Ventricular premature beats	Correct electrolyte deficits and decrease sympathetic tone	Potassium and magnesium replacement; beta-blockers
	Ventricular tachycardia	Prophylaxis against ventricular fibrillation, restoration of hemodynamic stability	Antiarrhythmic agents; cardioversion
	Ventricular fibrillation	Urgent reversion to sinus rhythm	Defibrillation
	Accelerated idioventricular rhythm	Observation unless hemodynamic function is compromised	Increase sinus rate (atropine, atrial pacing); antiarrhythmic agents
	Nonparoxysmal atrioventricular junctional tachycardia	Search for precipitating causes (e.g., digitalis intoxication); suppress arrhythmia only if hemodynamic function is compromised	Atrial overdrive pacing; antiarrhythmic agents; cardioversion relatively contraindicated if digitalis intoxication present
2. Pump failure/excessive sympathetic stimulation	Sinus tachycardia	Reduce heart rate to diminish myocardial oxygen demand	Antipyretics; analgesics; consider beta-blocker unless congestive heart failure present; treat latter with diuretics and afterload reduction
	Atrial fibrillation and/or atrial flutter	Control ventricular rate; restore sinus rhythm	Diltiazem, verapamil, digitalis; anticongestive measures (diuretics, afterload reduction); cardioversion; rapid atrial pacing (for atrial flutter)
	Paroxysmal supraventricular tachycardia	Reduce ventricular rate; restore sinus rhythm	Vagal maneuvers; verapamil, digitalis, beta-adrenergic blockers; cardioversion; rapid atrial pacing
3. Bradyarrhythmias and conduction disturbances	Sinus bradycardia	Acceleration of heart rate only if hemodynamic function is compromised	Atropine; atrial pacing
	Junctional escape rhythm	Acceleration of sinus rate only if loss of atrial "kick" causes hemodynamic compromise	Atropine; atrial pacing
	Atrioventricular block and intraventricular block	–	Ventricular pacing

Adapted from (17).

11.6. PROGNOSIS

The Thrombolysis in Myocardial Infarction (TIMI) risk score for ST-segment elevation STEMI is a simple tool for bedside risk assessment *(16)*. The elements of the TIMI score are shown in Fig. 3 and include history, physical examination, and electrocardiographic findings on presentation. The actual score is a summed weighted integer score based on eight characteristics. With current therapy, patients treated with early reperfusion therapy have a 4–6% hospital mortality and a 2–4% risk for death in the year following discharge. However, long-term prognosis is variable and depends on left ventricular function, ischemic burden, revascularization status, and co-morbidities.

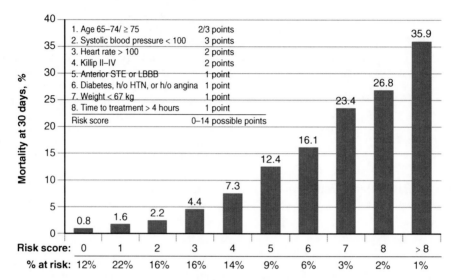

Fig. 3. Prediction of 30-day mortality with thrombolysis in myocardial infarction (TIMI) risk score after fibrinolytic therapy for STEMI *(16)*.

11.7. FOLLOW-UP

All patients should have a return clinic visit in 2–4 weeks and be considered for a cardiac rehabilitation program. Aspirin 81 mg daily should be continued for life. Clopidogrel 75 mg daily should be continued for 12 months. Oral anticoagulants should be given to patients who do not tolerate aspirin and clopidogrel and to those with clinical indications. Oral beta-blockers, ACE inhibitors or angiotensin receptor inhibitors, and statins should be administered to all patients without contraindications. Aldosterone blockade may be considered with left ventricular ejection fraction <40% and heart failure or diabetes, if the creatinine is <2.5 mg/dL in men and <2.0 mg/dL in women, and the potassium is ≤5.0 mEq/L. Elective stress testing can be performed as clinically indicated to evaluate patients with multivessel disease for elective coronary revascularization. Assessments for cardiac resynchronization therapy or implantation of an implantable cardioverter defibrillator are made after 1 month of treatment in patients with significant left ventricular dysfunction. All patients should receive yearly influenza immunizations.

Aggressive targets for managing hypertension (blood pressure <140/90 mmHg), diabetes mellitus (HbA1c <7.0%), and LDL-cholesterol (<70 mg/dL) have been established. Smoking cessation, diet, weight control, and aerobic exercise at least five times per week are important lifestyle interventions.

11.8. CASE STUDIES

11.8.1. Case 1

A 76-year-old man presents to the emergency department with a 2-h history of retrosternal chest tightness, lightheadedness, and nausea. Medications include aspirin, lisinopril, and simvastatin. On physical examination, the blood pressure is 100/60 mmHg, heart rate 50 bpm, and respirations 20 per min. The jugular venous pressure is 10 cm with a positive Kussmaul sign, the lungs are clear, the heart sounds are normal without extra sounds or murmurs, and degenerative joint disease is present in the hands and knees. The ECG shows sinus bradycardia, 3-mm ST-segment elevation in the inferior leads, 2-mm ST-segment depression in leads V_1–V_3, and 1-mm ST-segment elevation in lead V_4R. A diagnosis of acute inferior/right ventricular STEMI is made and the patient is immediately referred to the interventional cardiology laboratory for primary PCI. During the informed consent process, the patient states that he is scheduled for total knee replacement surgery in 1 month.

11.8.2. Management Decisions

Although the standard STEMI protocol includes administering nitroglycerin and morphine, these drugs should be withheld in a patient with right ventricular infarction because they decrease ventricular filling pressures. Adequate preload and maintenance of atrioventricular synchrony are important to assure hemodynamic stability.

The ECG would predict a large right coronary artery with a proximal occlusion and that was what angiography demonstrated. Although the patient was on chronic aspirin, an additional 325-mg dose would be reasonable. Prasugrel is a new thienopyridine agent. Compared with clopidogrel, it has faster onset of action, more complete platelet inhibition, and almost no non-responders, so it is an excellent option for primary PCI. The unanswered question is whether there would be additional benefit in adding a glycoprotein IIb/IIIa inhibitor as a third antiplatelet agent, or only increased risk for bleeding.

A guidewire was easily passed into the distal artery, and aspiration thrombectomy retrieved thrombotic material, restoring coronary blood flow. The ST-segment changes resolved quickly, suggesting microvascular reperfusion and salvage of ischemic myocardium. Stent implantation reduces the risk of infarct artery re-occlusion during the first days and weeks after PCI and decreases the risk of restenosis over the following months. Given the large diameter of the artery and the need for elective surgery in the near future, a bare metal stent was implanted without complication. Dual antiplatelet therapy can be discontinued in 4 weeks, and surgery can be performed 7 days after stopping prasugrel. Implantation of a drug-eluting stent would require at least 6 months of uninterrupted dual antiplatelet therapy, with 12 months considered preferable. When surgery is required in patients on dual antiplatelet therapy after stent implantation, the first option is to continue dual antiplatelet therapy, the second option is to stop only aspirin, and the last option is to stop both drugs. Therapy should be resumed as soon as possible after surgery to decrease the risk of subacute stent thrombosis.

11.8.3. Case 2

A 65-year-old woman collapses in a shopping mall after feeling ill for 30 min. A bystander notes the patient is apneic and pulseless, so starts cardiopulmonary resuscitation. An automated external defibrillator successfully restores her heart rate and consciousness, and she is emergently transported to the emergency department of a hospital without primary PCI capability. On physical examination, she is ashen and restless. Blood pressure is 80/40 mmHg, heart rate 115 bpm, respirations 32 per min, and oxygen saturation 85% on a face mask. Rales are heard in both lung bases, heart sounds are distant, and extremities are cool. The ECG shows ST-segment elevation in leads V_{2-6}, I, and aVL. A diagnosis of acute anterior STEMI complicated by cardiogenic shock is made.

11.8.3.1. MANAGEMENT DECISIONS

Several interventions must immediately be pursued to stabilize the patient. Oxygenation and airway support require tracheal intubation and mechanical ventilation. Rhythm control may require an external pacemaker for bradycardia or cardioversion/defibrillation for tachyarrhythmias. Inotropic support with dobutamine and vasopressor support with dopamine or norepinephrine should be titrated to maintain perfusion pressure. Nasogastric and urinary catheters need to be inserted. Initiation of intra-aortic balloon counterpulsation can offer mechanical support of the circulation.

Hospitals without PCI capability should give fibrinolytic therapy to patients with STEMI when interhospital transfer and primary PCI cannot be accomplished within 90 min. A transfer plan needs to be in place for patients needing rescue PCI or primary PCI when fibrinolytic contraindications are present. With cardiogenic shock, however, emergency transfer for PCI must occur regardless of treatment delays, unless further treatment is considered futile. Fibrinolytic therapy can be administered, but reperfusion rates are low because of hypotension. Only early revascularization with PCI or CABG has been shown to significantly decrease the mortality risk.

The hospital mortality rate with cardiogenic shock is approximately 50%. More than 80% of 1-year survivors are in NYHA functional class I or II. In addition to the routine recommendations for post-discharge care and additional treatment if heart failure is present, these patients require measurement of left ventricular ejection fraction at least 1 month after presentation; an implantable cardioverter–defibrillator is usually indicated for values less than 30%.

REFERENCES

1. American Heart Association. *Heart Disease and Stroke Statistics—2008 Update*. Dallas: American Heart Association. 2008. www.americanheart.org
2. Antman EM, Anbe DT, Armstrong PW, et al. ACC/AHA guidelines for the management of patients with ST-elevation myocardial infarction: a report of the American College of Cardiology/American Heart Association Task Force on Practice Guidelines (Committee to Revise the 1999 Guidelines for the Management of Patients with Acute Myocardial Infarction). *J Am Coll Cardiol*. 2004;44:e1–e211.
3. Antman EM, Hand M, Armstrong PW, et al. 2007 focused update of the ACC/AHA 2004 Guidelines for the Management of Patients with ST-Elevation Myocardial Infarction: a report of the American College of Cardiology/American Heart Association Task Force on Practice Guidelines (Writing Group to Review New Evidence and Update the ACC/AHA 2004 Guidelines for the Management of Patients with ST-Elevation Myocardial Infarction). *J Am Coll Cardiol*. 2008;51:210–247.
4. van de Werf F, Bax J, Betriu A, et al. Management of acute myocardial infarction in patients presenting with persistent ST-segment elevation: the Task Force on the Management of ST-Segment Elevation Acute Myocardial Infarction of the European Society of Cardiology. *Eur Heart J*. 2008;29:2909–2945.
5. Thygesen K, Alpert JS, White HD, on behalf of the Joint ESC/ACCF/AHA/WHF Task Force for the Redefinition of Myocardial Infarction. Universal definition of myocardial infarction. *Circulation*. 2007;116:2634–2653.
6. Bates ER, Kushner FG. ST-elevation myocardial infarction. In: Antman E, ed. *Cardiovascular Therapeutics, A Companion to Braunwald's Heart Disease*. 3rd ed. Philadelphia, PA: Elsevier Saunders; 2007:246–289.
7. Keeley EC, Boura JA, Grines CL. Primary angioplasty versus intravenous thrombolytic therapy for acute myocardial infarction: a quantitative review of 23 randomised trials. *Lancet*. 2003;136:13–20.
8. Wijeysundera HC, Vijayaraghavan R, Nallamothu BK, et al. Rescue angioplasty or repeat fibrinolysis after failed fibrinolytic therapy for ST-segment myocardial infarction: a meta-analysis of randomized trials. *J Am Coll Cardiol*. 2007;49:422–430.
9. Keeley EC, Boura JA, Grines CL. Comparison of primary and facilitated percutaneous coronary interventions for ST-elevation myocardial infarction: quantitative review of randomised trials. *Lancet*. 2006;367:579–588.
10. Sabatine MS, Cannon CP, Gibson CM, et al. Addition of clopidogrel to aspirin and fibrinolytic therapy for myocardial infarction with ST-segment elevation. *N Engl J Med*. 2005;352:1179–1189.
11. Stone GW, Witzenbichler B, Guagliumi G, et al. Bivalirudin during primary PCI in acute myocardial infarction. *N Engl J Med*. 2008;358:2218–2230.
12. Yusuf S, Mehta SR, Chrolavicius S, et al. Effects of fondaparinux on mortality and reinfarction in patients with acute ST-segment elevation myocardial infarction: the OASIS-6 randomized trial. *JAMA*. 2006;295:1519–1530.

13. Antman EM, Morrow DA, McCabe CH, et al. Enoxaparin versus unfractionated heparin with fibrinolysis for ST-elevation myocardial infarction. *N Engl J Med.* 2006;354:1477–1488.

14. Eikelboom JW, Quinlan DJ, Mehta SR, Turpie AG, Menown IB, Yusuf S. Unfractionated and low-molecular-weight heparin as adjuncts to thrombolysis in aspirin-treated patients with ST-elevation acute myocardial infarction: a meta-analysis of the randomized trials. *Circulation.* 2005;112:3855–3867.

15. Krumholz HM, Anderson JL, Bachelder BL, et al. ACC/AHA 2008 performance measures for adults with ST-elevation and non-ST-elevation myocardial infarction: a report of the American College of Cardiology/American Heart Association Task Force on Performance Measures (Writing Committee to develop performance measures for ST-elevation and non-ST-elevation myocardial infarction). *Circulation.* 2008;118:2596–2648.

16. Morrow DA, Antman EM, Charlesworth A, Cairns R, Murphy SA, de Lemos JA, Giugliano RP, McCabe CH, Braunwald E. TIMI risk score for ST-elevation myocardial infarction: a convenient, bedside, clinical score for risk assessment at presentation: an Intravenous nPA for Treatment of Infarcting Myocardium Early II Trial Substudy. *Circulation.* 2000;102:2031–2037.

17. Ryan TJ, Anderson JL, Antman EM, et al. ACC/AHA guidelines for the management of patients with acute myocardial infarction: a report of the American College of Cardiology/American Heart Association Task Force on Practice Guidelines (Committee on Management of Acute Myocardial Infarction). *J Am Coll Cardiol.* 1996;28:1328–1428.

12 Coronary Artery Stenting

Eric A. Heller and George D. Dangas

CONTENTS

Key Words: Angioplasty; Drug-eluting stent; Bare metal stent; In-stent thrombosis; Reperfusion.

KEY POINTS

- Coronary artery stenting is a form of percutaneous revascularization (PCI) that has revolutionized the treatment of coronary artery disease.
- PCI improves survival and prevents recurrent infarction in patients with acute MI.
- An early invasive strategy for ACS that includes PCI reduces major adverse coronary events.
- PCI in stable angina should be used as an adjunct to optimal medical therapy for symptom relief and ischemia reduction.
- PCI may be equivalent to CABG as the revascularization treatment of choice for selected patients with multivessel disease.
- Emerging evidence suggests the benefits of revascularization may be driven by ischemic burden and not symptom severity.
- In-stent restenosis (ISR) is the Achilles heel of PCI's efficacy and has been markedly reduced by drug-eluting stents (DES).
- Stent thrombosis is a rare but serious complication of PCI and is reduced by optimization of stent placement and adherence to dual antiplatelet therapy.

From: *Contemporary Cardiology: Comprehensive Cardiovascular Medicine in the Primary Care Setting*
Edited by: Peter P. Toth, Christopher P. Cannon, DOI 10.1007/978-1-60327-963-5_12
© Springer Science+Business Media, LLC 2010

12.1. INTRODUCTION

When Andreas Gruentzig performed the first percutaneous coronary angioplasty on an awake patient in 1977 (Zurich, Switzerland), he created the nascent field of interventional cardiology and ushered in a new era of coronary revascularization. Percutaneous coronary transluminal angioplasty (PTCA) was positioned to serve as an alternative and complement to coronary artery bypass grafting (CABG) and optimal medical therapy. As in many medical fields, the advancement of percutaneous coronary interventions (PCI) has been punctuated by innovations and pitfalls.

The refinement of PTCA for the treatment of ischemic coronary artery disease during the 1980s and 1990s led to a procedural success rate of >90%; however, while dilatation of the vessel wall led to improved clinical outcomes and augmented myocardial perfusion, PTCA also resulted in endothelial denudation, plaque modification, elastic recoil, and negative remodeling. The clinical correlates of controlled vessel injury were acute/subacute vessel closure (often requiring emergent CABG) and clinical restenosis (~30%). Laser angioplasty and directional or rotational atherectomy failed to improve on PTCA alone.

The concept of metal scaffolds that could prop open dilated arteries was conceived as early as 1912 by Nobel Laureate Alexis Carrel. The first human coronary stent was implanted after PTCA by Ulrich Sigwart in Lausanne, Switzerland (1986). Juan Palmaz and Richard Schatz, also pioneers in early stent design and implantation, worked with the concept that these scaffolds could help prevent abrupt/threatened vessel closure and restenosis. BENESTENT and STRESS, two pivotal trials published in 1994, demonstrated the improved clinical efficacy and significantly better restenosis rates as compared to PTCA *(1, 2)*. These data established bare metal stents (BMS) as the gold standard for PCI.

The major initial concern with BMS was an unacceptably high rate of acute and subacute stent thrombosis. The optimization of a dual antithrombotic regimen consisting of aspirin and a thienopyridine (clopidogrel or ticlopidine) helped reduce BMS thrombosis rates to <1%. The Achilles heel of BMS has proven to be in-stent restenosis—neointimal formation driven by smooth muscle cell proliferation. Restenosis rates of approximately 15% (further increased in patients with comorbidities such as diabetes mellitus and renal insufficiency) led to repeat revascularization, and, less often, acute coronary syndromes.

Drug-eluting stents (DES) were developed to reduce neointimal hyperplasia, thereby improving the efficacy while maintaining or improving the safety of PCI. Sirolimus and paclitaxel, drugs that inhibit smooth muscle proliferation and migration through different mechanisms, were the initial compounds used on these devices. These drugs are embedded into a polymer that is mounted onto a bare metal scaffold. Multiple randomized trials showed that DES markedly reduced target lesion revascularization (TLR), target vessel revascularization (TVR), and major adverse coronary events (MACE). DES restenosis rates were 7–8% at 1 year. Over the past several years, registry data and meta-analyses have pointed to an increased rate of stent thrombosis, particularly very late stent thrombosis (>1 year) with DES as compared to BMS. Controversy has arisen as to how this may affect stent safety, in particular death and myocardial infarction. In 2008, the FDA approved second-generation DES that utilize everolimus and zotarolimus as anti-proliferative agents. These compounds have been incorporated into stents with new polymers and bare metal platforms in a concerted effort to improve the safety and efficacy of PCI, (including bioabsorbable polymers and even bioabsorbable stents).

This chapter will review the state of PCI in the DES era, including indications, controversies, adjunctive pharmacology, and the role of intravascular imaging.

12.2. STENT TECHNIQUE

First-generation BMS, such as the Palmaz–Schatz and Gianturco–Roubin stents, have given way to second- and third-generation stents that exhibit superior conformability, flexibility, tracking, and positioning with a wider variety of diameters and lengths. This has resulted in higher procedural success for a wider variety and complexity of coronary lesion subsets including small vessels (<2.75 mm in diameter), diffuse disease, long lesions, bifurcation lesions, and chronic total occlusions.

Essentially all coronary stents are delivered and then deployed on balloons using guiding catheters and coronary guidewires. Femoral artery catheterization is most common, brachial artery technique is rare, while radial artery technique is growing secondary to potential benefits with respect to bleeding and vascular complications.

Although direct stenting may be performed in straightforward lesions, most coronary stenoses are pre-dilated with PTCA. High-pressure non-compliant balloons or rotational atherectomy may be used for plaque modification in "non-dilatable" (heavily calcified, diffusely diseased) lesions. Balloon inflation after stent deployment may be used to increase lumen diameter. Stent expansion, vessel apposition, and residual lumen stenosis are the most important factors in stent efficacy. These factors correlate directly with restenosis and thrombosis. The current *ACC/AHA Guidelines* recommend a residual stenosis of <20% *(3)*. Existing data have demonstrated a discrepancy between the trained eye of the interventionalist and quantitative coronary angiography in determining pre- and post-stent percentage of coronary stenosis. Intravascular ultrasound (IVUS) is a simple catheter based imaging technique that may be used for diagnostic and interventional purposes. IVUS images cross-sections of the arterial wall and can determine minimal lumen area, plaque burden, lesion length, plaque morphology, stent expansion, and stent apposition. In addition, IVUS may be used to diagnose complications of stenting such as coronary artery dissection and stent fracture. The benefit of routine IVUS guidance for stent placement remains controversial.

Coronary pressure wire derived fractional flow reserve (FFR) is a simple and safe way to determine the functional severity of a lesion or efficacy of stent deployment. FFR measures the coronary artery pressure distal to a given lesion relative to aortic pressure at maximal hyperemia (achieved with intracoronary or intravenous adenosine). Abnormal FFR is a significant predictor of adverse coronary events. Multiple studies support the deferral of intervention in hemodynamically significant lesions as measured by FFR (>0.80) or IVUS (>4.0 cm^2 for proximal epicardial vessels and >6.0 cm^2 for the left main artery) *(4–10)*. Preliminary data from the FAME trial suggest that FFR-guided PCI in multivessel coronary artery disease may be superior to angiographically guided interventions with respect to hard clinical outcomes such as death, MI, and repeat revascularization *(11)*.

12.3. PCI IN ACS

Unstable angina and biomarker-positive non-ST segment elevation MI represent a continuum on the spectrum of acute coronary syndromes. Both conservative and invasive treatment strategies have been developed for the treatment of ACS. The conservative strategy employs intensive medical therapy utilizing antithrombotic, antiplatelet, and anti-ischemic agents over a period of several days. If the patient responds, pharmacologic therapy is often followed by stress testing with myocardial perfusion imaging. Either a positive stress test or persistent/recurrent angina is followed by cardiac catheterization with revascularization.

An invasive strategy involves intensive therapy along with prompt cardiac catheterization and revascularization within 4–48 h following admission. The early invasive strategy involves targeting the culprit lesion, often with PCI, in hopes of limiting myocardial damage and improving overall prognosis.

Multiple randomized trials have compared conservative versus early invasive strategies in the treatment of ACS patients. The preponderance of the evidence supports early intervention. In FRISC II, TACTICS-TIMI 18, and RITA 3, an early invasive strategy in ACS was associated with a sustained reduction in death and MI, primarily driven by the latter endpoint *(12–14)*. An early invasive strategy was also associated with a reduction in angina and hospital readmission. Data from meta-analyses have been consistent with these trials *(15, 16)*. Subgroup analyses indicate that patients who may derive the most benefit from an early invasive strategy are those with positive troponin, new ST depression, LVEF

<40%, prior PCI within 6 months or CABG, new heart failure or worsening mitral regurgitation, and high TIMI or GRACE risk scores *(17)*.

The *ACC/AHA Guidelines* recommend that ACS patients who are hemodynamically unstable or have refractory angina, severe LV dysfunction, mechanical cardiac complications, or malignant ventricular arrhythmias undergo immediate catheterization and revascularization. Low-risk patients (i.e., TIMI risk score ≤2) may undergo a conservative strategy at the discretion of the caring physician (Table 1) *(17)*. Attention should be paid to intermediate risk (TIMI risk 3.4) females who may have increased bleeding complication with an invasive strategy *(12)*.

Table 1
Indications for Early Invasive and Conservative Strategies in the Treatment of ACS *(17)*

Preferred strategy	*Patient characteristics*
Invasive	Recurrent angina or ischemia at rest or with low-level activities despite intensive medical therapy
	Elevated cardiac biomarkers (TnT or TnI)
	New or presumably new ST-segment depression
	Signs or symptoms of HF or new or worsening mitral regurgitation
	High-risk findings from noninvasive testing
	Hemodynamic instability
	Sustained ventricular tachycardia
	PCI within 6 months
	Prior CABG
	High-risk score (e.g., TIMI, GRACE)
	Reduced LV function (LVEF less than 40%)
Conservative	Low-risk score (e.g., TIMI, GRACE)
	Patient or physician preference in absence of high-risk features

PCI is clearly indicated in ACS for the treatment of one vessel CAD; however, the majority of ACS patients will have multivessel disease. Multivessel stenting and complete revascularization are often preferred to culprit lesion PCI. There are no strong data to support this approach, although there is a wealth of data indicating complete revascularization is superior to incomplete revascularization regardless of the clinical setting *(12, 17, 18)*. Multivessel stenting is often staged to prevent a large amount of contrast dye or radiation in one sitting. There are scant and conflicting data as to whether PCI or CABG is preferable when both are viable options and most decisions are made on a case by case basis (patients' wishes, concomitant valvular disease, coronary anatomy, comorbidities). New data from the FAME Trial suggest that utilizing the invasive physiologic technique of fractional flow reserve (FFR) in multivessel stenting to guide stenting of ischemic lesions may improve long-term outcomes *(11)*. Drug-eluting stents appear to be safe in ACS and reduce restenosis and the need for repeat revascularization *(19)*.

12.4. ACUTE MYOCARDIAL INFARCTION

Primary PCI with stenting of the culprit lesion is the revascularization therapy of choice in acute MI with time to reperfusion resulting in incremental benefit. Multiple randomized trials have demonstrated the clinical benefit of primary stenting as opposed to thrombolysis *(20)*. The largest of these trials were DANAMI-2 and PRAGUE-2. DANAMI-2 randomized 1,572 AMI patients to primary PCI versus thrombolysis with alteplase *(21)*. Patients had to have a symptom duration <12 h and be transferred to a PCI center within 3 h of randomization. Primary PCI was associated with a significant reduction in death, MI, or stroke at 30 days. PRAGUE-2 randomized 850 AMI patients with a duration of symptoms <12 h to primary PCI versus thrombolysis with streptokinase *(22)*. Primary PCI was associated with a trend toward reduced mortality at 30 days and a significant reduction in all-cause mortality, recurrent MI, stroke, or repeat revascularization at 5 years. The *ACC/AHA Guidelines* recommend primary PCI as the preferred method of revascularization for patients within 12 h of symptom onset *(23)*. The guidelines also suggest that the preponderance of the evidence favors primary PCI in patients who present within 12–24 h of symptom onset and who have persistent angina, cardiogenic shock, malignant arrhythmias, or severe CHF. Primary PCI should only be performed on the culprit vessel. Intervention on other lesions is contraindicated unless a patient presents in cardiogenic shock.

Several randomized trials have demonstrated a significant decrease in repeat revascularization in primary PCI with no increase in stent thrombosis for DES as compared to BMS. Meta-analyses have shown similar results *(24, 25)*. HORIZONS AMI randomized 3,600 AMI patients to receive BMS versus paclitaxel-eluting stents *(26)*. DES were associated with a significant reduction in target lesion revascularization and no difference in the rate of stent thrombosis.

PCI following failure of thrombolysis (rescue PCI) has demonstrated clinical benefit. Facilitated PCI with full-dose thrombolytics is contraindicated and the same is true for repeat thombolysis *(27)*. The most recent *ACC/AHA Guidelines* recommend PCI as adjunctive therapy to fibrinolysis for patients with cardiogenic shock, recurrent MI, or significant post-infarct ischemia *(23)*. Adjunctive PCI may be reasonable in patients who develop malignant ventricular arrhythmias, CHF, have an ejection fraction <40%, or have a critical stenosis in an infarct-related artery >24 h after AMI.

12.5. STABLE CAD

12.5.1. Role and Limitations of Medical Therapy

The goals of therapy in stable CAD are to ameliorate symptoms and improve quality of life, delay/prevent/reverse progression of atherosclerotic coronary disease, and to prevent hard clinical endpoints such as death and myocardial infarction. All of these objectives can be accomplished with aggressive risk factor modification and secondary prevention with a medical regimen that includes aspirin (or clopidogrel), beta-blockers, ACE inhibitors/ARBs, statins, nitrates, calcium channel blockers, and aldosterone antagonists. Revascularization with PCI or CABG is indicated in select groups of patients, such as those whose angina is refractory to medical therapy, those who cannot tolerate medical therapy, and those in who the evidence supports a survival benefit with revascularization (left main disease, three vessel disease with decreased LV function).

A number of clinical trials have compared medical therapy to percutaneous and/or surgical revascularization; however, up until recently, these trials have had significant limitations. Most trial patients had focal coronary disease and preserved LV function, limiting generalizability. These trials either utilized PTCA alone as a means of percutaneous revascularization or used bare metal stents with anti-thrombotic regimens that would be considered substandard as compared with current *ACC/AHA Guidelines*. Finally, many studies utilized vein grafts exclusively for surgical revascularization as opposed to the accepted standard of an arterial conduit (i.e., internal mammary artery) to bypass the LAD vessel. Despite these limitations, CABG was associated with significant short and intermediate symptomatic improvement as compared to medical therapy in the CASS and VA cooperative studies *(28–30)*. More importantly, there was a survival benefit in subgroups of patients who had left main coronary artery disease or its equivalent, triple vessel disease, particularly with depressed LV function, and two vessel CAD with ≥75% stenosis in the proximal LAD (especially with impaired left ventricular function and/or evidence of myocardial ischemia by stress testing).

A number of trials compared PCI to "optimal" medical therapy, including RITA-2 and MASS II *(31, 32)* (Fig. 2, Table 2). These studies demonstrated a symptomatic improvement in favor of PCI or CABG, but no difference in death or myocardial infarction. ACIP was a small study in patients with silent ischemia which demonstrated favorable clinical outcomes with revascularization; however, all

Table 2
Patient Characteristics (a) and Results (b) of Randomized Trials Comparing PCI Versus Medical Therapy for the Treatment of Stable Angina (61)

	AVERT	RITA-2	TIME	MASS II	SWISS II	Courage
(a) Patient characteristics						
Patients, No.	341	1018	301	611	201	2287
Women, No. (%)	53(16)	183(18)	131(44)	187(31)	25(12)	338(15)
Mean age, y	59	58	80	60	55	62
Angina, Canadian class	Nearly all 0 to II	53% II, III, or IV	100% II, III, or IV	81% II or III	None (silent ischemia)	58% II or III
Prior MI No. (%)	136(40)	471(46)	141(47)	269(44)	201(100) (first in preceding 3 month)	836(38)
Diabetes, No. (%)	51(15)	90(9)	68(23)	177(29)	23(11)	766(34)
Mean LVEF. %	61	54	53	67	57	62
LVEF exclusion, %	<40	None	"Predominant CHF"	40	None	30; 35 if 3-vessel disease
Ischemia by treadmill test	Excluded	Not required	Not required	Required	Required	Required
Vessels diseased %[a]						
1	57	60	14	Excluded	1- or 2-vessel disease required	35
2	43	33	19	42	See above	39
3	Excluded	7	60	58	Excluded	25
Previous CABG or PCI	Excluded if PCI in last 6 month or if history of CABG	Excluded	18% PCI 20% MT	Excluded	Not reported	16% PCI 11% MT
(b) Results						
Primary end point	Ischemic event: cardiac death, cardiac resuscitation, nonfatal MI, stroke, CABG, PCI or angina with hospitalization	Death, nonfatal MI	Freedom from: MACI[b]	Death, nonfatal MI, or refractory angina requiring revascularization	Survival free of MACEs; cardiac death, nonfatal MI, or symptom-driven revascularization	Death, nonfatal MI

Results (most recent follow-up published)	PCI 21% MT 13% P = 0.048	PCI 14.5% MT 12.3% P = 0.21	Freedom from MACE INV 39% MT 20% P < 0.001; no difference in mortality or other quality-of-life measures at 4 year	PCI 32.7% MT 36% CABG 21.2% P = 0.003; pairwise comparison: no difference between PCI and MT	Adjusted HR (favoring PCI) 0.33; 95% CI. 0.20–0.55; P < 0.001 [using person-years])	PCI 19.0% MT 18.5% P = 0.62 and no difference in angina at 5 year
Main result for primary endpoint	Longer time to, and fewer ischemic events with MT + high-dose statin	No advantage of PCI over MT	Revascularization improves freedom from MACEs for the elderly no effect on mortality	If revascularization is needed, favor CABG	Patients with silent ischemia after MT may benefit from PCI	No advantage of PCI over MT

AVERT = Atorvastatin Versus Revascularization Treatment; CABG = coronary artery bypass grafting; CHF = congeslive heart failure; COURAGE = Clinical Outcomes Utilizing Revascularization and Aggressive Drug Evaluation; LVEF = left ventricular ejection fraction; MASS II = Medicine, Angioplasty, or Surgery Study; MI = myocardial infarction; MT = medical therapy; PCI = percutaneous coronary intervention; RITA-2 = Second Randomized Intervention Treatment of Angina; SWISSI II = Swiss Interventional Study on Silent Ischemia Trial II: TIME = Trial of Invasive Versus Medical Therapy in the Elderly; CI = confidence interval: HR = hazard ratio; INV = interventional arm, including percutaneous coronary intervention (PCI) and CABG; MACE = major adverse cardiac event; MASS II = Medicine Angioplasty, or Surgery Study; MI = myocardial infarction; MT = medical therapy; RITA-2 = Second Randomized Intervention Treatment of Angina: SWISSI II = Swiss Interventional Study on Silent Ischemia Trial; TIME = Trial of Invasive Versus Medical Therapy in the Elderly.

[a] In the TIME trial, the percentage of vessels diseased pertains only to individuals in PCI group; MT group not assessed.

[b] Initial primary outcome was improvement in measures of quality of life, including relief of angina and lower rates of MACEs (death, nonfatal MI, or hospitalization for angina or acute coronary syndrome a: 6 month). Freedom from MACEs was reported in the 1-year follow-up.

of these trials were performed before the drug-eluting stent era and before the advent of the current concept of optimal medical therapy.

COURAGE compared contemporary medical therapy to PCI. The COURAGE trial randomized 2,287 patients with stable CAD to optimal medical therapy (OMT) or OMT plus PCI with bare metal stenting (33). All subjects were required to have objective evidence of ischemia and angiographic evidence of significant CAD (stenosis ≥70%). The vast majority of patients (87%) were symptomatic and had Canadian Cardiovascular Society (CCS) Class II or III angina (58%). High-risk patients (LM disease ≥50%, EF <30%, high-risk stress test, CCS class IV angina) and those with unsuitable coronary anatomy for PCI were excluded from the trial.

At a mean follow-up of 4.6 years there was no significant difference in all-cause mortality or non-fatal MI (Table 3). There was also no significant difference in hospitalization for ACS. PCI was associated with decreased angina and improved quality of life up to 3 years; however, the results in the OMT group caught up thereafter. PCI was also associated with the ability to pare down a patient's anti-anginal pharmacologic regimen (calcium channel blockers, nitrates). Overall, the quality of life benefit in the PCI group was associated with more severe baseline ischemia.

Table 3
Results from the COURAGE Trial (Kaplan–Meier Curves) (33)

Outcome	Cumulative rate at 4.6 years		
	PCI (%)	Medical therapy (%)	p value
Death and MI	19	18.5	0.62
Death	7.6	8.3	0.38
MI	13.2	12.3	0.33
Hospitalization for ACS	12.4	11.8	0.56

The Courage Nuclear Substudy addressed whether a patient's quantitative ischemic burden during stress testing affected prognosis based upon treatment randomization (34). Three hundred and fourteen patients within the COURAGE study population received baseline myocardial perfusion scans before and then 6–18 months following randomization. PCI was associated with a significant reduction in ischemic myocardium as compared to OMT alone. Those patients with moderate to severe ischemia at baseline received the greatest benefit from PCI. Patients with ≥5% ischemia reduction had significantly lower unadjusted (but not adjusted) rates of death and myocardial infarction. This subgroup analysis suggests that the extent and severity of ischemic burden in patients with CAD should influence an initial strategy of OMT versus OMT plus PCI. Of note, almost one-third of patients in the OMT arm of COURAGE eventually crossed over to have PCI, and the results were analyzed on an intention-to-treat basis.

12.5.2. Multivessel Disease

Revascularization in multivessel coronary disease has traditionally fallen under the purview of CABG; however, with refinements and advancements of PCI, there have been multiple efforts to compare the percutaneous strategy to the surgical gold standard. In the mid-1990s, studies such as BARI, RITA, and CABRI compared CABG versus PTCA in multivessel disease (35–38). The ARTS I and SOS trials compared CABG to PCI with bare metal stents (39–42). These trials concluded that the hard clinical endpoints of death and myocardial infarction were similar between the two treatment strategies; however, PCI was associated with a significant increase in repeat revascularization which was ameliorated by the introduction of bare metal stents.

The ARTS II registry was conducted in the DES/GP IIB/IIIA era and compared 607 patients treated with sirolimus-eluting stents for multivessel disease with the ARTS I PCI and CABG populations

(43). At 1 year of follow-up, major adverse cardiovascular and cerebral events were similar between the ARTS II registry and ARTS I CABG populations; however, PCI with DES was associated with a statistically significant increase in repeat revascularization (8.4% versus 4.1%), but with much narrower gap than the one observed between Bare metal stents and CABG in ARTS- I trial.

Most recently, the SYNTAX trial made an ambitious attempt to compare PCI versus CABG in moderate- to high-risk patients with multivessel disease *(44)*. Eighteen hundred patients with three vessel or left main disease were randomized 1:1 to either CABG or PCI with paclitaxel-eluting stents (PES). Anatomy was suitable for either means of revascularization. At 12 months follow-up, PCI was associated with a statistically significant increase in death, MI, stroke, or repeat revascularization (17.8% versus 12.4%) (Table 4). The difference was driven by repeat revascularization (13.5% versus 5.9%), whereas there was no difference in death or MI and there was actually a statistically significant decrease in stroke in the PCI population (Table 4). There were similar rates of stent thrombosis and symptomatic graft occlusion. These results are consistent with those of the PTCA and BMS eras. Notably, there was a significant narrowing between PCI and CABG with respect to the rates of repeat revascularization as compared with BARI and RITA II. The left main SYNTAX substudy, the largest set of patients with left main disease randomized to CABG versus PCI to date, showed excellent results with PCI with no difference in death/MI, more repeat procedures and less stroke than CABG.

The SYNTAX score, a tool for angiographic risk stratification based upon disease burden and complexity, correlated highly with outcomes and may be used to guide a decision for surgical versus percutaneous revascularization. In the final analysis, the physician and patient must balance the surgical risk (including stroke) of CABG versus the risk of repeat revascularization with PCI when making a decision regarding revascularization for multivessel and high-risk CAD.

Table 4
Results of the SYNTAX Trial (Kaplan–Meier Curves) *(44)*

Outcome	12-Month follow-up		
	PCI (%)	CABG (%)	p value
Death, stroke, or MI	7.6	7.7	0.98
Death	4.4	3.5	0.37
Stroke	0.6	2.2	0.003
MI	4.8	3.3	0.11
Repeat revascularization	13.5	5.9	<0.001

12.5.3. Diabetic Patients

There has been particular interest in the optimal method of revascularization in diabetic patients. In the BARI trial, which compared CABG to PTCA, CABG was associated with significantly increased survival (58% versus 46% at 10 years) *(35)*. The survival benefit was most marked in insulin-requiring patients and observed only to those who received an internal mammary graft. The diabetic patients in the study had more severe and diffuse disease than the rest of the study population, a potential confounder especially since the chosen method of percutaneous revascularization was with PTCA. The CARDIA trial randomized diabetic patients with multivessel disease to either PCI or CABG. Preliminary results showed no difference in death, non-fatal stroke, and non-fatal MI at 1 year between surgical and percutaneous revascularization.

The BARI-2D trial studied stable diabetic patients with few symptoms or silent ischemia. The investigators concluded the following: (1) an initial medical stabilization therapy with reservation of a revascularization procedure can be undertaken safely and was utilized in about half of the patients studied; (2) as the ischemic risk and coronary heart disease burden increases, complete revascularization may offer significant clinical benefit even in survival; and (3) insulin-sensitizing therapy offers improved metabolic and lipid profiles to an insulin-providing therapy and this may translate to a clinical benefit in combination with revascularization in the higher risk patients *(45)*. This study included routine coronary angiography in all patients as a method to define risk and did not directly compare stenting with CABG. Furthermore, both bare metal and drug-eluting stent types were used in PCI procedures. Results indicated 1) no major difference between types of diabetic management, 2) not much difference in death or MI between revascularization and optimal therapy in the low risk cohort, 3) advantage with surgery over optimal medical therapy in the higher risk cohort.

The ongoing FREEDOM trial was designed to discern the optimal means of revascularization for higher risk (greater than that studied in BARI-2D) diabetic patients with multivessel CAD (Fig. 1). FREEDOM has randomized 1,901 patients with type I or type II diabetes and multivessel disease with angina or ischemia to CABG versus DES. The primary endpoint will be death, MI, or stroke at 3 years.

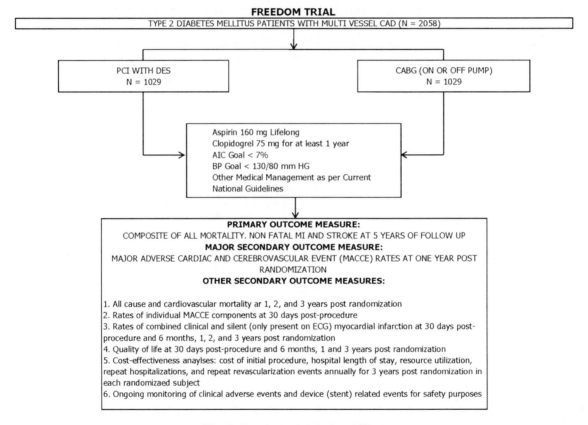

Fig. 1. Freedom trial design *(62)*.

12.6. ISCHEMIC BURDEN AND REVASCULARIZATION

Multiple lines of investigation in the cardiac imaging literature have correlated the quantitative ischemic burden in CAD patients with adverse cardiac outcomes. Invasive studies using fractional flow reserve (FFR) and intravascular ultrasound have demonstrated that certain cutoffs for hemodynamic flow reserve or lumen cross sectional area are associated with, and predictive for, future cardiac death and MI. Most recently, the COURAGE nuclear study, a hypothesis generating subgroup analysis, demonstrated that ischemic burden correlated with the degree of anginal relief following PCI *(34)*.

A mounting body of evidence supports targeting quantitative ischemic burden rather than symptoms with medical therapy and revascularization in an effort to reduce death, MI, and stroke. The latest in this series of studies is the FAME trial.

FAME was a multicenter trial that randomized 1,005 patients with stable CAD undergoing PCI with DES to angiographically versus FFR-guided revascularization (5). The former group underwent revascularization of all angiographically significant lesions. The latter group underwent revascularization of angiographically significant lesions only if the FFR was ≤ 0.8 (deemed hemodynamically significant). FFR-driven revascularization was associated with a significant reduction in the primary endpoint of death, MI or repeat revascularization at 1 year (Table 5). Future studies will address the primary targeting of ischemic burden and outcomes with revascularization and/medical therapy.

Table 5
Results from the FAME Trial (Kaplan–Meier Curves) (5)

Outcome	12-Month follow-up		
	Angiography group (%)	FFR group (%)	p value
Death, MI, or repeat revascularization	18.3	13.2	0.02
Death	3.0	1.8	0.19
MI	8.7	5.7	0.07
Repeat revascularization	9.5	6.5	0.08

12.6.1. Recommendations and Guidelines

The latest joint *ACC/AHA Guidelines for the Management of Stable of CAD* was published in 2009 (3, 46).

PCI has been deemed appropriate for patients with asymptomatic ischemia and/or CCS class I/II angina who (1) have significant lesion(s) in one to two coronary arteries that subtend a moderate to large area of viable myocardium on non-invasive testing and have a high likelihood of procedural success, (2) restenosis after PCI with a large area of viable myocardium at risk or high-risk features on non-invasive testing, and (3) left main disease in a patient who is not eligible for CABG.

PCI was deemed appropriate for patients with CCS Class III angina who (1) have single or multivessel disease, are receiving medical therapy, and have a high likelihood of procedural success with low morbidity/mortality; (2) have focal saphenous vein graft lesion(s); (3) have multiple lesions but are poor candidates for repeat CABG; and (4) have left main disease but are poor candidates for CABG. A 2009 guideline update indicates PCI as a IIb category for left main disease regardless of CABG eligibility.

PCI in multivessel disease may be considered particularly in patients with multi focal disease and preserved left ventricular ejection fractions, younger patients who may require multiple reoperations during the course of their lives, and older patients with multiple comorbidities that make the morbidity/mortality of CABG unacceptably high. These guidelines did not take into account the marked benefit of drug-eluting stents on target vessel revascularization and may be revised in the near future. Finally, all decisions regarding revascularization should take into account the educated opinions of the cardiologist and referring physicians as well as the particular concerns of the individual patient (Fig. 2).

Most recently the ACC, AHA, and numerous other professional organizations have published a consensus document regarding the appropriate criteria for percutaneous and/or surgical revascularization of patients in 180 different clinical scenarios (47). A more extensive discussion of these criteria and scenarios is beyond the scope of this chapter.

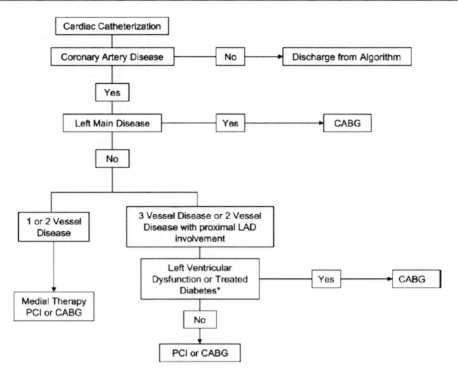

Fig. 2. Algorithm for surgical versus percutaneous revascularization for single and multivessel coronary artery disease *(17).*

12.7. POST-STENT CARE

Patients who have undergone uncomplicated PCI may be discharged the day after their procedure. The duration of dual antiplatelet therapy varies depending upon the type of stent placed. The current *ACC/AHA Guidelines* recommend treatment with aspirin and a thienopyridine for at least 1 month following placement of BMS and at least 1 year following DES *(48).* Dual antiplatelet therapy may be extended for patients with complex/high-risk lesions and/or major comorbidities. A patient's cardiologist should be consulted if dual antiplatelet therapy may be stopped prior to surgery or other circumstances. MRI appears to be safe for any patient with coronary stents.

Prasugrel has emerged as an alternative to clopidogrel, with higher antiplatelet efficacy (greater inhibition of the P2Y12 receptor), albeit more bleeding complications, due to which it is contraindicated in patients with low body weight, prior stroke (or transient ischemic attack), or age over 75 years. According to recent guidelines, it is indicated after stenting and can be particularly useful in patients with clopidogrel hyporesponsiveness due to generic polymorphism or other reason *(49, 50).*

12.7.1. Restenosis

Intracoronary stent restenosis has been the Achilles heel of PCI with respect to efficacy. Studies in the 1990s showed that PTCA alone was associated with a 30–40% rate of angiographic restenosis. First generation stents, such as the Palmaz–Schatz stents, were associated with a 20–30% rate of restenosis. The advent of second-generation bare metal stent platforms, better post-dilatation techniques, and a standardized anti-thrombotic regimen dramatically reduced the rates of clinical restenosis to 12–14% at 1 year. After 1 year, restenosis rates drop precipitously and recurrent angina and/or ischemia is more likely due to a de novo lesion. The mechanism underlying restenosis appears to be an inflammatory/wound healing response to the stent, smooth muscle cell proliferation and migration, and neointimal growth within the stent.

Drug-eluting stents brought great promise in combating restenosis. Paclitaxel and sirolimus are both drugs that inhibit vascular smooth muscle cell proliferation/migration and, therefore, were expected to reduce neointimal formation within the stent. First-generation DES reduced the rate of clinical restenosis to 6–7% at 1-year follow-up (target lesion revascularization). Second-generation DES, such as those containing everolimus or zotarolimus, hold promise for even greater reductions in the rates of clinical restenosis, also in association with biodegnadable polymers.

Restenosis may be focal or diffuse (intrastent, proliferative, occlusive) and the pattern of restenosis correlates with prognosis (Fig. 3) *(51)*. Independent procedural predictors include stent length, multiple stents, small vessel size, ostial lesions, prior restenosis at the stent site, post-procedural plaque burden, final minimal lumen diameter <3 mm, stent malapposition, and stent underexpansion. The latter two variables can be optimized by IVUS guidance. Independent clinical predictors include diabetes, renal insufficiency, hypertension, increased BMI, and multivessel disease.

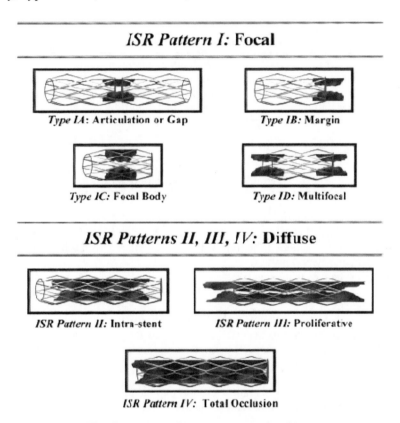

Fig. 3. Patterns of in-stent restenosis *(51)*.

Most cases of clinical restenosis present as new onset angina rather than an acute coronary syndrome or acute MI *(52)*. Treatment for in-stent restenosis includes DES placement or PTCA alone, often with IVUS guidance. Multiple randomized trials have confirmed the efficacy of treating BMS restenosis with DES *(53–56)*. CABG or intracoronary radiation is only considered with multiple restenoses or in high-risk clinical cases.

12.7.2. Stent Thrombosis

Stent thrombosis is the Achilles heel of PCI with respect to safety. Stent thrombosis is a rare, but often severe complication of PCI that may be fatal. Stent thrombosis often presents as an acute MI. Thrombosis may be characterized temporally as acute (≤24 h), subacute (1–30 days), late

(1 month–1 year), and very late (>1 year) (Table 6) *(57)*. Each case can be classified according to the consensus ARC definition as definite, probable, or possible (Table 7) *(58)*. Risk factors may be broadly characterized into patient, procedure, stent, or lesion related and are thought to stem from one of the three mechanisms: (1) hypoperfusion, (2) lack of subendothelialization of the stent surface, and (3) increased thrombogenicity. Specific risk factors include impaired LV function, emergent stent placement, increased stent length, stent underexpansion, residual plaque burden, small vessel caliber, residual thrombus or dissection, and medical non-compliance. The association of aspirin and/or clopidogrel non-responsiveness to stent thrombosis is under active investigation.

Dual antiplatelet therapy with aspirin and a thienopyridine (usually clopidogrel) markedly reduce the incidence of acute, subacute, and late stent thrombosis and may have an impact on very late stent thrombosis. The *ACC/AHA Guidelines* advocate for 1 month of dual antiplatelet therapy after BMS, at

Table 6
Temporal Categorization of Stent Thrombosis *(58)*

Acute stent thrombosis	0–24 h after stent implantation
Subacute stent thrombosis	>24 h to 30 days after stent implantation
Late stent thrombosis	>30 days to 1 year after stent implantation
Very late stent thrombosis	>1 year after stent implantation

Table 7
ARC Definitions of Stent Thrombosis *(58)*

Definite stent thrombosis
  Angiographic confirmation of stent thrombosis[a]
    The presence of a thrombus[b] that originates in the stent or in the segment 5 mm proximal or distal to the stent and presence of at least one of the following criteria within a 48-h time window:
    Acute onset of ischemic symptoms at rest
    New ischemic ECG changes that suggest acute ischemia
    Typical rise and fall in cardiac biomarkers (refer to definition of spontaneous MI)
    Nonocclusive thrombus
      Intracoronary thrombus is defined as a (spheric, ovoid, or irregular) noncalcified filling defect or lucency surrounded by contrast material (on three sides or within a coronary stenosis) seen in multiple projections, or persistence of contrast material within the lumen, or a visible embolization of intraluminal material downstream
    Occlusive thrombus
      TIMI 0 or TIMI 1 intrastent or proximal to a stent up to the most adjacent proximal side branch or main branch (if originates from the side branch)
  Pathological confirmation of stent thrombosis
    Evidence of recent thrombus within the stent determined at autopsy or via examination of tissue retrieved following thrombectomy
Probable stent thrombosis
  Clinical definition of probable stent thrombosis is considered to have occurred after intracoronary stenting in the following cases
  Any unexplained death within the first 30 days[c]
  Irrespective of the time after the index procedure, any MI that is related to documented acute ischemia in the territory of the implanted stent without angiographic confirmation of stent thrombosis and in the absence of any other obvious cause
Possible stent thrombosis
  Clinical definition of possible stent thrombosis is considered to have occurred with any unexplained death from 30 days after intracoronary stenting until end of trial follow-up

least 1 year of dual antiplatelet therapy with DES and indefinite aspirin therapy *(48)*. Longer duration of dual antiplatelet therapy may be indicated in situations that are deemed to be high risk such as left main stenting, multiple stents, chronic total occlusions, and bifurcation stenting. Some studies have shown that the addition of cilostazol to dual antiplatelet therapy may reduce the incidence of stent thrombosis in selected high-risk clinical scenarios *(57, 60)*.

Most (80%) stent thrombosis after placement of BMS occurs during the first 2 weeks; subacute stent thrombosis is less common, late stent thrombosis is rare, and very late stent thrombosis is almost never described. Notably, sensitivity over this very rare event was not present during BMS trials and this may have led to under-reporting. Meta-analyses of randomized trials have shown DES incurs approximately a 0.6% rate of stent thrombosis at 30 days and 0.75% at 1 year *(57)*. Very late stent thrombosis may occur at an annual rate of 0.6–0.9% after 1 year. Real-world registries show slightly higher rates of stent thrombosis. Very late stent thrombosis may occur several years following PCI at a very low rate. Ongoing studies are further characterizing the time course of this adverse event.

Pooled analyses of randomized trials and registries indicate the incidence of late stent thrombosis is equivalent between BMS and DES as long as guidelines for dual antiplatelet therapy are followed. There is an increased risk of very late stent thrombosis with DES as compared to BMS of approximately 0.5–0.6% per year. However, virtually every pooled analysis shows there is no difference in death or MI during this period of time. Individual risk/benefit analyses should be performed in every case to determine candidacy for BMS versus DES. If a patient has a history of clopidogrel intolerance, non-compliance with medication, or will be unable to obtain clopidogrel, strong consideration should be given to placement of a BMS rather than DES. Due to the extremely small incidence of stent thrombosis, any prospective study evaluating this phenomenon would require several thousand patients and long-term follow-up making feasibility extremely difficult.

Newer stent platforms, polymers, and drug formulations seek to maximize stent efficacy by abrogating restenosis while also maximizing safety through better prevention of stent thrombosis. As stated earlier, prasugrel can decrease stent thrombosis after DES and BMS compared to clopidogrel *(49, 50)*.

12.8. CASE STUDIES

12.8.1. Case Study 1

An active 57-year-old male with a history of type 2 diabetes on oral medication, hypertension, and hypercholesterolemia presents to his primary care physician complaining of exertional chest pain after walking 10 blocks. He is referred for an exercise stress test with a myocardial perfusion scan. The patient completes 8 min of Bruce protocol, achieving 87% of maximal predicted heart rate. He experiences the same exertional chest pain. There are no EKG changes. The myocardial perfusion scan reveals a moderate-sized area of anterior ischemia (moderate intensity). The patient is referred for cardiac catheterization, which reveals a 70% mid-LAD stenosis. What is the next step in management?

This case represents the plight of a typical patient who would fall within the realm of the COURAGE trial. It is the responsibility of the patient's cardiologist to explain that the LAD stenosis does not present an imminent risk for acute MI or acute coronary syndrome. The main goals of therapy should be symptomatic improvement, secondary prevention and risk factor reduction. First, the cardiologist must ensure that the patient is receiving optimal medical therapy. PCI would not reduce the patient's risk of death or MI, but would reduce the patient's angina and improve quality of life as compared to medical therapy in the short and intermediate terms. The risks of restenosis and stent thrombosis with PCI, as well as the requirement for dual antiplatelet therapy must be discussed. The decision for adding PCI to optimal medical therapy must be jointly made between the patient, primary care physician, and cardiologist.

12.8.2. Case Study 2

A 66-year-old female with a history of hypertension and hypercholesterolemia presents to her primary care physician complaining of exertional chest pain and dyspnea. The patient has no other medical problems. She is referred to a cardiologist who sends her for an exercise nuclear stress test. The patient performs 7 min of Bruce protocol, achieving 90% of maximal predicted heart rate for her age. She experiences chest pain but no EKG changes. Myocardial perfusion scanning reveals moderate sized, moderate intensity anterior and inferior defects. Cardiac catheterization reveals a 90% proximal LAD lesion, a 70% lesion of the first obtuse marginal artery, and an 80% mid-RCA lesion. All lesions are focal. Left ventriculography reveals an ejection fraction of 55% with no regional wall motion abnormalities. The patient is reluctant to undergo coronary bypass surgery but is not confident that multiple stents will be the best treatment. She desires the safest and most effective therapy. How should her cardiologist counsel her?

This patient has multivessel coronary disease with a normal ejection fraction. She is otherwise relatively healthy and has focal coronary disease that would be anatomically amenable to both CABG and PCI. A recommendation for this patient should take into account the data from numerous randomized trials in the literature comparing CABG with PCI in multivessel disease. The recent SYNTAX trial is of particular significance. A conversation with the patient would clarify that the extent and severity of her coronary disease would be amenable to both CABG and PCI. Given that she is relatively healthy, is not diabetic, and has normal LV function, either treatment modality would provide her with symptomatic improvement. With PCI, she would expect an increased likelihood of requiring repeat revascularization. Based on the lesion description, the SYNTAX score would be expected to be low and the repeat procedure rate after PCI not high. She would need to weigh the short-term morbidity of cardiac surgery (including a finite stoke risk) against that associated with subsequent hospitalization(s) for repeat PCI and the requirement of dual antiplatelet therapy for at least 1 year with DES. The patient's treatment plan should be individualized based upon her own thoughts and concerns regarding her health. She should have consultations with both an experienced interventional cardiologist and a cardiac surgeon. The ultimate plan should be a joint decision between the patient, her primary care physician, and clinical cardiologist—the physicians who know her the best. Typically such conversations might have preceded the catheterization procedure based on noninvasive studies and if an option of PCI was favored, this could have been performed at the same time as angiography.

REFERENCES

1. Fischman DL, Leon MB, Baim DS, et al. A randomized comparison of coronary-stent placement and balloon angioplasty in the treatment of coronary artery disease. Stent Restenosis Study Investigators. *N Engl J Med.* 1994;331: 496–501.
2. Serruys PW, de Jaegere P, Kiemeneij F, et al. A comparison of balloon-expandable-stent implantation with balloon angioplasty in patients with coronary artery disease. Benestent Study Group. *N Engl J Med.* 1994;331:489–495.
3. Smith SC Jr, Feldman TE, Hirshfeld JW Jr, et al. *ACC/AHA/SCAI 2005 Guideline* update for percutaneous coronary intervention—summary article: a report of the American College of Cardiology/American Heart Association Task Force on Practice Guidelines. ACC/AHA/SCAI Writing Committee to Update the *2001 Guidelines for Percutaneous Coronary Intervention. Circulation.* 2006;113:156–175.
4. Kern MJ, Donohue TJ, Aguirre FV, et al. Clinical outcome of deferring angioplasty in patients with normal translesional pressure-flow velocity measurements. *J Am Coll Cardiol.* 1995;25(1):178–187.
5. Pijls NH, De Bruyne B, Peels K, et al. Measurement of fractional flow reserve to assess the functional severity of coronary-artery stenoses. *N Engl J Med.* 1996;334:1703–1708.
6. Bech GJ, De Bruyne B, Bonnier HJ, et al. Long-term follow-up after deferral of percutaneous transluminal coronary angioplasty of intermediate stenosis on the basis of coronary pressure measurement. *J Am Coll Cardiol.* 1998;31: 841–847.
7. Bech GJ, Droste H, Pijls NH, et al. Value of fractional flow reserve in making decisions about bypass surgery for equivocal left main coronary artery disease. *Heart.* 2001;86:547–552.

8. Legalery P, Schiele F, Seronde MF, et al. One-year outcome of patients submitted to routine fractional flow reserve assessment to determine the need for angioplasty. *Eur Heart J.* 2005;26:2623–2629.

9. Tobis J, Azarbal B, Slavin L. Assessment of intermediate severity coronary lesions in the catheterization laboratory. *J Am Coll Cardiol.* 2007;49:839–848.

10. Pijls NH, van Schaardenburgh P, Manoharan G, et al. Percutaneous coronary intervention of functionally nonsignificant stenosis: 5-year follow-up of the DEFER Study. *J Am Coll Cardiol.* 2007;49:2105–2111.

11. Tonino PA, De Bruyne B, Pijls NH, et al. Fractional flow reserve versus angiography for guiding percutaneous coronary intervention. *N Engl J Med.* 2009;360:213–224.

12. Cannon CP, Weintraub WS, Demopoulos LA, et al. Comparison of early invasive and conservative strategies in patients with unstable coronary syndromes treated with the glycoprotein IIb/IIIa inhibitor tirofiban. *N Engl J Med.* 2001;344:1879–1887.

13. FRISC-II Investigators. Invasive compared with non-invasive treatment in unstable coronary-artery disease: FRISC II prospective randomised multicentre study. FRagmin and Fast Revascularisation during InStability in Coronary Artery Disease Investigators. *Lancet.* 1999;354:708–715.

14. Fox KA, Poole-Wilson PA, Henderson RA, et al. Interventional versus conservative treatment for patients with unstable angina or non-ST-elevation myocardial infarction: the British Heart Foundation RITA 3 Randomised Trial. Randomized Intervention Trial of Unstable Angina. *Lancet.* 2002;360:743–751.

15. Mehta SR, Cannon CP, Fox KA, et al. Routine vs selective invasive strategies in patients with acute coronary syndromes: a collaborative meta-analysis of randomized trials. *JAMA.* 2005;293:2908–2917.

16. Bavry AA, Kumbhani DJ, Rassi AN, Bhatt DL, Askari AT. Benefit of early invasive therapy in acute coronary syndromes: a meta-analysis of contemporary randomized clinical trials. *J Am Coll Cardiol.* 2006;48:1319–1325.

17. Anderson JL, Adams CD, Antman EM, et al. ACC/AHA 2007 guidelines for the management of patients with unstable angina/non ST-elevation myocardial infarction: a report of the American College of Cardiology/American Heart Association Task Force on Practice Guidelines (Writing Committee to Revise the *2002 Guidelines for the Management of Patients With Unstable Angina/Non ST-Elevation Myocardial Infarction*): developed in collaboration with the American College of Emergency Physicians, the Society for Cardiovascular Angiography and Interventions, and the Society of Thoracic Surgeons: endorsed by the American Association of Cardiovascular and Pulmonary Rehabilitation and the Society for Academic Emergency Medicine. *Circulation.* 2007;16:e148–e304.

18. Shishehbor MH, Lauer MS, Singh IM, et al. In unstable angina or non-ST-segment acute coronary syndrome, should patients with multivessel coronary artery disease undergo multivessel or culprit-only stenting? *J Am Coll Cardiol.* 2007;49:849–854.

19. Windecker S, Remondino A, Eberli FR, et al. Sirolimus-eluting and paclitaxel-eluting stents for coronary revascularization. *N Engl J Med.* 2005;353:653–662.

20. Weaver WD, Simes RJ, Betriu A, et al. Comparison of primary coronary angioplasty and intravenous thrombolytic therapy for acute myocardial infarction: a quantitative review. *JAMA.* 1997;278:2093–2098.

21. Andersen HR, Nielsen TT, Rasmussen K, et al. A comparison of coronary angioplasty with fibrinolytic therapy in acute myocardial infarction. *N Engl J Med.* 2003;349:733–742.

22. Thune JJ, Hoefsten DE, Lindholm MG, et al. Simple risk stratification at admission to identify patients with reduced mortality from primary angioplasty. *Circulation.* 2005;112:2017–2021.

23. Antman EM, Hand M, Armstrong PW, et al. 2007 focused update of the ACC/AHA 2004 Guidelines for the Management of Patients with ST-Elevation Myocardial Infarction: a report of the American College of Cardiology/American Heart Association Task Force on Practice Guidelines: developed in collaboration with the Canadian Cardiovascular Society endorsed by the American Academy of Family Physicians: 2007 Writing Group to Review New Evidence and Update the *ACC/AHA 2004 Guidelines for the Management of Patients with ST-Elevation Myocardial Infarction*, writing on behalf of the 2004 Writing Committee. *Circulation.* 2008;117:296–329.

24. Brar SS, Leon MB, Stone GW, et al. Use of drug-eluting stents in acute myocardial infarction: a systematic review and meta-analysis. *J Am Coll Cardiol.* 2009;53:1677–1689.

25. Kastrati A, Dibra A, Spaulding C, et al. Meta-analysis of randomized trials on drug-eluting stents vs. bare-metal stents in patients with acute myocardial infarction. *Eur Heart J.* 2007;28:2706–2713.

26. Stone GW, Witzenbichler B, Guagliumi G, et al. Bivalirudin during primary PCI in acute myocardial infarction. *N Engl J Med.* 2008;358:2218–2230.

27. Ellis SG, da Silva ER, Heyndrickx G, et al. Randomized comparison of rescue angioplasty with conservative management of patients with early failure of thrombolysis for acute anterior myocardial infarction. *Circulation.* 1994;90:2280–2284.

28. Investigators CASS. Coronary Artery Surgery Study (CASS): a randomized trial of coronary artery bypass surgery. Survival data. *Circulation.* 1983;68:939–950.

29. Detre K, Murphy ML, Hultgren H. Effect of coronary bypass surgery on longevity in high and low risk patients. Report from the V.A. Cooperative Coronary Surgery Study. *Lancet.* 1977;2:1243–1245.

30. Murphy ML, Hultgren HN, Detre K, Thomsen J, Takaro T. Treatment of chronic stable angina. A preliminary report of survival data of the Randomized Veterans Administration Cooperative Study. *N Engl J Med.* 1977;297: 621–627.

31. RITA-2 Investigators. Coronary angioplasty versus medical therapy for angina: the Second Randomised Intervention Treatment of Angina (RITA-2) Trial. RITA-2 trial participants. *Lancet.* 1997;350:461–468.

32. Hueb W, Soares PR, Gersh BJ, et al. The medicine, angioplasty, or surgery study (MASS-II): a randomized, controlled clinical trial of three therapeutic strategies for multivessel coronary artery disease: one-year results. *J Am Coll Cardiol.* 2004;43:1743–1751.

33. Boden WE, O'Rourke RA, Teo KK, et al. Optimal medical therapy with or without PCI for stable coronary disease. *N Engl J Med.* 2007;56:1503–1516.

34. Shaw LJ, Berman DS, Maron DJ, et al. Optimal medical therapy with or without percutaneous coronary intervention to reduce ischemic burden: results from the Clinical Outcomes Utilizing Revascularization and Aggressive Drug Evaluation (COURAGE) Trial Nuclear Substudy. *Circulation.* 2008;117:1283–1291.

35. Investigators BARI. Comparison of coronary bypass surgery with angioplasty in patients with multivessel disease. The Bypass Angioplasty Revascularization Investigation (BARI) Investigators. *N Engl J Med.* 1996;335:217–225.

36. Investigators RITA. Coronary angioplasty versus coronary artery bypass surgery: the Randomized Intervention Treatment of Angina (RITA) Trial. *Lancet.* 1993;341:573–580.

37. Sculpher MJ, Seed P, Henderson RA, et al. Health service costs of coronary angioplasty and coronary artery bypass surgery: the Randomised Intervention Treatment of Angina (RITA) Trial. *Lancet.* 1994;344:927–930.

38. Investigators CABRI. First-year results of CABRI (Coronary Angioplasty versus Bypass Revascularisation Investigation). CABRI Trial Participants. *Lancet.* 1995;346:1179–1184.

39. Serruys PW, Unger F, Sousa JE, et al. Comparison of coronary-artery bypass surgery and stenting for the treatment of multivessel disease. *N Engl J Med.* 2001;44:1117–1124.

40. Investigators SOS. Coronary artery bypass surgery versus percutaneous coronary intervention with stent implantation in patients with multivessel coronary artery disease (the Stent or Surgery Trial): a randomised controlled trial. *Lancet.* 2002;360:965–970.

41. van den Brand MJ, Rensing BJ, Morel MA, et al. The effect of completeness of revascularization on event-free survival at one year in the ARTS Trial. *J Am Coll Cardiol.* 2002;39:559–564.

42. Booth J, Clayton T, Pepper J, et al. Randomized, controlled trial of coronary artery bypass surgery versus percutaneous coronary intervention in patients with multivessel coronary artery disease: six-year follow-up from the Stent or Surgery Trial (SoS). *Circulation.* 2008;118:381–388.

43. Valgimigli M, Dawkins K, Macaya C, et al. Impact of stable versus unstable coronary artery disease on 1-year outcome in elective patients undergoing multivessel revascularization with sirolimus-eluting stents: A subanalysis of the ARTS II Trial. *J Am Coll Cardiol.* 2007;49:431–441.

44. Serruys PW, Morice MC, Kappetein AP, et al. Percutaneous coronary intervention versus coronary-artery bypass grafting for severe coronary artery disease. *N Engl J Med.* 2009;360:961–972.

45. TBDS Investigators. Group TBDS: a randomized trial of therapies for type 2 diabetes and coronary artery disease. *N Engl J Med.* 2009;360:2503–2515.

46. Kushner FG, Hand M, Smith SC, et al. Focused updates: ACC/AHA guidelines for the management of patients with ST-elevation myocardial infarction and ACC/AHA/SCAI guidelines on percutaneous coronary intervention. *J Am Coll Cardiol.* 2009;54:2205–2241.

47. Patel MR, Dehmer GJ, Hirshfeld JW, Smith PK, Spertus JA. ACCF/SCAI/STS/AATS/AHA/ASNC 2009 appropriateness criteria for coronary revascularization: a report of the American College of Cardiology Foundation Appropriateness Criteria Task Force, Society for Cardiovascular Angiography and Interventions, Society of Thoracic Surgeons, American Association for Thoracic Surgery, American Heart Association, and the American Society of Nuclear Cardiology. *Circulation.* 2009;119(9):1330–1352.

48. King SB 3rd, Smith SC Jr., Hirshfeld JW Jr, et al. 2007 focused update of the *ACC/AHA/SCAI 2005 Guideline Update for Percutaneous Coronary Intervention*: a report of the American College of Cardiology/American Heart Association Task Force on Practice Guidelines: 2007 Writing Group to Review New Evidence and Update the ACC/AHA/SCAI 2005 Guideline Update for Percutaneous Coronary Intervention, writing on behalf of the 2005 Writing Committee. *Circulation.* 2008;117:261–295.

49. Wiviott SD, Braunwald E, McCabe CH, et al. Prasugrel versus clopidogrel in patients with acute coronary syndromes. *N Engl J Med.* 2007;357:2001–2015.

50. Montalescot G, Wiviott SD, Braunwald E, et al. Prasugrel compared with clopidogrel in patients undergoing percutaneous coronary intervention for ST-segment elevation myocardial infarction (TRITON-TIMI 38): double-blind, randomized controlled trial. *Lancet.* 2009;373:723–731.

51. Mehran R, Dangas G, Abizaid AS, et al. Angiographic patterns of in-stent restenosis: classification and implications for long-term outcome. *Circulation.* 1999;100:1872–1878.

52. Stone GW, Ellis SG, Colombo A, et al. Offsetting impact of thrombosis and restenosis on the occurrence of death and myocardial infarction after paclitaxeleluting and bare metal stent implantation. *Circulation.* 2007;115:2842–2847.

53. Kastrati A, Mehilli J, von Beckerath N, et al. Sirolimus-eluting stent or paclitaxel-eluting stent vs balloon angioplasty for prevention of recurrences in patients with coronary in-stent restenosis: a randomized controlled trial. *JAMA.* 2005;293:165–171.

54. Alfonso F, Perez-Vizcayno MJ, Hernandez R, et al. A randomized comparison of sirolimus-eluting stent with balloon angioplasty in patients with in-stent restenosis: results of the Restenosis Intrastent: Balloon Angioplasty Versus Elective Sirolimus-Eluting Stenting (RIBS-II) Trial. *J Am Coll Cardiol.* 2006;47:2152–2160.

55. Migliorini A, Shehu M, Carrabba N, et al. Predictors of outcome after sirolimus-eluting stent implantation for complex in-stent restenosis. *Am J Cardiol.* 2005;96:1110–1112.

56. Silber S, Albertsson P, Aviles FF, et al. Guidelines for percutaneous coronary interventions. The Task Force for Percutaneous Coronary Interventions of the European Society of Cardiology. *Eur Heart J.* 2005;26:804–847.

57. Spaulding C, Daemen J, Boersma E, Cutlip DE, Serruys PW. A pooled analysis of data comparing sirolimus-eluting stents with bare-metal stents. *N Engl J Med.* 2007;356:989–997.

58. Cutlip DE, Windecker S, Mehran R, et al. Clinical end points in coronary stent trials: a case for standardized definitions. *Circulation.* 2007;115:2344–2351.

59. Lee SW, Park SW, Kim YH, et al. Drug-eluting stenting followed by cilostazol treatment reduces late restenosis in patients with diabetes mellitus the DECLARE-DIABETES Trial (a randomized comparison of triple antiplatelet therapy with dual antiplatelet therapy after drug-eluting stent implantation in diabetic patients). *J Am Coll Cardiol.* 2008;51:1181–1187.

60. Biondi-Zoccai GG, Lotrionte M, Anselmino M, et al. Systematic review and meta-analysis of randomized clinical trials appraising the impact of cilostazol after percutaneous coronary intervention. *Am Heart J.* 2008;155:1081–1089.

61. Coylewright M, Blumenthal RS, Post W. Placing COURAGE in context: review of the recent literature on managing stable coronary artery disease. *Mayo Clin Proc.* 2008;83:799–805.

62. Farkouh ME, Dangas G, Leon MB, et al. Design of the future revascularization evaluation in patients with diabetes mellitus: optimal management of Multivessel Disease (FREEDOM) Trial. *Am Heart J.* 2008;155:215–223.

13   Coronary Artery Bypass Surgery

Ramanan Umakanthan, Nataliya V. Solenkova,
Marzia Leacche, John G. Byrne,
and Rashid M. Ahmad

CONTENTS

Key Words: Cardiopulmonary bypass; Graft failure; Left main equivalent; Saphenous vein graft; Internal mammary artery.

KEY POINTS

- The primary care physician plays a very important role in providing the patient with treatment options and helping the patient make decisions regarding treatment based on the relative risks and interventions.
- The selection of the specific management strategy must incorporate the extent of the patient's coronary artery disease, co-morbidities, expected symptomatic relief, and survival benefits that have been established and quantitated by clinical trials.
- Current treatment options for coronary artery disease include medical management, percutaneous coronary intervention (PCI), and coronary artery bypass grafting (CABG).
- Several landmark studies performed at the Cleveland Clinic and other institutions from 1985 to 1996 have revealed the left internal mammary (LIMA) to left anterior descending (LAD) artery graft to result in excellent patency rates and outcomes after CABG, and this technique has led to major advances in CABG surgery.
- Trials comparing the outcomes of medical therapy with CABG have shown that in patients with multivessel disease, left ventricular (LV) dysfunction (LVEF less than 50%), and moderate-to-severe angina/ischemia, the survival benefits of CABG clearly exceed the benefits of medical therapy.
- Trials comparing the outcomes of medical therapy with PCI have shown that in patients with stable angina, PCI showed no benefit over medical management in terms of survival, MI, or freedom from

From: *Contemporary Cardiology: Comprehensive Cardiovascular Medicine in the Primary Care Setting*
Edited by: Peter P. Toth, Christopher P. Cannon, DOI 10.1007/978-1-60327-963-5_13
© Springer Science+Business Media, LLC 2010

subsequent revascularization and that all patients with stable angina should have a trial of optimized medical therapy prior to consideration of PCI.

- Trials comparing CABG to PCI and medical therapy consistently demonstrated that patients with proximal multivessel disease, diabetes mellitus, left main artery disease, left main artery equivalent disease (referring to combined proximal left anterior descending artery disease and proximal left circumflex artery disease), and LV dysfunction have better outcomes with CABG.
- The dominant theme demonstrating the superiority of CABG over medical management and PCI in the context of event-free survival, freedom from major adverse cardiac and cerebrovascular events (MACCE), and lower rates of repeat revascularization occurs in patients with left main disease, left main equivalent disease, multivessel disease, proximal vessel disease, diabetes, and LV dysfunction.
- It is important that a multidisciplinary approach be used to optimally tailor treatment options for the patient with CAD, and the primary care provider is in the unique position to advocate for the patient's best treatment option from an unbiased perspective.

13.1. BACKGROUND

Coronary artery bypass grafting (CABG) is one of the most common cardiac surgery procedures performed in the United States to treat coronary artery disease (CAD) and has evolved since its introduction in the 1960s *(1)*.

In 1962, Dr. Mason Sones at the Cleveland Clinic reported on a technique of coronary angiography *(2)*. He was able to place a catheter through an artery in the groin or the arm and directly injected contrast material into the coronary arteries. This technique laid the groundwork for the surgical treatment of coronary artery disease. Now surgeons would be able to see the exact location of blockages to perform coronary bypass surgery.

The concept of bypassing blocked or damaged arteries was emerging during the Korean War. Surgeons were commonly utilizing the greater saphenous vein, a superficial vein that runs from the groin to the ankle area, to bypass arteries in the leg that were injured or blocked *(3)*. As the concept began to gain acceptance, physicians began to consider using vein grafts to bypass blocked coronary arteries.

In 1967, Dr. René Favaloro, a surgeon from the Cleveland Clinic, used the saphenous vein to bypass stenoses of the right coronary artery in 15 patients *(4)*. Dr. Dudley Johnson then expanded the procedure and began grafting branches of the left coronary artery *(5)*. The following year, Dr. Charles Bailey and Dr. Teruo Hirose from New York published a report in which the internal mammary artery was used to bypass blockages in the right coronary artery in two patients *(6)*.

It was not until 1968 that Dr. George Green used the heart–lung machine to bypass a patient's left anterior descending artery (LAD) with the left internal mammary artery (LIMA), paving the path for one of the greatest milestones in the history of CABG *(7)*. The LIMA to LAD graft would subsequently emerge as a gold standard in the treatment of coronary artery disease due to its superiority for long-term patency and survival. Several landmark studies performed at the Cleveland Clinic and other institutions from 1985 to 1996 revealed the LIMA to LAD graft to result in superior early and long-term survival, event-free survival, and outcomes after CABG *(8–13)*. The superior biological characteristics, unparalleled long-term patency, and better clinical outcomes associated with the use of the LIMA conduit rendered it as the conduit of choice for all surgical coronary revascularization procedures.

During the 1970s and early 1980s, patient options for revascularization remained primarily surgical. In 1977, the era of interventional cardiology was born with the advent of the first percutaneous transluminal coronary angioplasty (PTCA) performed by Dr. Andreas Gruentzig from Zurich *(14)*. This technique continued to evolve and subsequently led to applications such as coronary atherectomy in 1986 and coronary stenting in 1987. By 1997, percutaneous coronary intervention (PCI) utilizing angioplasty or stenting had become one of the most common medical interventions in the world *(15)*.

The current treatments for CAD include medical management with beta blockers, angiotensin-converting enzyme inhibitors, statins, aspirin, long-acting nitrates, PCI, and surgical revascularization *(16)*. The primary care physician plays a very important role in providing the patient with treatment options and helping the patient make decisions regarding treatment based on the relative risks and interventions. The selection of the specific management strategy must incorporate extent of coronary artery disease, a patient's co-morbidities, expected symptomatic relief, and survival benefits that have been established and quantitated by large clinical trials.

Three major randomized studies, the Coronary Artery Surgery Study (CASS), the Veterans Administration Cooperative Study Group (VA), and the European Coronary Surgery Study (ECSS), and other smaller randomized trials conducted between 1972 and 1984, compared the outcomes of medical therapy with CABG *(17–24)*. These studies have shown that for patients with multivessel disease, left ventricular (LV) dysfunction (LVEF less than 50%), and moderate-to-severe angina/ischemia, the survival benefits of CABG clearly exceed the benefits of medical therapy. In 2005, a meta-analysis combining the results of these randomized trials demonstrated enhanced survival at 5, 7, and 10 years for patients with multivessel disease, left main coronary artery disease, left ventricular dysfunction, and moderate-to-severe angina/ischemia *(25)*. Specifically, the outcomes of 1,324 patients who were assigned CABG surgery and 1,325 patients who were assigned medical management between 1972 and 1984 were analyzed. The CABG group had significantly lower mortality than the medical treatment group at 5 years (10.2% versus 15.8%), 7 years (15.0% versus 21.7%), and 10 years (26.4% versus 30.5%).

With the advent of angioplasty in 1977 and percutaneous coronary stenting in 1987, the first trials compared the outcomes of medical therapy with PCI. Three major randomized studies, the ACME (A Comparison of Angioplasty with Medical Therapy) study, the Randomized Intervention Treatment of Angina-2 (RITA-2) study, the Atorvastatin versus Revascularization Trial (AVERT), conducted between 1992 and 2000, allowed direct comparison of the outcomes of medical therapy versus PCI *(26–30)*. These studies together suggested that in patients with stable angina, an initial trial of medical therapy is appropriate.

A meta-analysis of PCI versus medical management combining the results of ACME, AVERT, RITA-2, and several other randomized trials was published in 2005 *(31)*. In patients with stable angina, PCI showed no benefit over medical management in terms of survival, MI, or freedom from subsequent revascularization. This meta-analysis gave supporting evidence that all patients with stable angina should have a trial of optimized medical therapy prior to consideration of PCI. It also indicated that PCI does not decrease mortality except in the context of an acute ischemic episode. Several other recent trials have also been conducted and validate a trial of optimal medical therapy in patients with stable CAD *(32–34)*. The results of the Clinical Outcomes Utilizing Revascularization and Aggressive Drug Evaluation (COURAGE) trial, published in 2007, was a study that randomized patients with stable CAD to a regimen of optimal medical treatment alone or optimal medical treatment combined with PCI *(32)*. The results of the trial showed that there was no evidence of a better outcome for the PCI group over the medical group for the combined endpoints of death, MI, and stroke, for admission to the hospital for acute coronary syndrome, or for MI alone. Thus, both treatment strategies resulted in similar outcomes. The Bypass Angioplasty Revascularization Investigation 2 Diabetes (BARI 2D) trial, the results of which were published in 2009, was a randomized study designed to test the outcomes of optimal medical therapy versus revascularization (CABG or PCI) in type 2 diabetic patients with stable CAD *(33)*. Patients were assigned to a CABG or PCI stratum and underwent either medical therapy or revascularization. The study found that there was no significant difference in the rates of death at 5 years between the optimal medical treatment and revascularization. However, patients in the CABG stratum who were assigned to revascularization had significantly higher cardiovascular event-free survival at 5 years (77.6%) than did patients in the CABG stratum who were assigned to the medical therapy group (69.5%). In contrast, rates of cardiovascular events at 5 years among patients in the PCI stratum who were assigned to revascularization did not significantly differ from those in the PCI stratum who were assigned to medical therapy. The results of the Detection of Ischemia in Asymptomatic Diabetics (DIAD) study were published in 2009 *(34)*. This study sought to determine if screening for critical CAD with myocardial perfusion imaging in asymptomatic type 2 diabetics to identify patients who may benefit from prophylactic revascularization improves outcomes. This study found that in asymptomatic diabetic patients, the cardiac event rates were low (2.9% over an average follow-up of 4.8 years) and were not significantly reduced by such screening. Hence the DIAD study concluded that optimal medical treatment and close follow-up were appropriate in asymptomatic diabetic patients.

Most studies comparing CABG to PCI and medical therapy consistently demonstrated that patients with proximal multivessel disease, left main disease, left main equivalent disease, diabetes mellitus with symptomatic or multivessel CAD, and LV dysfunction have better outcomes with CABG *(35–38)*. In a multicenter study of patients with ejection fractions less than 40%, published in 1991, only 75% of the patients were still alive 2 years after multivessel angioplasty *(38)*. Overall, the outcomes of PCI are less favorable than CABG in patients with multivessel disease (greater than or equal to two-vessel disease) and many authors believe this to be a result of more complete revascularization obtained following CABG *(39, 40)*. In addition, the risks of proximal plaque rupture after PCI do not confer protection from low-grade plaques breaking loose that exist proximal to the stent. Hence in patients with multivessel CAD, data from large trials indicate that outcomes from CABG are superior to multivessel stenting. We shall briefly discuss the results of these trials.

In 2004, the results of the largest randomized trial performed at a single institution, the Medicine, Angioplasty, or Surgery Study (MASS-2), compared the relative efficacy of medical therapy, PCI, and CABG for patients with symptomatic multivessel CAD *(35)*. Six hundred and eleven patients with angiographically documented proximal multivessel coronary stenosis greater than 70% and confirmed ischemia were randomized to receive medical therapy, PCI, or CABG. The rate of event-free survival—namely the combined incidence of cardiac mortality, myocardial infarction (MI), or refractory angina requiring revascularization—was most favorable in the CABG group at 1 year. Patients assigned to the PCI group had more events (24%) than patients in the medical therapy group (14%) or CABG group (6%). Angina relief was superior in the CABG group (88%) compared to the PCI group (79%) or the medical therapy group (46%). The greatest difference noted among the three groups was the need for additional revascularization at 1-year follow-up. Only 0.5% of CABG group required additional intervention compared to 8% of the medical therapy group and 12% of the PCI group. The MASS-2 study showed CABG to be superior to PCI and medical therapy for event-free survival, angina relief, and freedom from additional revascularization in these patients with severe multivessel proximal coronary artery disease as seen by the above-mentioned results.

Randomized trials specifically comparing the outcomes of PCI versus CABG in patients with multivessel disease have been conducted *(36, 37)*. All have shown higher rates of repeat revascularization in the PCI groups as compared to patients undergoing CABG. In the Arterial Revascularization Therapy Study (ARTS), published in 2001, 1,205 patients with multivessel disease underwent CABG or PCI with bare-metal stents *(36)*. The rate of event-free survival at 1 year, defined as survival without cerebrovascular events, MI, or repeat revascularization, was significantly better in the CABG group versus the PCI group (87.8% versus 73.8%). At 1-year follow-up, the lowest rate of revascularization was seen in the CABG group (3.5%). In the PCI group, the rate was four times as high (16.8%).

Subgroup analysis of diabetic patients in the ARTS study was separately published in 2001 *(41)*. The outcomes of a subgroup of 112 diabetic patients who underwent PCI were compared to the outcomes of 96 diabetic patients who underwent CABG. At 1 year, patients assigned to CABG had a superior rate of event-free survival (84.4%) versus PCI (63.4%). Patients assigned to PCI had a higher incidence of combined major adverse cerebrovascular and cardiac events (MACCE) compared with CABG, regardless of diabetic status. A subgroup analysis of an earlier randomized trial in 1997, the Bypass Angioplasty Revascularization Investigation (BARI), had also demonstrated that diabetic patients with multivessel CAD had superior outcomes after CABG as compared to balloon angioplasty *(42)*. This subgroup analysis of the ARTS trial confirmed superiority of CABG as compared to PCI in diabetic patients with multivessel CAD *(41)*.

The second Argentine Randomized Trial of Coronary Angioplasty versus Bypass Surgery in Multivessel Disease (ERACI-2) was published in 2001 *(37)*. A total of 2,759 patients with multivessel coronary artery disease were screened at seven clinical sites, and 450 patients were randomized to undergo either PCI (225 patients) or CABG (225 patients). Repeat revascularization was more common in the PCI group during the following 33 months (16.8%) versus CABG (4.78%). In diabetics, repeat revascularization was reported at 22.3% in the PCI group versus 3.1% in the CABG group. However, in this study, the initial 30-day mortality was higher in the CABG group (5.7%) than in the PCI group (0.9%), even though there was no difference in survival at 5 years. These differences in early mortality were believed by the authors to be due to the fact that the study involved a large cohort of patients with a higher risk of in-hospital surgical morbidity and mortality. The study was not completely randomized. Only 16% of the patients were randomized to the two treatment arms and patients with greater co-morbidities were preferentially placed in the CABG group.

The findings of the Surgery or Stent (SOS) study, published in 2005, comparing the outcomes in 988 patients with multivessel disease, demonstrated higher rates of repeat revascularization with PCI (21%) versus CABG (6%) at a median follow-up time of 2 years *(43)*. Freedom from angina was higher in the CABG patients (79%) versus the PCI patients (66%) at 1 year.

Hannan et al. published the results of a large non-randomized, retrospective study in 2005 comparing the outcomes of PCI and CABG in patients with multivessel disease from 1997 to 2000 by accessing the New York Cardiac Registries *(44)*. Overall survival was observed to be higher among 37,212 patients who underwent CABG than among 22,102 patients who underwent stent placement after adjustment for known risk factors. Specifically, 3-year survival for CABG versus PCI was 93.3% versus 91.4% for patients with two-vessel disease without LAD disease; 92.1% versus 89.8% for patients with two-vessel disease with proximal LAD disease; and 89.3% versus 84.4% for patients with three-vessel disease with proximal LAD disease. A comparison of the Kaplein–Meier survival curves among the subgroups of patients is shown in Fig. 1. It is apparent in reviewing the graphs that patients with multivessel disease and proximal LAD disease derive greater benefit from CABG over PCI. The 3-year rates of revascularization were considerably higher in the PCI group (7.8% required subsequent CABG and 27.3% required subsequent PCI) versus the CABG group (0.3% required subsequent CABG and 4.6% required subsequent PCI).

With the introduction of drug-eluting stents (DES) in 2003, Hannan et al. published the results of a large non-randomized, retrospective study in 2008 comparing the outcomes of 9,963 patients receiving PCI using DES and 7,437 patients undergoing CABG from October 2003 to December 2004 *(45)*. All patients had multivessel disease. The study compared risk-adjusted adverse outcomes (death, myocardial infarction, or repeat revascularization). Patients with two- or three-vessel disease undergoing CABG were found to have a survival advantage, lower rates of myocardial infarction, and lower repeat revascularization when compared to DES at 18 months. Specifically, 18-month survival for CABG versus PCI was 96.0% versus 94.6% in patients with two-vessel disease and 94.0% versus 92.7% in patients with three-vessel disease. In, addition, 18-month survival free from myocardial infarction for CABG versus PCI was 94.5% versus 92.5% in patients with two-vessel disease and 92.1% versus 89.7% in patients with three-vessel disease. Figure 2 shows a comparison of the survival curves. Of patients who underwent PCI, 28.4% underwent repeat revascularization with PCI and 2.2% underwent repeat revascularization with CABG by 18 months. In contrast, of the CABG patients, only 5.1% underwent repeat revascularization with PCI and only 0.1% underwent repeat revascularization with CABG by 18 months.

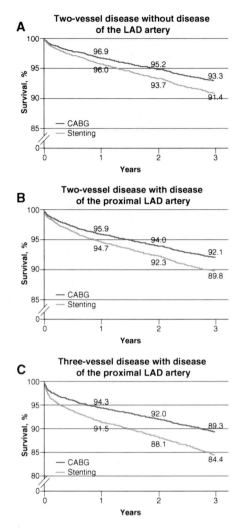

Fig. 1. Adjusted Kaplein–Meier survival curves in patients with two-vessel disease without involvement of the LAD artery (**a**); patients with two-vessel disease with involvement of the proximal LAD artery (**b**); and patients with three-vessel disease with involvement of the proximal LAD artery (**c**). Reproduced with permission from *(44)*.

A second study comparing the outcomes of CABG versus PCI with DES in 1,800 patients with multivessel coronary disease was published in 2009 *(46)*. This was a randomized controlled trial called the SYNergy between percutaneous coronary intervention with TAXus and cardiac surgery (SYNTAX). The study found that rates of MACCE at 12 months were significantly higher in the DES group (17.8%) versus the CABG group (12.4%).

In summary, the dominant theme demonstrating superiority of CABG in the context of event-free survival, freedom from MACCE, and lower rates of repeat revascularization occurs in the following groups: patients with left main disease, left main equivalent disease, multivessel disease, proximal vessel disease, diabetes, and LV dysfunction. Percutaneous coronary intervention has only been proven to be beneficial over medical therapy in patients with acute coronary syndromes (unstable angina, MI) and not in patients with stable CAD. For this reason, it is important that a multidisciplinary approach be used to optimally tailor treatment options for the patient with CAD. The primary care provider is

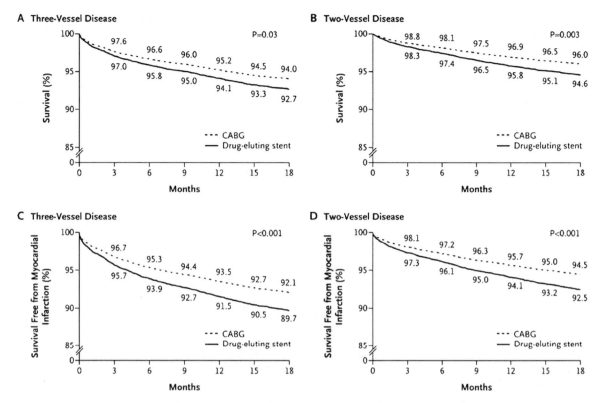

Fig. 2. Adjusted curves for long-term survival and survival free from myocardial infarction according to the number of diseased vessels. (**a–d**) Survival curves adjusted for age; sex; ejection fraction; hemodynamic state; history or no history of myocardial infarction before the procedure; the presence or the absence of cerebrovascular disease, peripheral arterial disease, congestive heart failure, chronic obstructive pulmonary disease, diabetes, and renal failure; and involvement of the proximal left anterior descending (LAD) artery. CABG denotes coronary artery bypass grafting. Reproduced with permission from *(45)*.

in a unique position to advocate for the patient's best treatment option from an unbiased perspective. Both the interventional cardiologist and the cardiac surgeon can skew the presentation to the patient. The primary care provider has the unique vantage point of maintaining equipoise in selecting the best treatment for the patient.

13.2. ASSESSMENT OF FUNCTIONAL STATUS

Although the quantification of the degree of CAD will be revealed by coronary angiography, it is important to develop an appreciation of the patient's functional status to help select the optimal treatment strategy.

The Canadian Cardiovascular Society (CCS) system for grading the clinical severity of angina pectoris has become widely accepted *(47)*. The CCS grading system of angina is as follows:

0, No angina
1, Angina only with strenuous or prolonged exertion
2, Angina with walking at a rapid pace at level, on a grade, or upstairs (slight limitation of normal activities)
3, Angina with walking at a normal pace less than two blocks or one flight of stairs (marked limitation)
4, Angina even with mild activity

However, due to the fact that angina is a subjective presentation, the prospective evaluation of the assessment of functional classification by the CCS criteria has demonstrated a reproducibility of only 73% *(48)*. In addition, there may be a poor correlation between the severity of symptoms and the magnitude of ischemia in diabetic patients who present with asymptomatic "silent ischemia."

There are several non-invasive tests of cardiac function that can be performed. Ideally, the patient should undergo a physical stress test. However, if there is a physical limitation, then a pharmacologically induced stress test can be utilized to assess functional status. In order to reach the appropriate stress level, a target heart rate of at least 85% of the maximal predicted heart rate based on the patient's age must be achieved.

An abnormal electrocardiogram (ECG) can be helpful in providing an assessment of the ischemic burden, while a normal ECG is a relatively reliable indicator of normal left ventricular function *(49, 50)*. The performance of an ECG under stress conditions can be a useful screening tool because it can provide information about the extent of ischemia and prognosis of the disease and is a simple and inexpensive test. Among patients with anatomically defined disease, stress ECG provides additional information about the severity of ischemia and the prognosis of the disease *(51–53)*. The sensitivity of the test increases with patient age, with the severity of the patient's disease, and with the magnitude of observed ST segment changes *(51)*. If ST segment depression is greater than 1 mm, stress ECG has a predictive value of 90% and a 2-mm change with accompanying angina is essentially diagnostic *(54)*. Early onset of ST segment depression and prolonged depression after discontinuation of exercise are strongly associated with significant multivessel disease.

Perfusion imaging with thallium or technetium tracer may be useful in patients with abnormal baseline ECGs. Reversible defects demonstrated by comparison of images obtained after injection of the tracer at peak stress with rest images are diagnostic of ischemia with viability. An irreversible defect indicates non-viable scarring *(55, 56)*. Both tracers have an average sensitivity and specificity of approximately 90 and 75% *(52)*. For patients with exercise limitations, pharmacologic vasodilators such as adenosine or dipyridamole may be used with similar sensitivity *(57–61)*.

The use of echocardiography during exercise or pharmacologically induced stress has also become increasingly popular. The accuracy of this method is similar to that of the perfusion studies *(52)*. Patients unable to exercise may be stressed with dipyridamole or dobutamine *(62, 63)*. An initial augmentation and subsequent loss of contractility is diagnostic of reversible ischemia, whereas failure to augment contractility suggests the presence of fibrotic tissue from a previous MI and irreversible ischemic changes *(64, 65)*. This test has the advantage of providing information on cardiac valvular function during the examination.

Cardiac magnetic resonance imaging (MRI) is another technique that has been useful in assessing myocardial viability in patients with CAD *(66)*. The ability to distinguish viable myocardium with dysfunction due to a reversible etiology (such as hibernation or stunning) from non-viable scar is critical for determining proper management of the patient. Cardiac MRI is a technique that has been observed to be useful for the detection of myocardial viability. Advancements in the field have shown promising developments that may soon make cardiac MRI the gold standard for viability assessment in select patients *(66)*.

Cardiac computed tomography (CT) scans have become popular as less invasive methods of imaging CAD. The 64-slice CT scans, first introduced in the United States in 2005 and initially tested at Johns Hopkins, showed that, on average, 91% of patients with blockages were detected by 64-CT and that the scans were able to diagnose 83% of patients without blockages *(67)*. Proponents are optimistic that the use of 64-CT scans will eventually dramatically improve our ability to detect and treat people with suspected coronary disease and chest pain much earlier in their disease. Investigations are ongoing.

13.3. CURRENT TREATMENT OPTIONS AND INDICATIONS FOR CABG

The current treatment options for coronary artery disease include are as follows:

- Optimal medical management (e.g., beta blocker, nitrates, calcium channel blockers, ACE inhibitors, statins, smoking cessation, blood sugar control in diabetic and insulin-resistant patients, weight control, and aspirin)
- Percutaneous coronary intervention (PCI)
- Coronary artery bypass grafting (CABG)
- Transmyocardial laser revascularization—a procedure used to relieve angina in patients with non-reconstructible CAD; a laser is used to drill a series of holes from the outside of the heart into the heart's pumping chamber in an effort to stimulate coronary angiogenesis. There is still limited follow-up data on long-term outcomes, however (68).

Definite indications for CABG as outlined by the American College of Cardiology (ACC) and American Heart Association (AHA) guidelines have been specified for different subgroups of patients (69).

For patients with asymptomatic/mild angina, the indications are as follows:

- Left main artery disease
- Proximal LAD and proximal circumflex artery disease
- Triple vessel disease (refers to disease involving all three major coronary vessels which are the left anterior descending artery, left circumflex artery, and right coronary artery)
- Proximal LAD artery and one-vessel disease
- One- or two-vessel disease not involving proximal LAD artery if a large territory is at risk on non-invasive studies or LVEF less than 50%

For patients with stable angina, the indications are as follows:

- Left main artery disease
- Proximal LAD artery and proximal circumflex artery disease
- Triple vessel disease
- Proximal LAD artery disease with one-vessel disease
- One- or two-vessel disease without proximal LAD artery disease but with a large territory at-risk and high-risk criteria on non-invasive testing
- Disabling angina refractory to medical therapy

For patients with unstable angina/non-ST segment elevation MI (NSTEMI), the indications are as follows:

- Left main artery disease
- Proximal LAD artery and proximal circumflex artery disease
- Ongoing ischemia not responsive to maximal non-surgical therapy
- Proximal LAD artery disease with one- or two-vessel disease
- One- or two-vessel disease without proximal LAD stenosis when PCI is not possible if a large territory is at risk

For patients with ST segment elevation (Q wave) MI, the indications are as follows:

- Failed PCI with persistent pain or hemodynamic instability and anatomically feasible
- Persistent or recurrent ischemia refractory to medical treatment with acceptable anatomy who have a significant territory at risk and not a candidate for PCI
- Require surgical repair of postinfarction ventricular septal rupture or mitral valve insufficiency

- Cardiogenic shock in patients less than 75 years of age who have ST segment elevation, left bundle branch block, or a posterior MI within 18 h of onset
- Life-threatening ventricular arrhythmias in the presence of ≥50% left main artery stenosis or triple vessel disease
- Patients who have failed fibrinolytics or PCI and are in the early stages (6–12 h) of an evolving STEMI

For patients with poor LV function (LVEF less than 50%), the indications are as follows:

- Left main artery disease
- Proximal LAD artery and proximal circumflex artery disease
- Proximal LAD disease and one- or two-vessel disease
- Significant viable territory and non-contractile myocardium

For patients with life-threatening ventricular arrhythmias, the indications are as follows:

- Left main artery disease
- Three-vessel disease
- Bypassable one- or two-vessel disease
- Proximal LAD disease and one-vessel disease

For patients who underwent a failed PCI, the indications are as follows:

- Ongoing ischemia with significant territory at risk
- Diffuse vessel disease not amenable to PCI
- Hemodynamic instability
- Foreign body in critical position
- Coronary artery rupture, dissection, or thrombosis after PCI

For patients with previous CABG, the indications are as follows:

- Disabling angina refractory to medical therapy
- Large territory at risk
- Vein grafts supplying LAD or large territory that have greater than 50% stenosis

Although the optimal treatment plan for each patient should be tailored on a case-by-case basis utilizing the aforementioned guidelines, the results of major trials reviewed thus far indicate that CABG is recommended in high-risk patients such as those with left main artery disease, left main equivalent disease (proximal LAD artery and proximal circumflex artery disease), three-vessel disease, two-vessel disease involving the proximal LAD, severe left ventricular dysfunction/low ejection fraction, and in diabetics with two- or more vessel disease.

13.4. PATENCY RATES OF CABG GRAFTS

The LIMA–LAD graft has shown excellent patency rates, which have correlated very well with increased event-free survival. Recent reports suggest a 5-year patency rate as high as 99% and at 10 years between 95 and 98% *(70–74)*. The LIMA–LAD graft is responsible for a significant portion of the benefit of CABG surgery and has proved to be a major milestone for the CABG procedure. Interestingly, with PCI, the location of a lesion in the proximal LAD has been identified as an independent risk factor for in-stent restenosis with rates between 19 and 44% *(75, 76)*. It is, of course, cardinal to note that with any revascularization procedure, a tailored plan of aggressive medical management with smoking cessation, exercise, and relief of insulin resistance must be adhered to in order to ensure maximal benefit.

The second most commonly used conduit after the LIMA to bypass non-LAD vessels is the saphenous vein graft (SVG). Failure rates for SVGs have been reported at 1 year between 1.6 and 30% with an average of 20% *(70–78)*. It is worth noting that the right internal mammary artery (RIMA) and radial artery (RA) have been used as alternative conduits in selected patients. A common use of the RIMA is to use the LIMA to bypass the LAD and the RIMA to bypass an obtuse marginal branch of the left circumflex artery through the transverse sinus *(79)*. However, due to anatomical considerations, surgeons may encounter difficulties getting the RIMA graft to reach distal obtuse marginal branches, particularly in patients with cardiomegaly *(80)*. Previous studies have demonstrated that patients who receive bilateral internal mammary artery grafts have better long-term survival, decreased myocardial infarction rates, and decreased revascularization rates than patients who receive a single internal mammary artery graft *(81–83)*. However, due to limitations with conduit length, this technique is not always employed. The use of the RA as a conduit for coronary bypass was originally described by Carpentier and associates in the early 1970s *(84)*. Spasm of the artery was common during surgery, and the initial results were disappointing with 32% of grafts occluded at 2 years *(85)*. Hence, the RA was initially abandoned as a conduit for CABG. Proponents of the RA have demonstrated encouraging results with a pedicled harvesting technique and pharmacologic manipulation to prevent artery vasospasm, and as a result, interest in the RA as a supplementary arterial conduit for coronary revascularization has been rekindled *(86–88)*. The radial artery graft is not superior to the vein graft in all circumstances. The patency of the radial graft is related to the severity of the target lesion stenosis. For example, a radial graft will have a shorter patency rate in a coronary lesion of 60% when compared to a vein graft. When lesions are greater than 90%, the radial graft patency will exceed vein graft patency.

A recent study published in July 2009 found that the implementation of 75 mg of daily clopidogrel in addition to 100 mg of daily aspirin in CABG patients increased graft patency at 12 months after CABG to 97.8% for LIMA grafts and 96.3% for saphenous vein grafts *(89)*.

In an aggressive effort to enhance the long-term patency of CABG grafts, we have implemented the use of clopidogrel in our CABG patients as well as the routine use of completion coronary angiogram at our institution. Our operating room (OR) has the facilities to perform completion coronary angiogram immediately after the completion of the CABG procedure. Defects in graft patency can be detected and addressed before the patient leaves the OR. We have seen that most cases of postoperative graft failure are related to conduit issues including vasospasm of the graft, graft kinking, and seldom due to technical error. We have found completion coronary angiography to be very useful in immediately detecting these defects and correcting them before the patient leaves the OR.

13.5. ALTERNATIVE APPROACHES

In the past few years, new surgical techniques without using the cardiopulmonary bypass (CPB) machine have been used to perform beating heart surgery as an alternative to standard CABG in selected patients. The development of improved cardiac stabilizers and intracoronary shunts has allowed refinement off-pump coronary artery bypass (OPCAB) techniques *(77)*. It is believed that avoidance of CPB decreases the intensity of the inflammatory response, which could result in a lower incidence of post-operative complications. Randomized trials have shown a reduction in the need for red blood cell transfusion, hemodynamic support, respiratory infections, and new onset atrial fibrillation with OPCAB *(77)*.

Minimally invasive techniques have also become popular for CABG. This helps to avoid the dangers of redo sternotomy in patients who have undergone previous cardiac surgery and require a second or third operation. Although redo sternotomy continues to be a common surgical approach in patients with a prior history of cardiac surgery who require CABG, re-operative median sternotomy can have associated risks such as injury to prior grafts and difficulty with exposure *(90–94)*.

For one-vessel revascularization of the left anterior descending coronary artery (LAD) using the left internal mammary artery (LIMA), the MIDCAB (minimally invasive direct coronary artery bypass) technique through a left anterior small thoracotomy has become widely employed *(95–98)*. The advantages and disadvantages relative to the median sternotomy approach have yet to be clearly defined.

Close-chest CABG surgery is another technique that has been performed with robotic systems and allows manipulation of tissues within thoracic ports through the use of fine instruments and peripheral institution of cardiopulmonary bypass. At a separate operating console, the surgeon controls the instruments while the operation is viewed stereoscopically (three-dimensional view). In 1998, Loulmet et al. introduced Totally Endoscopic Coronary Artery Bypass grafting (TECAB) of the LIMA–LAD using peripheral access for cardiopulmonary bypass *(99)*.

13.6. CASE STUDIES

Treatment for CAD has advanced during the past several decades. It is evident that CABG surgery has also advanced substantially over the decades with the use of the LIMA to LAD graft and has outcomes superior to PCI in select cases of patients with CAD. Based on the data, the utility of PCI is highest in patients with acute ischemia and treatment of a specific culprit lesion. Otherwise, surgical or optimal medical management should be considered.

It is equally important to note, however, that a thorough assessment of the patient's condition is appreciated before treatment decisions are made. There may exist the inclination to perform a less invasive procedure, such as PCI, over surgery on patients who are at high risk. Less invasive does not necessarily imply better outcomes. We shall briefly discuss two cases from our experience at the Vanderbilt Heart and Vascular Institute that clearly demonstrate this point.

13.6.1. Case Study 1

The first patient described is a 52-year-old male with a history of three-vessel CAD, stroke, type 2 diabetes mellitus, congestive heart failure, chronic obstructive pulmonary disease, and renal failure, who had undergone the placement of eight stents in his LAD, left circumflex artery, and right coronary artery 2 years prior. He had been informed initially that due to his multiple co-morbidities, his risk of mortality from CABG would be very high. Hence he had been advised to undergo PCI with stent placement for the treatment of his CAD. The patient presented approximately 2 years subsequent to his PCI with a complaint of the onset of severe chest pain associated with diaphoresis and shortness of breath over the course of the previous 3 days. Coronary angiography performed revealed severe three-vessel disease, which had developed despite the previously placed stents. The patient subsequently underwent three-vessel CABG and had no intraoperative complications. He did well post-operatively and was discharged home in good condition 4 days after his procedure.

13.6.2. Case Study 2

The second patient is a 62-year-old female with CAD of the proximal LAD and left circumflex artery and heart failure. The patient also had multiple co-morbidities including an ejection fraction of approximately 15%, very poor pulmonary function, moderate mitral regurgitation, and severe peripheral vascular disease. The patient had been referred for heart transplant but was deemed not a suitable candidate as she was a smoker. Given the patient's co-morbidities, surgical revascularization appeared to pose a relatively high risk. However, it was also equally apparent that the patient's progressive heart failure could eventually lead to her demise. After careful discussion and consideration of the risks and benefits involved, the patient opted to undergo CABG to address her CAD. Aggressive diuresis and an intra-aortic balloon pump were used to optimize her medical condition prior to performing her surgery. The patient subsequently underwent two-vessel CABG and tolerated the procedure well. She was extubated 5 h after her procedure and discharged from the hospital 5 days after her CABG and has done well.

The important lessons learned from cases such as these are that a thorough understanding of the presenting etiology is crucial to help decide whether a patient will be best treated by either PCI or CABG. There may be the misconception that higher risk patients who present emergently may benefit from a less invasive procedure. This clearly was not the case in the two scenarios described. Data from patients in the USA have revealed that other misconceptions also exist. In a recently published study, it was found that certain patients believed that PCI in stable angina was being performed as an emergency (33% of patients surveyed) and that it would prevent MI (71%) as well as extend lifespan (66%) *(100)*. Therefore, it is critical that all patients with CAD be evaluated by a multidisciplinary team to assess and inform them of what the best options are so that thoughtful and robust decisions are made with regard to their management.

REFERENCES

1. Góngora E, Sundt T. Myocardial Revascularization with Cardiopulmonary Bypass. In: Cohn LH, ed. *Cardiac Surgery in the Adult*. New York, NY: McGraw-Hill; 2008:599–632.
2. Sones FM, Shirey EK. Cine coronary arteriography. *Mod Concepts Cardiovasc Dis*. 1962;31:735–738.
3. Stephenson L, Rodengen J. Coronary Artery Disease and Treatment Options. *State of the Heart*. Fort Lauderdale: Write Stuff Enterprises; 1999:110–129.
4. Favalaro RG. Saphenous vein autograft replacement of severe segmental coronary artery occlusion. *Ann Thorac Surg*. 1968;5:334–339.
5. Johnson WD, Flemma RJ, Lepley D Jr, Ellison EH. Extended treatment of severe coronary artery disease: a total surgical approach. *Ann Surg*. 1969;170:460–470.
6. Bailey CP, Hirose T. Successful internal mammary-coronary arterial anastomosis using a "minivascular" suturing technic. *Int Surg*. 1968;49:416–427.
7. Green GE. Internal mammary artery-to-coronary artery anastomosis. Three-year experience with 165 patients. *Ann Thorac Surg*. 1972;14:260–271.
8. Cosgrove DM, Loop FD, Lytle BW, et al. Does mammary artery grafting increase surgical risk? *Circulation*. 1985;72(3 Pt 2):II170–II174.
9. Edwards FH, Clark RE, Schwartz M. Impact of internal mammary artery conduits on operative mortality in coronary revascularization. *Ann Thorac Surg*. 1994;57:27–32.
10. Grover FL, Johnson RR, Marshall G, et al. Impact of mammary grafts on coronary bypass operative mortality and morbidity. Department of Veterans Affairs Cardiac Surgeons. *Ann Thorac Surg*. 1994;57:559–568.
11. Sergeant P, Lesaffre E, Flameng W, et al. Internal mammary artery: methods of use and their effect on survival after coronary bypass surgery. *Eur J Cardiothorac Surg*. 1990;4:72–78.
12. Loop FD, Lytle BW, Cosgrove DM, et al. Influence of the internal-mammary-artery graft on 10-year survival and other cardiac events. *N Engl J Med*. 1986;314:1–6.
13. Cameron A, Davis KB, Green G, et al. Coronary bypass surgery with internal-thoracic-artery grafts—effects on survival over a 15-year period. *N Engl J Med*. 1996;334:216–219.
14. Gruntzig AR, Senning A, Siegenthaler WE. Nonoperative dilatation of coronary-artery stenosis: percutaneous transluminal coronary angioplasty. *N Engl J Med*. 1979;301:61–68.
15. Nirav J, Mehta MD, Ijaz A, Khan MD. Cardiology's 10 greatest discoveries of the 20th century. *Texas Heart Inst J*. 29(3):164–171.
16. Jameson JN, Kasper DL, Harrison TR, et al. *Harrison's Principles of Internal Medicine*. 16th ed. New York, NY: McGraw-Hill Medical Publishing Division; 2005.
17. CASS Principal Investigators and Their Associates. Coronary Artery Surgery Study (CASS): a randomized trial of coronary artery bypass surgery; survival data. *Circulation*. 1983;68:939–950.
18. Veterans Administration Coronary Artery Bypass Surgery Cooperative Study Group. Eleven-year survival in the Veterans Administration Randomized Trial of Coronary Bypass Surgery for Stable Angina. *N Engl J Med*.1984;311: 1333–1339.
19. Murphy ML, Hultgren HN, Detre K, et al. Treatment of chronic stable angina: a preliminary report of survival data of the randomized Veterans Administration Cooperative Study. *N Engl J Med*. 1997;1297:621–627.
20. Varnauskas E. European Coronary Surgery Study Group. Twelve-year follow-up of survival in the randomized European Coronary Surgery Study. *N Engl J Med*. 1988;319:332–337.

21. European Coronary Surgery Study Group. Prospective, randomized study of coronary artery bypass surgery in stable angina pectoris: second interim report. *Lancet.*1980;2:491–495.

22. Norris RM, Agnew TM, Brandt PWT, et al. Coronary surgery after recurrent myocardial infarction: progress of a trial comparing surgical and nonsurgical management for asymptomatic patients with advanced coronary disease. *Circulation.* 1981;63:788–792.

23. Mathur VS, Guinn GA. Prospective randomized study of the surgical therapy of stable angina. *Cardiovasc Clin.* 1977;8:131–144.

24. Kloster FE, Kremkau EL, Ritzman LW, et al. Coronary bypass for stable angina. *N Engl J Med.* 1979;300:149–157.

25. Yusuf S, Zucker D, Peduzzi P, et al. Effect of coronary artery bypass graft surgery on survival: overview of 10-year results from randomized trials by the Coronary Artery Bypass Graft Surgery Trialist Collaboration. *Lancet.* 1994;344:563–570.

26. Parisi AF, Folland ED, Hartigan P, on behalf of the Veterans Affairs ACME Investigators. A comparison of angioplasty with medical therapy in the treatment of single-vessel coronary artery disease. *N Engl J Med.* 1992;326:10–16.

27. Ryan TJ, Bauman WB, Kennedy J, et al. ACC/AHA Task Force Report: guidelines for percutaneous transluminal coronary angioplasty. A report of the American College of Cardiology/American Heart Association Task Force on Assessment of Diagnostic and Therapeutic Cardiovascular Procedures (Committee on Percutaneous Transluminal Angioplasty). *J Am Coll Cardiol.* 1993;22:2033–2054.

28. Folland ED, Hartigan PM, Parisi AF, for the Veterans Affairs ACME Investigators. Percutaneous transluminal coronary angioplasty versus medical therapy for stable angina pectoris: outcomes for patients with double-vessel versus single-vessel coronary artery disease in a Veterans Affairs cooperative randomized trial. *J Am Coll Cardiol.* 1997;29:1505–1511.

29. Pocock SJ, Henderson RA, Clayton T, et al. Quality of life after coronary angioplasty or continued medical treatment for angina: three-year follow-up in the RITA-2 trial. Randomized intervention treatment of angina. *J Am Coll Cardiol.* 2000;35:907–914.

30. Scandinavian Simvastatin Survival Study Group. Randomized trial of cholesterol lowering in 4444 patients with coronary heart disease: the Scandinavian Simvastatin Survival Study (4S). *Lancet.* 1994;344:1383–1389.

31. Katritsis DG, Ioannidis JP. Percutaneous coronary intervention versus conservative therapy in nonacute coronary artery disease: a meta-analysis. *Circulation.* 2005;111:2906–2912.

32. Boden WE, O'Rourke RA, Teo KK, et al. Optimal medical therapy with or without PCI for stable coronary disease. *N Engl J Med.* 2007;356:1503–1516.

33. Frye RL, August P, Brooks MM, et al. BARI 2D Study Group. A randomized trial of therapies for type 2 diabetes and coronary artery disease. *N Engl J Med.* 2009;360:2503–2515.

34. Young LH, Wackers FJ, Chyun DA, et al. DIAD Investigators. Cardiac outcomes after screening for asymptomatic coronary artery disease in patients with type 2 diabetes: the DIAD study: a randomized controlled trial. *JAMA.* 2009;301(15):1547–1555.

35. Hueb W, Soares PR, Gersh BJ, et al. The Medicine, Angioplasty, or Surgery Study (MASS-II): a randomized, controlled clinical trial of three therapeutic strategies for multivessel coronary artery disease: one-year results. *J Am Coll Cardiol.* 2004;43:1743–1751.

36. Serruys PW, Unger F, Sousa JE, et al. Arterial Revascularization Therapies Study Group: comparison of coronary-artery bypass surgery and stenting for the treatment of multivessel disease. *N Engl J Med.* 2001;344:1117–1124.

37. Rodriguez A, Bernardi V, Navia J, et al. ERACI II Investigators. Argentine Randomized Study: coronary angioplasty with stenting versus coronary bypass surgery in patients with multiple-vessel disease (ERACI II): 30-day and 1-year follow-up results. *J Am Coll Cardiol.* 2001;37:51–58.

38. Ellis SG, Cowley MJ, DiSciascio G, et al. Determinants of 2-year outcome after coronary angioplasty in patients with multivessel disease on the basis of comprehensive procedural evaluation: implications for patient selection. *Circulation.* 1991;83:1905–1914.

39. Weintraub WS, Jones EL, King SBIII, et al. Changing use of coronary angioplasty in coronary bypass surgery in the treatment of chronic coronary artery disease. *Am J Cardiol.* 1990;65:183–188.

40. Bell MR, Gersh BJ, Schaff HV, et al. Effect of completeness of revascularization on long-term outcome of patients with three-vessel disease undergoing coronary artery bypass surgery: a report from the Coronary Artery Surgery Study (CASS) registry. *Circulation.* 1992;86:446–457.

41. Abizaid A, Costa MA, Centemero M, et al. Arterial Revascularization Therapy Study Group. Clinical and economic impact of diabetes mellitus on percutaneous and surgical treatment of multivessel coronary disease patients: insights from the Arterial Revascularization Therapy Study (ARTS) trial. *Circulation.* 2001;104(5):533–538.

42. BARI Investigators. Comparison of coronary bypass surgery with angioplasty in patients with multivessel disease. The Bypass Angioplasty Revascularization Investigation (BARI) Investigators. *N Engl J Med.* 1996;335(4):217–225.

43. Zhang Z, Pertus JA, Mahoney EM, et al. The impact of acute coronary syndrome on clinical, economic, and cardiac-specific health status after coronary artery bypass surgery versus stent-assisted percutaneous coronary intervention: 1-year results from the stent or surgery (SoS) trial. *Am Heart J.* 2005;140:175–181.

44. Hannan EL, Racz MJ, Walford G, et al. Long-term outcomes of coronary-artery bypass grafting versus stent implantation. *N Engl J Med.* 2005;352:21742183.
45. Hannan E, Wu C, Walford G, et al. Drug-eluding stents vs. coronary artery bypass grafting in multivessel coronary disease. *N Engl J Med.* 2008;358:331–341.
46. Serruys PW, Morice M-C, Kappetein AP, et al. Percutaneous coronary intervention versus coronary-artery bypass grafting for severe coronary artery disease. *N Engl J Med.* 2009;360(10):961–972.
47. Campeau L. Grading of angina pectoris (letter). *Circulation.* 1976;54:522.
48. Goldman L, Hashimoto B, Cook EF, et al. Comparative reproducibility and validity of systems for assessing cardiovascular functional class: advantage of a new activity scale. *Circulation.* 1976;54:522–523.
49. Christian TF, Millder TD, Chareonthaitawee P, et al. Prevalence of normal resting left ventricular function with normal rest electrocardiograms. *Am J Cardiol.* 1997;79:1295–1298.
50. Rihal CS, Eagle KA, Gersh BJ. The utility of clinical, electrocardiographic, and roentgenographic criteria in the estimation of left ventricular function. *Am J Cardiol.* 1995;75:220–223.
51. Gibbons RJ, Chatterjee K, Daley J, et al. ACC/AHA/ACP-ASIM guidelines for the management of patients with chronic stable angina: a report for the American College of Cardiology/American Heart Association Task Force on Practice Guidelines. *J Am Coll Cardiol.* 1999;33:2092–2197.
52. Gibbons RJ, Balady GJ, Beasley JW, et al. ACC/AHA guidelines for exercise testing: a report of the American College of Cardiology/American Heart Association Task Force on Practice Guidelines (Committee on Exercise Testing). *J Am Coll Cardiol.* 1997;30:260–311.
53. Chang JA, Froelicher VF. Clinical and exercise test markers of prognosis in patients with stable coronary artery disease. *Curr Probl Cardiol.* 1994;19:533587.
54. Ribisl PM, Morris CK, Kawaguchi T, et al. Angiographic patterns and severe coronary artery disease: exercise test correlates. *Arch Intern Med.* 1992;152:1618–1624.
55. Pagley PR, Beller GA, Watson DD, et al. Improved outcome after coronary bypass surgery in patients with ischemic cardiomyopathy and residual myocardial viability. *Circulation.* 1997;96:793–800.
56. Bonow RO. Identification of viable myocardium (editorial). *Circulation.* 1996;94:2674–2680.
57. Ritchie JL, Bateman TM, Bonow RO, et al. Guidelines for clinical use of cardiac radionuclide imaging: report of the American College of Cardiology/American Heart Association Task Force on Assessment of Diagnostic and Therapeutic Cardiovascular Procedures (Committee on Radionuclide Imaging), developed in collaboration with the American Society of Nuclear Cardiology. *J Am Coll Cardiol.* 1995;25:521–547.
58. Iskandrian AS, Heo J, Lemlek J, et al. Identification of high-risk patients with left main and three-vessel coronary artery disease by adenosine-single photon emission computed tomographic thallium imaging. *Am Heart J.* 1993;125:1130–1135.
59. Taillefer R, Amyot R, Turpin S, et al. Comparison between dipyridamole and adenosine as pharmacologic coronary vasodilators in detection of coronary artery disease with thallium-201 imaging. *J Nucl Cardiol.* 1996;3:204–211.
60. Pennell DJ, Underwood SR, Ell PJ. Safety of dobutamine stress for thallium-201 myocardial perfusion tomography in patients with asthma. *Am J Cardiol.* 1993;71:1346–1350.
61. Calnon DA, Glover DK, Beller GA, et al. Effects of dobutamine stress on myocardial blood flow, ^{99m}Tc-sestamibi uptake, and systolic wall thickening in the presence of coronary artery stenoses: implications for dobutamine stress testing. *Circulation.* 1997;96:2353–2360.
62. Dagianti A, Penco M, Agati L, et al. Stress echocardiography: comparison of exercise, dipyridamole and dobutamine in detecting and predicting the extent of coronary artery disease. *J Am Coll Cardiol.* 1995;26:18–25.
63. Beleslin BD, Ostojic M, Stephanovic J, et al. Stress echocardiography in the detection of myocardial ischemia: head-to-head comparison of exercise, dobutamine, and dipyridamole tests. *Circulation.* 1994;90:1168–1176.
64. Perrone-Filardi P, Pace L, Prastaro M, et al. Assessment of myocardial 24-hour ^{201}Tl tomography versus dobutamine echocardiography. *Circulation.* 1996;94:2712–2719.
65. Bax JJ, Poldermans D, Elhendy A, et al. Improvement of left ventricular ejection fraction, heart failure symptoms and prognosis after revascularization in patients with chronic coronary artery disease: rest-4-hour-24-hour ^{201}Tl tomography versus dobutamine echocardiography. *Circulation.* 1999;34:163–169.
66. Lloyd SG, Gupta H. Assessment of myocardial viability by cardiovascular magnetic resonance. *Echocardiography.* 2005;22(2):179–193.
67. Girzadas M, Varga P, Dajani K. A single-center experience of detecting coronary anomalies on 64-slice computed tomography. *J Cardiovasc Med.* 2009; Epub ahead of print.
68. Briones E, Lacalle JR, Marin I. Transmyocardial laser revascularization versus medical therapy for refractory angina. *Cochrane Database Syst Rev.* 2009;21(1):CD003712. Review.
69. Eagle KA, Guyton RA, Davidoff R, et al. ACC/AHA 2004 guideline update for coronary artery bypass graft surgery: a report of the American College of Cardiology/American Heart Association Task Force on Practice Guidelines (Committee to Revise the 1999 Guidelines for Coronary Artery Bypass Graft Surgery). *Circulation.* 2004;110:e340–e437.

70. Alexander JH, Hafley G, Harrington RA, et al. Efficacy and safety of edifoligide, an E2F transcription factor decoy, for prevention of vein graft failure following coronary artery bypass graft surgery: PREVENT IV: a randomized controlled trial. *JAMA*. 2005;294:2446–2454.

71. BARI Investigators. The final 10-year follow-up results from the BARI randomized trial. *J Am Coll Cardiol*. 2007;49:1600–1606.

72. Kim KB, Cho KR, Jeong DS. Midterm angiographic follow-up after off-pump coronary artery bypass: serial comparison using early, 1-year, and 5-year postoperative angiograms. *J Thorac Cardiovasc Surg*. 2008;135:300–307.

73. Hayward PA, Buxton BF. Contemporary coronary graft patency: 5-year observational data from a randomized trial of conduits. *Ann Thorac Surg*. 2007;84:795–799.

74. Tatoulis J, Buxton BF, Fuller JA. Patencies of 2127 arterial to coronary conduits over 15 years. *Ann Thorac Surg*. 2004;77:93–101.

75. Versaci F, Gaspardone A, Tomai F, Crea F, Chiariello L, Gioffre PA. A comparison of coronary-artery stenting with angioplasty for isolated stenosis of the proximal left anterior descending coronary artery. *N Engl J Med*. 1997;336: 817–822.

76. Kastrati A, Schomig A, Elezi S, et al. Predictive factors of restenosis after coronary stent placement. *J Am Coll Cardiol*. 1997;30:1428–1436.

77. Puskas JD, Williams WH, Mahoney EM, et al. Off-pump vs conventional coronary artery bypass grafting: early and 1-year graft patency, cost, and quality-of-life outcomes: a randomized trial. *JAMA*. 2004;291:1841–1849.

78. Balacumaraswami L, Taggart DP. Intraoperative imaging techniques to assess coronary artery bypass graft patency. *Ann Thorac Surg*. 2007;83:2251–2257.

79. Vander Salm TJ, Chowdhary S, Okike ON, Pezzella AT, Pasque MK. Internal mammary artery grafts: the shortest route to the coronary arteries. *Ann Thorac Surg*. 1989;47:421–427.

80. Battellini R, Borger MA, Climente C, Mohr FW. Extending the in situ right internal mammary artery graft with retrocaval positioning. *Ann Thorac Surg*. 2003;75:1335–1336.

81. Lytle BW, Blackstone EH, Loop FD, et al. Two internal thoracic artery grafts are better than one. *J Thorac Cardiovasc Surg*. 1999;117:855–872.

82. Endo M, Nishida H, Tomizawa Y, Kasanuki H. Benefit of bilateral over single internal mammary artery grafts for multiple coronary artery bypass grafting. *Circulation*. 2001;104:2164–2170.

83. Taggart DP, D'Amico R, Altman DG. Effect of arterial revascularisation on survival: a systematic review of studies comparing bilateral and single internal mammary arteries. *Lancet*. 2001;358:870–875.

84. Carpentier A, Guermonprez JL, Deloche A, et al. The aorta-to-coronary radial artery bypass graft. A technique avoiding pathological changes in grafts. *Ann Thorac Surg*. 1973;16:111–121.

85. Carpenteier A. Selection of coronary bypass. Anatomic, physiological, and angiographic considerations of vein and mammary artery grafts. Discussion. *J Thorac Cardiovasc Surg*. 1975;70:414–431.

86. Iaco AL, Teodori G, Di Giammarco G, et al. Radial artery for myocardial revascularization: long-term clinical and angiographic results. *Ann Thorac Surg*. 2001;72:464–468.

87. Tatoulis J, Royse AG, Buxton BF, et al. The radial artery in coronary surgery: a 5-year experience—clinical and angiographic results. *Ann Thorac Surg*. 2002;73:143–147.

88. Possati G, Gaudino M, Alessandrini F, et al. Midterm clinical and angiographic results of radial artery grafts used for myocardial revascularization. *J Thorac Cardiovasc Surg*. 1998;116:1015–1021.

89. Gao C, Ren C, Li D, Li L. Clopidogrel and aspirin versus clopidogrel alone on graft patency after coronary artery bypass grafting. *Ann Thorac Surg*. 2009;88(1):59–62.

90. Dobell AR, Jain AK. Catastrophic hemorrhage during redo sternotomy. *Ann Thorac Surg*. 1984;37:273–278.

91. Ban T, Soga Y. [Resternotomy]. *Nippon Geka Gakkai Zasshi*. 1998;99:63–67.

92. Elami A, Laks H, Merin G. Technique for reoperative median sternotomy in the presence of a patent left internal mammary artery graft. *J Card Surg*. 1994;9:123–127.

93. English TA, Milstein BB. Repeat open intracardiac operation: analysis of fifty operations. *J Thorac Cardiovasc Surg*. 1978;76:56–60.

94. Macmanus Q, Okies JE, Phillips SJ, Starr A. Surgical considerations in patients undergoing repeat median sternotomy. *J Thorac Cardiovasc Surg*. 1975;69:138–143.

95. Calafiore AM, Di Giammarco G, Teodori G, et al. Left anterior descending coronary artery bypass grafting via left anterior small thoracotomy without cardiopulmonary bypass. *Ann Thorac Surg*. 1996;61: 1658–1663.

96. Cremer J, Struber M, Wittwer T, et al. Off-bypass coronary bypass grafting via minithoracotomy using mechanical epicardial stabilization. *Ann Thorac Surg*. 1997;63:S79–S83.

97. Subramanian VA, McCabe JC, Geiler CM. Minimally invasive direct coronary artery bypass grafting: two-year clinical experience. *Ann Thorac Surg*. 1997;64:1648–1653.

98. Diegeler A, Matin M, Kayser S, et al. Angiographic results after minimally invasive coronary bypass grafting using the minimally invasive direct coronary bypass grafting (MIDCAB) Approach. *Eur J Cardiothorac Surg.* 1999;15:680–684.

99. Loulmet D, Carpentier A, d'Attellis N, et al. Endoscopic coronary artery bypass grafting with the aid of robotic assisted instruments. *J Thorac Cardiovasc Surg.* 1999;118:4–10.

100. Lee JH, Chuu K, Spertus J, et al. Widespread patient misconceptions regarding the benefits of elective coronary percutaneous intervention. *Circulation.* 2008;118:S1161.

14 Cardiac Rehabilitation

William E. Kraus

CONTENTS

Key Words: Nutrition; Graded exercise testing; Smoking; Type A behavior; Transtheoretical model of behavior change.

KEY POINTS

- Changes in Medicare Reimbursement Guidelines, updating of program guidelines, expansion of the role of cardiac rehabilitation to all aspects of cardiac prevention, incorporation of the principles of exercise testing and behavior change into clinic encounters have made cardiac rehabilitation more powerful and effective.
- Although much is known about how patients respond to and benefit from regular exercise and therapeutic lifestyle changes, more work is needed relative to improving long-term compliance to known beneficial lifestyle and medical therapies, improving referral rates of eligible patients to secondary prevention programs, and improving retention of patients who are referred to and begin participation in cardiac rehabilitation.
- Despite cardiac rehabilitation representing a Class 1B guideline therapy for most patients with cardiovascular disease, gender, age, and race discrepancies persist in terms of program access and utilization.
- Like other therapies available to patients with cardiovascular disease, cardiac rehabilitation has a bright future for serving as a cost-effective strategy that improves mood, restores functional capacity, lessens or alleviates symptoms, and lowers the risk for and occurrence of subsequent clinical cardiovascular events, with all of the attendant social, economic, and medical benefits that ensue from its successes. The primary care physician who understands these principles can be an invaluable ally in this process.

From: *Contemporary Cardiology: Comprehensive Cardiovascular Medicine in the Primary Care Setting*
Edited by: Peter P. Toth, Christopher P. Cannon, DOI 10.1007/978-1-60327-963-5_14
© Springer Science+Business Media, LLC 2010

14.1. INTRODUCTION

Cardiac rehabilitation was developed in the mid-1970s as a mechanism to instruct and deliver exercise therapy to those having survived a recent acute coronary syndrome. Although the field of cardiac rehabilitation has a relatively short (25 years) history as evidence-based care for patients with cardiovascular disease, it continues to evolve. Changes in program scope have shifted the emphasis away from cardiac rehabilitation as a limited short-term intervention to one of a comprehensive secondary preventive strategy that targets the multiple medical, exercise, nutritional, and behavioral factors that place a patient at increased risk for a subsequent cardiac event. Consistent with this change in program scope, third party payers such as Medicare now recognize the importance of a comprehensive secondary prevention approach to the cardiac patient. In fact, the new national coverage policy from Medicare specifies that rehabilitation should not be solely an exercise program, but rather one that is multidisciplinary and aimed at reducing subsequent cardiovascular disease risk through intensive risk factor management and institution of therapeutic lifestyle changes.

For the physician and allied health professional interested in the secondary prevention of cardiovascular disease, a good summary of the secondary prevention goals and treatment guidelines can be found in a recent American Heart Association/American College of Cardiology (AHA/ACC) statement on this topic *(1)* and other associated statements from the American Association of Cardiovascular and Pulmonary Rehabilitation (AACVPR) *(2–5)*. Table 1 provides a summary of these goals. In addition, the (AACVPR) also has been a long-standing proponent of a multidisciplinary program for cardiac rehabilitation, such that programs address the broad scope of cardiovascular disease and its related risk-related morbidities (diabetes, hypertension, dyslipidemias, metabolic syndrome, psychosocial stress, and smoking behavior) through both medical and multi-component lifestyle interventions *(6, 7)*. In fact, both the ACC and the AACVPR, along with the American College of Sports Medicine, the American Hospital Association, and other organizations and individuals, were instrumental in providing the scientific evidence and opinion that led to the most recent changes in Medicare's national coverage policy *(8)*. A summary of these changes is outlined in Table 2. As is evident, Medicare now expects rehabilitation programs to extend service beyond exercise only, by using an interdisciplinary

Table 1

Summary of the American Heart Association/American College of Cardiology Goals for Secondary Prevention in Patients with Coronary and Other Atherosclerotic Vascular Disease *(1)*

Risk factor or therapy	Goal
Smoking	Complete cessation. No exposure to environmental tobacco smoke
Blood pressure	<140/90 or <130/80 mmHg if patient has diabetes or chronic kidney disease
Lipid management	LDL cholesterol <100 mg/dL; if triglycerides are $\geq$200 mg/dL then non-HDL cholesterol should be <130 mg/dL
Physical activity	30 min, 7 days/week (minimum 5 days/week)
Weight management	Body mass index: 18.5–24.9 kg/m^2
	Waist circumference: men <40 in. and women <35 in.
Diabetes management	HemoglobinA_{1c} <7%
Antiplatelet agents/anticoagulants	See full paper for treatment recommendations *(1)*
Renin–angiotensin–aldosterone system blockers	See full paper for treatment recommendations *(1)*
Beta-adrenergic blockers	See full paper for treatment recommendations *(1)*
Influenza vaccination	Patients with cardiovascular disease should be vaccinated

Table 2

Summary of Important Changes in Medicare National Coverage Decision Policy, March 2006, 1982 and March 2006, Present *(3)*

	March 2006, 1982	*March 26, 2006, Present*
Program components	Stipulated exercise only	Medical evaluation, risk factor modification, exercise and education
Program duration	36 visits in 12 weeks	36 visits in 18 weeks (following review, up to 72 visits in 36 weeks)
ECG rhythm strips	Required	Clinician determined need for ECG monitoring
Level of physician supervision	Proximal to exercise area	Hospital premises (within 250 yd for separate buildings on campus). Off-hospital campus then present and immediately available
"Incident to" physician	Unclear	Can vary based on setting of the services provided; however, ordering physician, primary care physician, or program medical director should all suffice as long as there is documentation in the medical record of interactions between the physician and rehabilitation staff concerning patient status
Indications	STEMI, NSTEMI, CABG, stable angina	NTEMI, STEMI, CABG, angina, PTCA, coronary stenting, heart valve surgery, and cardiac transplant

STEMI = ST segment elevation myocardial infarction, NSTEMI = non-ST segment elevation myocardial infarction, CABG = coronary artery bypass graft surgery, PTCA = percutaneous transluminal coronary angioplasty.

team approach to promoting recovery from an acute cardiac event and reducing the risk of subsequent events.

In this chapter, we will provide information that should be of use to practicing physicians who are considering referral to and interacting with a cardiac rehabilitation program. First, we will explore the utility and interpretation of the graded exercise tolerance test in the cardiac and noncardiac patients undergoing evaluation. Second, we explore the structure of a cardiac prevention strategy, whether it be conducted within a clinic setting, in cardiac rehabilitation, or in a combination of the two, where the cardiac rehabilitation program communicates with the referring physician to address the needs and progress of the cardiac rehabilitation participant. Finally, we will provide some example of patient cases of individuals that have gone through a cardiac rehabilitation program to illustrate these concepts.

14.2. THE GRADED EXERCISE TEST

In the primary care setting or in cardiac rehabilitation, a graded exercise test (GXT) might be obtained for risk stratification and prognostication, for diagnostic reasons (e.g., to test for residual ischemia in the setting of recurrent symptoms following an invasive therapeutic cardiovascular procedure), for therapeutic reasons (to develop an exercise prescription), or to quantify functional capacity—at baseline or in response to exercise training. It is important that the primary care provider be able to understand the reason for testing and the potential results that are obtained so as to be able to adequately address the needs and status of the cardiac patient.

Reasons for obtaining a GXT in cardiac rehabilitation:

1. Diagnosis—evaluation of ischemia and symptoms following event or procedure
2. Prognosis—following a cardiac event

3. Exercise prescription—when entering a CR program
4. Evaluation of functional capacity—following exercise training

14.2.1. The GXT for Diagnostic Purposes

In most settings, the primary reason for obtaining a graded exercise test (GXT), sometimes referred to as an exercise tolerance test (ETT), is to confirm or refute the diagnosis of functionally significant occlusive coronary artery disease when patients have symptoms suspicious for stable angina pectoris. The consensus guidelines and literature supporting this indication are thoroughly addressed in the official guidelines of the American Heart Association and American College of Cardiology *(9)* that are periodically updated. However, in the cardiac rehabilitation setting, only rarely is graded exercise testing performed for a de novo diagnosis of occlusive coronary artery disease. Rather, following an invasive procedure (percutaneous coronary intervention or coronary artery bypass grafting) for correction of occlusive disease, the cardiac patient might experience recurrent symptoms that are reminiscent or suggestive of angina. In such settings, it is reasonable to consider performing a graded exercise test with ECG monitoring in order to screen for exercise-induced ischemia. This may occur early in the setting of postevent rehabilitation and discharge, during a cardiac rehabilitation program (for example, indicative of incomplete revascularization) or later in the patient's course after cardiac rehabilitation (for example, restenosis following angioplasty or stenting). If ischemia is documented, often the patient should be referred for more extensive studies and perhaps a repeat revascularization procedure.

14.2.1.1. THE POSITIVE EXERCISE ECG TRACING

The diagnosis of functionally occlusive coronary artery disease is made on the basis of the exercise ECG. The following criteria are used to read the test as "positive" for such a condition. They are designed to optimize the balance between sensitivity and specificity in a population with a relatively high rate of cardiovascular risk factors. The ST segments have to be depressed 0.1 mV compared with the PR interval for the same beat, with a configuration that is downsloping or flat at a point in the complex that is 0.08 ms from the conclusion of the QRS complex in a lead tracing with no baseline ST depression. Additionally, this configuration has to be consistent and evident in at least three successive complexes to avoid findings due to motion artifacts. The finding must be in at least 1 of the 12 standard ECG leads other than III and aV_R. A lone finding in lead III is not considered to be valid, but rather it has to be accompanied by a similar finding in leads II or aV_F. In lead tracings with baseline ST depression, the tracing has to meet "double criteria" in order to be considered positive: where the ST tracing has to be depressed further than baseline by an additional 0.2 mV. That is, if the tracing is already 0.05 mV below the resting PR interval, then to meet double criteria the tracing has to be.25 mV below the PR interval (baseline) at 0.08 ms from the conclusion of the QRS complex.

There are several additional caveats. In order to reduce the prevalence of false positive tests, the exercise ECG is "uninterpretable" if there is baseline ST changes due to left ventricular hypertrophy or left bundle branch block or if the subject is taking digitalis and related medications. A test is considered interpretable in the lateral precordial leads (V_4–V_6) and in the limb leads in the presence of a right bundle branch block.

Note that there is a high prevalence of false positive tests in patients using exogenous estrogens. This is likely due to the fact that the chemical structure of estrogens resembles that of digitalis. Higher levels of endogenous estrogens are also likely the cause of the higher rate of false positive testing in middle-aged women, although this has never been conclusively proven. It might be prudent to proceed directly to a functional imaging study for diagnosis or exclusion of occlusive coronary artery disease in women on exogenous estrogen therapy instead of obtaining a simple GXT, given the relatively higher rate of false positive tests in this demographic, since progression to functional imaging studies might be required anyway. Many of these considerations are summarized in an excellent text by Ellestad on the subject dealing with the interpretation of the exercise electrocardiogram *(10)*.

Interpretations of the Exercise ECG:

1. Criteria for positive test

   a. ST segments depressed 0.1 mV in the absence of baseline changes

      - Three successive beats
      - Flat or down sloping 0.08 ms from the completion of the QRS complex
      - Any 1 or more of 10 leads, excluding III and aV_R

   b. Meets "double criteria" in presence of baseline ST depression

2. Uninterpretable in the presence of

   a. LBBB, LVH with strain, digitalis

3. High prevalence of false positives (i.e., use caution) in the presence of

   a. Exogenous estrogen used, LVH without strain, middle-aged women

14.2.2. The GXT for Prognostic Purposes

14.2.2.1. CARDIORESPIRATORY FITNESS

Cardiorespiratory fitness, as measured by a graded exercise tolerance test, provides strong and independent prognostic information about overall—and especially cardiovascular—morbidity and mortality. Cardiorespiratory fitness is a valid prognostic indicator in apparently healthy individuals, in at-risk individuals with diabetes mellitus, metabolic syndrome, and hypertension, and in patients with cardiovascular disease, such as present to cardiac rehabilitation programs *(11–17)*. However, despite the profoundly important prognostic information provided by simple clinical assessments of fitness, they are, unfortunately, rarely used in the clinical setting and often ignored in the exercise testing laboratory. There appears to be an undue emphasis—both on the part of the cardiac specialist and primary care physician—on the exercise ECG, the diagnostic interpretation that was just discussed. Tables 3 and 4 indicate, for women and men, the expected fitness level in METS, where 1 MET is the "metabolic equivalent" or energy utilized by a person at rest (approximated by 3.5 mL O_2/kg/min or 1 kcal/kg/min). Due to its increasingly recognized value, testing laboratories should report the fitness classification on clinical GXT reports. This can be used as a valuable marker to follow longitudinally the changes in risk stratification in individuals in cardiac rehabilitation programs.

Table 3
Cardiorespiratory Fitness Classifications for Women (METS) *(18)*

Age (year)	Low	Below average	Average	Above average	High
20–29	≤8.0	8.0–9.9	10.0 – 12.4	12.5–13.9	≥14.0
30–39	≤7.7	7.8–9.6	9.7 – 11.9	12.0–13.6	≥13.7
40–49	≤7.1	7.2–9.0	9.1 – 11.6	11.7–13.0	≥13.1
50–65	≤6.0	6.2–8.2	8.3 – 10.5	10.6–11.9	≥12.0

14.2.2.2. THE EXERCISE ECG FOR PROGNOSTIC PURPOSES

There is rich literature from the 1980s regarding the use of the exercise ECG—specifically, the time during the GXT at which it becomes abnormal—and the prognostic implications of this in clinical

Table 4
Cardiorespiratory Fitness Classifications for Men (METS) *(18)*

Age (year)	Low	Below average	Average	Above average	High
20–29	≤10.9	11.0–12.5	12.6–14.8	14.9–16.2	≥16.3
30–39	≤9.7	9.8–11.3	11.4–13.6	13.7–14.8	≥14.9
40–49	≤8.6	8.7–10.2	10.3–12.5	12.6–13.6	≥13.7
50–59	≤7.1	7.2–9.0	9.1–11.3	11.4–12.5	≥12.6
60–69	≤6.0	6.1–7.6	7.7–10.2	10.3–11.3	≥11.4

decision making. In one set of investigations, it was shown that after myocardial infarction, a submaximal test can be used to determine medium and long-term risk of recurrent ischemic events and cardiovascular death. Additionally, GXT information can be used to determine the likelihood of left main and three vessel coronary artery disease (sometimes referred to as "surgical disease").

In a publication during this period, the Duke Treadmill Score was developed and subsequently reached broad popularity for prognostic purposes *(15)*. It was observed that a limited GXT performed within the first several weeks following a myocardial infarction could help determine whether follow-up testing was indicated in order to identify patients who would benefit most from coronary artery bypass grafting (CABG). If the exercise ECG of a GXT was positive or symptoms developed before a HR of 120 beats per minute (bpm) was achieved, this indicated a 22% likelihood of the patient having three vessel occlusive coronary disease or left main coronary artery disease *(19)*. This would prompt further studies in the coronary catheterization laboratory with the anticipation that the patient will require CABG. Soon, these criteria were shown to be relevant for all individuals suspected of having occlusive coronary artery disease *(20)*. Unfortunately, with the ready availability of invasive diagnostic and therapeutic catheterization laboratories at many institutions, this practice has fallen out of favor and the GXT is rarely used today as a prognostic test when developing a therapeutic plan.

14.2.3. The Use of the GXT for Therapeutic Purposes—Modifying the Exercise Prescription

The GXT can also be used to follow a patient's progress and to adjust exercise training. It is for this purpose that the Center for Medicare and Medicaid Services (CMS) recognizes the need to reimburse for a GXT both prior to and following an approved period (36 sessions) of cardiac rehabilitation. The principles underlying this practice in the coronary patient are summarized in Fig. 1.

It is a basic principle of exercise physiology that there is a linear relationship between heart rate and workload from rest to the ventilatory threshold when the oxygen demands precipitated by the exercise workload exceeds the oxygen supply to working muscles. After a period of exercise training, there occur three observable physiologic responses that characterize the "training effect." These three responses are illustrated in Fig. 1: (1) resting bradycardia—where the resting heart rate is lower following exercise training; (2) a training bradycardia—a relative bradycardia at each successive workload to HR maximum; (3) an increase in maximum workload (measured as peak VO_2 with a metabolic cart). This physiology is particularly pertinent for individuals with occlusive coronary artery disease and angina pectoris. With a fixed lesion, the angina threshold (HR at which angina occurs) is reproducible and corresponds to a given workload. In the figure, before and following exercise training, the angina threshold is approximately 115 bpm. The maximum workload at the angina threshold is 6 METS prior to training and 10 METs following, representing a 66% increase in exercise tolerance following exercise training.

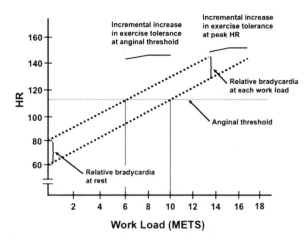

Fig. 1. The principles underlying graded exercise testing in the cardiac patient. For a full discussion of the principles, please see the text. The graphic depicts the linear response of heart rate (HR) to increasing workloads in metabolic equivalents (METS; multiples of resting energy expenditure) before and following an exercise training program (shown by the *dotted lines* where the pre-program line is higher and to the left of the post-program line). The three components of an exercise "training effect" are evident: decrease in resting heart rate (training bradycardia), a relative bradycardia at each workload, and an increase in maximum work tolerance. When angina from a fixed lesion reproducibly occurs at a heart rate of 115 bpm there is a similar increase in workload (from 6 to 8 METs) before the onset of angina, resulting in an effective increase in asymptomatic work tolerance with exercise training for the cardiac patient having stable exercise-induced angina.

It should be noted that these responses are specific to the muscles undergoing exercise training and, therefore, careful attention should be given to the exercise prescription and the muscle groups that will be commonly used in the activities of daily living when the angina threshold is likely to be exceeded. For example, if a patient works in a job that requires primarily upper body work, then consideration should be given to exercise training the upper body primarily during the cardiac rehabilitation period in order to provide the greatest increase in exercise tolerance in the work setting.

Thus, graded exercise testing is a useful clinical tool with prognostic, diagnostic, and therapeutic uses. Careful attention to the use of this tool in the cardiac rehabilitation program can increase the utility of program components to modify risk for subsequent events.

14.3. CARDIAC CARE IN THE OUTPATIENT SETTING: BEHAVIORAL AND THERAPEUTIC STRATEGIES

The assessment of global cardiovascular risk at baseline and in response to therapy is an important issue to assess during cardiac rehabilitation. Many cardiac rehabilitation programs assess the patient before and after a period of cardiac rehabilitation using established modifiable markers of cardiovascular risk, including each component of the lipid profile, blood pressure, metabolic syndrome, diabetes mellitus, central adiposity, cigarette smoking, depression, social support, and others. The goal is to modify the risk in order to prevent downstream cardiovascular morbidity and mortality. Although much is accomplished in the setting of the cardiac rehabilitation program itself, much can also be accomplished in the clinic-based visits with physicians and mid-level providers to reinforce messages from the cardiac rehabilitation program, to titrate and optimize medical therapy, and to further refine risk modification strategies when cardiac rehabilitation is completed. For lifestyle modification to be successful in the clinic setting, the provider must base the approach upon a behavioral construct that to the clinician makes sense and is one that can readily be employed. Many consider the standard Stages of Change behavioral change construct *(21)* to be the most useful. This is discussed below.

14.3.1. Assessment of Risk in the Cardiac Rehabilitation Setting

It is critical to assess modifiable cardiovascular risk factors prior to, and following, a course of cardiac rehabilitation. First, such an assessment can focus the attention of the patient and the CR staff on targeted areas of particular interest during the rehabilitation period. Follow-up assessments can demonstrate significant improvement when patients are compliant with prescribed therapeutic and lifestyle modifications. Second, such information can be shared as objective evidence of success to referring providers, thus becoming a reinforcing strategy for participant recruitment. Two case examples demonstrating these principles are presented later. Third, the CR staff can use these data to assess the effectiveness of the program and, in general, ineffective strategies can be modified and adapted to be more efficacious or abandoned if found to have no utility.

We have used the format illustrated in the case examples to collect relevant data on individual participants. Such data are shared with the referring health-care provider and can become part of the medical record of the individual. In addition, data are collected in a longitudinal database for subsequent program-wide assessments, as previously discussed.

14.3.2. Assessment and Modification of Risk in the Clinic Setting

As noted, the clinic visit, with either a member of the CR team or the referring physician, is an important ancillary component of cardiac rehabilitation. It is important to incorporate smoking, inactivity, and poor eating habits into a behavior change strategy. There are at least four steps to a successful intervention when trying to achieve behavioral change: (1) bringing attention to the behavior; (2) discussion of the behavior with the individual; (3) developing an effective strategy for changing behavior; and (4) following up with the progress of the strategy at the next encounter. It is clear, however, that such approaches take time and the pressures of current medical practice require that strategies to address behavior change in the outpatient setting be both effective and time-efficient.

Steps in successful clinic-based behavior change strategies:

1. Bring attention to the behavior—surveying
2. Discussion of importance of changing the behavior
3. Agreeing on plan and contracting
4. Follow-up

14.3.2.1. BRINGING ATTENTION TO THE BEHAVIOR

There are several methods to bring a particular behavior to the attention of a patient. When this comes from the physician, the individual becomes aware that the physician believes in its importance. For example, measuring a weight or waist circumference or asking about eating and physical activity behaviors are important components of drawing the patient's attention to the issue and stressing that the health-care provider believes that the issue is important enough to seek and record this information. Short surveys administered about eating and physical activity behaviors, administered in the waiting room while the individual is waiting to see the care giver, also provides an effective strategy for collecting this information. It is essential, however, in order for this strategy to be effective, that the information subsequently be addressed and referenced during the clinic encounter with the physician. Such data should also become part of the medical record, preferably in the clinic visit note.

14.3.2.2. DISCUSSION OF THE BEHAVIOR IN THE CLINIC WITH THE PATIENT

It is important, once the data are collected on a given behavior, to discuss the behavior with patients during the clinic encounter. That being said, it is clear, that not all behaviors of interest can be effectively addressed in each clinic visit. That is, it may be particularly ineffective to mention as a parting comment during a clinic encounter that the individual "should lose weight, eat better, and get more regular exercise." Although better than not acknowledging the problem at all, the absence of a detailed, if brief, discussion of important behavioral issues will rarely lead to significant or long-term behavior change. Rather, the provider must spend some time explaining the importance of the behavior under issue. Addressing *one* of the potentially four important cardiovascular behaviors in *each* visit is an efficient and effective means to promoting behavior change. In the prevention setting, the important behaviors that should be addressed are smoking, poor nutrition choices, lack of sufficient physical activity, and type A behavior (high mental stress levels due to excessive external demands as perceived by the individual). How does one choose which behavior to address in a given clinic visit?

14.3.2.2.1. Choosing Which Risk Factor to Address: The Transtheoretical Model of Behavioral Change. The transtheoretical model of behavior change is a common approach to instituting behavior change in the clinical setting. It can also be used to decide which behavior of several that could be chosen should be addressed in any given encounter. For example, should an individual be a smoker, have a poor diet, excessive job-related stress, and be physically inactive, one might ask which behavior might be best to address first. One approach might be to assess in which stage of pre-contemplation, contemplation, or planning the individual is in, by prompting with questions such as "Have you considered stopping smoking?" or "Have you made plans to stop smoking within the next several months?" Depending upon this survey of prospective behaviors, it might make sense first to address those behaviors to which the individual is willing or even eager to direct their attention. For example, in a patient that responds to such queries with "I enjoy smoking and do not wish to consider stopping at the present, but I do want to consider changing my diet and getting more exercise," it does not make sense to address first the smoking issue ahead of diet and exercise issues.

14.3.2.3. A SERIES OF CLINIC VISITS BECOME A PROGRAM FOR BEHAVIOR CHANGE

Given time constraints and limitations on the amount of information any one individual can absorb in one visit, it makes sense to address only one behavior in each visit and attempt to move the behavior change along the transtheoretical model spectrum (pre-contemplation, to contemplation, to planning, to action, to maintenance and reinforcement) in each clinic encounter. This typically may take from 5 to 15 min. Thus, in reality, *a series of clinic visits becomes a program of behavior change* and, for example, it may take up to 16 sequential clinic visits to address and promote effective behavior change in each of four distinct behaviors.

14.3.2.3.1. Developing a Behavior Change Plan. As noted, developing a behavior change plan is an essential step in the process of promoting lifestyle changes in the clinic setting. This may take as little as 5 min and as much as 15 min. Addressing the need to increase physical activity, for example, the clinician might probe the individual's lifestyle and suggest where within the normal routine of a day a patient may dedicate time for physical activity and exercise. As it does not require large changes in physical activity to make a significant difference in health parameters and modest changes in physical activity are relatively easy to institute, formulating a plan with an individual in the clinic setting is important. Often, for example, in order to promote daily, moderate levels of activity of about 30 min duration, we often suggest that patients walk the dog daily—whether he/she has one or not! Once a plan is made, it is important to document it in the clinic record for later reference.

14.3.2.4. FOLLOW-UP AT THE NEXT ENCOUNTER—THE IMPORTANCE OF CONTRACTING

The final essential step in a clinic-based process promoting behavior change is follow-up and reinforcement. By recording the plan in the clinic note, the clinician is prepared to query progress at the next visit. Contracting also is a useful approach. For example, if weight loss is a goal, one might agree on a target for a given amount of weight loss in the interim until the next visit (for example, agreeing on a 10 lb weight loss in 5 months). One might reinforce the understanding by contracting on the behavior (looking the patient in the eyes, shaking hands on the agreement, and recording it in the chart). This can be particularly effective in helping the individual recall the contract. The contract and progress in achieving the agreement are then reviewed at the next encounter and a new contract formed. When it is important to reinforce behavior when change is actively taking place, more as opposed to less frequent clinic visits should be arranged.

14.4. SUMMARY AND OUTSTANDING QUESTIONS

Assessing global cardiovascular risk is important in both the cardiac rehabilitation setting and in the cardiovascular disease prevention or primary care clinic that works in parallel. Assessing risk permits one to assess the effectiveness and make necessary adaptation of procedures and tactics for promoting lifestyle changes in these settings. In the clinic setting, promotion of lifestyle change is a progressive process, often based upon behavioral change strategies, such as the transtheoretical model, where a series of stepwise counseling can be considered a program. Although many of the suggestions presented in this summary are seemingly rational and self-evident, many questions are in need of scientific testing for efficacy in randomized trials. For example, an important question might be that, when multiple behaviors need to be addressed, whether it is better to address a behavior that the individual is open to change (i.e., contemplative) or one that potentially presents the greatest risk (e.g., smoking). Scientific studies addressing such questions will greatly assist those that promote lifestyle change strategies in the clinic setting.

14.5. SUMMARY

These are exciting times for professionals working in the field of cardiac rehabilitation and secondary prevention. Although much is known about how patients respond to and benefit from regular exercise and therapeutic lifestyle changes, more work is needed relative to improving long-term compliance to known beneficial lifestyle and medical therapies, improving referral rates of eligible patients to secondary prevention programs, and improving the retention of patients who are referred to and begin participation in cardiac rehabilitation. Despite cardiac rehabilitation representing a Class 1B guideline therapy for most patients with cardiovascular disease, gender, age, and racial discrepancies persist in terms of program access and utilization. Like other therapies available to patients with cardiovascular disease, cardiac rehabilitation is a cost-effective strategy that improves mood, restores functional capacity, lessens or alleviates symptoms, and lowers the risk for and occurrence of subsequent clinical cardiovascular events, with all of the attendant social, economic, and medical benefits that ensue from its successes. It is imperative that primary care physicians ally themselves with the multidisciplinary team approach which cardiac rehabilitation offers to patients who have sustained acute coronary syndromes or have undergone coronary revascularization.

DUKE CARDIAC REHABILITATION

| EXIT SUMMARY |

PATIENT'S NAME: Mr. XXXXX
MD: XXXXX   HISTORY NUMBER: XY0000
Program dates: 10.29.07 to 3.12.08   Number of sessions: 32/36

	Initial	Exit	%Change	Comments
Metabolic Syndrome	Yes	No		Diabetic; HTN
Smoking	No	No		
Hypertension				Average of first and last 3 BP readings
systolic	132	117	11%	
diastolic	74	67	9%	
Hyperlipidemia				
Total	138	113	18%	
LDL	57	32	44%	Goal for LDL is <70mg/dL
HDL	35	45	29%	Goal : >40mg/dL men, >50 mg/dL women
Triglycerides	228	179	21%	Goal for TG is <150 mg/dL
Diabetes				
HBA1C	6.7	6.2	7%	
Fasting glucose	183	110	40%	Average of first and last 3 fasting glucoses
Framingham 10 yr. CHD Risk	9%	6%	33%	
Exercise METS	3.6	9.5	164%	
6 Minute Walk (meters)	510.3	774.4	52%	
Waist Circumference (cm)	106.5	96	10%	Goal for men < 102 cm
Educational score	15	18	20%	20 total questions

MEDICATIONS AT DISCHARGE: Aspirin, 81 mg daily; Diovan, 160 mg daily; Plavix, 75 mg daily; Metformin, 500 mg twice daily; Avandia, 4 mg daily; Vytorin, 10/40 mg daily; Wellbutrin XL, 150 mg daily; Triamterene/HCTZ, 32.5/25 mg ½ daily

PROGRESSION TOWARD GOALS: Mr. XXXXX's goals coming into rehab were to lose 20 pounds and to run a 5k race in under 35 minutes. His weight at the beginning of rehab was 196.4 and on the last session of rehab his weight was 176. He recently competed in a race in Raleigh and finished the 3.2 miles in 31:40.

BEHAVIOR MODIFICATION: Mr. XXXXX saw great improvements in his lipids, blood glucose, exercise METS and waist measurement. He made significant lifestyle changes and seemed to do so in a way that he will be able to maintain. Throughout his participation in rehab, he appeared to handle his stress well and did not cite any anxiety or depressive symptoms.

NUTRITION COMPONENT: Mr. XXXXX attended the November classes and found he was eating more starches than needed and less vegetables than suggested. His weight loss is evidence of adopting positive eating habits.

OTHER SERVICES ATTENDED: Regular lecture attendance ☐   Stress Management series ☐   Relaxation/Meditation class ☐
Strength training ☐   Flexibility program ☐   Consistent exercise outside of cardiac rehab ☐

RECOMMENDED EXERCISE PLAN

	AEROBIC EXERCISE	STRENGTH	FLEXIBILITY
FREQUENCY	3 -4 times/week	2 – 3 times/week	After each exercise session
INTENSITY	120 – 144 bpm	Somewhat hard	Light
TYPE	Jogging; walking	Free weights	Stretches
TIME	30 – 50 minutes	20 -30 minutes	10 minutes
ENERGY EXPENDITURE	1200 calories/week		

_____
EXERCISE PHYSIOLOGIST

_____
MEDICAL DIRECTOR
If you have any concerns, please call our team at 660-6724.

Cardiac Rehab Plan
☐ Join the Fred Cobb Healing HEARTS program
☐ Join the Duke Health and Fitness Center
☒ Home exercise program
☐ Discharge to exercise facility of choice

Fig. 2. Patient example 1. The report provided to the referring physician about the course during participation in cardiac rehabilitation is shown here. Note the development of rigorous exercise habits, better nutrition, and 9 kg (20 lb) weight loss, with significant improvements in serum lipids, blood glucose control, fitness, and waist circumference. A recommended discharge treatment plan is provided.

DUKE CARDIAC REHABILITATION

PATIENT'S NAME: Ms. YYYYY
MD: YYYYY
HISTORY NUMBER: XY11111

EXIT SUMMARY

Program dates: 7-9 to 12-19-07   Number of sessions: 36

	Initial	Exit	% Change	Comments
Metabolic Syndrome	no	no		
Smoking	no	no		
Hypertension	no	no		Average of first and last 3 BP readings
systolic	96	106	-10%	
diastolic	62	68	-10%	
Hyperlipidemia	yes	yes		
Total	205	134	35%	
LDL	112	52	54%	Goal for LDL is <70mg/dL
HDL	77	73	-5%	Goal: >40mg/dL men, >50 mg/dL women
Triglycerides	79	45	43%	Goal for TG is <150 mg/dL
Diabetes	no	no		
HBA1C	5.8	n/a		
Fasting glucose	n/a	n/a		Average of first and last 3 fasting glucoses
Framingham 10 yr. CHD Risk	6%	4%	33%	
Exercise METS	4.0	5.8	45%	
6 Minute Walk (meters)	574.9	680.8	18%	
Waist Circumference (cm)	77	70.5	8%	Goal for women: <88cm
Educational score	13	17	31%	20 total questions

MEDICATIONS AT DISCHARGE: Plavix 75 mg daily, Axid 150 mg daily, Lipitor 20 mg daily, ASA 81 mg daily, Iron 325 mg daily, Vitamin C 250 mg tid, Lopressor 12.5 mg bid

PROGRESSION TOWARD GOALS: Ms. YYYYY's goals included exercising 3-5 days per week, learn meditation skills and to get to a goal weight of 130. She achieved all of her stated goals and plans on maintaining her current exercise program.

BEHAVIOR MODIFICATION: She is regularly meditating at home and is working on her primary stressor, which is her job.

NUTRITION COMPONENT: She attended the 4 hour nutrition class in December.

OTHER SERVICES ATTENDED: Regular lecture attendance ☒   Stress Management series ☐   Relaxation/Meditation class ☒
Strength training ☒   Flexibility program ☒   Consistent exercise outside of cardiac rehab ☒

RECOMMENDED EXERCISE PLAN

	AEROBIC EXERCISE	STRENGTH	FLEXIBILITY
FREQUENCY	3-5 days per week	2-3 days per week	After each exercise session
INTENSITY	TR: 96-123	1-3 sets; 10-15 reps	
TYPE	TM, EFX, biking		
TIME	30-60 minutes		
ENERGY EXPENDITURE	1000-1200 calories/week		

_____
EXERCISE PHYSIOLOGIST

_____
MEDICAL DIRECTOR
If you have any concerns, please call our team at 660-6724.

Cardiac Rehab Plan
☐ Join the Fred Cobb Healing HEARTS program
☒ Join the Duke Health and Fitness Center
☐ Home exercise program
☐ Discharge to exercise facility of choice

Fig. 3. Patient example 2. The report provided to the referring physician about the course during participation in cardiac rehabilitation is shown here. Note the improvement in serum lipids, Framingham risk factor score, exercise fitness level, 6-min walk, waist circumference, education level regarding cardiac risk, adoption of a regular exercise habit, better nutrition habits, and a plan for managing job-related stress. A recommended discharge treatment plan is provided.

14.6. PATIENT EXAMPLES

14.6.1. Patient Example 1

The patient is a 58-year-old gentleman referred to cardiac rehabilitation with a diagnosis of recurrent angina pectoris and status post-angioplasty. He has a history of coronary artery disease dating back 4 years when he presented with classical angina pectoris and underwent percutaneous coronary intervention with a stent to the right coronary artery (RCA). Now 4 years later he presented with an abnormal stress ECG and underwent coronary catheterization and stent placement for an in stent restenosis in the RCA and to a 90% new lesion in the large optional marginal 2 coronary artery. A 40% lesion in the proximal left anterior descending coronary artery was not stented. The patient carries cardiac co-morbidities and risk conditions including diabetes mellitus, dyslipidemia, hypertension, and depression. His medical regimen includes aspirin, simvastatin/ezetimibe40/10, valsartan, clopidogrel, triamterene/HCTZ, metformin, rosiglitazone, glipizide, and Wellbutrin XL.

The cardiac rehabilitation program report to his primary care doctor is presented here. One can see from the report that the patient was able to develop rigorous exercise habits, better nutrition habits, and lose 9 kg (20 lb) in the process so that he was able to participate in a 5 k race. As a consequence, there were significant improvements in serum lipids, blood glucose control, fitness, and waist circumference. A recommended discharge treatment plan is provided.

14.6.2. Patient Example 2

The patient is a 60-year-old lady referred to cardiac rehabilitation after bypass surgery for a single vessel coronary artery lesion. She had no significant past medical history before she presented to her primary doctor complaining of a history of chest discomfort and palpitations for several months that had been increasing in frequency. The chest discomfort was described as a pressure sensation without radiation, diaphoresis or shortness of breath, originally only associated with exertion but now also occurs at rest and upon awakening in the morning. Risk factor evaluation revealed a lipid panel of total cholesterol 251 mg/dL, LDL cholesterol of 154 mg/dL, triglycerides of 50 mg/dL, and HDL cholesterol of 78 mg/dL. A stress echocardiogram revealed evidence of stress-induced anteroseptal and apical wall motion abnormalities with a normal left ventricular ejection fraction. Cardiac catheterization revealed a 95% proximal left anterior descending (LAD) coronary artery lesion that was not approachable by percutaneous angioplasty and, therefore, the patient underwent single vessel coronary artery bypass grafting to the LAD. She was discharged home on aspirin, clopidogrel, metoprolol, atorvastatin, omega-3 fatty acids, and sublingual nitroglycerin as needed and referred to cardiac rehabilitation.

The patient's cardiac rehabilitation course is described in Fig. 3. She experienced improvement in serum lipids, Framingham risk factor score, exercise fitness level, 6 min walk, waist circumference, and education level regarding cardiac risk. She had also adopted a regular exercise habit, better nutrition habits, and a plan for managing job-related stress. A recommended discharge treatment plan is provided.

REFERENCES

1. Smith SC, Allen J, Blair SN, et al. AHA/ACC guidelines for secondary prevention for patients with coronary or other atherosclerotic vascular disease: 2006 update. *J Am Coll Cardiol.* 2006;47:2130–2139.
2. Balady GJ, Williams MA, Ades PA, et al. Core components of cardiac rehabilitation/secondary prevention programs: 2007 update: a scientific statement from the American Heart Association Exercise, Cardiac Rehabilitation, and Prevention Committee, the Council on Clinical Cardiology; the Councils on Cardiovascular Nursing, Epidemiology and Prevention, and Nutrition, Physical Activity, and Metabolism; and the American Association of Cardiovascular and Pulmonary Rehabilitation. *Circulation.* 2007;115:2675–2682. Epub 007 May 18.

3. King ML, Williams MA, Fletcher GF, et al. Medical director responsibilities for outpatient cardiac rehabilitation/secondary prevention programs: a scientific statement from the American Heart Association/American Association for Cardiovascular and Pulmonary Rehabilitation. *Circulation.* 2005;112:3354–3360.

4. Leon AS, Franklin BA, Costa F, et al. Cardiac rehabilitation and secondary prevention of coronary heart disease: an American Heart Association scientific statement from the Council on Clinical Cardiology (Subcommittee on Exercise, Cardiac Rehabilitation, and Prevention) and the Council on Nutrition, Physical Activity, and Metabolism (Subcommittee on Physical Activity), in collaboration with the American Association of Cardiovascular and Pulmonary Rehabilitation. Medical director responsibilities for outpatient cardiac rehabilitation/secondary prevention programs: a scientific statement from the American Heart Association/American Association for Cardiovascular and Pulmonary Rehabilitation. *Circulation.* 2005;111:369–376.

5. Thomas RJ, King M, Lui K, et al. AACVPR/ACC/AHA 2007 performance measures on cardiac rehabilitation for referral to and delivery of cardiac rehabilitation/secondary prevention services endorsed by the American College of Chest Physicians, American College of Sports Medicine, American Physical Therapy Association, Canadian Association of Cardiac Rehabilitation, European Association for Cardiovascular Prevention and Rehabilitation, Inter-American Heart Foundation, National Association of Clinical Nurse Specialists, Preventive Cardiovascular Nurses Association, and the Society of Thoracic Surgeons. *J Am Coll Cardiol.* 2007;50:1400–1433.

6. Kraus WE, Keteyian SJ. *Cardiac Rehabilitation.* Totowa, NJ: Humana Press; 2007.

7. American Asssociation of Cardiovascular and Pulmonary Rehabilitation. *Guidelines for Cardiac Rehabilitation and Secondary Prevention Programs.* 4th ed. Champaign, IL: Human Kinetics Publishers; 2004.

8. Medicare Coverage Database. Centers for Medicare and Medicaid Services. Decision memo for cardiac rehabilitation programs (CAG-00089R). Available at: www.cms.hhs.gov/mcd/viewdecisionmemo.asp?id-164 (Accessed 10/8/07).

9. AHA/ACC. ACC/AHA 2002 guideline update for exercise testing: summary article. A report of the American College of Cardiology/American Heart Association Task Force on Practice Guidelines (Committee to Update the 1997 Exercise Testing Guidelines). *Circulation.* 2002(106):1883–1892.

10. Ellestad MH, Selvester RH, Mishkin FS, James FW, Muzami K. *Exercise Electrocardiography.* 4th ed. Philadelphia, PA: F.A. Davis Company; 1996.

11. Blair SN, Kampert JB, Kohl HWI, et al. Influences of cardiorespiratory fitness and other precursors on cardiovascular disease and all-cause mortality in men and women. *JAMA.* 1996;276:205–210.

12. Blair SN, Kohl HWI, Paffenbarger RS Jr., Clark DG, Cooper KH, Gibbons LW. Physical fitness and all-cause mortality: a prospective study of healthy men and women. *JAMA.* 1989;262:2395–2401.

13. Kraus WE, Douglas PS. Where does fitness fit in? *N Engl J Med.* 2005;353:517–519.

14. Lee S, Kuk JL, Katzmarzyk PT, Blair SN, Church TS, Ross R. Cardiorespiratory fitness attenuates metabolic risk independent of abdominal subcutaneous and visceral fat in men. *Diabet Care.* 2005;28:895–901.

15. Mark DB, Hlatky MA, Harrell FE Jr., Lee KL, Califf RM, Pryor DB. Exercise treadmill score for predicting prognosis in coronary artery disease. *Ann Intern Med.* 1987;106:793–800.

16. Mark DB, Lauer MS. Exercise capacity: the prognostic variable that does not get enough respect. *Circulation.* 2003;108:1534–1535.

17. Morris CK, Myers J, Froelicher VF, Kawaguchi T, Ueshima K, Hideg A. Nomogram based on metabolic equivalents and age for assessing aerobic exercise capacity in men. *J Am Coll Cardiol.* 1993;22:175–182.

18. Mahler DA, Froelicher VF, Houston Miller N, York TD. *ACSM Guidelines for Exercise Testing and Prescription.* 7th ed. Baltimore, MD: William & Wilkins; 2006.

19. McNeer JF, Margolis JR, Lee KL, et al. The role of the exercise test in the evaluation of patients for ischemic heart disease. *Circulation.* 1978;57:64–70.

20. Abraham RD, Freedman SB, Dunn RF, et al. Prediction of multivessel coronary artery disease and prognosis early after acute myocardial infarction by exercise electrocardiography and thallium-201 myocardial perfusion scanning. *Am J Cardiol.* 1986;58:423–427.

21. Prochaska J, DiClemente C. Stages and processes of self-change for smoking: toward an integrative model of change. *J Consult Clin Psycho.* 1983;51:390–395.

III PERIPHERAL FORMS OF VENOUS AND ARTERIAL DISEASE

15 Carotid Artery Disease

Andreas Kastrup

Contents

Key Words: Angioplasty; Atherosclerosis; Endarterectomy; Transient ischemic attack; Stroke.

KEY POINTS

- In patients with carotid artery stenosis, risk factors such as hypertension, diabetes mellitus, hyperlipedemia, and smoking should be evaluated and treated aggressively.
- The use of prophylactic aspirin is recommended in all patients with carotid artery stenosis.
- Patients with an asymptomatic carotid stenosis should be educated about possible symptoms of transient ischemic attacks and should immediately contact a physician in case a transient ischemic attack occurs.
- In patients with an asymptomatic carotid stenosis, prophylactic carotid endarterectomy (CEA) can be recommended only in highly selected patients with high-grade stenosis performed by surgeons with established perioperative morbidity and mortality rates of <3%. With regard to carotid angioplasty and stenting (CAS), there is currently insufficient data to properly guide treatment decisions. If considered, CAS should be performed only by operators with established perioperative morbidity and mortality rates of <3%.
- Carotid endarterectomy should be considered in patients with recent TIA or ischemic stroke within the last 6 months and ipsilateral severe (>70%) carotid artery stenosis. In patients with recent symptomatic moderate (50–69%) carotid stenosis, CEA should be considered in men, in patients older than 74 years of age, and in patients with hemispheric symptoms rather than transient monocular blindness. CEA should be performed only by surgeons with established perioperative morbidity and mortality rates of <6%.

From: *Contemporary Cardiology: Comprehensive Cardiovascular Medicine in the Primary Care Setting*
Edited by: Peter P. Toth, Christopher P. Cannon, DOI 10.1007/978-1-60327-963-5_15
© Springer Science+Business Media, LLC 2010

- In patients with a recently symptomatic carotid artery stenosis, surgery should ideally be performed within 2 weeks.
- Carotid angioplasty and stenting may be considered in symptomatic patients with severe (>70%) carotid artery stenosis, in whom the stenosis is difficult to access surgically, in whom medical conditions are present that greatly increase the risk for surgery, or in patiencats with restenosis after CEA or radiation-induced stenosis. CAS should be performed only by operators with established perioperative morbidity and mortality rates of <6%.

15.1. INTRODUCTION

Stroke is one of the leading causes of morbidity and mortality in North America, affecting over half a million patients at a cost of over $30 billion a year. Depending on the population studied, extracranial internal carotid artery stenosis accounts for approximately 10–15% of ischemic strokes. Aside from these symptomatic cases, large population-based studies indicate that the prevalence of asymptomatic carotid artery stenosis is approximately 0.5% in the sixth decade and increases up to 10% in persons over 80 years of age *(1)*.

Carotid stenoses may result in brain ischemia either through direct hemodynamic impairment of the cerebral blood circulation or, more commonly, as a source of thromboembolic material arising from symptomatic carotid plaques. These mainly develop in regions of low vessel-wall shear stress such as the carotid bulb and are characterized by increased cellular proliferation, lipid accumulation, calcification, ulceration, hemorrhage, and thrombosis. Symptomatic carotid artery disease is commonly manifested by transient contralateral symptoms or ipsilateral monocular blindness and then detected during further diagnostic work-up, whereas patients with an asymptomatic carotid stenosis are most commonly found by physical examination of a carotid bruit.

The main approaches for treating patients with carotid artery disease include the stabilization of the carotid plaque through risk factor modification and medication as well as the removal of the stenosis through carotid endarterectomy (CEA) or carotid angioplasty and stenting (CAS).

15.2. DIAGNOSTIC TESTING

Obtaining a history and performing general medical (including auscultation of the neck for carotid bruits and transmitted murmurs) and neurological (to correlate neurological symptoms with an ischemic territory) examinations are crucial steps in selecting proper treatment for patients with carotid artery disease. The approach of any patient with carotid artery disease should also involve recognition of this disease as a specific manifestation of a generalized arteriopathy. Therefore, a thorough search should be made for other evidence of atherosclerosis, including cardiac and peripheral vascular disease. A clear separation between symptomatic and asymptomatic carotid artery stenosis is critical. Symptoms of a carotid artery stenosis typically include contralateral weakness or numbness, dysphasia, ipsilateral monocular blindness (amaurosis fugax), and, in rare instances, syncope, confusion, or seizures. Specific signs of left hemisphere ischemia include aphasia, while right hemisphere ischemia may be manifest by apraxia or visuospatial neglect. All of these symptoms may be transient, representing TIAs, or permanent, resulting in cerebral infarction. Non-specific symptoms such as a blurred vision or a subjective generalized weakness should not be considered as a symptomatic event. Laboratory testing should be performed to determine the presence of cardiovascular risk factors (e.g., unknown diabetes mellitus and hyperlipidemia). It is also useful in ruling out metabolic and hematologic causes of neurological symptoms such as hypoglycemia, hyponatremia, and thrombocytosis.

Patients with an asymptomatic carotid stenosis are most commonly found by physical examination of a carotid bruit. Although carotid bruits only have a limited value for the diagnosis of carotid artery disease, carotid auscultation should be part of the routine physical examination of patients with cardiovascular risk factors. While carotid auscultation is a sufficient screening test for asymptomatic patients, all patients with a TIA or stroke must be evaluated with duplex ultrasonography either alone or supplemented with digital subtraction angiography (DSA), computed tomographic angiography (CTA), magnetic resonance angiography (MRA), or contrast-enhanced MRA. *Duplex ultrasonography is the imaging tool of choice to screen for carotid artery stenosis.*

To date, conventional or digital subtraction cerebral angiography is still considered to be the gold standard for imaging the carotid arteries. In the large clinical trials, cerebral angiography was used to evaluate the entire carotid system, including the intracranial collateral circulation, and served as standard for defining the degree of carotid stenosis and for defining morphological features of the offending plaque. However, this technique is invasive, expensive, and is associated with a risk of serious neurological complications or death of approximately 0.5–1%. Therefore, it has largely been replaced by CTA or MRA. Nowadays, the latter techniques are mainly used as confirmatory tests after results of an ultrasound examination are suggestive of the presence of a carotid stenosis in most centers. Carotid duplex ultrasound is a non-invasive, safe, and inexpensive technique that has a high sensitivity and specificity in detecting a significant stenosis of the ICA. On the other hand, the accuracy of carotid ultrasound relies heavily upon the experience and expertise of the examiner and may be limited by features such as calcified, tortuous arteries, or far distal stenoses. In these cases, CTA may be particularly useful. With this technique, three-dimensional reconstruction allows relatively accurate measurements of the residual lumen diameter. MRA images are either based on two- or three-dimensional time-of-flight (TOF) or gadolinium-enhanced sequences. The contrast-enhanced techniques produce higher quality images that are less prone to artifacts. While MRA is less operator dependent than ultrasound, it is more expensive and time consuming and may not be performed if the patient has claustrophobia, a pacemaker, or ferromagnetic implants.

15.3. MEDICAL TREATMENT

The estimated annual risk of stroke in patients with an asymptomatic stenosis is approximately 1–2% *(2)* and 4–6% in patients with a symptomatic carotid stenosis *(3)*, respectively. Aside from considering a surgical removal or an interventional therapy for a carotid stenosis, primary and secondary medical therapies are clearly indicated, all the more considering that 20% of patients undergoing CEA for symptomatic carotid artery stenosis and 45% of patients undergoing CEA for asymptomatic carotid artery stenosis subsequently have strokes related to other etiologies *(4)*. While the concept of "best medical therapy" for patients with asymptomatic or symptomatic carotid artery disease mainly consisted of "stop smoking" and "take aspirin" in the large trials comparing CEA with medical therapy, major advances have been made in the past two decades regarding statin, antiplatelet, and antihypertensive therapies. Although several cardiovascular risk factor modifications and medical therapies have not been specifically evaluated in patients with severe carotid artery stenosis, they are generally recommended to limit progression of atherosclerosis and decrease clinical events, irrespective of carotid revascularization.

In patients with an asymptomatic carotid stenosis, antiplatelet therapy with aspirin is indicated for primary prevention mainly of cardiovascular events *(5)*. In patients with symptomatic carotid stenosis current recommendations are based on the results of large stroke prevention studies with mixed patient populations and include the use of aspirin, clopidogrel, or a fixed combination of aspirin with extended-release dipyridamole *(6, 7)*. There is no data to support the use of aspirin in doses grater than 325 mg day. Clopidogrel might be a more potent antiplatelet agent than aspirin, but due consideration must also be given to the risk of excess bleeding should the patient require surgery.

Although not specifically tested for in patients with carotid artery disease, there is a general consensus that a stringent control of blood pressure is the cornerstone of therapy to modify atherogenic risk factors, and the benefits of antihypertensive therapy extend to all patient subgroups, especially diabetic patients. For primary stroke prevention, a large meta-analysis found that regardless of the agent used, a 10 mmHg reduction in systolic blood pressure produced a 31% relative risk reduction for stroke *(8)*. For secondary stroke prevention, proven agents include angiotensin-converting enzyme inhibitors, angiotensin receptor blockers, and the combination of a thiazide diuretic with an angiotensin-converting enzyme inhibitor *(6, 7)*. Although there is emerging evidence that some antihypertensive medications may exert their beneficial effect in ways other than by reducing blood pressure, the primary goal of blood pressure therapy should be to achieve values of <140/90 mmHg for nondiabetic patients and <130/80 mmHg for patients with diabetes. The selection of drugs should therefore primarily be influenced by the presence of comorbid conditions such as diabetes mellitus, renal failure, or left ventricular dysfunction. Many patients will require multiple medications to achieve optimal blood pressure values.

Statins have assumed a prominent role in cerebrovascular and cardiovascular risk modification *(9, 10)*. The SPARCL Trial, which randomized 4,732 patients with recent stroke or TIA to atorvastatin 80 mg/day or placebo, reported a 16% relative risk reduction (RRR) in future stroke *(10)*. In a subgroup analysis of 1,007 patients with documented carotid stenosis patients taking atorvastatin 80 mg daily, the RRR for future stroke was 33%, 42% for major coronary events, and 56% for the need of carotid revascularization *(11)*. In a review of 180 patients undergoing CAS, a significantly higher 30-day rate of stroke, MI, or death was identified among patients who were not taking preprocedural statin therapy *(12)*. A similar result was obtained for symptomatic patients undergoing CEA *(13)*. In a further study of patients receiving medical treatment for severe carotid artery disease, statin use was associated with significantly lower rates of stroke, MI, or death *(14)*.

Smoking, physical inactivity, and eating habits are also important modifiable risk factors for the development and progression of carotid artery disease. While preventive medications are easy to prescribe, lifestyle modification should be considered as equally important. A combination of nicotine replacement therapy, social support, and skills training, for instance, has been shown to be effective in treating tobacco dependence.

In patients with carotid artery stenosis risk factors such as hypertension, diabetes mellitus, hyperlipedemia, and smoking should be evaluated and treated aggressively.

15.4. CAROTID ENDARTERECTOMY IN PATIENTS WITH SYMPTOMATIC CAROTID STENOSIS

The superiority of CEA over medical treatment in the management of symptomatic high-grade carotid artery stenosis has been established in two, large randomized trials: the North American Symptomatic Carotid Endarterectomy Trial (NASCET) *(3)* and the European Carotid Surgery Trial (ECST) *(15)*. A third trial was stopped prematurely when the results of NASCET were announced *(16)*.

In NASCET and ECST, all surgeons were screened for an acceptable operative record. Entry criteria for these trials included carotid artery stenosis (>30% reduction in the luminal diameter on conventional angiogram) and ipsilateral TIA, non-disabling stroke, or retinal infarction within 4–6 months. The main exclusion criteria included a probable cardiac source of embolism, serious disease likely to cause death within 5 years, or intracranial disease that was more significant than the carotid lesion. Both trials used different methods to measure carotid stenosis. While NASCET used the residual lumen diameter at the most stenotic portion of the vessel and compared this to the lumen diameter in a normal portion of the internal carotid artery distal to the stenosis to determine the degree of stenosis, ECST used the lumen diameter at the most stenotic portion of the vessel and compared this to the estimated probable original diameter at the most stenotic portion of the vessel. In the meantime, equivalent measurements for the two methods have been determined: a 50% stenosis with the NASCET method is equivalent to a 75% for ECST and a 70% stenosis with the NASCET method is equivalent to an 85% stenosis for ECST.

In NASCET and for patients with symptomatic carotid stenosis of 70–99% (measured by the NASCET method), CEA reduced the 2-year risk of ipsilateral stroke from 26% in the medical group ($n = 331$) to 9% in the surgical group ($n = 328$), yielding an absolute risk reduction of 17% ($p < 0.001$). The number needed to treat (NNT) to prevent one stroke was 6 (NNT $= 12$ at 1 year). A 5.8% incidence of perioperative stroke or death was reported for patients in the surgical arm. In patients with moderate degrees of stenosis (50–69%), the 5-year ipsilateral stroke risk was 22.2% in the medical arm and 15.7% in the surgical arm ($p < 0.045$). The NNT to prevent one stroke was 15 (NNT $= 77$ at 1 year). Benefit in the 50–60% stenosis group was best achieved in patients presenting with hemispheric, not retinal symptoms, with stroke rather than TIA, male sex, and intracranial carotid artery stenosis. In this group of patients, subgroup analysis did not demonstrate a benefit of CEA in women (NNT $= 125$ to prevent one major ipsilateral stroke in 5 years). Patients with <50% stenosis did not benefit from surgery.

The ECST reported a similar efficacy of CEA in the secondary prevention of stroke for patients with a high-grade carotid stenosis. In this trial, the frequency of a major stroke or death at 3 years was 26.5% in the control group ($n = 220$) versus 14.9% in the surgical group ($n = 356$), so that surgery was associated with an absolute benefit of 11.6% ($p < 0.001$). The NNT to prevent one stroke annually was 21. A 7.4% incidence of perioperative stroke or death was reported for patients in the surgical arm. The risk of these complications was not related to the severity of the stenosis.

Although NASCET and ECST have clearly demonstrated the superiority of CEA combined with medical therapy over medical management alone for symptomatic patients with carotid artery stenosis of >70% (NASCET) *(3)* or >80% (ECST) *(15)*, several post hoc analyses have been performed to identify subsets of patients who are most likely to benefit from surgery. In fact, the decision to treat individual patients with carotid artery disease surgically should not be exclusively based on the stenosis severity, but should also take into account age, gender, neurological symptoms, and other determining factors for subsequent stroke or surgical risk. In addition, patients who have severe comorbidities, patients with persistent disabling neurological deficits, and those with a total occlusion of the carotid artery are unlikely to benefit from CEA and should thus be treated with medical therapy.

The benefit of CEA increases steadily from 50 to 99% (NASCET method) as a consequence of an enhanced risk of ipsilateral stroke, proportional to the severity of the stenosis, while surgery-related morbidity does not vary substantially with the degree of stenosis *(17)*. A patient with a 90–99% symptomatic stenosis derives twice the benefit from CEA than one with a 70–79% stenosis.

Other factors that can be used to estimate the absolute risk of ipsilateral stroke for individual patients with symptomatic carotid stenosis who are candidates for CEA include patient age, gender, type of presenting event, plaque morphology, and time since last event *(18)*.

In a subgroup analysis of NASCET, the benefit of CEA for patients with a symptomatic carotid stenosis aged 75 years or older was compared with that for those aged 65–74 years and less than 65 years *(19)*. Among medically treated patients with 70–99% carotid stenosis the risk of ipsilateral ischemic stroke at 2 years was highest (36.5%) in patients aged 75 years or older. The rates of perioperative stroke and death were 7.9, 5.5, and 5.2% in patients younger than 65 years, 65–74 years, and >75 years, respectively. Because patients aged 75 years or older had the highest risk with medical treatment, the absolute risk reduction by CEA was greatest in this subgroup (28.9%). Only three patients had to undergo surgery to prevent one ipsilateral ischemic stroke at 2 years. Thus, elderly patients profited more from CEA than younger patients in this trial. Likewise, the ECST data has indicated that increasing age is associated with a greater benefit from CEA for symptomatic carotid stenosis *(20)*.

Men gain more benefit from CEA than women. The stroke risk reduction with CEA is highest in patients presenting with hemispherical TIAs or minor strokes compared to retinal symptoms. Plaque ulceration also confers an increased stroke risk on medically treated patients. Patients with recently symptomatic stenoses are at the highest risk of subsequent stroke and thus derive a substantial benefit from surgery. *Patients with a recently symptomatic carotid artery stenosis have a high early risk for subsequent stroke, so that expedited evaluation and surgery are of utmost importance to maximize benefit of treatment.*

In a combined 5-year analysis of the NASCET and ECST patients with a symptomatic carotid stenosis ($\geq$50%, NASCET method), the NNT to prevent one stroke was 9 for men and 36 for women, 5 for age $\geq$75 years and 18 for < 65 years, and 5 if randomized within 2 weeks of the last TIA and 125 if randomized > 12 weeks after the last TIA *(21)*.

According to current guidelines, CEA should be considered in patients with recent TIA or ischemic stroke within the last 6 months and ipsilateral severe (>70%, NASCET method) carotid artery stenosis *(6, 7)*. In patients with recent symptomatic moderate (50–69%, NASCET) carotid stenosis, CEA should be considered in men, in patients older than 74 years of age, and in patients with hemispheric symptoms rather than transient monocular blindness (Fig. 1).

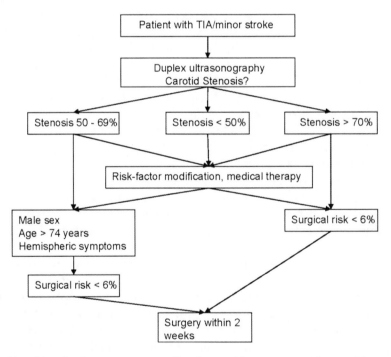

Fig. 1. Algorithm for the management of patients with a symptomatic carotid stenosis.

15.5. CAROTID ENDARTERECTOMY IN PATIENTS WITH ASYMPTOMATIC CAROTID STENOSIS

Altogether, there have been five randomized trials of endarterectomy for patients with asymptomatic extracranial carotid artery stenosis.

The Carotid Artery Surgery Asymptomatic Narrowing Operation Versus Aspirin (CASANOVA) Trial included 410 patients with an asymptomatic internal carotid artery stenosis of 50–90%, based on cerebral angiography *(22)*. Patients with more than 90% stenosis were excluded from this trial. All patients were treated with 330 mg aspirin daily and 75 mg dipyridamole three times daily. After a minimum of 3 years of follow-up for each patient, statistical analysis found no significant difference in the number of neurological deficits and deaths between both groups.

The Veterans Affairs Asymptomatic Carotid Endarterectomy Trial compared the outcomes of 211 surgically versus 233 medically treated patients with an asymptomatic angiographically proven carotid stenosis of 50–99% *(23)*. While the combined outcome of stroke and death was not significantly different between both treatment groups, the study showed a reduction in the relative risk of ipsilateral neurological events with surgery when TIA and stroke were included as composite endpoints.

The Mayo Asymptomatic Carotid Endarterectomy (MACE) Trial was terminated early due to a significantly higher number of TIAs and myocardial infarctions in the surgical group compared with the medical group, likely reflecting the avoidance of aspirin in the surgical group *(24)*.

The Asymptomatic Carotid Atherosclerosis Study (ACAS) evaluated the efficacy of endarterectomy in patients with a >60% diameter reduction (determined either by angiography or by Doppler ultrasound scanning) in asymptomatic carotid stenosis *(25)*. Patients were aged 40–79 years and had a life expectancy of at least 5 years. Approximately 30% of patients had other cerebrovascular symptoms. The event rate in surgically treated patients for the primary endpoint (ipsilateral stroke, perioperative stroke, or death) was 5.1% over 5 years. This included a 1.2% risk of angiography-related complications among the 424 patients undergoing postrandomization angiograms and an exceedingly low 1.1% surgical risk (2.3% aggregate perioperative stroke risk). The corresponding rate in medically treated patients was 11% (5.9% absolute risk reduction; NNT = 17; $p = 0.004$). The NNT to prevent one event was 83 at 1 year. The risk of major ipsilateral stroke or any perioperative stroke or death was not significantly different between both treatment groups (6.5% in the medical group versus 3.4% in the surgical group, $p = 0.12$). The benefits of CEA were greater for men than women (relative risk reduction in men 66% versus 17% in women, respectively), and perioperative complications were higher among women than men (3.6% versus 1.7%).

The recently published ACST confirmed the marginal benefit of CEA in patients with asymptomatic severe stenoses *(26)*. In this study, 3,120 asymptomatic patients with >60% carotid stenosis identified during ultrasonography were assigned to immediate CEA or deferral of surgery and were followed for a mean period of 3.4 years. The risk of stroke or death within 30 days of CEA was 3.1% in the CEA group and 0.8% in the deferral group, whereas 5-year risks of non-preoperative stroke were 3.1 and 11% ($p < 0.0001$). When the preoperative and non-perioperative stroke risk was combined, a significant 5.4% absolute risk reduction occurred, very similar to the ACAS results. The benefits were similar in males and females and were not substantially different with varying degrees of carotid stenosis. However, patients 75 years of age and older did not benefit. Despite the relatively low perioperative complication rate in ACST, the net benefit of CEA was delayed for about 2 years after surgery, so that CEA in asymptomatic patients should be considered a long-term investment.

In both the ACAS and the ACST, an extremely low perioperative stroke rate was achieved, without which there would be no benefit from surgical management of asymptomatic carotid artery stenoses. A combined analysis of ACAS and ACST suggests that CEA in asymptomatic patients with >60% carotid stenosis leads to a small but significant overall benefit if the surgery can be performed with low preoperative morbidity and mortality rates *(26)*. Especially in patients with an asymptomatic carotid stenosis the benefit of CEA is highly dependent on a low risk of procedural neurological complications and is eliminated when the combined 30-day stroke and death rates exceed approximately 3% *(27, 28)*. It should also be considered that the benefits of CEA in asymptomatic patients may generally be overestimated. In a subgroup analysis of NASCET the causes of stroke on the asymptomatic side of 1,800 patients was determined during follow-up. Nearly 50% of the strokes were lacunar or cardioembolic in origin and were thus not preventable by CEA *(2)*.

According to current guidelines, all patients having CEA for asymptomatic carotid stenosis should receive low-dose aspirin prior to surgery and for at least 3 months after surgery *(5)*. Prophylactic

CEA can be recommended in highly selected patients with high-grade asymptomatic carotid stenosis performed by surgeons with <3% morbidity and mortality rates. Patient selection should be guided by an assessment of comorbid conditions and especially life expectancy and should include a thorough discussion of the risks and benefits of the procedure with an understanding of patient preferences (Fig. 2).

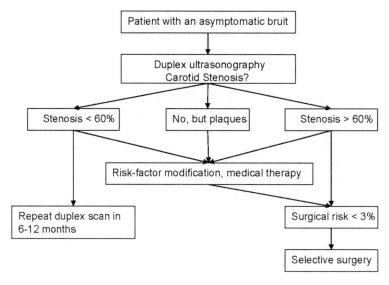

Fig. 2. Algorithm for the management of patients with an asymptomatic carotid stenosis.

15.6. CAROTID ANGIOPLASTY AND STENTING

While CEA is currently the accepted standard for the treatment of patients with high-grade symptomatic and for the treatment of selected patients with an asymptomatic internal carotid artery stenosis, carotid angioplasty and stenting (CAS) have increasingly been used as an alternative to CEA for the primary and secondary prevention of stroke related to carotid stenosis. Potential advantages over surgery include avoiding a surgical incision and its complications, including cranial nerve palsies and wound hematoma. Unlike CEA, which is limited to the cervical carotid artery, CAS can be performed in patients with distal or even intracranial lesions. It has also been argued that CAS does not require general anesthesia and may be associated with shorter hospitalization and thus lower costs. On the other hand, CAS has the major disadvantage of producing more emboli to the brain than CEA *(29)*.

To date, several large randomized single or multicenter trials comparing CAS with CEA and large stent registries have been published. In the large stent registries encompassing many thousands of patients the 30-day stroke, myocardial infarction, and death rates have varied from approximately 2–8% in mixed populations of asymptomatic and symptomatic patients *(30, 31)*. While these results clearly indicate that CAS can be performed with acceptable complication rates, randomized trials directly comparing CAS with CEA have produced conflicting results.

The very first, prospective, randomized trial comparing CAS with CEA was performed at a single university teaching hospital in Leicester and was stopped early by the Steering Committee after inclusion of only 17 patients with a symptomatic carotid stenosis (≥70%) due to an excessive complication rate in the CAS arm the trial (5 out of 7 CAS patients developed a stroke) *(32)*.

The Carotid and Vertebral Artery Transluminal Angioplasty Study (CAVATAS) was the first completed, prospective multicenter trial comparing endovascular (*n* = 251, mainly angioplasty alone) versus surgical treatment ($n = 253$) of patients with symptomatic (96.4%) and asymptomatic carotid stenosis *(33)*. Periprocedural stroke (symptoms > 7 days) and death rates were similar for endovascular treatment and surgery (10.0% versus 9.9%). After 3 years the rate of any stroke or death after 3 years was 14.3 in the endovascular group versus 14.2% in the surgical group indicating that the long-term results are also comparable between both procedures *(33)*.

The Wallstent study was a multicenter randomized trial comparing CAS ($n = 107$) with CEA ($n = 112$) in patients with a symptomatic carotid stenosis of at least 60% *(34)*. The cumulative incidence of ipsilateral stroke and procedure related or vascular death within 1 year was 12.1% for the stent group versus 3.6% for the endarterectomy group ($p < 0.05$). The incidence of any stroke or death within 30 days was significantly higher after CAS than CEA (12.2% versus 4.5%, $p < 0.05$).

Two prospective, single-center, randomized trials performed in a community hospital with either patients with a symptomatic carotid stenosis (CEA $n = 51$ versus CAS $n = 53$) or with an asymptomatic carotid stenosis (85 patients randomly assigned to CAS or CEA) have been published *(35, 36)*. In the trial dealing with symptomatic patients the composite outcome of any stroke or death within 30 days was 2% in patients treated with CEA and 0% in those treated with CAS, whereas no strokes or deaths occurred in both treatment arms of the asymptomatic trial.

The multicenter Stenting and Angioplasty with Protection in Patients at High Risk for Endartectomy (SAPPHIRE) study compared CEA with protected CAS in patients with a moderate to severe carotid stenosis (exceeding 80% in asymptomatic patients or 50% in symptomatic patients who also had comorbid conditions that might increase the risk of surgery (e.g., recent myocardial infarction, congestive heart failure, sever pulmonary disease, advanced age, and contralateral carotid occlusion) *(37)*. Excluded patients ($n = 404$) were entered into a registry and not randomized. The trial was terminated early after randomization of 334 patients because of an abrupt slowing in the pace of patient enrollment. The primary endpoint (composite of stroke, myocardial infarction, or death within 30 days or ipsilateral stroke between 31 days and 1 year) occurred in 20 CAS patients versus 32 CEA patients (12.2% versus 20.1%, $p = 0.004$ for non-inferiority and $p = 0.053$ for superiority). With respect to the subgroup of symptomatic patients the primary endpoint was similar between CAS and CEA (16.8% versus 16.5%).

The Endarterectomy Versus Stenting in Patients with Symptomatic Severe Carotid Stenosis Study (EVA-3S) compared CAS ($n = 261$) with CEA ($n = 259$) in patients with a symptomatic (amaurosis fugax, hemispherical transient ischemic attack, or minor stroke in the previous 120 days) carotid stenosis of 60–99% according to NASCET criteria *(38)*. The trial was stopped prematurely after the inclusion of 527 patients due to increased complication rates in the CAS group. The 30-day incidence of any stroke or death was 3.9% in surgical patients versus 9.6% in patients treated with CAS ($p < 0.05$). Thirty-day mortality was similar in both groups. The 30-day incidence of disabling stroke or death was 1.5% after CEA compared with 3.4% after CAS. The main prespecified secondary outcome (any periprocedural stroke or death and any ipsilateral stroke occurring in up to 4 years of follow-up) was also significantly higher with CAS than with CEA (11.1% versus 6.2%, $p < 0.05$). This difference was largely driven by the higher periprocedural complications rates associated with CAS, demonstrating a low risk of ipsilateral stroke after the periprocedural period, which was similar in both treatment groups.

The Stent-Protected Angioplasty versus Carotid Endarterectomy in Symptomatic Patients (SPACE) study compared CAS ($n = 605$) with CEA ($n = 595$) in symptomatic patients with a carotid stenosis of at least 70% (according to ECST criteria, corresponding to a stenosis of $\geq 50\%$ according to NASCET) *(39)*. High-risk patients with uncontrolled hypertension or severe concomitant disease and a poor prognosis were excluded from this trial. The use of embolic protection devices was optional (eventually 26.6% of the patients were treated with embolic protection devices during CAS). The primary endpoint was ipsilateral stroke (ischemic stroke or intracerebral hemorrhage or both, with symptoms lasting longer than 24 h) or death of any cause between randomization and 30 days after treatment. Using a predefined non-inferiority margin of 2.5% or more, this trial aimed to show that CAS is not worse than CEA. The primary endpoint occurred in 41 CAS patients versus 37 CEA patients (6.84% versus 6.34%, $p = 0.09$ for non-inferiority). Therefore, SPACE failed to prove the non-inferiority of CAS compared with CEA, expressed as the rate of ipsilateral stroke or death within 30 days. The rate of any stroke or death within 30 days was 7.68% in CAS patients compared to 6.51% in CEA patients. In a subgroup analysis, older age in the CAS group was significantly associated with an increased risk for ipsilateral stroke *(40)*. At 2 years follow-up, there was no statistically significant difference between CAS and CEA with respect to the composite endpoint of any periprocedural stroke or death and ipsilateral ischemic stroke (9.4% versus 7.8% using a per protocol analysis). However, recurrent carotid stenoses were significantly more frequent in the CAS group.

Taken together, the data of the randomized trials comparing CEA with CAS published to date demonstrate that CAS is associated with an increased risk of peri-interventional stroke or death. Therefore, CEA remains the treatment of choice for suitable carotid stenosis. On the other hand, CAS may be an acceptable option in selected patients considered to be high risk for CEA. Although much remains to be done to identify the factors related to patient characteristics, arterial anatomy, operator experience, and the procedure itself that are associated with an increased risk for stroke after CAS, certain subgroups of patients characterized by an increased surgical versus a low interventional risk have already been identified.

While patients with a symptomatic carotid stenosis in the presence of an occluded contralateral carotid artery have a risk of ipsilateral ischemic stroke (69% at 2 years) justifying aggressive treatment, CEA in this subgroup is associated with high 30-day stroke and death rates (14.3% in NASCET and 12.5% in ECST). In contrast to the surgical data, patients with and without contralateral carotid occlusion had comparable complication rates after CAS in several large case series or registries *(41–43)* and EVA-3S *(38)*. In addition to patients with a symptomatic carotid stenosis in the presence of an occluded contralateral carotid artery, those who develop early restenosis after CEA due to intimal hyperplasia, as well as those patients with prior neck irradiation, appear to be good candidates for CAS *(37)*.

15.7. SUMMARY

The approach to any patient with carotid artery disease should always involve recognition of this disease as a specific manifestation of a generalized arteriopathy.

In patients with a carotid artery disease, best medical management should be given scrupulous attention including control of blood pressure, reduction of atherogenic lipoproteins, glycemic control, smoking cessation, and control of heart disease if it develops. All patients should receive antithrombotic medication in the form of aspirin.

From an evidence-based point of view, CEA currently remains the treatment of choice for patients with a symptomatic carotid stenosis and selected patients with an asymptomatic carotid stenosis. However, the overall benefit of CEA strongly depends on the surgical risk. Therefore, appropriate patient selection remains a key issue for any physician to consider. Acceptable guidelines for operative risk are 3% for asymptomatic patients and 6% for those patients with a TIA or stroke due to a carotid stenosis. Current guideline recommendations and the positive data of the large surgical trials, should not be used to justify performing CEA without a clear medical indication or in centers with little experience and poor outcome data. It is becoming evident that CEA and CAS might have a complementary role, so that future treatment decisions will have to focus on the individual patient rather than being based on the belief that "one procedure fits all."

15.8. CASE STUDY

A 54-year-old man presented with two transient episodes of right-sided hemiparesis mainly involving the upper extremity combined with some slurring of his speech as well as difficulty finding appropriate words. Both episodes had occurred in the last 2 days and had lasted less than 10 min each. There were no further episodes of transient or permanent focal neurological deficits. The patient was taking no medications. He had a history of smoking (45 pack years). Except for a bruit in the left side of the neck, the neurological examination was normal on admission.

A computed tomography scan showed no signs of ischemia, whereas a diffusion-weighted MRI scan revealed multiple cortical signal abnormalities throughout the left hemisphere, as well as internal border zone regions consistent with multiple ischemic lesions of embolic and possibly also hemodynamic origin (Fig. 3). An extracranial Doppler and duplex sonography showed a severely ulcerated high-grade stenosis at the origin of the left internal carotid artery (ICA) (approximately 90%), which was confirmed by a contrast-enhanced magnetic resonance angiography. A post-stenotic flow pattern was seen in the left main segment of the middle cerebral artery with transcranial duplex sonography, all other detectable intracranial vessels revealed normal and symmetric flow signals. A cardiac source of embolism was ruled out by performing a 24-h electrocardiogram and transthoracic echocardiography. Diabetes mellitus and hyperlipidemia were ruled out.

Based on the clinical presentation and the results of the work-up, the diagnosis of a symptomatic high-grade stenosis of the left ICA with a lumen reduction of about 80–90% was made. The current

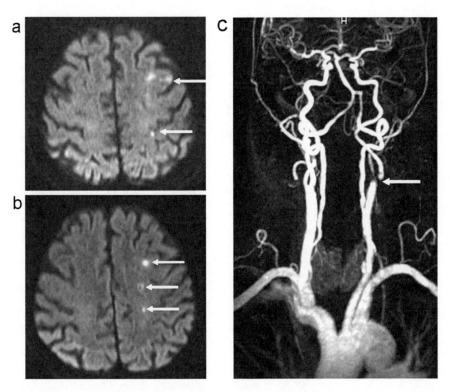

Fig. 3. Diffusion-weighted MR images (**a, b**) showing multiple embolic lesions throughout the left hemisphere (*arrows*), partially involving hemodynamic border zones. Contrast-enhanced magnetic resonance angiography revealing a high-grade stenosis at the origin of the left internal carotid artery.

American Heart Association guidelines for the care of patients with a TIA or minor stroke due to a high-grade carotid stenosis recommend risk factor modification, the use of antithrombotic medications, and endarterectomy. The risks and potential benefits of surgical removal of the ICA stenosis were discussed extensively with the patient and his family. Three days after admission the patient underwent uneventful carotid endarterectomy and was given aspirin indefinitely. In addition, he was encouraged to change his lifestyle (smoking cessation, regular exercise, and avoidance of excessive alcohol consumption).

REFERENCES

1. Prati P, Vanuzzo D, Casaroli M, et al. Prevalence and determinants of carotid atherosclerosis in a general population. *Stroke*. 1992;23(12):1705–1711.
2. Inzitari D, Eliasziw M, Gates P, et al. The causes and risk of stroke in patients with asymptomatic internal-carotid-artery stenosis. North American Symptomatic Carotid Endarterectomy Trial Collaborators. *N Engl J Med*. 2000;342(23):1693–1700.
3. North American Symptomatic Carotid Endarterectomy Trial Collaborators. Beneficial effect of carotid endarterectomy in symptomatic patients with high-grade carotid stenosis. *N Engl J Med*. 1991;325(7):445–453.
4. Barnett HJ, Gunton RW, Eliasziw M, et al. Causes and severity of ischemic stroke in patients with internal carotid artery stenosis. *JAMA*. 2000;283(11):1429–1436.
5. Goldstein LB, Adams R, Alberts MJ, et al. Primary prevention of ischemic stroke: a guideline from the American Heart Association/American Stroke Association Stroke Council: cosponsored by the Atherosclerotic Peripheral Vascular Disease Interdisciplinary Working Group; Cardiovascular Nursing Council; Clinical Cardiology Council; Nutrition, Physical Activity, and Metabolism Council; and the Quality of Care and Outcomes Research Interdisciplinary Working Group. *Circulation*. 2006;113(24):e873–e923.
6. Adams RJ, Albers G, Alberts MJ, et al. Update to the AHA/ASA recommendations for the prevention of stroke in patients with stroke and transient ischemic attack. *Stroke*. 2008;39(5):1647–1652.
7. Sacco RL, Adams R, Albers G, et al. Guidelines for prevention of stroke in patients with ischemic stroke or transient ischemic attack: a statement for healthcare professionals from the American Heart Association/American Stroke Association Council on Stroke: co-sponsored by the Council on Cardiovascular Radiology and Intervention: the American Academy of Neurology affirms the value of this guideline. *Stroke*. 2006;37(2):577–617.
8. Lawes CM, Bennett DA, Feigin VL, Rodgers A. Blood pressure and stroke: an overview of published reviews. *Stroke*. 2004;35(4):1024.
9. Amarenco P, Labreuche J, Lavallee P, Touboul PJ. Statins in stroke prevention and carotid atherosclerosis: systematic review and up-to-date meta-analysis. *Stroke*. 2004;35(12):2902–2909.
10. Amarenco P, Bogousslavsky J, Callahan AIII, et al. High-dose atorvastatin after stroke or transient ischemic attack. *N Engl J Med*. 2006;355(6):549–559.
11. Sillesen H, Amarenco P, Hennerici MG, et al. Atorvastatin reduces the risk of cardiovascular events in patients with carotid atherosclerosis: a secondary analysis of the Stroke Prevention by Aggressive Reduction in Cholesterol Levels (SPARCL) trial. *Stroke*. 2008;39(12):3297–3302.
12. Groschel K, Ernemann U, Schulz JB, Nagele T, Terborg C, Kastrup A. Statin therapy at carotid angioplasty and stent placement: effect on procedure-related stroke, myocardial infarction, and death. *Radiology*. 2006;240(1):145–151.
13. Kennedy J, Quan H, Buchan AM, Ghali WA, Feasby TE. Statins are associated with better outcomes after carotid endarterectomy in symptomatic patients. *Stroke*. 2005;36(10):2072–2076.
14. Ravipati G, Aronow WS, Ahn C, Channamsetty V, Sekhri V. Incidence of new stroke or new myocardial infarction or death in patients with severe carotid arterial disease treated with and without statins. *Am J Cardiol*. 2006;98(9):1170–1171.
15. European Carotid Surgery Trialists' Collaborative Group. Randomised trial of endarterectomy for recently symptomatic carotid stenosis: final results of the MRC European Carotid Surgery Trial (ECST). *Lancet*. 1998;351(9113):1379–1387.
16. Mayberg MR, Wilson SE, Yatsu F, et al. Carotid endarterectomy and prevention of cerebral ischemia in symptomatic carotid stenosis. Veterans Affairs Cooperative Studies Program 309 Trialist Group. *JAMA*. 1991;266(23):3289–3294.
17. Rothwell PM, Eliasziw M, Gutnikov SA, et al. Analysis of pooled data from the randomised controlled trials of endarterectomy for symptomatic carotid stenosis. *Lancet*. 2003;361(9352):107–116.
18. Rothwell PM. Risk modeling to identify patients with symptomatic carotid stenosis most at risk of stroke. *Neurol Res*. 2005;27(Suppl 1):S18–S28.
19. Alamowitch S, Eliasziw M, Algra A, Meldrum H, Barnett HJ. Risk, causes, and prevention of ischaemic stroke in elderly patients with symptomatic internal-carotid-artery stenosis. *Lancet*. 2001;357(9263):1154–1160.

20. Rothwell PM, Warlow CP. Prediction of benefit from carotid endarterectomy in individual patients: a risk-modelling study. European Carotid Surgery Trialists' Collaborative Group. *Lancet.* 1999;353(9170):2105–2110.

21. Rothwell PM, Eliasziw M, Gutnikov SA, Warlow CP, Barnett HJ. Endarterectomy for symptomatic carotid stenosis in relation to clinical subgroups and timing of surgery. *Lancet.* 2004;363(9413):915–924.

22. The CASANOVA Study Group. Carotid surgery versus medical therapy in asymptomatic carotid stenosis. *Stroke.* 1991;22(10):1229–1235.

23. Hobson RW, Weiss DG, Fields WS, et al. Efficacy of carotid endarterectomy for asymptomatic carotid stenosis. The Veterans Affairs Cooperative Study Group. *N Engl J Med.* 1993;328(4):221–227.

24. Mayo Asymptomatic Carotid Endarterectomy Study Group. Results of a randomized controlled trial of carotid endarterectomy for asymptomatic carotid stenosis. *Mayo Clin Proc.* 1992;67(6):513–518.

25. Executive Committee for the Asymptomatic Carotid Atherosclerosis Study. Endarterectomy for asymptomatic carotid artery stenosis. *JAMA.* 1995;273(18):1421–1428.

26. Halliday A, Mansfield A, Marro J, et al. Prevention of disabling and fatal strokes by successful carotid endarterectomy in patients without recent neurological symptoms: randomised controlled trial. *Lancet.* 2004;363(9420):1491–1502.

27. Abbott AL, Chambers BR, Stork JL, Levi CR, Bladin CF, Donnan GA. Embolic signals and prediction of ipsilateral stroke or transient ischemic attack in asymptomatic carotid stenosis: a multicenter prospective cohort study. *Stroke.* 2005;36(6):1128–1133.

28. Biller J, Feinberg WM, Castaldo JE, et al. Guidelines for carotid endarterectomy: a statement for healthcare professionals from a special writing group of the Stroke Council, American Heart Association. *Stroke.* 1998;29(2):554–562.

29. Schnaudigel S, Groschel K, Pilgram SM, Kastrup A. New brain lesions after carotid stenting versus carotid endarterectomy. a systematic review of the literature. *Stroke.* 2008;39(6):1911–1919.

30. Barrett KM, Brott TG. Carotid endarterectomy versus angioplasty/stenting for carotid stenosis. *Curr Atheroscler Rep.* 2007;9(4):333–340.

31. Bates ER, Babb JD, Casey DE Jr., et al. ACCF/SCAI/SVMB/SIR/ASITN 2007 clinical expert consensus document on carotid stenting: a report of the American College of Cardiology Foundation Task Force on Clinical Expert Consensus Documents (ACCF/SCAI/SVMB/SIR/ASITN Clinical Expert Consensus Document Committee on Carotid Stenting). *J Am Coll Cardiol.* 2007;49(1):126–170.

32. Naylor AR, Bolia A, Abbott RJ, et al. Randomized study of carotid angioplasty and stenting versus carotid endarterectomy: a stopped trial. *J Vasc Surg.* 1998;28(2):326–334.

33. CAVATAS Investigators. Endovascular versus surgical treatment in patients with carotid stenosis in the Carotid and Vertebral Transluminal Angioplasty Study (CAVATAS): a randomised trial. *Lancet.* 2001;357:1729–1737.

34. Alberts MJ, for the publication committee of WALLSTENT. Results of a multicenter prospective randomized trial of carotid stenting vs. carotid endarterectomy. *Stroke.* 2001;32:325.

35. Brooks WH, McClure RR, Jones MR, Coleman TC, Breathitt L. Carotid angioplasty and stenting versus carotid endarterectomy: randomized trial in a community hospital. *J Am Coll Cardiol.* 2001;38(6):1589–1595.

36. Brooks WH, McClure RR, Jones MR, Coleman TL, Breathitt L. Carotid angioplasty and stenting versus carotid endarterectomy for treatment of asymptomatic carotid stenosis: a randomized trial in a community hospital. *Neurosurgery.* 2004;54(2):318–324.

37. Yadav JS, Wholey MH, Kuntz RE, et al. Protected carotid-artery stenting versus endarterectomy in high-risk patients. *N Engl J Med.* 2004;351(15):1493–1501.

38. Mas JL, Chatellier G, Beyssen B, et al. Endarterectomy versus stenting in patients with symptomatic severe carotid stenosis. *N Engl J Med.* 2006;355(16):1660–1671.

39. Ringleb PA, Allenberg J, Brückmann H, et al. 30 day results from the SPACE trial of stent-protected angioplasty versus carotid endarterectomy in symptomatic patients: a randomised non-inferiority trial. *Lancet.* 2006;368(9543):1239–1247.

40. Stingele R, Berger J, Alfke K, et al. Clinical and angiographic risk factors for stroke and death within 30 days after carotid endarterectomy and stent-protected angioplasty: a subanalysis of the SPACE study. *Lancet Neurol.* 2008;7(3):216–222.

41. Hofmann R, Niessner A, Kypta A, et al. Risk score for peri-interventional complications of carotid artery stenting. *Stroke.* 2006;37(10):2557–2561.

42. Safian RD, Bresnahan JF, Jaff MR, et al. Protected carotid stenting in high-risk patients with severe carotid artery stenosis. *J Am Coll Cardiol.* 2006;47(12):2384–2389.

43. White CJ, Iyer SS, Hopkins LN, Katzen BT, Russell ME. Carotid stenting with distal protection in high surgical risk patients: the BEACH trial 30 day results. *Catheter Cardiovasc Interv.* 2006;67(4):503–512.

16 Peripheral Arterial Disease

Jay Giri and Emile R. Mohler III

CONTENTS

KEY POINTS
INTRODUCTION
PROGNOSIS
DIAGNOSIS
MEDICAL MANAGEMENT OF PAD
CASE STUDIES
REFERENCES

Key Words: Amputation; Angioplasty; Atherosclerosis; Bypass surgery; Claudication; Gangrene.

KEY POINTS

- Peripheral arterial disease (PAD) is common and highly underdiagnosed.
- Patients with PAD have a higher rate of cardiovascular events than the highest risk groups predicted by the Framingham risk score, up to 20% over 5 years.
- Over half of PAD patients have concomitant coronary artery disease.
- The National Cholesterol Education Program recognizes PAD as a coronary heart disease (CHD) risk equivalent, which defines these patients as being at high risk for CHD-related events, such as myocardial infarction and death.
- Only one-third of patients with PAD have typical calf symptoms of claudication.
- All patients at risk of PAD should be screened with the simple, non-invasive, inexpensive ankle–brachial index (ABI). The ABI is 95% sensitive and 99% specific for the diagnosis of PAD.
- Management of PAD involves two paths: aggressive treatment of cardiovascular risk factors to decrease cardiovascular events and mortality as well as treatment of lower extremity symptoms.
- Lower extremity revascularization is never indicated in the asymptomatic patient. However, aggressive risk factor modification should be undertaken in all PAD patients.
- Consensus guidelines for PAD are produced by two major societies, the American College of Cardiology/American Heart Association (ACC/AHA) and the Trans-Atlantic Intersociety Consensus Working Group (TASC-II). Recommendations from the two societies are largely concordant.

16.1. INTRODUCTION

For the purposes of this chapter, peripheral arterial disease (PAD) refers to the development and progression of atherosclerotic disease in the arteries of the lower extremities. A broader definition of peripheral arterial disease would encompass the aorta and all its major visceral branches (carotid

From: *Contemporary Cardiology: Comprehensive Cardiovascular Medicine in the Primary Care Setting*
Edited by: Peter P. Toth, Christopher P. Cannon, DOI 10.1007/978-1-60327-963-5_16
© Springer Science+Business Media, LLC 2010

arteries, mesenteric arteries, renal arteries, and extremity arteries). This chapter will not cover therapeutic considerations related to disease in each of these arterial beds.

16.1.1. Pathophysiology

While there are several uncommon causes of lower extremity arterial disease, the predominant
pathophysiologic process in the majority of PAD cases is atherosclerosis. The uptake and oxidation of low-density lipoprotein (LDL) in the vessel wall is a key-triggering event for atherosclerosis
(1–4). The oxidation of LDL leads to a cascade of inflammatory and proatherogenic events that result
in increased LDL uptake by macrophages with foam cell formation, smooth muscle proliferation and
migration, arterial stenosis, and, when an atheromatous plaque ruptures, in situ thrombosis *(5–15)*.
While these principles provide a framework for a general understanding of atherosclerosis, factors
specific to the peripheral arteries have not been well studied. It is uncommon for patients to suddenly develop claudication symptoms. Claudication is typically an insidious process. It is unclear if
plaque rupture and thrombosis results in claudication symptoms. For this reason, PAD is currently best
thought of as progressive arterial stenosis of the lower extremity arteries due to atherosclerotic plaque
formation, with subsequent development of exertional skeletal muscle and other tissue ischemia.

16.1.2. Prevalence

PAD is highly prevalent. In selected populations of elderly patients or those with major risk factors
for cardiovascular disease, the prevalence of PAD ranges from one in three to one in eight patients.
In the PAD Awareness, Risk, and Treatment: New Resources for Survival (PARTNERS) study, a large
observational study of patients over 70 years old or aged 50–69 with a history of diabetes mellitus or
smoking, the prevalence of PAD, as defined by an ankle–brachial index (ABI) of less than 0.9, was
29% *(16)*. An analysis of data from the National Health and Nutrition Examination Survey (NHANES)
revealed that, in patients over the age of 40, the prevalence of PAD was 4.3%. However in patients over
age 70, the prevalence increased to 14.5% *(17)*. The prevalence of PAD dramatically increases with
age and is common in both men and women *(18, 19)*. Epidemiologic studies have suggested that
African-Americans may have the highest prevalence of PAD of any racial group *(20)*.

16.1.3. Risk Factors

Risk factors for PAD are familiar, as they are those that underlie atherosclerosis more generally.
These include age, smoking, diabetes mellitus, hypertension, hypercholesterolemia, and chronic renal
insufficiency. Based on epidemiologic studies of patients with PAD, various risk groups have been
identified. An American College of Cardiology/American Heart Association (ACC/AHA) consensus
working group has identified an at-risk population for PAD *(21)*. This population is defined as having
any one of the following characteristics:

1. Known atherosclerotic coronary, carotid, or renal arterial disease
2. Age >70
3. Age >50 with risk factors of diabetes mellitus or smoking
4. Age <50 with diabetes mellitus and an additional cardiovascular risk factor (smoking, hypertension,
   hyperlipidemia)
5. Abnormal lower extremity pulse examination
6. Exertional leg symptoms

The value of aggressively screening for PAD became apparent in a primary care practice-based
screening study. In the PARTNERS study, patients over the age of 70 or those over 50 with a history of
diabetes mellitus or smoking were screened for PAD with an ABI measurement. Twenty-nine percent

of those screened had PAD. Importantly, greater than half of those patients found to have PAD had evidence of concomitant coronary artery disease *(16)*.

In order to confirm the diagnosis of PAD, patients who meet any of the above criteria should be studied with the simple, non-invasive ankle–brachial index (ABI). The ABI is an office-based measurement that is 95% sensitive and 99% specific for the presence of PAD (see below) *(21)*.

16.2. PROGNOSIS

16.2.1. Limb Outcomes

In patients diagnosed with PAD, regardless of their initial symptoms (or lack thereof), nearly all will become symptomatic over 5 years. Roughly 70–80% will develop stable claudication symptoms, 10–20% will develop accelerating claudication symptoms, and less than 2% will progress to critical limb ischemia (CLI) *(21)*. The intermediate-term outcomes for patients who develop critical limb ischemia, defined as ischemic rest pain, gangrene, or non-healing ulcers, are dismal. An analysis of patients with CLI treated medically showed a 6-month amputation rate of 35% and, even more worrisome, a 6-month mortality rate of 20% *(22)*.

16.2.2. Cardiovascular Events

PAD patients are at significantly higher risk of myocardial infarction than those in the highest risk category predicted by the Framingham risk score. Specifically, epidemiological studies have shown that the risk of myocardial infarction in patients with ABI <0.7 is nearly 20% at 5 years. For those in the mild PAD risk category, with ABI of 0.7–0.9, the risk is 10% at 5 years *(23)*. For comparison, high-risk Framingham patients have 10-year event rates of 20%. Additionally, a recent meta-analysis demonstrated a doubling of Framingham-predicted cardiovascular risk in patients with ABI <0.9 *(24)*. Importantly, regardless of the clinical presentation, cardiovascular events occur more frequently in PAD patients than ischemic limb events.

16.2.3. Death

Overall, intermediate- and long-term mortality risk in PAD is high. In patients with PAD, yearly mortality rates range from 3 to 6%. All-cause mortality reliably increases with ABI less than 1.00 or greater than 1.30 *(25)*. Patients with diabetes and co-existent PAD fare particularly poorly. In one cohort of men with a mean age of 68 followed longitudinally, 2-year mortality rates in this subset of patients approached 40% *(26)*.

16.3. DIAGNOSIS

16.3.1. History and Physical

Evaluation of patients for PAD should begin with a careful history and physical examination. A comprehensive vascular examination includes palpation of the carotid, radial, femoral, popliteal, posterior tibialis, and dorsalis pedis pulses (Table 1). The measurement of bilateral arm blood pressures, examination for aortic aneurysm, careful inspection of the feet, and auscultation over the various arteries for bruits are also part of the complete vascular examination. By history, the classic presentation of lower extremity peripheral artery disease is one of intermittent claudication, the onset of calf pain with walking that is relieved by rest. Examination findings in the patient with PAD include diminished or absent lower extremity pulses. Arterial bruits, brittle lower extremity nails, prolonged (greater than 10 s) pallor after leg elevation for 1 min, and dependent rubor also point to the diagnosis. While it is important to identify these characteristics if they exist, their sensitivity for PAD detection is poor.

Table 1
Physical Examination Findings of Lower Extremity Arterial
Disease

Diminished or absent pulses
Brittle nails
Pallor with leg elevation
Dependent rubor
Non-healing, punched-out ulcers
Gangrene

Population studies have shown that only 15–30% of patients present with typical symptoms of claudication. A large percentage of patients, as many as 50%, have more atypical presentation of leg pain that is not so closely tied to exertion. Many have no symptoms at all, perhaps due to collateralization of arteries in the lower extremities. A small minority of patients (~1%) present with CLI. And, unlike in the coronary or cerebrovascular circulations where acute coronary syndrome and cerebrovascular accident are common initial manifestations of the underlying disease, acute limb ischemia is a relatively rare presentation of PAD, accounting for less than 2% of initial diagnoses. Thus, it is important to conduct a careful vascular review of symptoms in patients at risk for PAD. This should include specific questioning regarding the presence of any discomfort in the lower extremity, from the buttocks to the foot. Limitation of activity due to the discomfort and its relationship to exertion must be assessed. Patients may describe the discomfort associated with PAD in various terms including pain, achiness, numbness, tingling, or fatigue *(21)*.

As for the examination findings, a diminished or absent pedal pulse has been shown to have relatively poor sensitivity and positive predictive value for the diagnosis of PAD *(27, 28)*. Thus, in patients in the risk groups described above, it is important that the ABI is used as the screening test for PAD (Fig. 1).

16.3.2. Performing an ABI Test

The ABI examination should be performed with the patient in the supine position. Appropriately sized blood pressure cuffs must be used on the upper arm and ankle. An ultrasound probe should be used to identify the strongest arterial signal over the brachial arteries bilaterally. Bilateral systolic brachial artery blood pressures should be obtained. Next, the probe should be used to identify the strongest posterior tibial and dorsalis pedis pulses bilaterally. The systolic blood pressure should be obtained using the probe in all four extremities. The higher of the posterior tibial or dorsalis pedis pressures in a given leg is used as the ankle systolic blood pressure for that leg. In order to calculate the left-leg ABI, divide the left ankle systolic pressure by the highest brachial systolic pressure. The same calculation can be used to obtain the right-leg ABI, again using the highest brachial systolic pressure (Table 2).

$$ABI = \frac{\text{ankle systolic blood pressure (higher of DP/PT)}}{\text{higher brachial artery systolic pressure}}$$

There are some circumstances in which the ABI is limited in its ability to properly diagnose PAD. The most common case is in the patient with an ABI >1.3. These patients have poorly compressible arteries due to medial artery calcification. This finding is not uncommon in patients with diabetes mellitus, renal failure, or advanced age. An ABI over 1.3 should not be considered normal, but rather uninterpretable. A toe–brachial index (TBI) can sometimes be effective in evaluating for the presence

Diagnostic algorithm for PAD

Individuals at risk for lower extremity pad
• Age less than 50 years with diabetes and one other atherosclerosis risk factor (smoking, dyslipidemia, hypertension, or hyperhomocysteinemia)
• Age 50 to 69 years and history of smoking or diabetes
• Age 70 years and older
• Leg symptoms with exertion (suggestive of claudication) or ischemic rest pain
• Abnormal lower extremity pulse examination
• Known atherosclerotic coronary, carotid, or renal arterial disease

Obtain history of walking impairment and/or limb ischemic symptoms:
Obtain a vascular review of symptoms:
• Leg discomfort with exertion
• Leg pain at rest; nonhealing wound; gangrene

| No leg pain | "Atypical" leg-pain* | Classic claudication symptoms: Exertional fatigue, discomfort, or frank pain localized to leg muscle groups that consistently resolves with rest | • Ischemic leg pain at rest • Nonhealing wound • Gangrene | Sudden onset ischemic leg symptoms or signs of acute limb ischemia: The five "Ps" [†] |

Perform a resting ankle-brachial index measurement

| ABI greater than 1.30 (abnormal) | ABI 0.91 to 1.30 (borderline & normal) | ABI less than or equal to .90 (abnormal) | Obtain vascular medicine consultation |

Pulse volume recording toe-brachial index (Duplex ultrasonography*)

Measure ankle-brachial index after exercise test

Normal results: No peripheral arterial disease

Abnormal results

Normal post-exercise ankle-brachial index: No peripheral arterial disease

Decreased post-exercise ankle-brachial index

Evaluate other causes of leg symptoms[†]

Confirmation of PAD diagnosis

Risk factor normalization:
• Immediate smoking cessation
• Treat hypertension: JNC-7 guidelines
• Treat lipids: NCEP ATP III guidelines
• Treat diabetes mellitus: HbA_{1c} Less than 7%[‡]

Pharmacological risk reduction:
• Antiplatelet therapy
• ACE inhibition: Class IIb, LOE C

Fig. 1. Diagnostic algorithm for PAD. Adapted from *(21)*.

Table 2
Interpretation of ABI Measurements

>1.30 uninterpretable
1.00–1.29 normal
0.91–0.99 borderline
0.71–0.90 mild PAD
0.41–0.70 moderate PAD
<0.40 severe PAD

of PAD in those with a supranormal ABI. A specially designed cuff is placed around the great toe to obtain the systolic arterial pressure there. This is divided by the highest brachial arterial systolic pressure to derive a TBI. Values of <0.7 have been found to be sensitive for the diagnosis of PAD *(21)*.

In some cases, patients may have a normal resting ABI but develop an abnormal ABI with exercise. Thus, performing an ABI after a treadmill exercise test can help to clarify functional status as well as confirm the diagnosis of PAD in patients in whom a high suspicion for disease exists despite a normal resting ABI. Important additional information regarding a patient's PAD can be provided with segmental pressures and pulse volume recordings. These are non-invasive tests performed in vascular laboratories that allow for evaluation of level of disease in lower extremities. Segmental pressures are typically performed by placing four blood pressure cuffs sequentially down each leg, two at the thigh, as well as the calf and ankle, and measuring systolic blood pressures at each leg segment. Pulse volume recordings are non-invasive recordings of the arterial wave forms representing blood flow at the same levels where pressures are obtained. A metatarsal or toe pressure cuff may also be applied for evaluation of pedal vessels. Abnormally low pressures or abnormally shaped pulse volume waveforms in a given portion of the leg allow interpreters to localize lower extremity arterial stenoses. One drawback to segmental pressures and pulse volume recordings is that the techniques do not allow for precise localization of the exact area of stenosis.

Some laboratories do an initial ABI and, if abnormal, do an extensive ultrasound evaluation of the lower extremity arterial system. More expensive imaging technologies such as computed tomographic angiography (CTA) and magnetic resonance angiography (MRA) are primarily useful for planning of initial vascular interventions and surveillance of prior interventions. The initial diagnosis of PAD is made cheaply, effectively, and in a risk-free fashion with the ABI, segmental pressures, and pulse volume recordings.

16.4. MEDICAL MANAGEMENT OF PAD

16.4.1. Diabetes Management

The ACC/AHA and Trans-Atlantic Intersociety Consensus Working Group (TASC-II) guidelines recommend aggressive treatment of diabetes mellitus with lowering of the HBA1c to less than 7%. TASC-II takes a particularly aggressive stance, arguing for attempted lowering to as close to 6% as possible *(21, 22)*. A common complication in diabetics with PAD is foot ulcerations. Thus, it is important that proper foot care is emphasized in this patient group with daily self-inspections of the feet as well as semi-annual podiatry visits. Additionally, lesions and ulcerations on the feet should be addressed urgently when they arise.

16.4.2. Smoking Cessation

It is also important to aggressively address smoking cessation in patients with PAD. Cigarette smoking is highly correlated with the development and progression of PAD. Smoking cessation should be undertaken in a comprehensive fashion that includes counseling, behavioral techniques, nicotine replacement therapy, or other pharmocological approaches including buproprion or vareni-cline administration. Smoking cessation has been associated with a rapid decrease in symptomatic claudication *(29)*.

16.4.3. Lipid Lowering Therapies

A post hoc analysis of the Heart Protection Study suggested a substantial reduction in cardiovascular events among those patients with PAD who were treated with 40 mg of simvastatin *(30)*. This benefit was seen even in patients without diagnosed coronary artery disease. In addition to the benefits seen in cardiovascular events, statins have been shown in two randomized trials and in one prospective cohort to modestly improve leg functioning in PAD patients *(31–33)*. The ACC/AHA recommends using statin therapy to target an LDL <10 mg/dL in all patients with PAD. If a patient has disease in multiple vascular beds (i.e., coronary, renal, carotid, or mesenteric disease), a more aggressive target of LDL <70 mg/dL is recommended.

16.4.4. Hypertension

Blood pressure control is important in PAD management, and guidelines recommend values less than 140/90 mmHg *(34)*. ACE inhibitors and thiazide diuretics are generally the first-line therapies to control BP in patients with PAD. Post hoc analysis of the Heart Outcomes Prevention Evaluation (HOPE) trial demonstrated a 15% mortality reduction in symptomatic PAD patients treated with ramipril as opposed to placebo. The mortality benefit in asymptomatic PAD patients treated with ramipril was also significant, 19–42% *(35)*. Preliminary investigations also suggest that ramipril may have positive effects on leg functioning in PAD patients, in addition to their overall decrease in cardiovascular events *(36)*. It is important also to recognize that beta-blockers are safe in PAD patients. There had been initial concerns regarding compromise of lower extremity perfusion in claudication patients on beta-blockers *(37–39)*. These fears have been disproven by multiple studies including a meta-analysis of 11 placebo-controlled trials failing to show an association between beta-blocker use and impaired leg function in patients with claudication *(40)*. Therefore, when required, particularly in patients with concomitant coronary artery disease, beta-blockers should be used without hesitation in PAD patients.

16.4.5. Antithrombotic Therapy

Anti-platelet therapy with aspirin or clopidogrel is a core feature of the medical management of PAD. Specifically, in the large Antithrombotic Trialist's Collaboration meta-analysis, patients treated with anti-platelet therapy had a relative risk reduction of 23% for subsequent serious vascular events *(41)*. Post hoc analysis of the Clopidogrel vs. Aspirin in Patients at Risk of Recurrent Ischemic Events (CAPRIE) Trial showed a 24% risk reduction in stroke, MI, or cardiovascular death in a population of patients with known PAD who were treated with clopidogrel as opposed to aspirin *(42, 43)*. This result raised the question about the potential superiority of clopidogrel over aspirin in PAD patients. This has yet to be fully investigated, and current guideline recommendations by the ACC/AHA and TASC-II consensus groups recommend using either agent. Importantly, aspirin therapy may not provide significant clinical benefit in asymptomatic PAD patients who do not have a history of myocardial infarction, stroke, or claudication. The Prevention Of Progression Of Arterial Disease And Diabetes (POPADAD) Trial showed no difference in outcomes in a diabetic population with asymptomatic PAD treated with aspirin versus placebo, though it was criticized for being underpowered *(44)*. Dual anti-platelet therapy does not yet have a defined role in patients with PAD. As a primary prevention strategy in patients with cardiovascular disease or multiple cardiac risk factors, the combination of aspirin and clopidogrel has not shown significant cardiovascular benefit over aspirin alone but has resulted in increased bleeding complications *(45, 46)*. It remains to be seen whether specific higher risk populations such as those with a history of polyvascular disease, myocardial infarction, or stroke might benefit from dual anti-platelet therapy. Finally, chronic anticoagulation therapy with warfarin does not have a role in the medical management of PAD. The Warfarin Antiplatelet Vascular Evaluation (WAVE) Trial demonstrated increased rates of life-threatening bleeding among PAD patients treated with a combination of warfarin and an anti-platelet agent compared to lone anti-platelet therapy *(47, 48)*.

16.4.6. Symptomatic Therapy

In addition to the goal of reducing cardiovascular events through risk factor modification via the techniques above, therapies exist for the treatment of symptomatic claudication. First, supervised exercise rehabilitation improves pain-free walking distance in patients with PAD *(49–53)*. Additionally, patients with PAD and significant physical activity in their daily lives have decreased cardiovascular events compared to their more sedentary counterparts *(54)*. As for pharmaceutical agents, a 3- to 6-month trial of cilostazol in dosages of 50–100 mg twice daily is recommended by the AHA/ACC for relief of symptomatic claudication *(55)*. In a meta-analysis of six randomized trials of cilostazol versus placebo in patients with PAD, patients taking cilostazol had improvements of 34% in both maximal treadmill walking distance and calf pain severity after 3–6 months on the drug. Patients taking placebo had improvements of 21 and 24%, respectively, in the two outcomes. An important caveat to use of this drug is its contraindication in patients with a history of congestive heart failure. This warning is based on studies showing potential adverse effects of other phosphodiesterase inhibitors in heart failure patients. Additionally, emerging data reveal ACE inhibitors and statins to have effects on functional leg outcomes in PAD in addition to their core role as risk factor modifiers *(31–33, 36)*. Although still prescribed, currently, the use of pentoxifylline for claudication is not strongly supported by evidence *(56)*.

16.4.7. Interventional Therapy

When life-altering symptoms persist despite optimal medical therapy, revascularization of the lower extremity can be considered. Importantly, lower extremity revascularization is never indicated in the asymptomatic patient, regardless of the severity of PAD as measured by hemodynamic or imaging techniques *(21)*. However, in symptomatic patients with significant disability who have failed exercise rehabilitation and pharmacologic therapies and in whom significant functional benefit is anticipated, there are a few different options for revascularization. These options include percutatenous transluminal angioplasty, endovascular stenting, and lower extremity bypass surgery. The recommendations for specific types of procedures vary based on patient and stenotic lesion characteristics. When considering lower extremity revascularization for a patient, seek consultation from an experienced vascular medicine specialist.

16.4.8. Acute Limb Ischemia

Acute limb ischemia refers to a sudden (less than 2-week duration) and rapidly progressive decrease in perfusion to a limb, usually threatening its viability. This can occur in patients with pre-existing severe peripheral arterial disease who show the sudden onset of signs of critical limb ischemia. Atheromatous plaque rupture with overlying thrombosis and luminal obstruction of an at-risk arterial segment is often the mechanism for this syndrome. Alternatively, embolism of a lower extremity can cause the development of acute limb ischemia. This is of particular concern in patients with atrial fibrillation who are not adequately anticoagulated. The classic symptoms of acute limb ischemia are illustrated by the 5 P's: pain, pallor, pulselessness, paresthesia, and paralysis. When acute limb ischemia is suspected, urgent consultation with a vascular medicine specialist should be obtained. Parenteral anticoagulation should be initiated. If limb viability is in question, possible modalities for urgent revascularization include thrombolytic administration, endovascular intervention, and open surgical bypass grafting *(22)*.

16.5. CASE STUDIES

16.5.1. Case 1

A 62-year-old man with a history of hypertension presents to his primary care physician with a complaint of some mild discomfort in his proximal left lower extremity. The discomfort is sometimes but not always related to exertion. He describes it as an ache that occurs unpredictably, sometimes when sitting on the couch. His overall exertional tolerance is good; he is able to walk three blocks without difficulty. He is a 35-pack/year smoker with a family history of coronary artery disease in his father.

Up to 70% of patients with PAD do not present with typical exertional claudication, calf or thigh pain exacerbated by exercise and relieved by rest. Atypical leg pain or no symptoms characterize the majority of the PAD population. The patient above has atypical leg symptoms and is over 50 years old and has a history of smoking. For this reason, the first step in the evaluation of his symptoms (after a physical examination) is the easy, inexpensive, office-based ABI. Patients over 50 with a history of diabetes mellitus or smoking should be screened for PAD with an ABI. Diabetics under 50 with an additional major cardiovascular risk factor, patients over age 70, patients with known vascular disease, and patients with exertional leg symptoms or abnormal pulse examinations should also be routinely screened.

Bilateral ABI is performed revealing an ABI of 0.56 on the left and 0.63 on the right. Segmental pressures and pulse volume recordings are shown in Fig. 2.

Based on his ABI measurements, the patient has moderate left lower extremity PAD and moderate right lower extremity PAD. The segmental pressures performed in a vascular laboratory are typically accompanied by pulse volume recordings (PVR). This helps to localize the lesion. A thigh to brachial index of >1.1 is considered normal, whereas a calf to brachial index of >1.0 is normal. In this patient's case, the study revealed left iliac disease and probable right iliac disease. At this point, two parallel lines of medical management should begin: intensive risk factor modification and treatment of claudication symptoms. The risk factor modification should be initiated to decrease the patient's risk of future cardiovascular events and progression of PAD. Specifically, if he is found to have diabetes it should be aggressively managed with a target HBA1c of 7% or less. Also, one should initiate comprehensive smoking cessation therapy that includes nicotine replacement therapy, behavioral techniques, and wellbutrin or varenicline if necessary. His blood pressure should be treated initially with an ACE inhibitor. Hydrochlorothiazide is also a reasonable first- or second-line agent in management of his hypertension. A fasting cholesterol panel should be obtained and a statin should be initiated with a goal LDL of less than 100 mg/dL. Finally, he should be started on either aspirin or clopidogrel as anti-platelet therapy.

The other important approach in this patient is treatment of claudication symptoms. He should be referred, if possible, to a formalized, exercise rehabilitation program. If this is unavailable, as is the case in many areas, he should be counseled to begin a home walking exercise program. A 3-month trial of 100 mg of cilostazol can be initiated as this patient does not have a history of congestive heart failure. He should be followed up regularly for monitoring of his symptoms and risk factors. Medications should be titrated and added as needed in order for the patient to meet national guideline-specified goals for his various risk factors.

The patient exhibits good medication compliance and appropriately increases his level of physical activity. His blood pressure and LDL cholesterol are well controlled. Unfortunately, he continues to

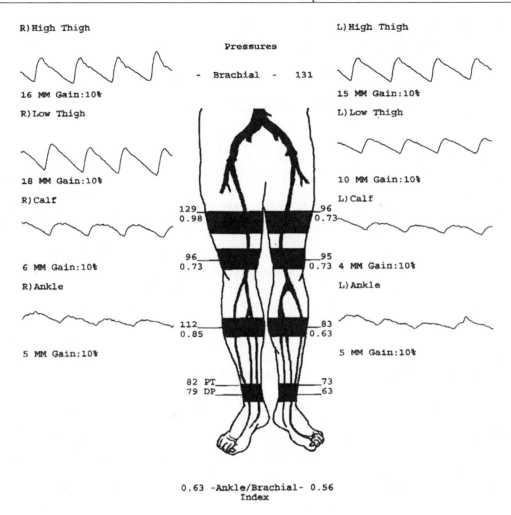

R) High Thigh
16 MM Gain:10%

R) Low Thigh
18 MM Gain:10%

R) Calf
6 MM Gain:10%

R) Ankle
5 MM Gain:10%

Pressures

- Brachial - 131

L) High Thigh
15 MM Gain:10%

L) Low Thigh
10 MM Gain:10%

L) Calf
4 MM Gain:10%

L) Ankle
5 MM Gain:10%

129 0.98   96 0.73

96 0.73   95 0.73

112 0.85   83 0.63

82 PT   73
79 DP   63

0.63 -Ankle/Brachial- 0.56
Index

Fig. 2. Segmental pressures and pulse volume recordings.

smoke. He notices initial improvement in his symptoms but insidiously, over the course of 3 years, his left lower extremity symptoms become worse eventually causing him difficulty at his job as a bellman that requires him to walk hotel guests to their rooms while carrying luggage.

The patient noticed improvements initially, but now appears to be failing medical therapy. Additionally, his symptoms are interfering with his daily life and making him more sedentary, increasing his risk for future cardiovascular events. At this point, it would be appropriate to refer him to a vascular medicine specialist to consider further interventional options to treat his claudication.

He is seen by a vascular medicine specialist who orders a CTA showing severe left iliac disease and moderate right iliac disease with good three-vessel run-off (evidence of patent anterior tibial, posterior tibial, and peroneal arteries). He undergoes percutaneous balloon angioplasty followed by implantation of a nitinol stent to his left iliac artery and notices significant relief of his symptoms. He vows to stop smoking.

16.5.2. Case 2

A 74-year-old man with a history of diabetes mellitus and hypertension comes to the primary care office with complaints of a sore foot for 2 weeks. The patient was diagnosed with claudication secondary to PAD 3 years earlier. The patient was urged to quit smoking at that time but, unfortunately, was unable to comply. The physical examination reveals an ulceration on the great toe of the right lower extremity. Laboratory testing reveals a mildly elevated fasting glucose level of 110 mg/dL. His laboratory testing along with the finding of a waist circumference greater than 40 in. is consistent with metabolic syndrome. The patient is referred to the vascular laboratory where he is found to have a right ankle–brachial index of 0.3 and a left ankle–brachial index of 0.6.

The annual incidence of critical limb ischemia is approximately 500–1,000 persons per million of population in North America and Europe *(22)*. The natural history of patients with claudication over 5 years for development of CLI is relatively low at approximately 1%. However, risk factors such as persistent smoking and metabolic syndrome increase this risk. The patient described above warrants immediate medical attention for evaluation of possible revascularization in order to provide enough blood flow and tissue oxygenation to heal the wound. Consultation from a vascular medicine specialist should be obtained.

The patient underwent lower extremity angiography and was found to have a 5-cm-long soft superficial femoral artery atherosclerotic lesion that resulted in complete occlusion of the vessel. This was opened with a guidewire and balloon angioplasty. An 80% occlusion of the popliteal artery was also noted and this vessel was also opened with an angioplasty balloon. Two of the three vessels below the popliteal artery were patent bilaterally. Although clinical trial data regarding combination anti-platelet therapy after peripheral percutaneous revascularization are very limited, the patient was given both aspirin and clopidogrel in order to maintain vessel patency and prevent thrombosis.

Guideline recommendations for treating patients after percutaneous revascularization for CLI include anti-platelet therapy, which decreases the rate of future vascular events. It is presumed that anti-platelet therapy also improves long-term patency of arterial segments that have been intervened upon, though this has not been rigorously studied in the lower extremities *(22)*.

Over the course of 4 weeks the patient's lower extremity pain resolved and he no longer needed analgesic pain relief. He was given prescriptions for a supervised exercise claudication program as well as consultation with a nutritionist. The patient again underwent counseling regarding smoking cessation.

REFERENCES

1. Ross R. Atherosclerosis—an inflammatory disease. *N Engl J Med.* 1999;340:115–126.
2. Schwenke DC. Comparison of aorta and pulmonary artery: II. LDL transport and metabolism correlate with susceptibility to atherosclerosis. *Circ Res.* 1997;81:346–354.
3. Schwenke DC. Comparison of aorta and pulmonary artery: I. Early cholesterol accumulation and relative susceptibility to atheromatous lesions. *Circ Res.* 1997;81:338–345.
4. Camejo G, Hurt-Camejo E, Wiklund O, Bondjers G. Association of apo B lipoproteins with arterial proteoglycans: pathological significance and molecular basis. *Atherosclerosis.* 1998;139:205–222.
5. Steinberg D. Atherogenesis in perspective: hypercholesterolemia and inflammation as partners in crime. *Nat Med.* 2002;8:1211–1217.
6. Navab M, Hama SY, Reddy ST, et al. Oxidized lipids as mediators of coronary heart disease. *Curr Opin Lipidol.* 2002;13:363–372. Erratum appears in *Curr Opin Lipidol.* 2002 Oct;13(5):589.
7. Dansky HM, Barlow CB, Lominska C, et al. Adhesion of monocytes to arterial endothelium and initiation of atherosclerosis are critically dependent on vascular cell adhesion molecule-1 gene dosage. *Arterioscler Thromb Vasc Biol.* 2001;21:1662–1667.
8. Cybulsky MI, Gimbrone MA Jr.. Endothelial expression of a mononuclear leukocyte adhesion molecule during atherogenesis. *Science.* 1991;251:788–791.
9. Cybulsky MI, Iiyama K, Li H, et al. A major role for VCAM-1, but not ICAM-1, in early atherosclerosis. *J Clin Invest.* 2001;107:1255–1262.
10. Collins RG, Velji R, Guevara NV, Hicks MJ, Chan L, Beaudet AL. P-Selectin or intercellular adhesion molecule (ICAM)-1 deficiency substantially protects against atherosclerosis in apolipoprotein E-deficient mice. *J Exp Med.* 2000;191:189–194.

11. Boring L, Gosling J, Cleary M, Charo IF. Decreased lesion formation in CCR2–/– mice reveals a role for chemokines in the initiation of atherosclerosis. *Nature.* 1998;394:894–897.
12. Gu L, Okada Y, Clinton SK, et al. Absence of monocyte chemoattractant protein-1 reduces atherosclerosis in low density lipoprotein receptor-deficient mice. *Mol Cell.* 1998;2:275–281.
13. Gosling J, Slaymaker S, Gu L, et al. MCP-1 deficiency reduces susceptibility to atherosclerosis in mice that overexpress human apolipoprotein B. *J Clin Invest.* 1999;103:773–778.
14. Smith JD, Trogan E, Ginsberg M, et al. Decreased atherosclerosis in mice deficient in both macrophage colony-stimulating factor (op) and apolipoprotein E. *Proc Natl Acad Sci USA.* 1995;92:8264–8268.
15. Rajavashisth TB, Andalibi A, Territo MC, et al. Induction of endothelial cell expression of granulocyte and macrophage colony-stimulating factors by modified low-density lipoproteins. *Nature.* 1990;344:254–257.
16. Hirsch AT, Criqui MH, Treat-Jacobson D, et al. Peripheral arterial disease detection, awareness, and treatment in primary care. *JAMA.* 2001;286(11):1317–1324.
17. Selvin E, Erlinger TP. Prevalence of and risk factors for peripheral arterial disease in the United States: results from the national health and nutrition examination survey, 1999–2000. *Circulation.* 2004;110(6):738–743.
18. Meijer WT, Hoes AW, Rutgers D, Bots ML, Hofman A, Grobbee DE. Peripheral arterial disease in the elderly: the Rotterdam Study. *Arterioscler Thromb Vasc Biol.* 1998;18(2):185–192.
19. Diehm C, Schuster A, Allenberg H, et al. High prevalence of peripheral arterial disease and comorbidity in 6880 primary care patients: cross sectional study. *Atherosclerosis.* 2004;172:95–105.
20. Criqui MH, Vargas V, Denenberg JO, et al. Ethnicity and peripheral arterial disease: the san Diego population study. *Circulation.* 2005;112(17):2703–2707.
21. Hirsch AT, Haskal ZJ, Hertzer NR, et al. ACC/AHA 2005 guidelines for the management of patients with peripheral arterial disease (lower extremity, renal, mesenteric, and abdominal aortic): executive summary a collaborative report from the American Association for Vascular Surgery/Society for Vascular Surgery, Society for Cardiovascular Angiography and Interventions, Society for Vascular Medicine and Biology, Society of Interventional Radiology, and the ACC/AHA Task Force on Practice Guidelines (Writing Committee to Develop Guidelines for the Management of Patients with Peripheral Arterial Disease) endorsed by the American Association of Cardiovascular and Pulmonary Rehabilitation; National Heart, Lung, and Blood Institute; Society for Vascular Nursing; TransAtlantic Inter-Society Consensus; and Vascular Disease Foundation. *J Am Coll Cardiol.* 2006;47(6):1239–1312.
22. Norgren L, Hiatt WR, Dormandy JA, et al. Inter-society consensus for the management of peripheral arterial disease (TASC II). *J Vasc Surg.* 2007;45(Suppl S):S5–S67.
23. Leng GC, Fowkes FG, Lee AJ, Dunbar J, Housley E, Ruckley CV. Use of ankle brachial pressure index to predict cardiovascular events and death: a cohort study. *BMJ.* 1996;313(7070):1440–1444.
24. Fowkes FG, Murray GD, Butcher I, et al. Ankle brachial index combined with Framingham risk score to predict cardiovascular events and mortality: a meta-analysis. *JAMA.* 2008;300:197–208.
25. O'Hare AM, Katz R, Shlipak MG, Cushman M, Newman AB. Mortality and cardiovascular risk across the ankle-arm index spectrum: results from the cardiovascular health study. *Circulation.* 2006;113(3):388–393.
26. Ogren M, Hedblad B, Engstrom G, Janzon L. Prevalence and prognostic significance of asymptomatic peripheral arterial disease in 68-year-old men with diabetes. Results from the population study "men born in 1914" from Malmo, Sweden. *Eur J Vasc Endovasc Surg.* 2005;29(2):182–189.
27. Criqui MH, Fronek A, Klauber MR, Barrett-Connor E, Gabriel S. The sensitivity, specificity, and predictive value of traditional clinical evaluation of peripheral arterial disease: results from noninvasive testing in a defined population. *Circulation.* 1985;71(3):516–522.
28. Hiatt WR, Marshall JA, Baxter J, et al. Diagnostic methods for peripheral arterial disease in the san Luis valley diabetes study. *J Clin Epidemiol.* 1990;43(6):597–606.
29. Criqui MH. Peripheral arterial disease—epidemiological aspects. *Vascular Medicine.* 2001;6(3 Suppl):3–7.
30. MRC/BHF Heart Protection Study of cholesterol lowering with simvastatin in 20,536 high-risk individuals: a randomised placebo-controlled trial. *Lancet.* 2002;360(9326):7–22.
31. Giri J, McDermott MM, Greenland P, et al. Statin use and functional decline in patients with and without peripheral arterial disease. *J Am Coll Cardiol.* 2006 Mar;47(5):998–1004.
32. Mohler ER 3rd, Hiatt WR, Creager MA. Cholesterol reduction with atorvastatin improves walking distance in patients with peripheral arterial disease. *Circulation.* 2003;108(12):1481–1486.
33. Mondillo S, Ballo P, Barbati R, et al. Effects of simvastatin on walking performance and symptoms of intermittent claudication in hypercholesterolemic patients with peripheral vascular disease. *Am J Med.* 2003;114(5):359–364.
34. Chobanian AV, Bakris GL, Black HR, et al. The seventh report of the Joint National Committee on Prevention, Detection, Evaluation, and Treatment of High Blood Pressure: the JNC 7 report. *JAMA.* 2003;289(19):2560–2572. Erratum appears in *JAMA.* 2003;290(2):197.
35. Yusuf S, Sleight P, Pogue J, et al. Effects of an angiotensin-converting-enzyme inhibitor, ramipril, on cardiovascular events in high-risk patients. The Heart Outcomes Prevention Evaluation Study Investigators. *N Engl J Med.* 2000;342(3):145–153. Erratum appears in *N Engl J Med.* 2000;342(18):1376.

36. Ahimastos AA, Lawler A, Reid CM, et al. Brief communication: ramipril markedly improves walking ability in patients with peripheral arterial disease: a randomized trial. *Ann Intern Med.* 2006;144(9):660–664. Summary for patients in *Ann Intern Med.* 2006;144(9):I24;PMID:16670129.

37. Fogoros RN. Exacerbation of intermittent claudication by propranolol. *N Engl J Med.* 1980;302(19):1089.

38. Ingram DM, House AK, Thompson GH, et al. Beta-adrenergic blockade and peripheral vascular disease. *Med J Aust.* 1998;1(12):509–511.

39. Smith RS, Warren DJ. Effect of beta-blocking drugs on peripheral blood flow in intermittent claudication. *J Cardiovasc Pharmacol.* 1982;4(1):2–4.

40. Radack K, Deck C. Beta-adrenergic blocker therapy does not worsen intermittent claudication in subjects with peripheral arterial disease. A meta-analysis of randomized controlled trials. *Arch Intern Med.* 1991;151(9):1769–1776.

41. Antithrombotic Trialists C. Collaborative meta-analysis of randomised trials of antiplatelet therapy for prevention of death, myocardial infarction, and stroke in high risk patients. *BMJ.* 2002;324(7329):71–86. Erratum appears in *BMJ.* 2002;324(7330):141.

42. Creager MA. Results of the CAPRIE Trial: efficacy and safety of clopidogrel. Clopidogrel versus aspirin in patients at risk of ischaemic events. *Vasc Med.* 1998;3(3):257–260.

43. Steering Committee CAPRIE. A randomised, blinded, trial of clopidogrel versus aspirin in patients at risk of ischaemic events (CAPRIE). *Lancet.* 1996;348(9038):1329–1339.

44. Belch J, MacCuish A, Campbell I, et al. The Prevention and Progression of Arterial Disease and Diabetes (POPADAD) Trial: factorial randomized placebo controlled trial of aspirin and antioxidants in patients with diabetes and asymptomatic peripheral arterial disease. *BMJ.* 2008;337:a1840.

45. Bhatt DL, Flather MD, Hacke W, et al. Patients with prior myocardial infarction, stroke, or symptomatic peripheral arterial disease in the CHARISMA Trial. *J Am Coll Cardiol.* 2007;49(19):1982–1988.

46. Bhatt DL, Fox KA, Hacke W, et al. Clopidogrel and aspirin versus aspirin alone for the prevention of atherothrombotic events. *N Engl J Med.* 2006;354(16):1706–1717.

47. Anand S, Yusuf S, Xie C, et al. Oral anticoagulant and antiplatelet therapy and peripheral arterial disease. *N Engl J Med.* 2007;357(3):217–227.

48. Mohler ER III.. Atherothrombosis—wave goodbye to combined anticoagulation and antiplatelet therapy? *N Engl J Med.* 2007;357(3):293–296.

49. Gardner AW, Poehlman ET. Exercise rehabilitation programs for the treatment of claudication pain. A meta-analysis. *JAMA.* 1995;274(12):975–980.

50. Hiatt WR, Regensteiner JG, Hargarten ME, et al. Benefit of exercise conditioning for patients with peripheral arterial disease. *Circulation.* 1990;81(2):602–609.

51. Hiatt WR, Wolfel EE, Meier RH, et al. Superiority of treadmill walking exercise versus strength training for patients with peripheral arterial disease. Implications for the mechanism of the training response. *Circulation.* 1994;90(4):1866–1874.

52. Regensteiner JG. Exercise in the treatment of claudication: assessment and treatment of functional impairment. *Vasc Med.* 1997;2(3):238–242.

53. Regensteiner JG, Meyer TJ, Krupski WC, et al. Hospital vs home-based exercise rehabilitation for patients with peripheral arterial occlusive disease. *Angiology.* 1997;48(4):291–300.

54. Garg PK, Tian L, Criqui MH, et al. Physical activity during daily life and mortality in patients with peripheral arterial disease. *Circulation.* 2006;114(3):242–248.

55. Regensteiner JG, Ware JE Jr., McCarthy WJ, et al. Effect of cilostazol on treadmill walking, community-based walking ability, and health-related quality of life in patients with intermittent claudication due to peripheral arterial disease: meta-analysis of six randomized controlled trials. *J AmGeriat Soc.* 2002;50(12):1939–1946.

56. Ernst E. Pentoxifylline for intermittent claudication: a critical review. *Angiology.* 1994;45:339–345.

17 Deep Venous Thrombosis and Pulmonary Embolism

Adam C. Schaffer and Sylvia C. W. McKean

CONTENTS

Key Words: Enoxaparin; Pulmonary embolism; Thrombosis; Warfarin; Wells score.

KEY POINTS

- DVT and PE are interrelated diseases.

- The majority of VTE diagnoses are made in the ambulatory setting, though a significant number of these patients will have been recently hospitalized.

- Vigilance is required on the part of primary care physicians to suspect VTE when at-risk medically ill patients are treated in the outpatient setting or seen following hospital discharge.

- Based on patient-specific risk factors and disease-specific risk factors—such as acute hospitalization, immobilization at home, cancer, or central venous access—clinicians can determine the likelihood of VTE.

From: *Contemporary Cardiology: Comprehensive Cardiovascular Medicine in the Primary Care Setting*
Edited by: Peter P. Toth, Christopher P. Cannon, DOI 10.1007/978-1-60327-963-5_17
© Springer Science+Business Media, LLC 2010

- Although the signs and symptoms of VTE may be non-specific, clinicians should specifically inquire and look for clues suggesting the diagnosis in at-risk patients.

- Common symptoms seen in patients with PE include dyspnea (at rest or with exertion), pleuritic chest pain, cough, orthopnea, wheezing, and non-pleuritic chest pain, as well as signs and symptoms of DVT.

17.1. INTRODUCTION

Venous thromboembolism (VTE), a term encompassing both deep vein thrombosis (DVT) and pulmonary embolus (PE), is a common problem, estimated to occur in about 1 in 1,000 adults annually *(1)*. DVT and PE are interrelated diseases. Not only do they share many risk factors, but in one autopsy series of 195 patients who died of PE, DVT was identified in 83% of patients *(2)*, and risk of PE from DVT is at least 40% *(3, 4)*. VTE is an extremely serious condition, with a 3-month mortality rate of 8.65% among patients who presented with symptomatic VTE *(5)*.

Although prior hospitalization or surgery is common among patients diagnosed with VTE, a majority of VTE diagnoses are made in ambulatory patients, necessitating vigilance on the part of primary care providers *(6)*. Moreover, there is a trend toward outpatient treatment of DVT, which, while it appears to be effective and reduces costs, will require intensive involvement by primary care providers *(7)*.

17.2. EPIDEMIOLOGY

Based on data from a predominantly Caucasian cohort from Minnesota, the average annual incidence of venous thromboembolism is about 117 per 100,000 person-years. There are over 275,000 new VTE cases annually in the United States *(8)*. Among patients with first-time VTE, about one-third present with PE and two-thirds with DVT *(9)*. One of the most striking epidemiological features of DVT and PE is that the incidence of these events increases with age (Fig. 1) *(10)*. Thus PE and DVT are predominantly diseases of the elderly. As patients age, the proportion of VTE that are PE also increases. VTE incidence rates in those over age 45 years show a slight male predominance *(11)*. An exception to the tendency for VTE to affect older individuals is the elevated risk of VTE among pregnant women, in whom the incidence is almost 200 per 100,000 person-years. The increase in risk begins in the first trimester, though the risk is even higher among post-partum women than among pregnant women *(12)*. Compared to Caucasians, the incidence of first-time, idiopathic DVT appears to be higher in African-Americans, lower in Hispanics, and markedly lower in Asian or Pacific Islanders. Part of the reason for the difference in the incidence of DVT among different ethnic groups may be a result of differences in the rate of underlying genetic thrombophilias. For instance, the rate of the factor V Leiden mutation is known to be lower in Asian-Americans than in Caucasians. However, African-Americans also have a lower rate of the factor V Leiden mutation than Caucasians and nonetheless have a higher incidence of DVT *(1, 13, 14)*.

17.3. RISK FACTORS

Many factors have been identified as increasing the risk of DVT and PE, with those conferring the greatest risk relating to injury or hospitalization. Some of the strongest risk factors include surgery—especially orthopedic surgery—trauma, and spinal cord injury *(15)*. Figure 2 shows the magnitude of the effect of different risk factors, based on data from a cohort of 625 patients with first lifetime VTE *(16)*. Although many of these risk factors relate to hospitalization, they are crucially important to outpatient practice, since, among those patients diagnosed with VTE in the outpatient setting, a significant number will have been recently hospitalized.

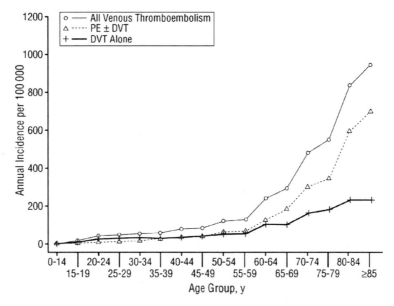

Fig. 1. Annual incidence of all venous thromboembolism, deep vein thrombosis (DVT) alone, and pulmonary embolism (PE) with or without deep vein thrombosis (PE ± DVT) among residents of Olmsted County, Minnesota, from 1966 to 1990, by age. Reprinted from *(10)*.

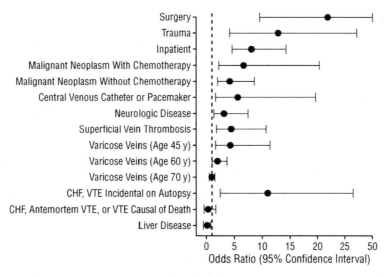

Fig. 2. Odds ratio (and 95% confidence intervals) of risk factors for definite deep vein thrombosis or pulmonary embolism among Olmsted County, Minnesota, residents with a first lifetime venous thromboembolism (VTE) diagnosed from 1976 through 1990. Reprinted from *(16)*.

One study examined 1,897 patients in the Worcester, Massachusetts, area identified as having VTE. Nearly three-quarters of patients with VTE developed it in the outpatient setting—defined as ambulatory patients presenting with signs and symptoms consistent with VTE, or diagnosed within 24 h of presentation to the hospital. Among the patients who developed VTE in the outpatient setting, 36.8% of these patients had been hospitalized in the preceding 3 months, and 23.1% had undergone surgery within the preceding 3 months. This study also points out the important nexus between inpatient care and outpatient VTE. Among those patients who were diagnosed with VTE in the outpatient setting following hospitalization, only 59.2% had received any VTE prophylaxis while an inpatient, and only 42.8% had received anticoagulant prophylaxis. Although risk factors—such as antecedent hospitalization—are important, 29.5% of these patients who developed VTE in the outpatient setting had no identifiable risk factors (6, 17).

Among patients presenting with VTE who have recently been hospitalized, if they received heparin during the hospitalization, heparin-induced thrombocytopenia (HIT) as a cause of the VTE should be a consideration. HIT occurs due to the formation of platelet factor 4–heparin antibody complexes, which induce platelet activation and thrombosis (18). Any patient who has thrombosis (including DVT, PE, or thrombosis at another site) while on heparin (either prophylactic or treatment doses) or within 2 weeks of receiving heparin should undergo diagnostic testing for HIT, consisting of serologic testing for platelet factor 4–heparin antibodies. A fall in the platelet count by $\geq 50\%$ in a patient who is on heparin should also raise a concern for HIT, though this may not always occur prior to the thrombosis. Most commonly, HIT occurs 5–14 days after heparin is begun in patients who have either never been treated with heparin in the past or have not received heparin for at least 100 days. However, in patients who have been treated with heparin within the previous 100 days, HIT may develop within hours of starting heparin, as a result of pre-existing platelet factor 4–heparin antibodies. In patients in whom there is a strong suspicion for HIT, or who have been diagnosed with HIT, unfractionated heparin and low molecular weight heparin should be avoided, as should warfarin in the acute phase of HIT, due to the risk of further thrombosis and digital gangrene (19, 20). In the case of patients with known or suspected HIT, hematology consultation should be obtained.

An important risk factor for VTE not captured in studies of first-time VTE is previous VTE. A history of previous VTE significantly increases the risk for a subsequent VTE. In a prospectively followed cohort of 738 patients with DVT, 5 years after the initial DVT, the rate of a recurrent VTE was 21.5%. Factors increasing the risk of a recurrent VTE included a proximal DVT and cancer. Conversely, patients whose initial DVT occurred in the postoperative setting were less likely to have a recurrent VTE (21). Use of oral contraceptives after an initial VTE also increases the risk of another VTE, and so women should be advised to discontinue oral contraceptives after an initial VTE (22).

A case–control study conducted by Samama involving 1,272 patients determined risk factors for lower extremity DVT among outpatients seeing general practitioners and excluded patients who had recently undergone surgery (23). Dividing risk factors into those that are permanent (or "intrinsic") and those that are transient (or "triggering"), this study found a number of risk factors to be significant, as shown in Table 1. Of the DVT risk factors listed, obesity is notable for being one that is potentially modifiable. Similarly, homocysteine has received attention as a VTE risk factor that could be subject to intervention (1). No trial has specifically examined whether weight loss reduces the risk of VTE. In two trials that assessed whether efforts to lower homocysteine levels using supplementation with folic acid, pyridoxine (vitamin B_6), and cyanocobalamin (vitamin B_{12}) would decrease the incidence of VTE, this intervention was not found to be effective for either the primary prevention (24) or secondary prevention (25) of VTE.

Thrombophilias—which may be inherited, such as the factor V Leiden mutation, prothrombin mutation G20210A, protein C deficiency, and protein S deficiency, or acquired, such as antiphospholipid syndrome—are also risk factors for VTE. Factor V Leiden and prothrombin mutation G20210A are the most common genetic thrombophilias. The increase in the risk conferred by the presence of these thrombophilias is, in general, greater for initial VTE than for recurrent VTE. For example, the relative risk of initial VTE in patients with the heterozygous factor V Leiden mutation in different studies ranges from 3 to 10, whereas the relative risk for recurrent VTE ranges from 1.1 to 1.4 (26). The role of testing for thrombophilias in clinical management is discussed later.

Table 1
Risk Factors for DVT in an Outpatient Medical Population
in Descending Order of Importance

Risk factors	Odds ratio (95% CI)	p
Intrinsic factors		
History of DVT or PE	15.6 (6.77–35.89)	<0.001
Venous insufficiency	4.45 (3.10–6.38)	<0.001
Chronic heart failure	2.93 (1.55–5.56)	0.001
Obesity	2.39 (1.48–3.87)	<0.001
Standing position >6 h/day	1.85 (1.12–3.06)	0.02
History of less than three pregnancies	1.74 (1.06–2.87)	0.03
Triggering factors		
Pregnancy	11.41 (1.40–93.29)	0.02
Violent effort or muscular trauma	7.59 (2.95–19.53)	<0.001
Deterioration in general condition	5.75 (2.20–15.01)	<0.001
Immobilization	5.61 (2.30–13.67)	<0.001
Long-distance travel	2.35 (1.45–3.80)	<0.001
Infectious disease	1.95 (1.31–2.92)	0.001

Risk factors for DVT in an outpatient medical population, in descending order of importance.

Taken from *(23)*.

17.4. THROMBOPHILIA TESTING

There is a lack of consensus regarding the role of testing for thrombophilias (sometimes referred to as a "hypercoagulability workup") in the management of VTE. Neither of the two major VTE guidelines, from the American College of Chest Physicians *(27)* and from the American College of Physicians *(28)*, addresses when or if testing for thrombophilias should be undertaken.

Arguments against routine testing for thrombophilias are based on the reasoning that, although a thrombophilia is a substantial risk factor for an initial VTE, the presence of a thrombophilia in patients who have already had an initial VTE confers only a slightly increased risk of recurrent VTE *(26)*. Broad testing for thrombophilias in unselected patients without VTE is clearly not feasible. In patients in whom VTE is diagnosed, who are often considered candidates for thrombophilia testing, diagnosing a thrombophilia means that they are at only modestly increased risk for a recurrent VTE relative to those patients who have an initial VTE and no thrombophilia. In patients with an initial VTE, those with a thrombophilic abnormality have a statistically non-significant 1.4-fold increase in the risk of recurrent VTE *(22)*. Opponents of routine testing for thrombophilias in patients with an initial VTE argue that, since identifying a thrombophilia in these patients means their risk of recurrence is only slightly increased compared to those patients with an initial VTE and no thrombophilia, routine testing in these patients is not indicated *(22, 26, 29, 30)*.

Illustrating the lack of consensus on this issue, other authors assert that thrombophilia testing should be performed in many patients who are diagnosed with a VTE. Proponents of thrombophilia testing say that the diagnosis of a thrombophilia may affect the duration of anticoagulation, and it might lead to the use of thromboprophylaxis in patients diagnosed with a thrombophilia who will be transiently at further elevated risk (e.g., extended air travel). Moreover, the diagnosis of a thrombophilia has implications for first-degree relatives and may prompt them to undergo thrombophilia testing. Of course, the diagnosis of a genetic thrombophilia may have other ramifications, on such matters as health insurance, which need to be discussed with the patient. Table 2 lists some of the more common thrombophilias

Table 2
Common Thrombophilic Disorders

Disorder	Prevalence in normals	Frequency in patients with VTE (%)	Relative risk of first episode of VTE
Factor V Leiden (heterozygous)	4.8% (in Caucasians)	18.8	7
	1.23% (in African-Americans)		
Factor V Leiden (homozygous)	0.02%		80
Prothrombin mutation G20210A	2.7% (in Caucasians)	7.1	2.8
	0.06% (in Africans or Asians)		
Antithrombin III deficiency	0.02%	1.9	20
Protein C deficiency	0.2–0.4%	3.7	6.5
Protein S deficiency	0.003%	2.3	5.0
Hyperhomocysteinemia (>18.5 µmol/L)	5–7%	10	2.95
Elevated factor VIII levels	11%	25	4.8

Adapted from *(31)*.

that can be included as part of the laboratory evaluation for hypercoagulability. In addition to those disorders listed in Table 2, factors IX and XI activity can be checked, and an assessment for antiphospholipid antibodies should be performed—including testing for lupus anticoagulant, anticardiolipin antibody, and anti-β(beta)$_2$-glycoprotein I *(31–33)*. Whitlatch and Ortel, proponents of thrombophilia testing, suggest testing under the following circumstances: idiopathic VTE in those aged ≤50 years; history of recurrent thromboses; thromboses at unusual sites (e.g., mesenteric or hepatic); thrombosis in a first-degree relative, especially age ≤50 years; thrombosis during pregnancy; or thrombosis while on oral contraceptive pills *(32)*.

One issue on which there is more uniformity of opinion is thrombophilia testing in women with a family or personal history of VTE who are considering oral contraceptive agents. The presence of a thrombophilia significantly increases the risk of VTE in women taking oral contraceptives. Women with a deficiency of either protein C, protein S, or antithrombin who took oral contraceptive agents had a relative risk of VTE of 9.7, as compared to women taking oral contraceptive agents without one of these deficiencies *(34)*. Therefore, women with either a personal or family history of VTE who want to take oral contraceptive agents should be tested for thrombophilias, and if one is found, women should be strongly advised not to use oral contraceptive agents *(26, 34)*. Routine testing for thrombophilias in women without a family or personal history of VTE who are about to start oral contraceptive agents is not recommended *(34, 35)*.

Therapy for VTE may interfere with the testing for thrombophilias that the VTE diagnosis prompts. Warfarin therapy can result in decreased serum levels of proteins C and S, both of which are vitamin K dependent. Heparin may cause inaccurate results when testing for antithrombin levels and lupus anticoagulant titers *(32)*. Thrombosis itself may lead to decreased antithrombin and protein S levels. Liver disease may result in decreased levels of protein C, protein S, and antithrombin secondary to reduced hepatic production *(36)*.

17.5. MALIGNANCY TESTING

As with thrombophilia testing and VTE, the major guidelines offer no recommendations on the role of cancer screening in patients with VTE. There is a definite association between VTE and malignancy. The highest risk of VTE is seen in patients with malignancies of the bones, ovary, brain, and pancreas *(37)*. Not only are patients with malignancies more likely to have a VTE, but patients with an idiopathic VTE are also at increased risk of subsequently being diagnosed with a malignancy. Compared to patients with secondary VTE, the odds ratio of a malignancy being diagnosed in patients with idiopathic VTE is 2.3 over a 2-year follow-up period. The odds ratio in patients with recurrent idiopathic VTE is 9.8 *(38)*. Therefore, patients diagnosed with an idiopathic VTE should undergo all age appropriate cancer screening and should be evaluated for any signs or symptoms of an underlying malignancy *(32)*.

17.6. DIAGNOSIS OF DVT

The American Academy of Family Physicians and the American College of Physicians have formulated a joint guideline, released in 2007, on the diagnosis of VTE in primary care (hereafter *AAFP/ACP Diagnosis of VTE Guidelines*), on which this discussion is based *(39)*. The first step in diagnosing a lower extremity DVT is to determine the pretest probability, which can be done using clinical prediction rules. Wells et al. have developed clinical prediction rules for both DVT and PE, which are commonly referred to as the Wells score. The Wells scoring system for lower extremity DVT is shown in Table 3 *(40)*. A score ≤0 denotes low probability of having a DVT, a score of 1–2 denotes intermediate probability of DVT, and a score of ≥3 denotes high probability *(39, 40)*. The incidence of DVT in the low, intermediate, and high groups is 5, 17, and 53%, respectively *(41, 42)*.

Table 3
The Wells Clinical Prediction Rule for DVT

Clinical feature	Score
Active cancer (treatment ongoing, within previous 6 months, or palliative)	1
Paralysis, paresis, or recent plaster immobilization of the lower extremities	1
Recently bedridden >3 days or major surgery within 12 weeks requiring general or regional anesthesia	1
Localized tenderness along the distribution of the deep venous system	1
Entire leg swollen	1
Calf swelling 3 cm larger than asymptomatic side (measured 10 cm below tibial tuberosity)	1
Pitting edema confined to the symptomatic leg	1
Collateral superficial veins (non-varicose)	1
Alternative diagnosis at least as likely as deep venous thrombosis	−2

Taken from *(39)*. Based on a rule in *(40)*.

Patients with a low pretest probability of DVT should have a D-dimer assay checked. An elevated D-dimer is results from endogenous lysis of the fibrin in a thrombus *(43)*. Patients in whom there is a low pretest probability of DVT who have a negative high-sensitivity D-dimer (sensitivity ≥96%, generally an ELISA) usually do not need to undergo further testing to exclude lower extremity DVT. Patients who have a positive D-dimer should undergo lower extremity ultrasound examination. If the ultrasound is negative, then the diagnosis of DVT has been reasonably excluded. If the ultrasound is positive, then the patient is diagnosed with DVT and should be treated accordingly. If the ultrasound is non-diagnostic, then it should be repeated, or contrast venography, which remains the gold standard test, should be considered. This approach is illustrated in Fig. 3 *(41)*.

A number of caveats apply when it comes to the use of the Wells score and the D-dimer assay. The Wells score may perform less well in patients who are elderly and who have many comorbidities *(39, 44)*. The D-dimer assay also may be a less accurate tool in the elderly (primarily because of a poor specificity) and in patients who have longstanding symptoms suggestive of VTE *(39, 43, 45)*.

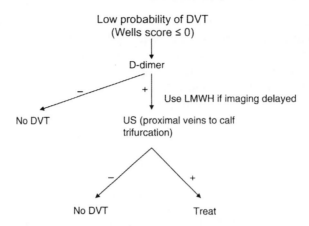

Fig. 3. Diagnostic approach to the patient with a low pretest probability of DVT. Reprinted, with alterations, from *(41)* with permission from Wiley–Blackwell. DVT = deep vein thrombosis, LMWH = low molecular weight heparin, US = ultrasound.

Conditions other than VTE can lead to an elevated D-dimer assay, including infection, inflammation, cancer, and pregnancy. This results in the D-dimer assay having a high sensitivity (86–99%) but a low specificity (34–44%) *(43, 46)*. Therefore, clinical judgment must be exercised when applying this and other algorithms, especially when they are used with patients who meet those conditions in which Wells criteria and the D-dimer assay perform less well. However, a systematic review has concluded that a low pretest probability using the Wells score in conjunction with a negative high-sensitivity D-dimer assay can effectively rule out DVT *(47)*.

Patients with a Wells score of ≥1, who therefore have an intermediate or high pretest probability of DVT, need to undergo ultrasound evaluation of the lower extremity to assess for DVT. If the lower extremity ultrasound is positive for DVT, then the diagnosis is made. The *AAFP/ACP Diagnosis of VTE Guidelines*, however, provides limited guidance regarding under what circumstances, when the lower extremity ultrasound is negative, should the ultrasound be repeated to adequately rule out DVT. Previously, it had been recommended that a negative ultrasound be repeated in a week to adequately exclude the diagnosis of DVT *(48)*. The guidelines say the ultrasound may need to be repeated if it is suspected the DVT is in the calf, an area for which ultrasound diagnosis is less sensitive, or if the ultrasound is technically limited or equivocal. It is important to remember that the sensitivity of the lower extremity ultrasound is dependent on the vascular technician performing the study. The use of the D-dimer in this setting of patients with an intermediate or high pretest probability of DVT, while inadequate to exclude the diagnosis of DVT, can help determine whether a repeat ultrasound 1 week after an initial negative ultrasound is necessary. Patients with a negative D-dimer and negative ultrasound have had the diagnosis of DVT effectively excluded, so a repeat ultrasound after 1 week is not necessary *(41, 49, 50)*. Patients with a positive D-dimer and an initial negative ultrasound should have this ultrasound repeated in 1 week to adequately exclude DVT. If there is going to be a delay in obtaining the initial ultrasound, then treating the patient with low molecular weight heparin should be considered until the initial ultrasound is obtained, depending on the level of clinical suspicion. This approach is illustrated in Fig. 4 *(41)*. In interpreting the ultrasound report, one potential pitfall to be avoided concerns the superficial femoral vein, which, despite its name, is part of the deep venous system *(51)*. Hence a thrombus detected in the superficial femoral vein should be treated as a DVT.

It should be noted that this discussion adheres to the AAFP/ACP guidelines in which a patient's pretest probability is categorized as low risk (Wells score ≤0), intermediate risk (Wells score 1–2), or high risk (Wells score ≥3). Some authors, including Wells, advocate a dichotomous categorization of pretest probability, in which the pretest probability of a DVT is considered unlikely with a Wells score

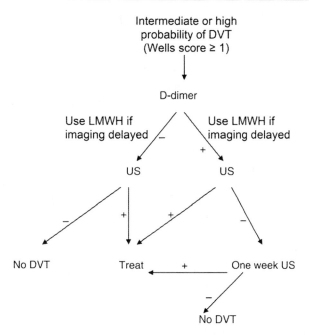

Fig. 4. Diagnostic approach to the patient with intermediate or high pretest probability of DVT. Reprinted, with alterations, from *(41)* with permission from Wiley–Blackwell. DVT = deep vein thrombosis, LMWH = low molecular weight heparin, US = ultrasound.

≤1 and likely with a Wells score ≥2. Under this scheme, patients with a Wells score ≤1 are generally evaluated like the patients with a low pretest probability under the *AAFP/ACP Diagnosis of VTE Guidelines*, and patients with a Wells score ≥2 are generally evaluated like patients with intermediate or high pretest probabilities under the *AAFP/ACP Diagnosis of VTE Guidelines (41, 52)*.

17.7. TREATMENT OF DVT

Two major guidelines exist addressing the treatment of VTE. One, released in 2008 by the American College of Chest Physicians (ACCP), is exhaustive in scope *(27)*. The second, released in 2007 by the American College of Physicians (ACP), is less comprehensive and more straightforward *(28, 53)*. Both will be referenced during this discussion.

17.7.1. Initial Treatment

For the initial treatment of a confirmed lower extremity DVT, although either IV unfractionated heparin (UFH) or subcutaneous (SC) low molecular weight heparin (LMWH) may be used *(27)*, LMWH is preferred *(28)*. The basis for the preference for LMWH is twofold. First, given the dosing complexities of IV UFH, its use often results in inadequate initial anticoagulation *(54)*. Second, compared to IV UFH, use of LMWH results in better outcomes, including lower mortality rates *(55–57)*.

An additional benefit of LMWH compared to IV UFH is that the incidence of heparin-induced thrombocytopenia (HIT) is lower with LMWH, though this decreased HIT incidence with LMWH has been demonstrated more clearly in patients receiving prophylactic doses rather than treatment doses of heparin *(58, 59)*. A meta-analysis of 15 studies found a reduction in the incidence of HIT with LMWH thromboprophylaxis as compared to UFH, with an overall odds ratio of 0.47 ($p = 0.06$). When only the randomized controlled trials were considered, the odds ratio was 0.10 ($p = 0.03$) *(58)*.

There is little data on the relative efficacy of different LMWHs compared to one another in treating DVT. One analysis suggested that dalteparin had a lower rate of major hemorrhage but a higher rate of DVT recurrence *(60)*. In general, LMWH therapy is inappropriate in patients with significant renal insufficiency (e.g., creatinine clearance ≤60 mL/min), who should instead be treated with IV UFH *(27, 61)*. One exception is enoxaparin, which has a dosing adjustment for patients with renal insufficiency. Another option for initial treatment of DVT is SC fondaparinux, which, along with LMWH and IV UFH, is also considered first-line treatment for DVT in the *ACCP VTE Treatment Guidelines (27)*. Fondaparinux—which binds antithrombin, resulting in inhibition of factor Xa and reduced activation of prothrombin *(62)*—at a dose of 7.5 mg/sc daily for patients weighing 50–100 kg has been shown to be at least as effective as the LMWH enoxaparin for the initial treatment of DVT *(63)*. Anticoagulation dosing, including dosing in patients with renal insufficiency, is discussed below in a separate section.

In general, warfarin should be started concomitantly with heparin. When using LMWH, the routine checking of anti-factor Xa levels to monitor the level of anticoagulation is not necessary. When transitioning a patient from heparin (either LMWH of IV UFH) to warfarin, the heparin should be continued for at least 5 days and until the INR has been between 2.0 and 3.0 for at least 24 h *(27)*. Long-term LMWH (rather than initial LMWH followed by a transition to warfarin) may be used in the treatment of DVT. Long-term LMWH may be preferred in patients with cancer, given data showing that in patients with VTE and cancer, patients who received 5–7 days of LMWH as a transition to warfarin had a higher rate of recurrent VTE than those patients treated with long-term LMWH *(28, 64)*. The *ACCP VTE Treatment Guidelines* also list monitored SC UFH and fixed-dose SC UFH as first-line options for initial treatment to DVT *(27)*. However, these are less commonly used in practice than LMWH and IV UFH, and we recommend LMWH for initial treatment of DVT.

17.7.2. Duration of Anticoagulation

Regarding duration of anticoagulation, an initial DVT that is idiopathic, without evident risk factor, should be anticoagulated for at least 3 months, according to the *ACCP VTE Treatment Guidelines (27)*. We believe that anticoagulation for an idiopathic DVT should be for at least 6 months and that serious consideration should be given to long-term anticoagulation with ongoing assessment of the risks and benefits, which is what is recommended by the *ACP VTE Treatment Guidelines (28)*. Demonstrating the benefit of extended anticoagulation for initial idiopathic DVT, Kearon et al. randomized 162 patients with a first episode of idiopathic DVT who had already been anticoagulated for 3 months either to further anticoagulation with coumadin (INR goal 2.0–3.0) for an additional 24 months or to placebo. This trial was terminated early due to a rate of recurrent VTE of 27.4% per patient-year in the placebo group compared to 1.3% per patient-year in the coumadin group ($p < 0.001$). The rate of bleeding was higher in the coumadin group at 3.8% per patient-year compared to 0% per patient-year in the placebo group ($p = 0.09$), though none of the bleeding events were fatal *(65)*.

Patients with an initial DVT in the setting of a transient risk factor, such as recent surgery, should be anticoagulated for 3–6 months. One prospective study that addressed this issue enrolled 165 patients with an initial DVT due to a transient risk factor and compared 1 month of anticoagulation with 3 months of anticoagulation. Over a mean duration of follow-up of 10.5 months, the group that was anticoagulated for 3 months had a lower rate of recurrent VTE (3.7%) than the group that was anticoagulated for 1 month (6.0%). There were no major bleeding events in either group *(66)*.

Patients who have a recurrent DVT should be anticoagulated indefinitely. This issue was studied in a multicenter trial in which 227 patients with a second episode of VTE were enrolled (193 DVT and 34 PE) *(67)*. Patients were randomized to 6 months of anticoagulation or indefinite anticoagulation. Anticoagulation was with coumadin with a goal INR of 2.0–2.85. Over a follow-up period of 4 years, 2.6% of patients in the indefinite anticoagulation group experienced a recurrent VTE, compared to 20.7% in the group who received 6 months of anticoagulation, yielding a relative risk of 8.0. There was a trend toward an increased risk of hemorrhage in the group receiving indefinite anticoagulation and no significant overall mortality difference between the two groups.

Table 4 shows the recommended duration of anticoagulation in different situations as recommended by the *American College of Chest Physicians VTE Treatment Guidelines* and the *American College of Physicians VTE Treatment Guidelines*.

Table 4
Recommended Duration of Anticoagulation

	Per ACCP guidelines	*Per ACP guidelines*
DVT due to transient risk factor (e.g., recent surgery)	3 months	3–6 months
Initial idiopathic (unprovoked) DVT	≥3 months seriously consider long-term anticoagulation	Consider extended-duration anticoagulation
Recurrent idiopathic (unprovoked) DVT	Long-term anticoagulation	≥12 months. Consider extended-duration anticoagulation
DVT and cancer	For as long as cancer is active. LMWH should be used for first 3–6 months	

ACCP guidelines *(27)*, ACP guidelines *(28)*.

17.7.3. Outpatient Treatment of DVT

One important advantage of LMWH is that it allows for patients to be treated for DVT with either a brief hospital stay or as an outpatient. Programs designed to allow outpatient treatment of acute DVT with LMWH have been successful, with important elements of such programs including patient education, careful monitoring at home with frequent (e.g., twice daily) home visits by a visiting nurse, and close follow-up with the patient's primary care physician *(68)*. Randomized trials of inpatient IV UFH versus outpatient LMWH *(69, 70)* and of inpatient LMWH versus outpatient LMWH *(71)* have shown outpatient LMWH to be at least as safe and effective as inpatient treatment. Moreover, treatment with outpatient LMWH results in cost savings, with one study concluding that the use of enoxaparin led to cost savings of $1,151 per patient *(72)*, and is associated with increased patient quality of life *(73)*. Potential contraindications to outpatient treatment of DVT include concern for PE, risk factors for active bleeding, past DVT, hypercoagulability, pregnancy, high risk for falls, barriers to compliance (such as dementia), and other acute conditions (such as cellulitis or dehydration) *(68)*. Although many of the trials of outpatient LMWH for treatment of DVT have excluded patients with cancer, in the absence of other factors preventing outpatient treatment, cancer is not an absolute contraindication to outpatient management of DVT *(74)*.

17.7.4. Thrombolysis

In addition to anticoagulation, thrombolysis is another potential treatment for acute DVT. One randomized trial found that thrombolysis performed on patients with DVT less than 10 days old, followed by anticoagulation, achieved greater rates of venous patency than anticoagulation alone *(75)*. The clinical implications of higher patency rates with thrombolysis are not entirely clear *(76)*. There are some retrospective data that suggest thrombolysis, in addition to anticoagulation, and may result in fewer symptoms of post-thrombotic syndrome and improved overall physical functioning compared to anticoagulation alone *(77)*. The *ACCP VTE Treatment Guidelines* state that patients with extensive proximal DVT <14 days old, good functional status, life expectancy >1 year, and a low bleeding risk can be considered for catheter-directed thrombolysis *(27)*. The *ACP VTE Treatment Guidelines* conclude that there are too little data to make recommendations on the role of thrombolysis in the treatment of DVT *(28)*.

17.7.5. Isolated Calf DVT

A DVT that is isolated to the calf (i.e., a distal DVT) is less hazardous than a more proximal DVT involving the thigh *(78)*. A study using venography in patients with symptomatic DVT found that 23% of them were isolated to the calf vein *(79)*. There is a risk that a calf DVT could extend more proximally, estimated in one study to occur in about 10% of cases *(80)*. This risk is part of the reason for the practice of performing repeat ultrasounds when evaluating patients for DVT *(81)*.

One analysis compared pooled data from studies in which the decision to anticoagulate was based on whether a DVT was detected using ultrasound examination of the proximal veins with studies using ultrasound examination of both the proximal and distal veins. Ultrasound examination of both the proximal and distal veins, thereby allowing detection and treatment of distal DVT, did not lead to a significantly lower 3-month thromboembolic rate than examination of the proximal veins alone (0.4 versus 0.6%). This finding raises the question of whether the benefits outweigh the risks for anticoagulation of isolated distal DVT *(80, 81)*. The importance of diagnosing distal DVT is a matter of debate *(82, 83)*, and the absence of prospective randomized trials on the issue precludes firm conclusions. Current guidelines from the American College of Chest Physicians recommend 3 months of anticoagulation for a spontaneous isolated distal DVT *(27)*. In certain patients, such as those with bilateral distal DVT, consideration should be given to treating as if the patient had a proximal DVT, given data suggesting that patients with bilateral distal DVT have similar outcomes to patients with proximal DVT *(84)*. Post-thrombotic syndrome (discussed below) can be seen with distal DVT *(85)*, providing additional impetus to treat them.

17.8. POST-THROMBOTIC SYNDROME

One potential complication of DVT is the post-thrombotic syndrome. Common symptoms of post-thrombotic syndrome include leg heaviness, pain, paresthesias, and cramps, with accompanying signs including edema, hyperpigmentation, erythema, and ulcers. Symptoms may be worse with activity *(86)*. In a cohort of 180 patients with an initial DVT, who were randomized to below-knee compression stockings or no stockings for 2 years, in addition to standard anticoagulation treatment, post-thrombotic syndrome developed in 49% of the control patients who did not wear the stockings. These symptoms were severe in 11% of the control patients. In contrast, among the patients who wore the stockings, post-thrombotic syndrome symptoms developed in 26% of patients and were severe in 3% of patients *(87)*. Other studies have also found a benefit to the use of elastic compression stockings in preventing post-thrombotic syndrome *(88)*. Therefore, as recommended in both the *ACP Treatment Guidelines* and *ACCP VTE Treatment Guidelines*, elastic compression stockings (pressure 30–40 mmHg at the ankle) should be used as soon as possible after a DVT has been diagnosed and anticoagulation started, and definitely within 1 month of diagnosis, and should be continued for at least 2 years *(27, 28)*.

17.9. VTE PROPHYLAXIS IN HOSPITALIZED PATIENTS

It is important to take appropriate measures to prevent VTE among hospitalized patients—known as thromboprophylaxis. Thromboprophylaxis is underutilized among hospitalized patients, with only 54% of patients receiving any VTE prophylaxis and only 33% of patients receiving low-dose unfractionated heparin (LDUH) or LMWH *(89)*. A recent meta-analysis of 36 studies examined different approaches to pharmacological thromboprophylaxis among hospitalized medical patients. This study found that both LDUH and LMWH significantly reduced the risk of DVT. LDUH at a dose of 5,000 units sc tid was more effective than 5,000 units sc bid. Compared to LDUH, LMWH was more effective in preventing DVT and had a lower incidence of injection site hematoma. There was no difference in the bleeding rate between the two agents. Neither LDUH nor LMWH demonstrated a reduction in mortality *(90)*. Options for LMWH include enoxaparin 40 mg sc once daily and dalteparin 5,000 U sc once daily *(91)*. Fondaparinux 2.5 mg sc once daily is also effective for thromboprophylaxis in hospitalized medical patients *(92)*. Patients with renal failure present a challenge. LDUH is probably preferred to LMWH is patients with significant renal insufficiency *(93)*. One study found that dalteparin 5,000 IU sc once daily did not lead to excessive anticoagulant effect in a population of 138 critical care patients with severe renal insufficiency (creatinine clearance <30 mL/min) *(94)*. Table 5 shows levels of VTE risk for hospitalized patients and the recommended thromboprophylaxis measures for the different risk levels *(95)*.

Table 5
VTE Risk and Recommended Thromboprophylaxis for Hospitalized Patients

Levels of risk	Approximate DVT risk without thromboprophylaxis (%)	Suggested thromboprophylaxis options
Low risk		
Minor surgery in mobile patients	<10	No specific thromboprophylaxis
Medical patients who are fully mobile		Early and "aggressive" ambulation
Moderate risk		
Most general, open gynecologic or urologic surgery patient	10–40	LMWH (at recommended doses), LDUH bid or tid, fondaparinux
Medical patients, bed rest, or sick		
Moderate VTE risk plus high bleeding risk		Mechanical thromboprophylaxis
High risk		
Hip or knee arthroplasty, HFS	40–80	LMWH (at recommended doses),
Major trauma, SCI		fondaparinux, oral VKA (INR 2–3)
High VTE risk plus high bleeding risk		Mechanical thromboprophylaxis

Mechanical thromboprophylaxis includes intermittent pneumatic compression devices and graduated compression stockings.

Taken from *(95)*.

HFS = hip fracture surgery, SCI = spinal cord injury, LMWH = low molecular weight heparin, LDUH = low-dose unfractionated heparin, VKA = vitamin K antagonist.

Statins may decrease the rate of VTE. The Justification for the Use of Statins in Prevention: An Intervention Trial Evaluating Rosuvastatin (JUPITER) trial enrolled nearly 18,000 subjects with low LDL levels (<130 mg/dL) and elevated C-reactive protein levels (>2.0 mg/L), who were randomized to rosuvastatin 20 mg daily or placebo, and had as its primary endpoint cardiac events *(96)*. A pre-specified secondary endpoint was a first occurrence of VTE. Over a median follow-up period of 1.9 years, the overall rate of VTE was 0.18 events per 100 person-years of follow-up in the group that received rosuvastatin, compared to 0.32 events per 100 person-years of follow-up in the placebo group ($p = 0.007$). The rates of unprovoked VTE were 0.10 and 0.17 in the rosuvastatin and placebo groups, respectively ($p = 0.09$), and the corresponding rates for provoked VTE were 0.08 and 0.16 ($p = 0.03$). A greater effect was seen in the prevention of DVT than in the prevention of PE *(97)*.

17.10. DIAGNOSIS OF PE

PE can be a challenging diagnosis to make, with the most common symptoms being dyspnea (at rest or with exertion), pleuritic chest pain, cough, orthopnea, wheezing, and non-pleuritic chest pain. In assessing a patient for PE, attention must be paid to symptoms of DVT, as calf or thigh pain and swelling are common symptoms in patients with PE *(98, 99)*. The first step in diagnosing PE involves determining pretest probability. The most commonly used clinical prediction rule for PE, also developed by Wells, is shown in Table 6 *(100)*. Following a diagnostic approach set forth by van Belle et al. *(101)*, patients with scores of ≤4 points are categorized as unlikely to have a PE, whereas patients with scores of ≥5 points are categorized as likely to have a PE. Patients categorized as unlikely to have PE can then undergo D-dimer testing, which, if negative, reasonably excludes PE. Patients initially categorized as unlikely to have PE but with a positive D-dimer and patients initially categorized as likely to have PE should undergo a PE-protocol CT using a multidetector CT scanner (PE CT). In most patients in whom the CT scan is negative, PE has been reasonably excluded. There is controversy over whether patients in whom there is a high clinical suspicion of PE can be considered to have the diagnosis of PE excluded by a negative PE CT scan alone. This issue is discussed further below.

Table 6
The Wells clinical prediction rule for PE

Clinical feature	*Score*
Clinical signs and symptoms of DVT (minimum of leg swelling and pain with palpation of the deep veins)	3.0
An alternative diagnosis is less likely than PE	3.0
Heart rate greater than 100 bpm	1.5
Immobilization or surgery in the previous 4 weeks	1.5
Previous DVT/PE	1.5
Hemoptysis	1.0
Malignancy (on treatment, treated in the last 6 months, or palliative)	1.0

Taken from *(100)*.

Patients with a PE CT scan positive for PE should be treated for a PE. Patients in whom the PE CT scan is non-diagnostic should undergo additional testing, with options including pulmonary angiography, ventilation–perfusion (V/Q) scanning, or magnetic resonance angiography. This approach is summarized in Fig. 5 *(101)*. In a study cohort of 3,306 patients (82% of whom were outpatients) validating this approach, the primary endpoint was VTE in patients during a 3-month follow-up period. This endpoint was reached in 0.5% of patients, categorized as PE unlikely and with a negative D-dimer, and in 1.3% of patients who had PE excluded on the basis of a negative PE CT scan *(101)*. The conditions under which this approach was validated included using a high-sensitivity D-dimer assay, with a cutoff between positive and negative of 500 ng/mL, and multidetector row CT scanning. This approach may not be applicable under different conditions, and the local radiological expertise in diagnosing PE using CT scanning needs to be taken into account. High respiratory rates, obesity, timing of the contrast bolus, age of the pulmonary embolism, and the expertise of the radiologist may influence the result. *The AAFP/ACP Diagnosis of VTE Guidelines* provide only limited guidance on the diagnosis of PE. The guidelines advocate use of the Wells prediction rule for PE and suggest that patients who are felt to be at intermediate (Wells score 2–6) or high (Wells score ≥7) clinical probability for PE undergo diagnostic imaging, with options including a V/Q scan, PE CT scan, or pulmonary angiography. The guidelines express a concern over whether the sensitivity of PE CT scanning is adequate to exclude PE in patients who are felt to have a high pretest probability of PE *(39)*. In patients in whom there is a high clinical probability for PE, whether a negative PE CT scan is

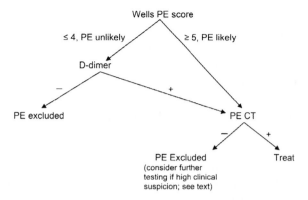

Fig. 5. Diagnostic approach to the patient with suspected PE. Based on the algorithm set forth in *(101)*. PE = pulmonary embolism, PE CT = pulmonary embolism protocol CT.

adequate to exclude a PE is controversial *(102, 103)*. In a thoughtful analysis of this issue, recent European guidelines on the diagnosis of PE conclude that this matter is "not settled" *(104)*. Therefore, in patients in whom there is a high clinical probability of PE but a negative PE CT scan, serious consideration should be given to obtaining additional testing. Options for additional testing include a V/Q scan, pulmonary angiography, and serial ultrasounds *(102)*. Magnetic resonance angiography is also an option *(105, 106)*.

17.11. TREATMENT OF PE

Many of the same considerations apply to the treatment of PE as to DVT. Indeed, some of the clinical trials on which PE treatment recommendations are based were conducted in patients with VTE, inclusive of both PE and DVT *(55)*.

17.11.1. Initial Treatment

Anticoagulation is the principal treatment for PE, and, if the suspicion for PE is high, should be started while diagnostic testing is under way, taking into consideration the risk of bleeding. For patients with submassive (i.e., hemodynamically stable) PE, anticoagulation may be initiated with either IV UFH or LMWH. Trials comparing IV UFH and LMWH have demonstrated that LMWH is at least as good as IV UFH for treatment of PE *(107–109)*, and possibly superior to IV UFH *(57, 110)*. In patients with significant renal insufficiency, IV UFH is preferred over LMWH due to the possibility of excessive anticoagulation from accumulation of LMWH when the level of anticoagulation is not monitored. A trial comparing fondaparinux with IV UFH in treatment of PE concluded that fondaparinux was at least as effective as IV UFH *(111)*. Therefore, either IV UFH, LMWH, or fondaparinux are considered first-line treatments for acute PE *(27, 104)*. Although, as discussed in an earlier section, there are data to suggest that LMWH may be superior to IV UFH in the treatment of acute DVT, extensive data are lacking that LMWH is superior to IV UFH for treatment of acute PE *(57)*. The *ACCP VTE Treatment Guidelines* also consider monitored SC UFH and fixed-dose SC UFH as treatment options for PE, though these are not suggested by recent European guidelines *(104)*. Monitored SC UFH and fixed-dose SC UFH are less commonly used in practice than the other anticoagulation options listed, and we do not recommend them. The outpatient treatment of PE, which has been suggested *(112)*, is not advisable at this time, given our limited ability to accurately risk stratify patients with PE and the fact that we do not have substantial prospective clinic trial data to support this approach *(113)*. Certain biomarkers do have prognostic value in acute pulmonary embolism. For example, elevated troponin levels are associated with worse short-term outcomes in patients with acute PE *(114)*, as are markedly elevated BNP *(115, 116)*, and D-dimer values *(117)*. In this setting, the elevated troponins and BNP are probably indicative of right heart dysfunction from severe PE, and the D-dimer a marker for the embolic burden *(115–118)*. The use of these biomarkers in the development of prognostic models is an active area of investigation *(118)*.

Some different issues need to be considered in patients with massive PE, which is defined as a PE resulting in hypotension. Some authors prefer IV UFH in the treatment of massive PE, since the trials demonstrating the efficacy of LMWH generally excluded massive PE *(104)*. Even more importantly, patients with massive PE should be considered for thrombolysis. Patients who have cardiogenic shock resulting from a PE should undergo rapid thrombolysis, unless contraindicated due to the bleeding risk *(4, 27, 119)*. Consultation with subspecialists, such as a cardiologist or pulmonologist, should be promptly obtained in cases of massive PE.

The transition from heparin to coumadin in acute PE is similar to that with acute DVT. Patients should be started on coumadin at the same time they are started on heparin. The patient should be continued on heparin for at least 5 days and for at least 24 h with an INR between 2.0 and 3.0. As with DVT, there are data suggesting that patients with cancer and acute PE should be treated with LMWH for at least 6 months because this results in a lower rate of recurrent VTE than treatment with LMWH for only 5–7 days before transitioning to Coumadin *(64)*.

17.11.2. *Duration of Anticoagulation*

The recommended duration of anticoagulation for PE is similar to that for DVT. For patients with a PE due to a transient risk factor, the *ACCP VTE Treatment Guidelines* recommend anticoagulation for 3 months *(27)*, whereas the *ACP VTE Treatment Guidelines* recommend 3–6 months *(28)*. We believe anticoagulation for at least 6 months is appropriate in cases of PE attributable to a transient risk factor. For patients with an idiopathic PE, anticoagulation should be for at least 3 months and should probably be long term, subject to an assessment of the patient's bleeding risk. For patients with a recurrent PE, anticoagulation should be long term. For patients with PE in the setting of cancer, they should be anticoagulated until the cancer has gone into remission, and, if possible, should receive LMWH rather than coumadin for at least the first 6 months of their anticoagulation *(27, 104)*.

Even more so with PE than for DVT, long-term anticoagulation should be considered in patients with a first episode of idiopathic PE, because when a patient has a recurrent VTE, the patient tends to have the same type of VTE. Patients whose initial VTE is a DVT are more likely to have another DVT as their recurrent VTE, and patients whose initial VTE is a PE are more likely to have another PE as their recurrent VTE *(120)*. For patient receiving long-term anticoagulation, there must be an ongoing assessment of this risks and benefits of continuing anticoagulation.

17.12. ANTICOAGULATION DOSING

The LMWH agents used in treatment of VTE include enoxaparin, dalteparin, and tinzaparin. Fondaparinux may also be used. The doses discussed in this section apply to VTE treatment, not VTE prophylaxis.

The recommended dose of enoxaparin for treatment of VTE is 1 mg/kg sc every 12 h or 1.5 mg/kg sc once daily *(121)*. In a trial involving 900 patients with symptomatic lower extremity DVT, the once-daily and twice-daily enoxaparin dosing was found to be equally effective as unfractionated heparin. There was a statistically non-significant trend toward higher rates of recurrent VTE in obese patients and patients with cancer who received the once-daily dosing of enoxaparin as compared to the twice-daily dosing *(107)*. Therefore, in these two patient populations, the twice-daily dosing of enoxaparin is preferred. In patients with severe renal impairment (creatinine clearance <30 mL/min), the dose should be adjusted to enoxaparin 1 mg/kg sc once daily (122). There is a lack of consensus about the best way to dose enoxaparin in obese patients. Some authors assert that no dosage adjustment is necessary when using enoxaparin in obese patients (123). However, when using enoxaparin or any of the LMWHs in obese patients, anti-factor Xa levels should be monitored with the assistance of pharmacy or hematology consultants. Patients at the opposite extreme, with a low body weight (women <45 kg and men <57 kg), are at increased risk of bleeding, and the monitoring of anti-factor Xa levels should also be considered (122).

The usual dose for dalteparin in the treatment of VTE is 200 units/kg sc once daily for 1 month, and then 150 units/kg sc once daily thereafter (studied for up to 5 months) (64). The maximum recommended dose is 18,000 units daily (124). The efficacy of dalteparin in treating VTE is based on one study in cancer patients (64). There is little human data on which to base recommendations for renal dosing of dalteparin, and so it should be used cautiously in patients with renal insufficiency (125). If it is used in patients with impaired renal function, anti-Xa levels should be monitored so that the proper dose can be determined (124). Dalteparin should also be used with caution in patients weighing <45 kg or >90 kg, and monitoring of anti-Xa levels should be undertaken (126). Although the package insert recommends not exceeding a dose of 18,000 units daily (124), one group has reported using dalteparin 200 units/kg sc once daily for 5–7 days based on the actual weight of 193 obese patients weighing >90 kg with no bleeding events related to the dalteparin (127).

The recommended dose of tinzaparin in the treatment of VTE is 175 units/kg sc once daily (121, 128). A study of tinzaparin in 37 obese subjects concluded that dosing based on body weight was appropriate in this population (129), which is what the manufacturer recommends (128). Furthermore, the manufacturer recommends against the use of tinzaparin in patients 90 years of age or older, or in patients with creatinine clearance ≤60 mL/min (128).

Fondaparinux is dosed at 7.5 mg sc daily for patients weighing between 50 and 100 kg. Fondaparinux should be dosed at 5 mg sc daily in patients weighing <50 kg and 10 mg sc daily in patients weighing >100 kg (63). Fondaparinux should not be used in patients with creatinine clearance <30 mL/min (130).

When using IV UFH heparin for the treatment of DVT, an initial bolus should be used (80 U/kg or 5,000 U) followed by a continuous infusion (initially at a dose of 18 U/kg/h or 1,300 U/h) (27). Thereafter, the dose should be adjusted based on the activated partial thromboplastin time (APTT). A standard nomogram for adjusting the dose of IV UFH is shown below in Table 7 (27, 131). Institution-specific heparin nomograms should be used when available, given variability in reagents used for APTT measurement and other factors.

Table 7
Standard nomogram for adjusting the dose of IV UFH

APTT (s)	Repeat bolus dose (U)	Stop infusion (min)	Change rate (dose) of infusion, mL/h at 40 U/mL (U/24 h)	Time of next APTT (h)
<50	5,000	0	+3 (+2,880)	6
50–59	0	0	+3 (+2,880)	6
60–85	0	0	0 (0)	Next morning
86–95	0	0	−2 (−1,920)	Next morning
96–120	0	30	−2 (−1,920)	6
>120	0	60	−4 (−3,840)	6

Taken from (27). Based on nomogram in (131).

17.13. INFERIOR VENA CAVA FILTERS

Accepted indications for inferior vena cava (IVC) filters in the management of patients with VTE include patients with an absolute contraindication to anticoagulation, patients who need to stop their anticoagulation due to bleeding complications, and patients with pulmonary hypertension due to chronic PE (27, 132). Providing the only prospective clinic trial data on the use of IVC filters, the Prevention du Risque d'Embolie Pulmonaire par Interruption Cave (PREPIC) study randomized 400 patients with proximal DVT to either an IVC filter or no filter, in addition to standard anticoagulation. After 2 years (133) and 8 years of follow-up (134), the patients who received IVC filters had a decreased risk of PE, but an increased risk of recurrent DVT. There was no significant difference in survival between the two groups. Therefore, the routine placement of an IVC filter in patients with DVT who can safely receive anticoagulation is not recommended. Moreover, in patients with DVT who had IVC filters placed due to an inability to safely receive anticoagulation, if they are able to safely receive anticoagulation in the future, they should be anticoagulated for a standard period, because the filter increases the risk of recurrent DVT, even while decreasing the risk of PE (27). Recently, retrievable IVC filters have become available, though their clinical role is not clear. In patients in whom the indication for the IVC filter is temporary (e.g., the risk of DVT or the contraindication to anticoagulation is transient), the use of retrievable IVC filters seems reasonable. However, risks of the retrievable IVC filters include an inability to remove them, which occurs in 9% of patients (135), an observed pattern of them not being removed for unclear reasons (136), and clinicians being less rigorous in considering the indications for placement of filters that they believe will only be temporary (132).

17.14. VTE AND TRAVEL

The possibility of VTE in the setting of airline travel—so-called economy class syndrome—is a concern among patients. Indeed, this concern extends to medical professionals. In a survey at a conference of thrombosis experts, 80% of them reported using some sort of measure to prevent VTE when flying (137). The absolute risk of VTE associated with air travel is modest (95). In a cohort study of almost 9,000 people who took flights lasting >4 h, the absolute risk of symptomatic VTE was one episode per 4,656 flights (138). Another study, designed to determine the relative risk of travel, found that travel confers an approximately twofold increased risk of VTE compared to controls (139). Some of the greatest risk factors for VTE with travel include the factor V Leiden mutation, BMI >30, and the use of oral contraceptives. The risk of VTE is not limited to air travel and also exists with other modes of travel in which there is an extended period of immobility, such as travel by bus, car, or train (139). The longer the distance traveled, the greater the risk of VTE. A study conducted looking at travel-associated PE found that the risk was much higher in persons traveling >5,000 km (3,100 mi) (140). Most people who develop VTE associated with travel have additional risk factors for thrombosis (95).

Of the interventions that have been tried to prevent travel-associated VTE, the most widely studied is the use of compression stockings. A review of the studies in this area concluded that compression stockings reduce the incidence of asymptomatic DVT and leg edema. The data were inadequate to determine whether compression stockings affect the rate of symptomatic DVT, PE, or death (141). One study randomized 300 subjects at elevated risk for DVT taking long-haul flights to either no intervention, aspirin, or LMWH. The rate of DVT in the LMWH group was significantly lower than in the no intervention or aspirin groups (142).

The ACCP, in its guidelines on prevention of VTE, makes the following recommendations. All people taking flights lasting >8 h should be advised to avoid constrictive clothing, keep well hydrated, and frequently move their calf muscles. In addition to the above measures, in patients with additional risk factors for VTE, one can consider prescribing graduated compression stockings (providing

15–30 mmHg at the ankle) or a single dose of LMWH prior to the flight. Aspirin is not recommended for prophylaxis against travel-associated VTE *(95)*.

17.15. CASE STUDIES

17.15.1. Case 1

A 65-year-old female is seen in her primary care physician's office for follow-up after a 5-day hospitalization for an exacerbation of chronic obstructive lung disease. She has stopped smoking. She now reports that she is no longer producing sputum and her fever has resolved, but that she has developed progressive shortness of breath of sudden onset.

During her hospitalization 10 days ago, her admission CBC revealed a WBC of 13,000 per mm^3 with a mild left shift, a hematocrit of 36%, and a platelet count of 415,000 per mm^3. She was treated with levofloxacin for 5 days, unfractionated heparin 5,000 units subcutaneously three times a day and nebulizers as needed. In the hospital she had transient left calf pain, which she did not mention to her care providers because she assumed that it was from a pulled muscle. She did not receive extended thromboprophylaxis post-discharge.

On examination, her vital signs are notable for a blood pressure of 110/80 mmHg, pulse of 98 bpm, respiratory rate of 20 breaths/min, temperature of 98.2°F, and a room air oxygen saturation of 92% at rest. She has rales at her left base, but otherwise her lungs are clear. Her heart sounds are regular and there is a soft I/VI systolic murmur.

An EKG is notable for a regular heart rhythm, rate of 99 bpm, absence of changes of ischemia or of right heart strain, and non-specific ST–T wave abnormalities.

Chest x-ray (PA and lateral) performed in the office reveals resolving peripheral left lower lobe pneumonia and changes suggestive of chronic lung disease.

1. What is this patient's risk for hospital-acquired venous thromboembolism (VTE)?

The majority of VTE diagnoses are made in the ambulatory setting. This necessitates vigilance on the part of primary care providers whenever they see patients after discharge from inpatient facilities *(6)*. Of note, the three major trials—MEDENOX *(143)*, PREVENT *(144)*, and ARTEMIS *(92)*—showed that pharmacologic thromboprophylaxis in medical patients significantly reduced the overall incidence of VTE, with a low (but not 0) risk of bleeding. Current ACCP guidelines recommend pharmacologic thromboprophylaxis *(95)*, which this patient received.

This patient had a number of risk factors for VTE, including the following:

- Recent acute hospitalization. The precipitating situation is the most important factor to consider when assigning VTE risk *(16)*.
- Immobilization in the hospital and at discharge *(16)*.
- COPD at hospital admission. An independent predictor of the development of clinical VTE, COPD at hospital admission poses an overall relative risk of 1.92 for pulmonary embolism and 1.30 for deep venous thrombosis (DVT) *(145)*.
- Acute Infections. This patient had acute pneumonia, which increases the risk of her developing VTE *(23)*.

Based on her risk factors, this patient was at moderate risk of developing hospital-acquired VTE, possibly as high as 50%. VTE prophylaxis in the hospital with a pharmacologic agent in appropriate dose might be expected to reduce her risk by about 50%.

2. In a patient who is suspected of having a pulmonary embolism, what signs on physical examination should the examiner look for?

The history and physical examination provide important information in assessing whether a patient has a pulmonary embolism (PE). Historical clues to the possibility of acute PE include recent hospitalization, the development of rapid onset of shortness of breath at rest, and calf pain. According to the Prospective Investigation of Pulmonary Embolism Diagnosis (PIOPED) II study, the most common symptoms of acute PE are sudden dyspnea (at rest or with exertion), pleuritic chest pain, non-pleuritic chest pain, and cough, as well as symptoms of DVT, such as calf or thigh pain (98, 99). One should personally count the respiratory rate because tachypnea is a common sign of PE (98). Examine for signs of right heart strain (distended neck veins, a right ventricular heave, accentuated P_2, and a new soft systolic murmur of tricuspid regurgitation), and carefully examine the legs for cords or any evidence of DVT.

3. For patients with confirmed VTE following hospitalization, what test(s) should be performed?

Regarding laboratory tests, a complete blood count should always be checked in the setting of a suspicion for acute VTE, and a baseline serum creatinine if the patient is going to undergo a contrast PE-protocol CT. Among previously hospitalized patients, a significant number of patients may not have received appropriate thromboprophylaxis (146). Of those that did receive heparin within the previous 90–120 days, especially in prophylactic doses, heparin-induced thrombocytopenia may be a consideration, in addition to treatment failure. If there is a prior heparin exposure in the appropriate time frame, the presence of thrombocytopenia or a 50% reduction in the platelet count might be a clue to the complication of HIT (19).

4. How should this patient be treated?

This patient's hospital-acquired VTE was confirmed by a PE-protocol CT, which revealed bilateral PE and she was referred back to the hospital for admission. Retrospective chart review revealed that she had missed some of her doses of prophylactic subcutaneous unfractionated heparin (UFH) (requiring administration three times a day) during the index hospitalization when she was off the floor for testing. There was a low index of suspicion for HIT given her platelet count of 355,000 per mm^3 and further testing for HIT or underlying hypercoagulable states was not performed.

For hemodynamically stable patients, low molecular weight heparin (LMWH) is preferred to UFH for the treatment of VTE, including acute PE. This has to do with the ease of dosing that more reliably achieves therapeutic levels within 24 h, consideration of outpatient therapy, and lower incidence of HIT. LMWH or fondaparinux in therapeutic dosing is equally efficacious as IV UFH in the treatment of PE (111). One of these drugs should be prescribed to overlap with warfarin for a minimum of 5 days, and until the INR has been in the therapeutic range of 2.0–3.0 for at least 24 h (27).

Because this patient had no evidence of right ventricular failure on physical examination, negative biologic markers (e.g., troponin, BNP), which when elevated have been associated with adverse outcomes (114–116), and normal cardiac function, she was able to be discharged after an abbreviated hospital stay for further outpatient treatment of her PE with LMWH as a bridge to therapeutic anticoagulation with warfarin. 5 mg of warfarin was initially prescribed with the plan to adjust the dosage according to the INR for a total duration of 6 months.

17.15.2. Case 2

A 78-year-old man with myelodysplasia, spinal stenosis, osteoarthritis, and congestive heart failure from hypertensive heart disease presents to his primary care physician's office with a new problem, a swollen right leg. He recently had banged his left shin against a car door. Concerned about a possible infection, he saw a covering physician who prescribed cephalexin and advised him to keep his leg elevated as much as possible. For the last week, he has been sitting in a recliner for most of the day and would get up mainly for meals and to use the bathroom.

On examination, he appears his stated age. His vital signs are notable for a blood pressure of 110/80 mmHg, pulse of 92 bpm, a respiratory rate of 20 bpm, temperature of 98.2°F, and a room air oxygen saturation of 97% at rest. His physical examination is notable for bilateral leg swelling, more prominent in the right lower extremity.

1. What is this patient's risk for VTE?

This patient has a number of risk factors for VTE including the following:

- Age >75 years. Risk of VTE increases with age. Age >75 years is an independent risk factor for VTE *(147, 148)*.
- Myelodysplasia. The presence of a malignancy puts the patient at increased risk of VTE *(37)*.
- Congestive heart failure. Following worsening heart failure, death from cardiac arrhythmias, myocardial infarction, and stroke, PE has been reported as the fifth most common cause of death among CHF patients *(149)*. For hospitalized medical patients, the presence of heart failure is an independent risk factor for VTE with more than double the risk compared to patients without heart failure *(150)*.
- Immobility. Immobility may further exacerbate the circulatory stasis that may be present in this patient due to his history of heart failure *(16)*.
- Acute infection. Infections, such as urinary tract infection and respiratory tract infection, confer a roughly twofold increased risk of DVT *(151)*.

Based on his risk factors, this patient was at moderate risk for developing acute VTE as a complication of his treatment, which included instructions to keep his leg elevated at all times.

2. In a patient who is suspected of having a DVT, what signs on physical examination should the examiner look for?

On physical examination, a non-ambulatory patient may not have the usual symptoms of a DVT, such as a cramp or pulling sensation in the lower calf aggravated by walking. The absence of signs and symptoms of DVT in this patient population necessitates vigilance on the part of primary care providers to consider risk factors and perform a targeted physical examination. When a patient complains of a swollen leg, however, there may be clues to the presence of DVT. The practitioner should examine the lower extremities for asymmetry. When the deep venous system is involved, the saphenous veins may function as collaterals. There may be overlying erythema, warmth, and tenderness. There may be evidence of chronic venous insufficiency. When there is extensive clotting, as may occur in association with malignancy, the limb may appear cyanotic and the posterior tibial pulsations may be reduced or absent (phlegmasia cerulea dolens) *(152)*. In this patient, examining the lower extremities might reveal a palpable cord or evidence of venous collateralization.

3. How would you treat this patient?

The initial evaluation of the patient with suspected DVT requires confirmation by lower extremity noninvasive examination. Lower extremity ultrasound confirmed the presence of bilateral DVT involving the right superficial femoral vein and the left popliteal vein. Given his myelodysplasia, a CBC should be performed to check for severe anemia and thrombocytopenia. A platelet count <50,000 per mm^3 would greatly increase the risk of bleeding with therapeutic anticoagulation. Serum creatinine should be checked to estimate the creatinine clearance. Because the kidneys primarily clear anticoagulants, the dosage needs to be adjusted in patients with significant renal insufficiency. Otherwise, anticoagulants may accumulate and increase the risk of bleeding. The goals of DVT treatment are to prevent thrombus extension, early and late recurrent thromboembolism, and the post-thrombotic syndrome. LMWH is more effective than UFH because it has been reported to reduce symptomatic thromboembolic complications, bleeding, and mortality compared with UFH. Fondaparinux, a synthetic pentasaccharide, is an alternative agent that has the advantage of once-daily dosing *(63)*. Heparin should be overlapped with coumadin for at least 5 days and for at least 24 h with a therapeutic INR of 2.0–3.0 *(27)*. The duration of anticoagulation is not straightforward in this patient. His recent immobility increased his risk of DVT and hence he may have a reversible cause of his DVT. Nevertheless, myelodysplasia significantly increased his risk of recurrent DVT as well as bleeding should he develop significant thrombocytopenia. His clinicians elected to prescribe LMWH for 3 months time. Shortly after discontinuing LMWH, he developed recurrent DVT, and so LMWH was resumed. As for the majority of VTE patients, VTE was a lifelong disease for this patient.

4. In patients with confirmed deep venous thromboembolism (DVT), how do you decide which patients require hospital admission?

Because LMWH can be administered subcutaneously, it can be used as outpatient therapy. Appropriately selected patients may receive some or all of their DVT treatment in the outpatient setting, at substantially reduced cost, coupled with improved patient satisfaction, as compared with inpatient therapy *(153–155)*. Multiple studies have compared treatment with LMWH versus UFH for patients with VTE. Some of the studies included patients who were briefly admitted prior to randomization to the outpatient group, and all of the studies required patient education and home care support with close monitoring. Two randomized controlled trials comparing the effectiveness and safety of LMWH given on an outpatient basis subcutaneously twice daily with continuous IV UFH in the hospital found no difference in mortality, recurrence of DVT, development of thrombocytopenia, or bleeding complications *(69, 70)*. The ACP and the AAFP developed joint guidelines for the initial management of DVT, which state that LMWH rather than UFH is the preferred agent. Treatment of DVT as an outpatient with LMWH is safe and economical for selected patients and can be considered if adequate support services are available *(28)*. Patient selection for the outpatient management of VTE is based on compendium of randomized controlled trials and observational studies. Absolute contraindications include the following:

- Symptoms or signs of pulmonary embolism (shortness of breath, chest pain, syncope, elevated respiratory rate, new right-sided flow murmur or accentuated P_2).
- Symptoms or signs of arterial insufficiency (unable to walk secondary to severe pain, reduced or asymmetric peripheral pulses, or the presence of cerulea phlegmasia dolens).
- Active bleeding, positive stool guaiac, or recent GI bleeding.
- History of major surgery, trauma, or stroke within the previous 2 weeks.
- Severe renal dysfunction, hypertensive emergency, history of heparin sensitivity or HIT, suspected HIT with thrombosis, thrombocytopenia (<100,000).
- Active or major coexisting illness that may complicate outpatient LMWH treatment.
- Social or socioeconomic factors—e.g., homelessness, inability to understand what is going on, concerns about adherence, inability to purchase LMWH for outpatient use.

Relative contraindications include the following:

- High risk of bleeding complications (underlying liver disorder, history of familial bleeding disorder).
- Pregnancy.
- Morbid obesity.
- Advanced age (>75 years).
- Iliofemoral DVT.
- Acquired or congenital hypercoagulable states.

Because this patient did not have the presence of massive DVT, suspicion of heparin-induced thrombocytopenia with thrombosis, presence of symptomatic pulmonary embolism, high risk of bleeding with anticoagulant therapy, or the presence of comorbid conditions or other factors that require hospitalization, the plan was outpatient treatment of his DVT with LMWH. His estimated creatinine clearance was >30 mL/min. Support services, including an anticoagulation clinic, were available to this patient, who also had a primary care physician. Appropriate ancillary measures included are as follows:

- A prescription for below-knee compression stockings (30–40 mmHg), which have been shown to reduce the frequency of the post-thrombotic syndrome.
- Written and verbal instructions, given with an interpreter if the patient is non-English speaking, at the patient's educational level. The patient was asked to repeat back the information provided, including the name and telephone number of whom to call should problems arise (VNA and MD). The patient was

advised to limit activity to what is comfortable, elevate his feet 7–10° above the hips from time to time, and never place pillows under the popliteal fossa.

- A follow-up appointment in 5–7 days.
- Outreach calls by a nurse or physician to be sure that the patient is not having difficulty with the injections.

REFERENCES

1. Cushman M. Epidemiology and risk factors for venous thrombosis. *Semin Hematol.* 2007;44:62–69.
2. Sandler DA, Martin JF. Autopsy proven pulmonary embolism in hospital patients: are we detecting enough deep vein thrombosis? *J R Soc Med.* 1989;82:203–205.
3. Moser KM, Fedullo PF, LitteJohn JK, Crawford R. Frequent asymptomatic pulmonary embolism in patients with deep venous thrombosis. *JAMA.* 1994;271:223–225.
4. Tapson VF. Acute pulmonary embolism. *N Engl J Med.* 2008;358:1037–1052.
5. Laporte S, Mismetti P, Decousus H, et al. Clinical predictors for fatal pulmonary embolism in 15,520 patients with venous thromboembolism: findings from the Registro Informatizado de la Enfermedad TromboEmbolica venosa (RIETE) registry. *Circulation.* 2008;117:1711–1716.
6. Spencer FA, Lessard D, Emery C, Reed G, Goldberg RJ. Venous thromboembolism in the outpatient setting. *Arch Intern Med.* 2007;167:1471–1475.
7. Othieno R, Abu Affan M, Okpo E. Home versus in-patient treatment for deep vein thrombosis. *Cochrane Database Syst Rev.* 2007;3:CD003076.
8. Heit JA. The epidemiology of venous thromboembolism in the community: implications for prevention and management. *J Thromb Thrombolysis.* 2006;21:23–29.
9. White RH. The epidemiology of venous thromboembolism. *Circulation.* 2003;107:I4–I8.
10. Silverstein MD, Heit JA, Mohr DN, Petterson TM, O'Fallon WM, Melton LJ 3rd. Trends in the incidence of deep vein thrombosis and pulmonary embolism: a 25-year population-based study. *Arch Intern Med.* 1998;158:585–593.
11. Heit JA. The epidemiology of venous thromboembolism in the community. *Arterioscler Thromb Vasc Bio.* 2008;28:370–372.
12. Heit JA, Kobbervig CE, James AH, Petterson TM, Bailey KR, Melton LJ 3rd. Trends in the incidence of venous thromboembolism during pregnancy or postpartum: a 30-year population-based study. *Ann Intern Med.* 2005;143: 697–706.
13. White RH, Zhou H, Romano PS. Incidence of idiopathic deep venous thrombosis and secondary thromboembolism among ethnic groups in California. *Ann Intern Med.* 1998;128:737–740.
14. Ridker PM, Miletich JP, Hennekens CH, Buring JE. Ethnic distribution of factor V Leiden in 4047 men and women. Implications for venous thromboembolism screening. *JAMA.* 1997;277:1305–1307.
15. Anderson FA Jr., Spencer FA. Risk factors for venous thromboembolism. *Circulation.* 2003;107:I9–I16.
16. Heit JA, Silverstein MD, Mohr DN, Petterson TM, O'Fallon WM, Melton LJ 3rd. Risk factors for deep vein thrombosis and pulmonary embolism: a population-based case-control study. *Arch Intern Med.* 2000;160:809–815.
17. Goldhaber SZ. Outpatient venous thromboembolism: the importance of optimum prophylaxis. *Nat Clin Pract Cardiovasc Med.* 2008;5:12–13.
18. Levy JH, Hursting MJ. Heparin-induced thrombocytopenia, a prothrombotic disease. *Hematol–Oncol Clin N Am.* 2007;21:65–88.
19. Warkentin TE, Greinacher A, Koster A, Lincoff AM. Treatment and prevention of heparin-induced thrombocytopenia: American College of Chest Physicians Evidence-Based Clinical Practice Guidelines (8th ed.). *Chest.* 2008;133: 340S–380S.
20. Arepally GM, Ortel TL. Clinical practice. Heparin-induced thrombocytopenia. *N Engl J Med.* 2006;355:809–817.
21. Hansson PO, Sorbo J, Eriksson H. Recurrent venous thromboembolism after deep vein thrombosis: incidence and risk factors. *Arch Intern Med.* 2000;160:769–774.
22. Christiansen SC, Cannegieter SC, Koster T, Vandenbroucke JP, Rosendaal FR. Thrombophilia, clinical factors, and recurrent venous thrombotic events. *JAMA.* 2005;293:2352–2361.
23. Samama MM. An epidemiologic study of risk factors for deep vein thrombosis in medical outpatients: the Sirius study. *Arch Intern Med.* 2000;160:3415–3420.
24. Ray JG, Kearon C, Yi Q, Sheridan P, Lonn E. Homocysteine-lowering therapy and risk for venous thromboembolism: a randomized trial. *Ann Intern Med.* 2007;146:761–767.
25. den Heijer M, Willems HPJ, Blom HJ, et al. Homocysteine lowering by B vitamins and the secondary prevention of deep vein thrombosis and pulmonary embolism: a randomized, placebo-controlled, double-blind trial. *Blood.* 2007;109:139–144.

26. Dalen JE. Should patients with venous thromboembolism be screened for thrombophilia? *Am J Med.* 2008;121: 458–463.

27. Kearon C, Kahn SR, Agnelli G, et al. Antithrombotic therapy for venous thromboembolic disease: American College of Chest Physicians Evidence-Based Clinical Practice Guidelines (8th ed). *Chest.* 2008;133:454S–545S.

28. Snow V, Qaseem A, Barry P, et al. Management of venous thromboembolism: a clinical practice guideline from the American College of Physicians and the American Academy of Family Physicians. *Ann Intern Med.* 2007;146: 204–210.

29. Baglin T, Luddington R, Brown K, Baglin C. Incidence of recurrent venous thromboembolism in relation to clinical and thrombophilic risk factors: prospective cohort study. *Lancet.* 2003;362:523–526.

30. Ho WK, Hankey GJ, Quinlan DJ, Eikelboom JW. Risk of recurrent venous thromboembolism in patients with common thrombophilia: a systematic review. *Arch Intern Med.* 2006;166:729–736.

31. Perry SL, Ortel TL. Clinical and laboratory evaluation of thrombophilia. *Clin Chest Med.* 2003;24:153–170.

32. Whitlatch NL, Ortel TL. Thrombophilias: when should we test and how does it help?. *Semin Respir Crit Care Med.* 2008;29:25–39.

33. Bauer KA, Rosendaal FR, Heit JA. Hypercoagulability: too many tests, too much conflicting data. *Hematology.* 2002:353–368.

34. van Vlijmen EFW, Brouwer J-L P, Veeger NJGM, Eskes TKAB, de Graeff PA, van der Meer J. Oral contraceptives and the absolute risk of venous thromboembolism in women with single or multiple thrombophilic defects: results from a retrospective family cohort study. *Arch Intern Med.* 2007;167:282–289.

35. Petitti DB. Clinical practice. Combination estrogen-progestin oral contraceptives. *N Engl J Med.* 2003;349:1443–1450.

36. Moll S. Thrombophilias—practical implications and testing caveats. *J Thromb.* 2006;21:7–15.

37. Blom JW, Vanderschoot JPM, Oostindier MJ, Osanto S, van der Meer FJM, Rosendaal FR. Incidence of venous thrombosis in a large cohort of 66,329 cancer patients: results of a record linkage study. *J Thromb Haemost.* 2006;4: 529–535.

38. Prandoni P, Lensing AW, Buller HR, et al. Deep-vein thrombosis and the incidence of subsequent symptomatic cancer. *N Engl J Med.* 1992;327:1128–1133.

39. Qaseem A, Snow V, Barry P, et al. Current diagnosis of venous thromboembolism in primary care: a clinical practice guideline from the American Academy of Family Physicians and the American College of Physicians. *Ann Fam Med.* 2007;5:57–62.

40. Wells PS, Anderson DR, Bormanis J, et al. Value of assessment of pretest probability of deep-vein thrombosis in clinical management. *Lancet.* 1997;350:1795–1798.

41. Wells PS. Integrated strategies for the diagnosis of venous thromboembolism. *J Thromb Haemost.* 2007;5(Suppl 1): 41–50.

42. Wells PS, Owen C, Doucette S, et al. Does this patient have deep vein thrombosis? *JAMA.* 2006;295:199–207.

43. Righini M, Perrier A, De Moerloose P, Bounameaux H. D-Dimer for venous thromboembolism diagnosis: 20 years later. *J Thromb Haemost.* 2008;6:1059–1071.

44. Oudega R, Hoes AW, Moons KGM. The Wells rule does not adequately rule out deep venous thrombosis in primary care patients. *Ann Intern Med.* 2005;143:100–107.

45. Aguilar C, del Villar V. Diagnostic performance of D-dimer is lower in elderly outpatients with suspected deep venous thrombosis. *Br J Haematol.* 2005;130:803–804.

46. Mountain D, Jacobs I, Haig A. The VIDAS D-dimer test for venous thromboembolism: a prospective surveillance study shows maintenance of sensitivity and specificity when used in normal clinical practice. *Am J Emerg Med.* 2007;25: 464–471.

47. Fancher TL, White RH, Kravitz RL. Combined use of rapid D-dimer testing and estimation of clinical probability in the diagnosis of deep vein thrombosis: systematic review. *BMJ.* 2004;329:821.

48. Kearon C, Ginsberg JS, Hirsh J. The role of venous ultrasonography in the diagnosis of suspected deep venous thrombosis and pulmonary embolism. *Ann Intern Med.* 1998;129:1044–1049.

49. Wells PS, Anderson DR, Rodger M, et al. Evaluation of D-dimer in the diagnosis of suspected deep-vein thrombosis. *N Engl J Med.* 2003;349:1227–1235.

50. Kraaijenhagen RA, Piovella F, Bernardi E, et al. Simplification of the diagnostic management of suspected deep vein thrombosis. *Arch Intern Med.* 2002;162:907–911.

51. Bundens WP, Bergan JJ, Halasz NA, Murray J, Drehobl M. The superficial femoral vein. A potentially lethal misnomer. *JAMA.* 1995;274:1296–1298.

52. Scarvelis D, Wells PS. Diagnosis and treatment of deep-vein thrombosis. *CMAJ.* 2006;175:1087–1092.

53. Segal JB, Streiff MB, Hofmann LV, Thornton K, Bass EB. Management of venous thromboembolism: a systematic review for a practice guideline. *Ann Intern Med.* 2007;146:211–222.

54. Wheeler AP, Jaquiss RD, Newman JH. Physician practices in the treatment of pulmonary embolism and deep venous thrombosis. *Arch Intern Med.* 1988;148:1321–1325.

55. Hettiarachchi RJ, Prins MH, Lensing AW, Buller HR. Low molecular weight heparin versus unfractionated heparin in the initial treatment of venous thromboembolism. *Curr Opin Pulm Med.* 1998;4:220–225.

56. Gould MK, Dembitzer AD, Doyle RL, Hastie TJ, Garber AM. Low-molecular-weight heparins compared with unfractionated heparin for treatment of acute deep venous thrombosis. A meta-analysis of randomized, controlled trials. *Ann Intern Med.* 1999;130:800–809.

57. van Dongen CJJ, van den Belt AGM, Prins MH, Lensing AWA. Fixed dose subcutaneous low molecular weight heparins versus adjusted dose unfractionated heparin for venous thromboembolism. *Cochrane Database Syst Rev.* 2004;4:CD001100.

58. Martel N, Lee J, Wells PS. Risk for heparin-induced thrombocytopenia with unfractionated and low-molecular-weight heparin thromboprophylaxis: a meta-analysis. *Blood.* 2005;106:2710–2715.

59. Warkentin TE, Greinacher A. So, does low-molecular-weight heparin cause less heparin-induced thrombocytopenia than unfractionated heparin or not?. *Chest.* 2007;132:1108–1110.

60. van der Heijden JF, Prins MH, Buller HR. For the initial treatment of venous thromboembolism: are all low-molecular-weight heparin compounds the same? *Thromb Res.* 2000;100:V121–V130.

61. Nagge J, Crowther M, Hirsh J. Is impaired renal function a contraindication to the use of low-molecular-weight heparin? *Arch Intern Med.* 2002;162:2605–2609.

62. Turpie AG, Gallus AS, Hoek JA. A synthetic pentasaccharide for the prevention of deep-vein thrombosis after total hip replacement. *N Engl J Med.* 2001;344:619–625.

63. Buller HR, Davidson BL, Decousus H, et al. Fondaparinux or enoxaparin for the initial treatment of symptomatic deep venous thrombosis: a randomized trial. *Ann Intern Med.* 2004;140:867–873.

64. Lee AYY, Levine MN, Baker RI, et al. Low-molecular-weight heparin versus a coumarin for the prevention of recurrent venous thromboembolism in patients with cancer. *N Engl J Med.* 2003;349:146–153.

65. Kearon C, Gent M, Hirsh J, et al. A comparison of three months of anticoagulation with extended anticoagulation for a first episode of idiopathic venous thromboembolism. *N Engl J Med.* 1999;340:901–907.

66. Kearon C, Ginsberg JS, Anderson DR, et al. Comparison of 1 month with 3 months of anticoagulation for a first episode of venous thromboembolism associated with a transient risk factor. *J Thromb Haemost.* 2004;2:743–749.

67. Schulman S, Granqvist S, Holmstrom M, et al. The duration of oral anticoagulant therapy after a second episode of venous thromboembolism. The Duration of Anticoagulation Trial Study Group. *N Engl J Med.* 1997;336:393–398.

68. Pearson SD, Blair R, Halpert A, Eddy E, McKean S. An outpatient program to treat deep venous thrombosis with low-molecular-weight heparin. *Eff Clin Pract.* 1999;2:210–217.

69. Koopman MM, Prandoni P, Piovella F, et al. Treatment of venous thrombosis with intravenous unfractionated heparin administered in the hospital as compared with subcutaneous low-molecular-weight heparin administered at home. The Tasman Study Group. *N Engl J Med.* 1996;334:682–687.

70. Levine M, Gent M, Hirsh J, et al. A comparison of low-molecular-weight heparin administered primarily at home with unfractionated heparin administered in the hospital for proximal deep-vein thrombosis. *N Engl J Med.* 1996;334:677–681.

71. Boccalon H, Elias A, Chale JJ, Cadene A, Gabriel S. Clinical outcome and cost of hospital vs home treatment of proximal deep vein thrombosis with a low-molecular-weight heparin: the Vascular Midi-Pyrenees study. *Arch Intern Med.* 2000;160:1769–1773.

72. Huse DM, Cummins G, Taylor DCA, Russell MW. Outpatient treatment of venous thromboembolism with low-molecular-weight heparin: an economic evaluation. *Am J Manag Care.* 2002;8:S10–S16.

73. Groce JB. Initial management of deep venous thrombosis in the outpatient setting. *Am J Health Syst Pharm.* 2008;65:866–874.

74. Ageno W, Steidl L, Marchesi C, et al. Selecting patients for home treatment of deep vein thrombosis: the problem of cancer. *Haematologica.* 2002;87:286–291.

75. Elsharawy M, Elzayat E. Early results of thrombolysis vs anticoagulation in iliofemoral venous thrombosis. A randomised clinical trial. *Eur J Vasc Endovasc Surg.* 2002;24:209–214.

76. Bjarnason H, Kruse JR, Asinger DA, et al. Iliofemoral deep venous thrombosis: safety and efficacy outcome during 5 years of catheter-directed thrombolytic therapy. *J Vasc Interv Radiol.* 1997;8:405–418.

77. Comerota AJ, Throm RC, Mathias SD, Haughton S, Mewissen M. Catheter-directed thrombolysis for iliofemoral deep venous thrombosis improves health-related quality of life. *J Vasc Surg.* 2000;32:130–137.

78. Monreal M, Ruiz J, Olazabal A, Arias A, Roca J. Deep venous thrombosis and the risk of pulmonary embolism. A systematic study. *Chest.* 1992;102:677–681.

79. Cogo A, Lensing AW, Prandoni P, Hirsh J. Distribution of thrombosis in patients with symptomatic deep vein thrombosis. Implications for simplifying the diagnostic process with compression ultrasound. *Arch Intern Med.* 1993;153:2777–2780.

80. Righini M, Paris S, Le Gal G, et al. Clinical relevance of distal deep vein thrombosis. Review of literature data. *J Thromb Haemost.* 2006;95:56–64.

81. Righini M, Bounameaux H. Clinical relevance of distal deep vein thrombosis. *Curr Opin Pulm Med.* 2008;14:408–413.

82. Righini M. Is it worth diagnosing and treating distal deep vein thrombosis? No. *J Thromb Haemost.* 2007;5 (Suppl 1):55–59.

83. Schellong SM, Distal DVT. worth diagnosing? Yes. *J Thromb Haemost.* 2007;5(Suppl 1):51–54.

84. Seinturier C, Bosson JL, Colonna M, Imbert B, Carpentier PH. Site and clinical outcome of deep vein thrombosis of the lower limbs: an epidemiological study. *J Thromb Haemost.* 2005;3:1362–1367.

85. Labropoulos N, Webb KM, Kang SS, et al. Patterns and distribution of isolated calf deep vein thrombosis. *J Vasc Surg.* 1999;30:787–791.

86. Kahn SR. The post-thrombotic syndrome: progress and pitfalls. *Br J Haematol.* 2006;134:357–365.

87. Prandoni P, Lensing AWA, Prins MH, et al. Below-knee elastic compression stockings to prevent the post-thrombotic syndrome: a randomized, controlled trial. *Ann Intern Med.* 2004;141:249–256.

88. Kolbach DN, Sandbrink MW, Hamulyak K, et al. Non-pharmaceutical measures for prevention of post-thrombotic syndrome. *Cochrane Database Syst Rev.* 2004;1:CD004174.

89. Tapson VF, Decousus H, Pini M, et al. Venous thromboembolism prophylaxis in acutely ill hospitalized medical patients: findings from the International Medical Prevention Registry on Venous Thromboembolism. *Chest.* 2007;132:936–945.

90. Wein L, Wein S, Haas SJ, Shaw J, Krum H. Pharmacological venous thromboembolism prophylaxis in hospitalized medical patients: a meta-analysis of randomized controlled trials. *Arch Intern Med.* 2007;167:1476–1486.

91. Francis CW. Clinical practice. Prophylaxis for thromboembolism in hospitalized medical patients. *N Engl J Med.* 2007;356:1438–1444.

92. Cohen AT, Davidson BL, Gallus AS, et al. Efficacy and safety of fondaparinux for the prevention of venous thromboembolism in older acute medical patients: randomised placebo controlled trial. *BMJ.* 2006;332:325–329.

93. Douketis JD. Prevention of venous thromboembolism in hospitalized medical patients: addressing some practical questions. *Curr Opin Pulm Med.* 2008;14:381–388.

94. Douketis J, Cook D, Meade M, et al. Prophylaxis against deep vein thrombosis in critically ill patients with severe renal insufficiency with the low-molecular-weight heparin dalteparin: an assessment of safety and pharmacodynamics: the DIRECT study. *Arch Intern Med.* 2008;168:1805–1812.

95. Geerts WH, Bergqvist D, Pineo GF, et al. Prevention of venous thromboembolism: American College of Chest Physicians Evidence-Based Clinical Practice Guidelines (8th ed). *Chest.* 2008;133:381S–453S.

96. Ridker PM, Danielson E, Fonseca FAH, et al. Rosuvastatin to prevent vascular events in men and women with elevated C-reactive protein. *N Engl J Med.* 2008;359:2195–2207.

97. Glynn RJ, Danielson E, Fonseca FAH, et al. A randomized trial of rosuvastatin in the prevention of venous thromboembolism. *N Engl J Med.* 2009;360.

98. Stein PD, Beemath A, Matta F, et al. Clinical characteristics of patients with acute pulmonary embolism: data from PIOPED II. *Am J Med.* 2007;120:871–879.

99. Goldhaber SZ. Diagnosis of acute pulmonary embolism: always be vigilant. *Am J Med.* 2007;120:827–828.

100. Wells PS, Anderson DR, Rodger M, et al. Derivation of a simple clinical model to categorize patients probability of pulmonary embolism: increasing the models utility with the SimpliRED D-dimer. *J Thromb Haemost.* 2000;83: 416–420.

101. van Belle A, Buller HR, Huisman MV, et al. Effectiveness of managing suspected pulmonary embolism using an algorithm combining clinical probability, D-dimer testing, and computed tomography. *JAMA.* 2006;295:172–179.

102. Stein PD, Woodard PK, Weg JG, et al. Diagnostic pathways in acute pulmonary embolism: recommendations of the PIOPED II Investigators. *Radiology.* 2007;242:15–21.

103. Douma RA, Kamphuisen PW, Huisman MV, Buller HR. On Behalf of the Christopher Study Investigators. False normal results on multidetector-row spiral computed tomography in patients with high clinical probability of pulmonary embolism. *J Thromb Haemost.* 2008;6:1978–1979.

104. Torbicki A, Perrier A, Konstantinides S, et al. Guidelines on the diagnosis and management of acute pulmonary embolism: the Task Force for the Diagnosis and Management of Acute Pulmonary Embolism of the European Society of Cardiology (ESC). *Eur Heart J.* 2008;29:2276–2315.

105. Meaney JF, Weg JG, Chenevert TL, Stafford-Johnson D, Hamilton BH, Prince MR. Diagnosis of pulmonary embolism with magnetic resonance angiography. *N Engl J Med.* 1997;336:1422–1427.

106. Stein PD, Woodard PK, Hull RD, et al. Gadolinium-enhanced magnetic resonance angiography for detection of acute pulmonary embolism: an in-depth review. *Chest.* 2003;124:2324–2328.

107. Merli G, Spiro TE, Olsson CG, et al. Subcutaneous enoxaparin once or twice daily compared with intravenous unfractionated heparin for treatment of venous thromboembolic disease. *Ann Intern Med.* 2001;134:191–202.

108. Simonneau G, Sors H, Charbonnier B, et al. A comparison of low-molecular-weight heparin with unfractionated heparin for acute pulmonary embolism. The THESEE Study Group. Tinzaparine ou heparine standard: evaluations dans l'embolie pulmonaire. *N Engl J Med.* 1997;337:663–669.

109. The Columbus Investigators. Low-molecular-weight heparin in the treatment of patients with venous thromboembolism. *N Engl J Med.* 1997;337:657–662.

110. Hull RD, Raskob GE, Brant RF, et al. Low-molecular-weight heparin vs heparin in the treatment of patients with pulmonary embolism. American–Canadian Thrombosis Study Group. *Arch Intern Med.* 2000;160:229–236.

111. Buller HR, Davidson BL, Decousus H, et al. Subcutaneous fondaparinux versus intravenous unfractionated heparin in the initial treatment of pulmonary embolism. *N Engl J Med.* 2003;349:1695–1702.

112. Beer JH, Burger M, Gretener S, Bernard-Bagattini S, Bounameaux H. Outpatient treatment of pulmonary embolism is feasible and safe in a substantial proportion of patients. *J Thromb Haemost.* 2003;1:186–187.

113. Tapson VF, Huisman MV. Home at last? Early discharge for acute pulmonary embolism. *Eur Respir J.* 2007;30: 613–615.

114. Becattini C, Vedovati MC, Agnelli G. Prognostic value of troponins in acute pulmonary embolism: a meta-analysis. *Circulation.* 2007;116:427–433.

115. Kucher N, Goldhaber SZ. Cardiac biomarkers for risk stratification of patients with acute pulmonary embolism. *Circulation.* 2003;108:2191–2194.

116. Piazza G, Goldhaber SZ. Acute pulmonary embolism: part II: treatment and prophylaxis. *Circulation.* 2006;114: e42–e47.

117. Grau E, Tenias JM, Soto MJ, et al. D-dimer levels correlate with mortality in patients with acute pulmonary embolism: findings from the RIETE registry. *Crit Care Med.* 2007;35:1937–1941.

118. Jimenez D, Yusen RD. Prognostic models for selecting patients with acute pulmonary embolism for initial outpatient therapy. *Curr Opin Pulm Med.* 2008;14:414–421.

119. Wan S, Quinlan DJ, Agnelli G, Eikelboom JW. Thrombolysis compared with heparin for the initial treatment of pulmonary embolism: a meta-analysis of the randomized controlled trials. *Circulation.* 2004;110:744–749.

120. Murin S, Romano PS, White RH. Comparison of outcomes after hospitalization for deep venous thrombosis or pulmonary embolism. *J Thromb Haemost.* 2002;88:407–414.

121. Nutescu EA. Assessing, preventing, and treating venous thromboembolism: evidence-based approaches. *Am J Health Syst Pharm.* 2007;64:S5–S13.

122. Enoxaparin sodium injection [package insert]. Accessed November 24, 2008, at http://products.sanofi-aventis.us/lovenox/lovenox.html

123. Bazinet A, Almanric K, Brunet C, et al. Dosage of enoxaparin among obese and renal impairment patients. *Thromb Res.* 2005;116:41–50.

124. Dalteparin sodium injection package insert. Accessed November 25, 2008, at http://media.pfizer.com/files/products/uspi_fragmin.pdf

125. Shprecher AR, Cheng-Lai A, Madsen EM, et al. Peak antifactor xa activity produced by dalteparin treatment in patients with renal impairment compared with controls. *Pharmacotherapy.* 2005;25:817–822.

126. Smith J, Canton EM. Weight-based administration of dalteparin in obese patients. *Am J Health Syst Pharm.* 2003;60:683–687.

127. Al-Yaseen E, Wells PS, Anderson J, Martin J, Kovacs MJ. The safety of dosing dalteparin based on actual body weight for the treatment of acute venous thromboembolism in obese patients. *J Thromb Haemost.* 2005;3:100–102.

128. Tinzaparin sodium injection [package insert]. Accessed November 25, 2008, at http://www.innohepusa.com/innohepus/FullPrescribingInformationforInnohep.pdf

129. Hainer JW, Barrett JS, Assaid CA, et al. Dosing in heavy-weight/obese patients with the LMWH, tinzaparin: a pharmacodynamic study. *J Thromb Haemost.* 2002;87:817–823.

130. Fondaparinux sodium [package insert]. Accessed December 1, 2008, at http://us.gsk.com/products/assets/us_arixtra.pdf

131. Cruickshank MK, Levine MN, Hirsh J, Roberts R, Siguenza M. A standard heparin nomogram for the management of heparin therapy. *Arch Intern Med.* 1991;151:333–337.

132. Crowther MA. Inferior vena cava filters in the management of venous thromboembolism. *Am J Med.* 2007;120: S13–S17.

133. Decousus H, Leizorovicz A, Parent F, et al. A clinical trial of vena caval filters in the prevention of pulmonary embolism in patients with proximal deep-vein thrombosis. Prevention du Risque d'Embolie Pulmonaire par Interruption Cave Study Group. *N Engl J Med.* 1998;338:409–415.

134. Prepic Study Group. Eight-year follow-up of patients with permanent vena cava filters in the prevention of pulmonary embolism: the PREPIC (Prevention du Risque d'Embolie Pulmonaire par Interruption Cave) randomized study. *Circulation.* 2005;112:416–422.

135. Stein PD, Alnas M, Skaf E, et al. Outcome and complications of retrievable inferior vena cava filters. *Am J Cardiol.* 2004;94:1090–1093.

136. Kirilcuk NN, Herget EJ, Dicker RA, Spain DA, Hellinger JC, Brundage SI. Are temporary inferior vena cava filters really temporary? *Am J Surg.* 2005;190:858–863.

137. Kuipers S, Cannegieter SC, Middeldorp S, Rosendaal FR, Buller HR. Use of preventive measures for air travel-related venous thrombosis in professionals who attend medical conferences. *J Thromb Haemost.* 2006;4:2373–2376.
138. Kuipers S, Cannegieter SC, Middeldorp S, Robyn L, Buller HR, Rosendaal FR. The absolute risk of venous thrombosis after air travel: a cohort study of 8,755 employees of international organisations. *PLoS Med.* 2007;4:e290.
139. Cannegieter SC, Doggen CJ, van Houwelingen HC, et al. Travel-related venous thrombosis: results from a large population-based case control study (MEGA study). *PLoS Med.* 2006;3:e307.
140. Lapostolle F, Surget V, Borron SW, et al. Severe pulmonary embolism associated with air travel. *N Engl J Med.* 2001;345:779–783.
141. Clarke M, Hopewell S, Juszczak E, Eisinga A, Kjeldstrom M. Compression stockings for preventing deep vein thrombosis in airline passengers. *Cochrane Database Syst Rev.* 2006;2:CD004002.
142. Cesarone MR, Belcaro G, Nicolaides AN, et al. Venous thrombosis from air travel: the LONFLIT3 study—prevention with aspirin vs low-molecular-weight heparin (LMWH) in high-risk subjects: a randomized trial. *Angiology.* 2002;53:1–6.
143. Samama MM, Cohen AT, Darmon JY, et al. A comparison of enoxaparin with placebo for the prevention of venous thromboembolism in acutely ill medical patients. Prophylaxis in Medical Patients with Enoxaparin Study Group. *N Engl J Med.* 1999;341:793–800.
144. Leizorovicz A, Cohen AT, Turpie AGG, et al. Randomized, placebo-controlled trial of dalteparin for the prevention of venous thromboembolism in acutely ill medical patients. *Circulation.* 2004;110:874–879.
145. Stein PD, Beemath A, Meyers FA, Olson RE. Pulmonary embolism and deep venous thrombosis in hospitalized adults with chronic obstructive pulmonary disease. *J Cardiovasc Med.* 2007;8:253–257.
146. Cohen AT, Tapson VF, Bergmann J-F, et al. Venous thromboembolism risk and prophylaxis in the acute hospital care setting (ENDORSE study): a multinational cross-sectional study. *Lancet.* 2008;371:387–394.
147. Anderson FA Jr, Wheeler HB, Goldberg RJ, et al. A population-based perspective of the hospital incidence and case-fatality rates of deep vein thrombosis and pulmonary embolism. The Worcester DVT Study. *Arch Intern Med.* 1991;151:933–938.
148. Spyropoulos AC, Merli G. Management of venous thromboembolism in the elderly. *Drugs Aging.* 2006;23:651–671.
149. Garg R, Yusuf S. Overview of randomized trials of angiotensin-converting enzyme inhibitors on mortality and morbidity in patients with heart failure. Collaborative Group on ACE Inhibitor Trials. *JAMA.* 1995;273:1450–1456.
150. Beemath A, Stein PD, Skaf E, Al Sibae MR, Alesh I. Risk of venous thromboembolism in patients hospitalized with heart failure. *Am J Cardiol.* 2006;98:793–795.
151. Smeeth L, Cook C, Thomas S, Hall AJ, Hubbard R, Vallance P. Risk of deep vein thrombosis and pulmonary embolism after acute infection in a community setting. *Lancet.* 2006;367:1075–1079.
152. Barham K, Shah T. Images in clinical medicine. Phlegmasia cerulea dolens. *N Engl J Med.* 2007;356:e3.
153. Heaton D, Pearce M. Low molecular weight versus unfractionated heparin. A clinical and economic appraisal. *Pharmacoeconomics.* 1995;8:91–99.
154. Dedden P, Chang B, Nagel D. Pharmacy-managed program for home treatment of deep vein thrombosis with enoxaparin. *Am J Health Syst Pharm.* 1997;54:1968–1972.
155. Hull RD, Raskob GE, Rosenbloom D, et al. Treatment of proximal vein thrombosis with subcutaneous low-molecular-weight heparin vs intravenous heparin. An economic perspective. *Arch Intern Med.* 1997;157:289–294.

18 Pulmonary Hypertension and Cor Pulmonale

Mary P. Mullen and Michael J. Landzberg

CONTENTS

Key Words: Pulmonary hypertension; Cor pulmonale; Prostacyclin; Inhaled nitric oxide; Sildenafil; Endothelin; Endothelin receptor antagonists; Atrial septostomy; Lung transplantation; Atrial septostomy; Dyspnea.

KEY POINTS

- Pulmonary hypertension is defined as mean PA pressure > 25 mmHg at cardiac catheterization with PCWp ≤ 15 mmHg and PVR > 3 Wood units.
- Common pathological findings include endothelial hyperplasia, smooth muscle hypertrophy, thrombus formation, and plexiform lesions.
- Echocardiogram is the most appropriate screening modality.
- Thorough work-up to elucidate underlying cause is essential.

From: *Contemporary Cardiology: Comprehensive Cardiovascular Medicine in the Primary Care Setting*
Edited by: Peter P. Toth, Christopher P. Cannon, DOI 10.1007/978-1-60327-963-5_18
© Springer Science+Business Media, LLC 2010

- Cardiac catheterization is used for confirmation of diagnosis as well as to assess response to therapy.
- Prognostic factors include right atrial pressure, cardiac index, right ventricular function, BNP, functional class, and exercise capacity.
- Determination of therapy is based on pulmonary vasodilator testing during cardiac catheterization followed by evidence-based clinical algorithm.
- Therapeutic objectives include symptom improvement, survival, and quality of life.

18.1. INTRODUCTION

Pulmonary hypertension is a clinically heterogeneous, progressive disease. Tremendous recent advances in diagnosis and treatment options have improved clinical outcomes and survival (1, 2). Key to appropriate patient management is categorization of disease and treatment of underlying associated pathology. An expanded array of diagnostic tests allow for better characterization of clinical status; however, cardiac catheterization remains essential for assessment of disease severity, determination of prognosis, and choice of appropriate treatment. Multiple therapies for pulmonary hypertension have emerged in the past decade. These strategies provide more patient choice, are better tolerated, and result in improved functional class, decreased symptoms, and enhanced quality of life.

18.2. SCIENTIFIC FRAMEWORK

The pulmonary circulation, normally a site of low resistance and high capacitance, is subject to physiologic and pathologic alteration. Pulmonary hypertension is a condition associated with vasoconstriction and vascular remodeling limiting blood flow through pulmonary arteries, resulting in increased pulmonary vascular resistance and eventually causing right ventricular failure (3). Common pathological findings include endothelial hyperplasia, smooth muscle hypertrophy, adventitial thickening, thrombus formation, and the development of plexiform lesions (4, 5). Numerous contributing factors are now recognized as participating in the clinical presentation of pulmonary hypertension. However, a number of interrelated cellular mechanisms may play key roles common to the development of disease. Gains in molecular biology have defined pathways that serve as important regulators of pulmonary vascular function (3). A variety of mediators may be involved in the pathogenesis of pulmonary hypertension and are summarized in Table 1. These pathways give rise to potential targets for therapeutic intervention.

18.3. CLASSIFICATION

Pulmonary hypertension is classified according to the WHO revised clinical classification (Table 2). This divides patients according to etiology and clinical causes. Group 1, pulmonary arterial hypertension or PAH, includes both idiopathic (IPAH) and familial causes, as well as other associated diseases (APAH) that share common clinical features or exhibit similar response to therapy. Importantly, this group includes patients with collagen vascular disease (6), congenital heart disease and left-to-right shunt lesions (7), portal hypertension, and HIV disease (8). Diagnosis of PAH is confirmed via hemodynamic measurements obtained during catheterization showing a mean PAP greater than 25 mmHg at rest or 30 with exercise, PVR > 3 Wood units, and normal left heart filling pressure determined by pulmonary capillary wedge pressure of 15 mmHg or less. Group 2 includes patients with left-sided heart disease and Group 3 with pulmonary hypertension associated with lung disease. Group 4 consists of patients with chronic thromboembolic pulmonary hypertension and Group

Table 1
Factors Mediating Pulmonary Hypertension *(76)*

Factor	Pulmonary vascular tone effects	Hemostatic effects	Cellular effects	Clinical observations
Prostacyclin	Vasodilator	Inhibits platelet activation	Antiproliferative	Prostacyclin synthase decreased in pulmonary arteries in PAH
Thromboxane A2	Vasoconstrictor		Promotes proliferation	
Endothelin-1	Vasoconstrictor		Stimulates pulmonary artery smooth muscle cell proliferation	Plasma levels increased in PAH
Serotonin	Vasoconstrictor		Promotes pulmonary artery smooth muscle hypertrophy and hyperplasia	
Vasoactive intestinal peptide	Vasodilator	Inhibits platelet activation	Decreased pulmonary artery smooth muscle cell proliferation	Levels decreased in PAH patients
Nitric oxide (NO)	Vasodilator	Inhibits platelet activation	Inhibits vascular smooth muscle cell proliferation	Decreased NO synthase in PAH

Adapted with Permission from Mullen, MP, Pulmonary Hypertension in Keane JF, et al., eds. Nadas' Pediatric Cardiology, Copyright Elsevier, 2006. p. 114.

5 miscellaneous causes. Patients are also classified according to functional ability (Table 3). These performance measures have been used as outcomes in clinical trials and have been shown to reflect prognosis.

18.4. EPIDEMIOLOGY

Estimates suggest a prevalence of pulmonary arterial hypertension between 2 and 15 patients per million *(9–11)*. There is a clear female predominance estimated at 1.7–1, and the largest proportion of all patients is diagnosed in the third and fourth decade of life. Race and ethnicity are similar to that of the general population. Many patients are noted to have a significant delay in diagnosis with mean time of 2 years since initial development of symptoms. A recent French study found that the majority of PAH patients present with advanced disease—80% of patients present with WHO Functional Class III or IV symptoms *(9)*. Increasingly, pulmonary hypertension has been diagnosed in the elderly. Population studies suggest an age-related increase in pulmonary artery pressure associated with increasing left heart diastolic pressures and systemic blood vessel stiffening *(12)*.

18.5. FAMILIAL PULMONARY ARTERY HYPERTENSION

A genetic basis for some forms of pulmonary arterial hypertension had long been assumed, as registries had shown that 6% of patients had an affected family member *(10)*. This was confirmed by the finding of mutations in two genes in the transforming growth factor receptor pathway, BMPR2 and ALK1, found in patients with hereditary hemorrhagic telangiectiasia (HHT) *(13–15)*. Inheritance is autosomal dominant with variable and incomplete penetrance. Sixty percent of patients with familial

Table 2
WHO Classification of Pulmonary Hypertension (3)

1. Pulmonary arterial hypertension (PAH)
    1.1. Idiopathic (IPAH)
    1.2. Familial (FPAH)
    1.3. Associated with (APAH)
        1.3.1. Connective tissue disorder
        1.3.2. Congenital systemic-to-pulmonary shunts
        1.3.3. Portal hypertension
        1.3.4. HIV infection
        1.3.5. Drugs and toxins
        1.3.6. Others (thyroid disorders, glycogen storage disease, Gaucher disease, hereditary hemorrhagic telangiectasia, hemoglobinopathies, chronic myeloproliferative disorders, splenectomy)
    1.4. Associated with significant venous or capillary involvement
        1.4.1. Pulmonary veno-occlusive disease
        1.4.2. Pulmonary capillary hemangiomatosis
    1.5. Persistent pulmonary hypertension of the newborn
2. Pulmonary hypertension with left heart disease
    2.1. Left-sided atrial or ventricular heart disease
    2.2. Left-sided valvular heart disease
3. Pulmonary hypertension associated with lung diseases or hypoxemia
    3.1. Chronic obstructive pulmonary disease
    3.2. Interstitial lung disease
    3.3. Sleep-disordered breathing
    3.4. Alveolar hypoventilation disorders
    3.5. Chronic exposure to high altitude
    3.6. Developmental abnormalities
4. Pulmonary hypertension due to chronic thrombotic and/or embolic disease
    4.1. Thromboembolic obstruction of proximal pulmonary arteries
    4.2. Thromboembolic obstruction of distal pulmonary arteries
    4.3. Non-thrombotic pulmonary embolism (tumor parasites, foreign material)
5. Miscellaneous
    Sarcoidosis, histiocytosis X, lymphangiomatosis, compression of pulmonary vessels (adenopathy, tumor, fibrosing mediastinitis)

Reprinted with Permission Circulation. 2009; 199:3350–2294, copyright 2009 American Heart Association, Inc.

Table 3
WHO Functional Classification for Pulmonary Hypertension (78)

Class I	No limitation
Class II	Slight limitation of physical activity, ordinary physical activity causes shortness of breath, fatigue, chest pain, or near syncope
Class III	Marked limitation of physical activity, less than ordinary activity causes shortness of breath, fatigue, chest pain, or near syncope
Class IV	Inability to carry out any physical activity without symptoms and have right heart failure. Shortness of breath or fatigue may be present at rest

PAH and 20% of patients with idiopathic PAH have been found to have BMPR2 mutations. Genetic anticipation—worsening of the disease and earlier presentation with subsequent generations—has been found in families with BMPR2 mutations. The product of these genes affects intracellular signal transduction leading to alterations in vascular cell growth (3).

18.6. PATIENT ASSESSMENT

PAH may be suspected in patients identified through report of symptoms, with physical exam findings or who undergo screening due to risk factors for the development of pulmonary hypertension. Reported symptoms of pulmonary hypertension may include shortness of breath with exertion, fatigue, chest pain, and syncope along with others. Additional complaints such as rash, arthralgias, snoring, or daytime somnolence may direct the provider to associated causes of pulmonary hypertension.

18.6.1. Screening

Current indications for screening for pulmonary hypertension include the presence of a first-degree relative with known genetic mutation predisposing to pulmonary hypertension or idiopathic pulmonary hypertension, scleroderma, portal hypertension, congenital heart disease with systemic-to-pulmonary shunt lesions, and sickle cell disease *(16)*. Diagnostic echocardiogram may be appropriate for symptoms suggestive of pulmonary hypertension in patients with documented obstructive sleep-disordered breathing, other forms of collagen vascular disease, hemoglobinopathies, HIV, and prior appetite suppressant use. Current recommendations for PH screening are summarized in Table 4 *(3)*.

Table 4
Indications for Screening in Suspected PAH *(3)*

Indication	Recommended screening	Rationale
BMPR2 mutation	Annual echocardiogram	Early detection; 20% chance of developing PAH
First-degree relative of patient with BMPR2 mutation	Genetic counseling and BMPR2 genotyping, annual echocardiogram if positive	
Scleroderma	Annual echocardiogram	8–27% PAH in scleroderma
HIV infection	Echocardiogram if symptoms or signs of PH	0.5% prevalence of PAH
Portal hypertension	Echocardiogram if liver transplant considered	4% prevalence of PAH in candidates for liver transplant
Sickle cell	Annual echocardiogram	30% develop PH, 10% PAH

Adapted with Permission Circulation. 2009; 199:3350–2294, copyright 2009 American Heart Association, Inc.

18.6.2. Diagnostic Algorithm

Patients suspected of pulmonary hypertension should undergo a complete work-up with goals of pulmonary hypertension diagnosis, delineation of hemodynamics, and identification of associated, potentially causative disorders for therapeutic correction. The diagnostic algorithm utilized by the Boston Adult Congenital Heart (BACH) and Pulmonary Hypertension Service is summarized in Fig. 1.

18.6.3. History

Evaluation of the patient with pulmonary hypertension is initiated with a complete history including childhood and congenital illnesses, respiratory diseases, genetic syndromes, connective tissue disorders, anorexigen intake, smoking, substance use, hypercoagulable disorders, liver disease, neurologic disease, airway anomalies, sleep disorders, cardiovascular risk assessment, reproductive history, and

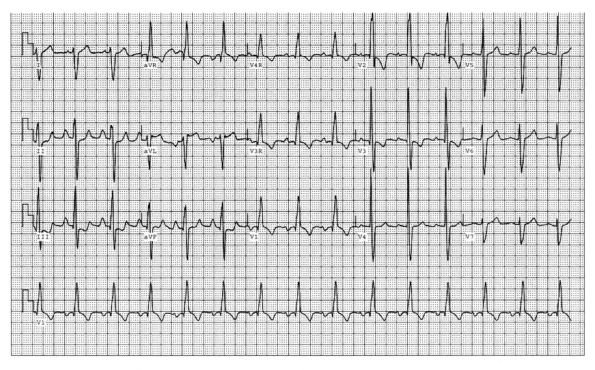

Fig. 1. EKG in patient with severe PAH.

residence at altitude. Each patient should undergo a comprehensive family history including account
of undiagnosed perinatal losses and sudden cardiac deaths.

18.6.4. Physical Exam

Physical exam findings associated with pulmonary hypertension include elevated jugular venous
pressure, murmur of tricuspid regurgitation, right ventricular heave, loud pulmonic component of

Table 5
Physical Exam Findings in Pulmonary
Hypertension *(16, 22)*

Loud pulmonary component of S2
Pansystolic murmur of tricuspid regurgitation
Diastolic murmur of pulmonary regurgitation
Right ventricular heave
Right ventricular S3
Right-sided S4
Early systolic ejection click
Prominent jugular a wave
Elevated jugular venous pulsation
Hepatojugular reflux
Liver enlargement
Pulsatile liver
Lower extremity edema
Ascites
Cool extremities
Cyanosis

second heart sound, hepatomegaly, ascites, and pedal edema. Additional physical exam findings are summarized in Table 5 *(16)*.

18.6.5. Electrocardiogram

The electrocardiogram is essential in the evaluation of a patient with pulmonary hypertension to document normal sinus rhythm and to assess for right ventricular strain and chamber enlargement. Findings of PAH may include sinus tachycardia or bradycardia, right axis deviation, right atrial enlargement, right ventricular hypertrophy, right bundle branch block or conduction delay, and right ventricular strain pattern. An EKG from a patient with severe PAH is shown in Fig. 2.

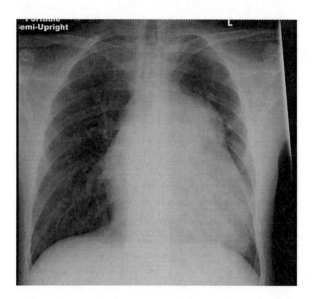

Fig. 2. Chest X-ray in patient with idiopathic pulmonary hypertension.

18.6.6. Chest X-Ray

CXR findings, seen in Fig. 3, may include cardiomegaly, right ventricular hypertrophy, and enlargement of the pulmonary arteries. In PAH, there may be a paucity of markings in the peripheral lung fields

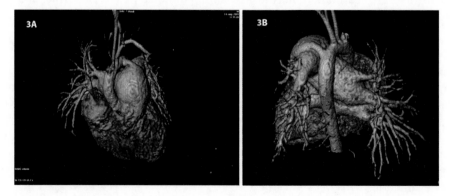

Fig. 3. MRI image of patient with severe PAH and small PDA. (**a**) Anterior view demonstrating dilated main pulmonary artery. (**b**) Posterior view showing dilated right and left PA, "pruning of distal vessels," descending aorta, and small PDA. Courtesy of O. Benavidez, MD, MPH.

due to limited pulmonary blood flow. In addition, the chest radiograph may be useful for diagnosing or excluding concomitant lung disease.

18.6.7. Echocardiogram

Transthoracic echocardiography is an extremely useful screening tool for the diagnosis of pulmonary hypertension and should be performed in all patients in whom the diagnosis is suspected. Goals of the study are to confirm the presence of elevated pulmonary artery pressures and determine extent of elevation, provide estimation of right ventricular size and function, and exclude the presence of other structural heart disease *(17)*. In the absence of pulmonary stenosis, right ventricular systolic pressure equals pulmonary artery pressure and is measured by the modified Bernoulli equation RVSP + $4 v^2$ + RAP where *v* represents systolic tricuspid regurgitant flow. In settings where there is insufficient tricuspid regurgitation to accurately measure the regurgitant jet, right ventricular pressure can be estimated by interventricular septal position. Additional non-invasive measures may estimate diastolic and mean PA pressure, as well as vascular impedance.

Echocardiography can provide information about right ventricular size and function; however, due to the geometric configuration of the right ventricle, accurate assessment may be challenging. Newer echocardiographic techniques that may be used to evaluate right ventricular function include the Tei index, three-dimensional echo, and tricuspid annular plane excursion (TAPSE) *(18–20)*.

It is essential to exclude the presence of concomitant structural heart disease during the assessment of the patient with pulmonary hypertension. Two-dimensional echocardiography is an excellent modality for diagnosing the presence of left-to-right shunt lesions such as atrial septal defect, ventricular septal defect, or patent ductus arteriosus; assessing valvular pathology; and determining left heart size and function. In the setting of pulmonary hypertension and unexplained cyanosis, contrast echocardiography may be used to determine presence of a patent foramen ovale allowing right-to-left atrial level shunt.

18.6.8. Functional Assessment

Patients with pulmonary hypertension should have assessment of exercise capacity during initial evaluation if physically capable as well as at periodic intervals to assess response to therapy. The 6-min walk test is an easily performed, reproducible test that correlates inversely with functional class and pulmonary vascular resistance and directly with maximal oxygen consumption obtained during exercise testing *(21, 22)*. The 6-min walk test serves as an endpoint for many therapeutic PH drug trials, has prognostic value, and is an independent predictor of survival *(21)*. Many centers facile in the management of severe heart failure may utilize cardiopulmonary exercise testing and gas exchange analysis in addition to the 6-min walk test.

18.6.9. Additional Diagnostic Work-Up

After a diagnosis of pulmonary hypertension, it is essential that each patient undergo extensive evaluation to elicit treatable underlying or co-existing conditions that may lead to correction or improvement in the degree of pulmonary vascular disease (see Fig. 4). Assessment must include evaluation of respiratory status including chest computed tomography, pulmonary function tests, and sleep study. HIV should be excluded by history and laboratory evaluation. Portal hypertension should be considered and evaluated by liver function tests, right upper quadrant ultrasound, MRI, and/or liver biopsy as appropriate. Collagen vascular diseases should be investigated by history, physical exam, and laboratory evaluation.

Since pulmonary hypertension due to chronic thromboembolic disease would receive specific management strategies, this diagnosis should be considered for each patient *(23, 24)*. V/Q scan is sensitive for the detection of thrombus but lacks specificity. High-resolution chest CT may be to exclude the

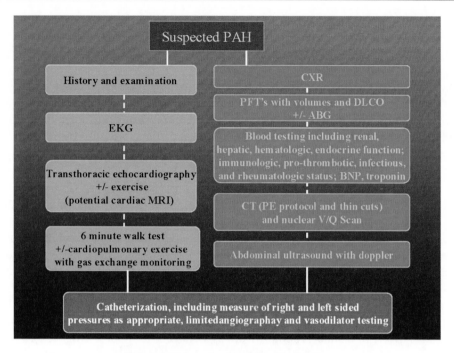

Fig. 4. Diagnostic algorithm for PAH.

diagnosis of chronic thromboembolism. D-Dimer and evaluation for lower extremity thrombus by ultrasound or CT should be performed if clinically indicated. Each patient should undergo a work-up for hypercoagulability including protein C and S, antithrombin III, lupus anticoagulant, factor V Leiden, homocysteine levels, and the assessment for the prothrombin gene mutation.

18.6.10. Laboratory Evaluation

Screening laboratory evaluation for the patient with pulmonary hypertension should include serum electrolytes, complete blood count, sedimentation, measures of rheumatologic or inflammatory activity, liver and renal function tests, HIV serologies, thyroid function tests, and biomarkers associated with RV failure include plasma brain natriuretic peptide (BNP), N-terminal pro-BNP, and troponin. If clinically indicated and after appropriate counseling, genetic testing for mutations in genes associated with familial pulmonary hypertension should be performed.

18.6.11. Cardiac MRI

Recent advances in cardiac MRI techniques have increased the utility of this imaging modality in patients with pulmonary hypertension (25). MRI provides a three-dimensional view of the heart and great vessels with excellent imaging quality (Fig. 3) and may provide accurate assessment of right ventricular size, function, and scarring. Increasingly, right ventricular function measured by MRI has been used as an outcome in clinical trials.

18.6.12. Cardiac Catheterization and Pulmonary Vasodilator Testing

Cardiac catheterization is essential in the diagnostic work-up of patients with pulmonary hypertension to confirm presence of elevated pressures, diagnose structural or left-sided heart disease, and assess response to pulmonary vasodilator testing (26). Hemodynamic measures obtained include right atrial pressure, right ventricular pressure, pulmonary artery pressure, pulmonary capillary wedge pressure, cardiac index, and pulmonary vascular resistance. Catheterization findings may be used to exclude other co-existing congenital or structural heart disease such as left-to-right shunt lesions, pulmonary vein stenosis, mitral valve stenosis, pericardial disease, and left heart systolic or diastolic dysfunction. Angiography may be performed providing important information about the distal pulmonary bed, pulmonary veins, and presence of collateral vessels.

Pulmonary vasodilator testing is performed using short-acting agents to predict response to calcium channel blocker therapy and to provide assessment of prognosis (27). Medications used for testing in the catheterization laboratory include inhaled nitric oxide, intravenous prostacyclin, and/or IV adenosine. The definition of response is a fall in mean pulmonary artery pressure by 10 mmHg to attain a mean PA pressure less than 40 mmHg with normal or high cardiac output.

18.6.13. Prognostic Indicators

Predictors of mortality in pulmonary hypertension include decreased functional class and impaired performance in 6-min walk test (28). Associated disease may portend prognosis, with PAH of the scleroderma spectrum having higher risk of death than IPAH (29). Registry studies have predicted increased risk of death associated with hemodynamic findings at cardiac catheterization including elevated mean right atrial pressure (mRAP), increased mean pulmonary artery pressure (mPAP), and decreased cardiac index (30). The presence of a pericardial effusion conveys a worse prognosis (31). Response to acute vasodilator challenge in the catheterization laboratory suggests improved long-term survival (10). In addition, MRI indices of decreased right ventricular function (32) and elevation in biomarkers pro-NT BNP, BNP, and Troponin T are associated with poorer prognosis (33–35).

18.7. MANAGEMENT OF PULMONARY HYPERTENSION

Therapies for the pulmonary hypertension are complex and warrant referral to centers with multidisciplinary teams and substantial experience in the disease. Medications for the treatment of pulmonary hypertension fall into the following general categories.

18.7.1. General Supportive Care

This group includes supplemental oxygen for the treatment of hypoxia, potential use of digoxin for right ventricular failure, diuretics, and low-salt diet for optimizing volume status and coumadin. Theoretically, coumadin prevents in situ thrombosis in distal pulmonary arteries, guards against systemic thromboembolism in the setting of right-to-left shunting, and improves long-term survival (10, 35, 36). The use of coumadin in patients with pulmonary hypertension should be balanced against the potential for bleeding in patients with multiple co-morbidities.

18.7.2. Pulmonary Vasodilator Therapies

18.7.2.1. Calcium Channel Blockers

Calcium channel blocker therapy is safe and efficacious in PAH patients responding to acute vasodilator testing, conveying >95% 5-year survival (10). However, less than 15% of adults are noted to be acute responders; patients with known BMPR2 mutations (37) or with PAH due to scleroderma (38) are unlikely to show acute response. In addition, patients initially felt to be responders may not sustain this over the long term and require close watching to verify improvement on therapy. The drugs most frequently used in this class include nifedipine, diltiazem, and amlodipine.

18.7.2.2. Prostanoid Therapies

Endogenous prostacyclin is known to be reduced in patients with pulmonary vascular disease. Treatment of PAH was revolutionized by the demonstration of improved exercise tolerance, hemodynamics, quality of life, and survival in patients with PAH treated with intravenous epoprostenol (28). Administered by continuous intravenous route, epoprostenol therapy is hampered by short half-life, requirement for central venous access, and side effects including rash, first bite jaw pain, headache, and diarrhea. Additional prostanoid formulations have been developed including iloprost and the longer acting treprostinil, approved for intravenous, subcutaneous, and inhaled use. Inhaled iloprost is delivered via a dedicated nebulizer and was found to improve functional class and 6-min walk distance compared with placebo (39). Of note, inhalation systems for prostanoid delivery continue to advance in ease of and timing required for administration. Regarding treprostinil, initial studies have shown comparable efficacy and side effect profile during conversion from intravenous epoprostenol to treprostinil; however, higher doses of treprostinil (up to two times) were required (40).

18.7.2.3. ENDOTHELIN RECEPTOR ANTAGONISTS

Circulating endothelin-1 is a potent vasoconstrictor that also stimulates smooth muscle cell growth. The dual endothelin-1 receptor antagonist bosentan was studied in PAH patients versus placebo, demonstrating improved 6-min walk distance and delayed time to clinical worsening (41). Recent studies have suggested improved survival with bosentan over historical controls. This drug has also been evaluated in patients with pulmonary hypertension related to Eisenmenger physiology, improving hemodynamics, and increasing exercise capacity without decreasing oxygen saturation (42). Side effects include flushing, elevated liver function tests, edema, and potential teratogenicity. Selective endothelin-1 receptor blockers include ambrisentan (43) and sitaxsentan with clinical trials showing improved 6-min walk tests with side effects similar to bosentan.

18.7.2.4. PHOSPHODIESTERASE INHIBITORS

Cyclic GMP, synthesized by nitric oxide-dependent soluble guanylate cyclase, produces vasodilation and inhibition of smooth muscle cell proliferation. It is degraded enzymatically by phosphodiesterase V found abundantly in lung tissue. Inhibition of phosphodiesterase V by drugs such as sildenafil or the longer acting tadalafil can increase intracellular cyclic GMP and potentiate blood vessel relaxation. The outpatient randomized placebo-controlled trial of sildenafil (44, 45) showed improved 6-min walk distance, hemodynamics, and reasonable safety profile. Recently, tadalafil was demonstrated to increase 6-min walk distance, delay time to clinical worsening, and improve quality of life in treatment naïve patients with PAH (46).

18.8. TREATMENT ALGORITHM

Therapy for pulmonary hypertension is determined according to evidence-based treatment algorithms (Fig. 5) (3). Patients are initially optimized with supplemental oxygen titrated to keep oxygen saturations greater than 90%. Volume status is optimized with diuretics according to clinical criteria and taking care to avoid hypovolemia. First choice of agent is usually a loop diuretic with spironolactone added secondarily to assist in the management of fluctuating potassium requirements. Coumadin therapy may be initiated, and INR should be maintained at 1.5–2.5. Acute vasodilator therapy is performed during diagnostic cardiac catheterization. Responders to vasodilator challenge are trialed on oral calcium channel blockers according to established protocols. Patients who demonstrate longstanding response are continued on this therapy.

Non-responders are divided according to functional class and severity of illness into lower and higher risk groups (Fig. 5) (3). Those at lower risk may initiate therapy with endothelin receptor antagonists or phophodiesterase-5 inhibitors. Other treatments including intravenous prostanoids, inhaled iloprost, or subcutaneous treprostinil may be considered as second-line agents. Patients with more severe disease or functional limitation (higher risk) should be treated first with intravenous prostanoids. Several recent studies have evaluated the utility of combination therapy for patients with PAH as well as the benefit of therapeutic interventions early in the recognized course of disease (47–49). Current guidelines suggest that combination therapy should be undertaken for inadequate response to initial treatment strategy.

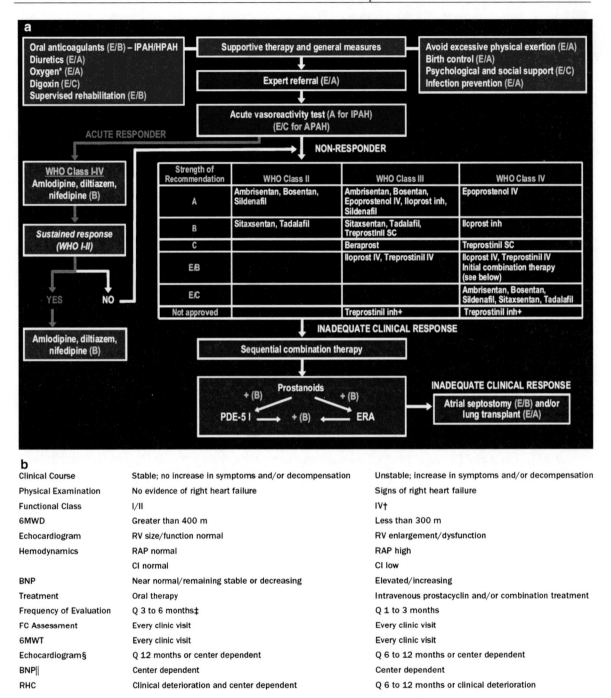

Fig. 5. (a) Acute treatment algorithm for PAH *(77)*. **(b)** Chronic treatment algorithm for PAH. From McLaughlin *(3)*.
Reprinted with Permission, *J Am Coll Cardiol*. 2009:54(1 Suppl) Barst RJ, et al. Updated evidence-based treatment algorithm in pulmonary arterial hypertension, S78–S84, copyright 2009 with permission from Elsevier.
Reprinted with Permission Circulation. 2009; 199:2250–2294, copyright 2009 American Heart Association, Inc.

18.9. ATRIAL SEPTOSTOMY

For patients with advanced disease refractory to medical therapy, transcatheter atrial septostomy using balloon or blade may decrease right atrial pressure, augment cardiac output, lessen symptoms, and improve functional class (50, 51). However, in addition to procedural risks, this intervention carries potential risk for thromboembolism associated with right-to-left shunting. In general, atrial septostomy is reserved for patients with recurrent syncope or recalcitrant right-sided heart failure on optimized medical regimen and as a bridge to lung transplant.

18.10. LUNG TRANSPLANTATION

Lung transplantation has been used for patients with pulmonary hypertension who fail to respond to medical therapy (52). Candidacy for lung transplant is determined according to established guidelines, balancing risks of severe pulmonary hypertension with benefits and consequences of transplantation. Indications include WHO functional Class III or IV while receiving optimized medical therapy, low (<350 m) or decreasing 6-min walk test, failing therapy with intravenous prostanoid, cardiac index < 2 L/min/m^2, and elevated right atrial pressure (53). Recent data for patients transplanted with the diagnosis of primary pulmonary hypertension show survival rates of 77 and 53.6% at 1 and 5 years (54). Complications of lung transplantation include chronic rejection, infection, and complications of long-term immunosuppression.

18.11. NON-CARDIAC SURGERY AND ANESTHETIC MANAGEMENT

General surgery carries increased perioperative risk in patients with pulmonary arterial hypertension, with estimates of perioperative mortality up to 7% (55). Thoracic and orthopedic procedures may have the highest morbidity. Additionally, patient characteristics comparable to those predictive of survival, i.e., lower WHO functional class, increased right atrial pressure, and depressed right ventricular function, convey increased perioperative risk (55). Prior to elective surgery, patients should undergo careful preoperative planning and consultation by an anesthesia team experienced in the management of patients with pulmonary hypertension. Clinical parameters including volume and respiratory status should be optimized before surgery, if possible. Induction and anesthetic agents should be selected with attention to ensuring hemodynamic stability. Procedures involving significant fluid shifts may require invasive monitoring with arterial or central venous catheters. The use of low-dose inotropy should be considered in the setting of right ventricular dysfunction or refractory hypotension. Patients should continue baseline pulmonary vasodilator therapies during surgery if feasible. As relatively short-acting pulmonary vasodilator with potential for improving V/Q mismatch and oxygenation, inhaled nitric oxide or inhaled epoprostenol may be beneficial both intraoperatively and postoperatively in the setting of prolonged mechanical ventilation. After surgery, close attention to adequacy of ventilation, pain control, fluid management, arrhythmia monitoring, and prevention of venous thromboembolism are essential.

18.12. HEALTH MAINTENANCE IN PAH

Patients with pulmonary hypertension benefit from close follow-up by primary medical providers. At high risk from respiratory infections, they should receive prophylactic influenza and pneumococcal vaccinations as well as prompt evaluation and treatment of community acquired illnesses. Cyanotic patients, those with indwelling central lines or other structural heart lesions, may require antibiotic prophylaxis according to established guidelines for the prevention of subacute bacterial endocarditis. Females of childbearing age should be advised of the significant maternal and fetal risks associated with pulmonary hypertension and provided with appropriate contraceptive counseling (56). Travel may pose challenges to patients with pulmonary hypertension. In general, trips to mountainous areas greater than 1,000 m should be avoided due to potential for increased vasoconstriction at high altitude in the setting of decreased partial pressure of oxygen. Patients may be advised to utilize supplemental oxygen during airplane flights; in addition, they should be cautioned to remain well hydrated and to avoid prolonged immobilization during travel to decrease risk of deep venous thrombosis.

Patients with pulmonary hypertension may be at risk for syncope and sudden death with exercise and should be counseled to self-limit during physical activity, avoiding strenuous exertion and resting when fatigued. However, patients should be encouraged to engage in low-level activities as tolerated. A recent study suggests that supervised exercise and respiratory training improves quality of life, WHO functional class, and peak oxygen consumption in a group of medically stabilized patients with pulmonary hypertension *(57)*.

Table 6
Therapies for Pulmonary Hypertension

Drug class	Drug	Route of administration	Dosing	Most common adversities
Prostanoids	Epoprostenol	Intravenous	ng/kg/min	Flushing, hypotension, nausea, vomiting, diarrhea, boney aches, rash
	Treprostinil	Subcutaneous, intravenous, inhaled	ng/kg/min	See above, when used SQ: local site redness and pain
	Iloprost	Inhaled	mcg	See above, though less
Endothelin receptor antagonists	Bosentan (A+B)	Oral	62.5–125 mg bid	Liver function abnormalities, volume retention, anemia
	Ambrisentan (A)	Oral	5–10 mg qd	See above, potentially fewer LFT changes
	Sitaxsentan (A)	Oral	100 mg qd	See above, similar to ambrisentan
Phosphodiesterase inhibitors	Sildenafil (PDE5)	Oral	20–80 mg tid	Headache, hypotension, visual changes, hearing changes
	Tadalafil (PDE5)	Oral	40 mg qd	See above

18.13. COR PULMONALE

The enlarged, failing right ventricle due to pulmonary hypertension in the setting of respiratory disease is known as cor pulmonale. Pulmonary hypertension and resultant right heart failure are known complications of severe chronic obstructive pulmonary disease with estimated prevalence of 20–35% *(58–63)*. Elevation of pulmonary artery pressure is associated with decreased resting PaO_2 in patients with COPD *(61, 64)* and use of supplemental oxygen therapy has been shown to improve survival in hypoxemic subjects *(65, 66)*.

There is also increased recognition of pulmonary hypertension in patients with interstitial lung diseases (ILD) *(67)*, pulmonary Langerhans cell histiocytosis, connective tissue-associated interstitial lung disease including scleroderma and Crest syndrome, sarcoidosis *(68)*, idiopathic pulmonary fibrosis, and the pneumoconiosis asbestosis and silicosis *(69)*. In contrast to COPD, pulmonary hypertension in ILD may not be associated with resting hypoxemia or decreased pulmonary function *(67)* but carries a poorer prognosis. Etiology of PAH in patients with ILD is likely multifactorial but may include vascular remodeling, vessel obstruction, inflammatory changes, and fibrosis.

Clinicians should maintain a low threshold for screening for PH in the presence of COPD or ILD; early symptoms of shortness of breath or exertional fatigue may be easily confused with those associated with the lung disease itself. Later, patients may present with lower extremity edema and volume overload associated with right heart failure. All patients diagnosed with pulmonary hypertension in the setting of chronic lung disease should undergo a full screening work-up for additional causes for pulmonary hypertension.

Therapeutic strategies in patients with COPD or ILD and pulmonary hypertension begin with optimal management of the underlying disease *(67)*. In some patients, lung biopsy may be required for more precise characterization of the interstitial lung process. Antiproliferative, anti-inflammatory, and immunosuppressive therapies for the treatment of ILD should be used according to established guidelines. Supplemental oxygen should be provided in the setting of hypoxemia; digoxin, diuretics, and low-salt diet may be of benefit in the treatment of volume loading associated with right heart dysfunction. Particularly in the setting of lower extremity edema, anticoagulant therapy to prevent venous thrombus and pulmonary arterial in situ thrombosis may be of benefit but there are no data clearly associated with benefit for anticoagulation in patients with PAH and COPD/ILD.

Pulmonary vasodilator therapy in ILD has been studied, with some benefit in a number of small series *(70–72)*; however, intravenous prostanoids may cause the development of worsening hypoxemia in the setting of increased ventilation–perfusion mismatch *(70)*. Patients should be closely followed with functional assessment both pre- and post-initiation of therapy. Lung transplant should be reserved for those without response to treatment.

18.14. QUALITY OF LIFE IN PULMONARY HYPERTENSION

Although significant advances have been made in understanding both the underlying pathophysiology and therapeutic options in pulmonary hypertension, patients must cope with issues of life-threatening illness, complicated treatments, medical uncertainty, and chronic disease. Few studies have addressed the psychosocial impact of the diagnosis of pulmonary hypertension on patients and their families. Anxiety and depression have been noted to occur more frequently in patients with pulmonary hypertension *(73)* and patients receiving prostacyclin therapy for pulmonary hypertension have reported decreases in emotional and social aspects of quality of life *(74)*. In addition, patients may encounter economic difficulties, family disruption, and social isolation as a consequence of their disease *(75)*. There is increased interest in the utilization of quality of life measures as endpoints in clinical trials for pulmonary hypertension. Primary care specialists are in a unique position to appreciate the psychosocial challenges faced by patients with pulmonary hypertension and to provide timely support and referral.

18.15. CASE STUDY

A 45-year-old lawyer presents with fatigue, worsening shortness of breath with exercise, and recent syncope. Five years ago she underwent fertility evaluation. She was found to be hypothyroid, and treatment was initiated. Dyspnea began 4 years prior to presentation, with insidious progression to current inability to perform routine activities around the home without shortness of breath (WHO functional Class III). Recent presentation to a primary care physician found normal liver and renal function and normal TSH. Weight was stable with BMI 25. Spirometry was normal. A program of exercise training and cataloguing of symptoms was prescribed, as well as strengthening of emotional supports.

Symptoms continued. A sense of chest pressure and lightheadedness developed after short periods of exercise, followed by acute syncope without sensed tachycardia, led to representation. Chest X-ray showed markedly enlarged pulmonary arteries. Echocardiography revealed severe right ventricular enlargement with moderately decreased function. Tricuspid regurgitation velocity suggested an RV pressure that was 100 mm, equal to her brachial arm cuff systemic blood pressure. The patient was admitted to hospital.

There was no history of alcohol, stimulant, or anorexigen use. No atherosclerotic risks were present. There was no family history of thrombosis. A family history of SLE was noted. Additionally, an otherwise well first-degree cousin had died in her thirties of unexplained heart failure. The patient and her family denied history of sleep-disordered breathing.

In hospital, initial evaluation included lung scintigraphy (V/Q scan), and PE-protocol CT, with 1 mm imaging. No pulmonary arterial obstruction was noted, and the lung parenchyma was normal. A 6-min walk was performed, during which time the patient was able to achieve a distance of 300 m, stopping with profound dyspnea and chest fullness. Cardiac catheterization was performed: epicardial coronary arteries were unobstructed, central filling pressure, and pulmonary capillary wedge (left atrial pressure) were normal. No oximetric shunt was present, and resting cardiac output was extremely low (1.5 L/min/m^2). Pulmonary artery systolic pressure was equal to systemic arterial systolic pressure, with PA pressure noted as 100/45/65. Pulmonary vascular resistance was calculated as "> 30 indexed Wood units" (normal < 2–4 indexed Wood units). The patient underwent acute vasodilator challenge with inhaled nitric oxide. Her PA pressure dropped to 50/20/30, with brachial arterial pressure unchanged at 100/70/80.

The patient was taught extensively about the pathophysiology, treated outcomes, and potential therapies for pulmonary hypertension. Dose titration with oral nifedipine was performed, and a home regimen was prescribed. After 6 months of medical therapy combined with supervised exercise training, the patient returns for a follow-up visit. She feels that her functional capacity has returned to 90% of her initial status. She is, however, aware that she has a chronic disease that may threaten her well-being unexpectedly. She has developed close relationships with primary and specialty care providers and presents for discussions about future therapies.

REFERENCES

1. McGoon MD, Kane GC. Pulmonary hypertension: diagnosis and management. *Mayo Clin Proc.* 2009;84(2):191–207.
2. Humbert M. Update in pulmonary hypertension 2008. *Am J Resp Crit Care Med.* 2009;179(8):650–656.
3. McLaughlin VV, Archer SL, Badesch DB, et al. ACCF/AHA 2009 expert consensus document on pulmonary hypertension: a report of the American College of Cardiology Foundation Task Force on Expert Consensus Documents and the American Heart Association: developed in collaboration with the American College of Chest Physicians, American Thoracic Society, Inc., and the Pulmonary Hypertension Association. *Circulation.* 2009;119(16):2250–2294.
4. Farber HW, Loscalzo J. Pulmonary arterial hypertension. *N Engl J Med.* 2004;351(16):1655–1665.
5. Heath D, Edwards JE. The pathology of hypertensive pulmonary vascular disease; a description of six grades of structural changes in the pulmonary arteries with special reference to congenital cardiac septal defects. *Circulation.* 1958;18(4 Part 1):533–547.
6. Condliffe R, Kiely DG, Peacock AJ, et al. Connective tissue disease-associated pulmonary arterial hypertension in the modern treatment era. *Am J Resp Crit Care Med.* 2009;179(2):151–157.
7. Diller GP, Gatzoulis MA. Pulmonary vascular disease in adults with congenital heart disease. *Circulation.* 2007;115(8):1039–1050.
8. Lederman MM, Sereni D, Simonneau G, Voelkel NF. Pulmonary arterial hypertension and its association with HIV infection: an overview. *AIDS.* 2008;22(Suppl 3):S1–S6.
9. Humbert M, Sitbon O, Chaouat A, et al. Pulmonary arterial hypertension in France: results from a national registry. *Am J Resp Crit Care Med.* 2006;173(9):1023–1030.
10. Rich S, Dantzker DR, Ayres SM, et al. Primary pulmonary hypertension. A national prospective study. *Ann Intern Med.* 1987;107(2):216–223.
11. Taichman DB, Mandel J. Epidemiology of pulmonary arterial hypertension. *Clin Chest Med.* 2007;28(1):1.
12. Lam CSP, Borlaug BA, Kane GC, Enders FT, Rodeheffer RJ, Redfield MM. Age-associated increases in pulmonary artery systolic pressure in the general population. *Circulation.* 2009;119(20):2663–2670.

13. Deng Z, Morse JH, Slager SL, et al. Familial primary pulmonary hypertension (gene PPH1) is caused by mutations in the bone morphogenetic protein receptor-II gene. *Am J Human Genetics*. 2000;67(3):737–744.

14. Lane KB, Machado RD, Pauciulo MW, et al. Heterozygous germline mutations in BMPR2, encoding a TGF-beta receptor, cause familial primary pulmonary hypertension. The International PPH Consortium. *Nat Genet*. 2000;26(1):81–84.

15. Trembath RC, Thomson JR, Machado RD, et al. Clinical and molecular genetic features of pulmonary hypertension in patients with hereditary hemorrhagic telangiectasia. *N Engl J Med*. 2001;345(5):325–334.

16. Barst RJ, McGoon M, Torbicki A, et al. Diagnosis and differential assessment of pulmonary arterial hypertension. *J Am Coll Cardiol*. 2004;43(12 Suppl S):S40–S47.

17. McLure LER, Peacock AJ. Imaging of the heart in pulmonary hypertension. *Int J Clin Pract Suppl*. 2007;156:15–26.

18. Tei C, Dujardin KS, Hodge DO, et al. Doppler echocardiographic index for assessment of global right ventricular function. *J Am Soc Echocard*. 1996;9(6):838–847.

19. Apfel HD, Shen Z, Gopal AS, et al. Quantitative three dimensional echocardiography in patients with pulmonary hypertension and compressed left ventricles: comparison with cross sectional echocardiography and magnetic resonance imaging. *Heart*. 1996;76(4):350–354.

20. Forfia PR, Fisher MR, Mathai SC, et al. Tricuspid annular displacement predicts survival in pulmonary hypertension. *Am J Resp Crit Care Med*. 2006;174(9):1034–1041.

21. Miyamoto S, Nagaya N, Satoh T, et al. Clinical correlates and prognostic significance of six-minute walk test in patients with primary pulmonary hypertension. Comparison with cardiopulmonary exercise testing. *Am J Resp Crit Care Med*. 2000;161(2 Pt 1):487–492.

22. McGoon M, Gutterman D, Steen V, et al. Screening, early detection, and diagnosis of pulmonary arterial hypertension: ACCP evidence-based clinical practice guidelines. *Chest*. 2004;126(1 Suppl):14S–34S.

23. Hoeper MM, Mayer E, Simonneau G, Rubin LJ. Chronic thromboembolic pulmonary hypertension. *Circulation*. 2006;113(16):2011–2020.

24. Bonderman D, Wilkens H, Wakounig S, et al. Risk factors for chronic thromboembolic pulmonary hypertension. *Euro Resp J*. 2009;33(2):325–331.

25. Benza R, Biederman R, Murali S, Gupta H. Role of cardiac magnetic resonance imaging in the management of patients with pulmonary arterial hypertension. *J Am Coll Cardiol*. 2008;52(21):1683–1692.

26. Hemnes AR, Forfia PR, Champion HC. Assessment of pulmonary vasculature and right heart by invasive haemodynamics and echocardiography. *Int J Clin Pract Suppl*. 2009;162:4–19.

27. Rich S, Kaufmann E, Levy PS. The effect of high doses of calcium-channel blockers on survival in primary pulmonary hypertension. *N Engl J Med*. 1992;327(2):76–81.

28. Barst RJ, Rubin LJ, Long WA, et al. A comparison of continuous intravenous epoprostenol (prostacyclin) with conventional therapy for primary pulmonary hypertension. The Primary Pulmonary Hypertension Study Group. *N Engl J Med*. 1996;334(5):296–302.

29. Kawut SM, Taichman DB, Archer-Chicko CL, Palevsky HI, Kimmel SE. Hemodynamics and survival in patients with pulmonary arterial hypertension related to systemic sclerosis. *Chest*. 2003;123(2):344–350.

30. D'Alonzo GE, Barst RJ, Ayres SM, et al. Survival in patients with primary pulmonary hypertension. Results from a national prospective registry. *Ann Intern Med*. 1991;15(5):343–349.

31. Eysmann SB, Palevsky HI, Reichek N, Hackney K, Douglas PS. Two-dimensional and Doppler-echocardiographic and cardiac catheterization correlates of survival in primary pulmonary hypertension. *Circulation*. 1989;80(2):353–360.

32. van Wolferen SA, Marcus JT, Boonstra A, et al. Prognostic value of right ventricular mass, volume, and function in idiopathic pulmonary arterial hypertension. *Euro Heart J*. 2007;28(10):1250–1257.

33. Nagaya N, Nishikimi T, Uematsu M, et al. Plasma brain natriuretic peptide as a prognostic indicator in patients with primary pulmonary hypertension. *Circulation*. 2000;102(8):865–870.

34. Fijalkowska A, Kurzyna M, Torbicki A, et al. Serum N-terminal brain natriuretic peptide as a prognostic parameter in patients with pulmonary hypertension. *Chest*. 2006;129(5):1313–1321.

35. Torbicki A, Kurzyna M, Kuca P, et al. Detectable serum cardiac troponin T as a marker of poor prognosis among patients with chronic precapillary pulmonary hypertension. *Circulation*. 2003;108(7):844–848.

36. Fuster V, Steele PM, Edwards WD, Gersh BJ, McGoon MD, Frye RL. Primary pulmonary hypertension: natural history and the importance of thrombosis. *Circulation*. 1984;70(4):580–587.

37. Elliott CG, Glissmeyer EW, Havlena GT, et al. Relationship of BMPR2 mutations to vasoreactivity in pulmonary arterial hypertension. *Circulation*. 2006;113(21):2509–2515.

38. Klings ES, Hill NS, Ieong MH, Simms RW, Korn JH, Farber HW. Systemic sclerosis-associated pulmonary hypertension: short- and long-term effects of epoprostenol (prostacyclin). *Arthr Rheuma*. 1999;42(12):2638–2645.

39. Olschewski H, Simonneau G, Galie N, et al. Inhaled iloprost for severe pulmonary hypertension. *N Engl J Med*. 2002;347(5):322–329.

40. Gomberg-Maitland M, Tapson VF, Benza RL, et al. Transition from intravenous epoprostenol to intravenous treprostinil in pulmonary hypertension. *Am J Resp Crit Care Med*. 2005;172(12):1586–1589.

41. Rubin LJ, Badesch DB, Barst RJ, et al. Bosentan therapy for pulmonary arterial hypertension. *N Engl J Med.* 2002;346(12):896–903.

42. Galie N, Beghetti M, Gatzoulis MA, et al. Bosentan therapy in patients with Eisenmenger syndrome: a multicenter, double-blind, randomized, placebo-controlled study. *Circulation.* 2006;114(1):48–54.

43. Galie N, Olschewski H, Oudiz RJ, et al. Ambrisentan for the treatment of pulmonary arterial hypertension: results of the ambrisentan in pulmonary arterial hypertension, randomized, double-blind, placebo-controlled, multicenter, efficacy (ARIES) study 1 and 2. *Circulation.* 2008;117(23):3010–3019.

44. Galie N, Ghofrani HA, Torbicki A, et al. Sildenafil citrate therapy for pulmonary arterial hypertension. *N Engl J Med.* 2005;353(20):2148–2157.

45. Barst RJ, Langleben D, Badesch D, et al. Treatment of pulmonary arterial hypertension with the selective endothelin-A receptor antagonist sitaxsentan. *J Am Coll Cardiol.* 2006;47(10):2049–2056.

46. Galie N, Brundage BH, Ghofrani HA, et al. Tadalafil therapy for pulmonary arterial hypertension. *Circulation.* 2009;119(22):2894–2903.

47. McLaughlin VV, Oudiz RJ, Frost A, et al. Randomized study of adding inhaled iloprost to existing bosentan in pulmonary arterial hypertension. *Am J Resp Crit Care Med.* 2006;174(11):1257–1263.

48. Hoeper MM, Leuchte H, Halank M, et al. Combining inhaled iloprost with bosentan in patients with idiopathic pulmonary arterial hypertension. *Euro Resp J.* 2006;28(4):691–694.

49. Simonneau G, Rubin LJ, Galie N, et al. Addition of sildenafil to long-term intravenous epoprostenol therapy in patients with pulmonary arterial hypertension: a randomized trial. *Ann Intern Med.* 2008;149(8):521–530.

50. Law MA, Grifka RG, Mullins CE, Nihill MR. Atrial septostomy improves survival in select patients with pulmonary hypertension. *Am Heart J.* 2007;153(5):779–784.

51. Kerstein D, Levy PS, Hsu DT, Hordof AJ, Gersony WM, Barst RJ. Blade balloon atrial septostomy in patients with severe primary pulmonary hypertension. *Circulation.* 1995;91(7):2028–2035.

52. Orens JB. Lung transplantation for pulmonary hypertension. *Int J Clin Prac Suppl.* 2007;158:4–9.

53. Orens JB, Estenne M, Arcasoy S, et al. International guidelines for the selection of lung transplant candidates: 2006 update—a consensus report from the Pulmonary Scientific Council of the International Society for Heart and Lung Transplantation. *J Heart Lung Transpl.* 2006;25(7):745–755.

54. Orens JB, Shearon TH, Freudenberger RS, Conte JV, Bhorade SM, Ardehali A. Thoracic organ transplantation in the United States, 1995–2004. *Am J Transpl.* 2006;6(5 Pt 2):1188–1197.

55. Ramakrishna G, Sprung J, Ravi BS, Chandrasekaran K, McGoon MD. Impact of pulmonary hypertension on the outcomes of noncardiac surgery: predictors of perioperative morbidity and mortality. *J Am Coll Cardiol.* 2005;45(10):1691–1699.

56. Weiss BM, Zemp L, Seifert B, Hess OM. Outcome of pulmonary vascular disease in pregnancy: a systematic overview from 1978 through 1996. *J Am Coll Cardiol.* 1998;31(7):1650–1657.

57. Mereles D, Ehlken N, Kreuscher S, et al. Exercise and respiratory training improve exercise capacity and quality of life in patients with severe chronic pulmonary hypertension. *Circulation.* 2006;114(14):1482–1489.

58. Burrows B, Kettel LJ, Niden AH, Rabinowitz M, Diener CF. Patterns of cardiovascular dysfunction in chronic obstructive lung disease. *N Engl J Med.* 1972;286(17):912–918.

59. Weitzenblum E, Sautegeau A, Ehrhart M, Mammosser M, Hirth C, Roegel E. Long-term course of pulmonary arterial pressure in chronic obstructive pulmonary disease. *Am Rev Resp Dis.* 1984;130(6):993–998.

60. Naeije R. Pulmonary hypertension and right heart failure in chronic obstructive pulmonary disease. *Proc Am Thoracic Soc.* 2005;2(1):20–22.

61. Presberg KW, Dincer HE. Pathophysiology of pulmonary hypertension due to lung disease. *Curr Opin Pul Med.* 2003;9(2):131–138.

62. Chaouat A, Naeije R, Weitzenblum E. Pulmonary hypertension in COPD. *Euro Resp J.* 2008;32(5):1371–1385.

63. Chaouat A, Bugnet AS, Kadaoui N, et al. Severe pulmonary hypertension and chronic obstructive pulmonary disease. *Am J Resp Crit Care Med.* 2005;172(2):189–194.

64. Kessler R, Faller M, Weitzenblum E, et al. "Natural history" of pulmonary hypertension in a series of 131 patients with chronic obstructive lung disease. *Am J Resp Crit Care Med.* 2001;164(2):219–224.

65. Nocturnal Oxygen Therapy Trial Group. Continuous or nocturnal oxygen therapy in hypoxemic chronic obstructive lung disease: a clinical trial. *Ann Intern Med.* 1980;93(3):391–398.

66. Timms RM, Khaja FU, Williams GW. Hemodynamic response to oxygen therapy in chronic obstructive pulmonary disease. *Ann Intern Med.* 1985;102(1):29–36.

67. Ryu JH, Krowka MJ, Pellikka PA, Swanson KL, McGoon MD. Pulmonary hypertension in patients with interstitial lung diseases. *Mayo Clin Proc.* 2007;82(3):342–350.

68. Shorr AF, Helman DL, Davies DB, Nathan SD. Pulmonary hypertension in advanced sarcoidosis: epidemiology and clinical characteristics. *Euro Resp J.* 2005;25(5):783–788.

69. Tomasini M, Chiappino G. Hemodynamics of pulmonary circulation in asbestosis: study of 16 cases. *Am J Indust Med.* 1981;2(2):167–174.
70. Strange C, Bolster M, Mazur J, Taylor M, Gossage JR, Silver R. Hemodynamic effects of epoprostenol in patients with systemic sclerosis and pulmonary hypertension. *Chest.* 2000;118(4):1077–1082.
71. Ghofrani HA, Wiedemann R, Rose F, et al. Sildenafil for treatment of lung fibrosis and pulmonary hypertension: a randomised controlled trial. *Lancet.* 2002;360(9337):895–900.
72. Fisher KA, Serlin DM, Wilson KC, Walter RE, Berman JS, Farber HW. Sarcoidosis-associated pulmonary hypertension: outcome with long-term epoprostenol treatment. *Chest.* 2006;130(5):1481–1488.
73. Lowe B, Grafe K, Ufer C, et al. Anxiety and depression in patients with pulmonary hypertension. *Psychosom Med.* 2004;66(6):831–836.
74. Peloquin J, Robichaud-Ekstrand S, Pepin J. Quality of life perception by women suffering from stage III or IV primary pulmonary hypertension and receiving prostacyclin treatment. *Can J Nurs Res.* 1998;30(1):113–136.
75. Wryobeck JM, Lippo G, McLaughlin V, Riba M, Rubenfire M. Psychosocial aspects of pulmonary hypertension: a review. *Psychosomatics.* 2007;48(6):467–475.
76. Mullen MP, Pulmonary H. In: Keene JF, Lock JE, Fyler DC, eds. *Nadas' Pediatric Cardiology.* 2nd ed. Philadelphia, PA: Saunders Elsevier; 2006:113–126.
77. Barst RJ, Gibbs JS, Ghofrani HA, et al. Updated evidence-based treatment algorithm in pulmonary arterial hypertension. *J Am Coll Cardiol.* 2009;54(1 Suppl):S78–S84.
78. Rubin LJ. Diagnosis and management of pulmonary arterial hypertension: ACCP Evidence-based clinical practice guidelines. *Chest.* 2004;126:7S–10S.

19   Diagnosis and Management of Ischemic Stroke

Aslam M. Khaja

CONTENTS

Keywords: Aphasia; Cerebral ischemia; Cerebral perfusion; Seizure; Stroke; Tissue plasminogen activator.

KEY POINTS

- The clinical diagnosis of acute ischemic stroke in the emergency room is based on clinical history, physical examination, and neuroimaging.
- Intravenous recombinant tissue plasminogen activator (tPA) is FDA approved for the treatment of acute ischemic stroke within 3 h of symptom onset, but is likely beneficial up to 4.5 h after onset.
- Hypoxia, fever, hypotension, hypertension, and hyperglycemia are associated with worse outcomes after ischemic stroke and should be managed appropriately.
- The in-patient evaluation consists of vascular imaging, echocardiography, and risk factor identification/management.
- Decompressive hemicraniectomy is a lifesaving procedure and should be considered in patients with large strokes involving more than two-thirds of the cerebral hemisphere.
- The first line of secondary stroke prevention is antiplatelet therapy.
- Management of risk factors such as hypertension, diabetes mellitus, dyslipidemia, and smoking is necessary to reduce the risk of recurrent cardiovascular events.
- Stroke patients with atrial fibrillation should be anticoagulated; if warfarin is contraindicated, then therapy with antiplatelet agents should be utilized.

From: *Contemporary Cardiology: Comprehensive Cardiovascular Medicine in the Primary Care Setting*
Edited by: Peter P. Toth, Christopher P. Cannon, DOI 10.1007/978-1-60327-963-5_19
© Springer Science+Business Media, LLC 2010

- Carotid endarterectomy should be considered in symptomatic stenosis >50% and asymptomatic stenosis >60%.
- Carotid artery stenting has not been proven superior to endarterectomy.

19.1. INTRODUCTION

Until relatively recently, ischemic stroke management was a classic example of "diagnose and adios." Care of patients presenting to the hospital or clinic with symptoms of stroke consisted of aspirin followed by rehabilitation, with few disease-specific strategies directed toward optimal treatment and outcomes. The past two decades have witnessed an explosion of research into ischemic stroke. We now have specific therapies and management strategies to reduce morbidity and mortality. This chapter will first discuss the identification of patients with ischemic stroke, followed by acute treatment, in-patient management, and secondary stroke prevention.

19.2. DIAGNOSIS

The clinical assessment remains the most efficient method to diagnose ischemic stroke in the emergency room. The history, general examination, and neurologic examination can almost always reliably determine the location of the infarct, even without the aid of neuroimaging. The goal of the initial evaluation is to diagnose an ischemic stroke and evaluate the appropriateness for any emergency treatments.

The first component of the clinical assessment is the history. The deficits are usually sudden in onset, during normal daily activities or upon awakening from sleep. Progression of symptoms over days or weeks is less common. Since patients presenting within the first few hours after onset can be eligible for acute reperfusion therapies, the time of onset is critical. Many times the patient can identify when the symptoms began. If the patient suffers from aphasia or has altered mental status, then determining the exact time of onset can be difficult. In this setting, the time of onset is considered the time the patient was last seen normal. For example, if the symptoms were present upon awakening from sleep, then the time the patient went to sleep the night before is considered the time of onset. Additional components of the history should focus on concurrent medical problems and medications, particularly the use of anticoagulants.

The general examination is similar to other patients and begins with the "ABCs" of airway, breathing, and circulation. Vital signs including temperature and oxygen saturation are important. Examination of the head and neck can reveal signs of trauma, seizure, or carotid artery disease. The cardiac examination should focus on identifying acute MI, atrial fibrillation, or aortic dissection. The skin exam can elucidate significant systemic disease, such as a coagulopathy or hepatic dysfunction (1).

The main purpose of the neurologic examination is to localize the lesion. Patients with ischemic stroke usually present with focal neurologic signs and symptoms that fit a recognized neuro-anatomic pattern. The pattern of deficits can be utilized by practitioners to localize the lesion and determine appropriate testing.

Common patterns of deficits in patients with ischemic stroke appear in Table 1. Since the left side of the brain controls the right side of the body, the stroke in the brain is typically on the opposite side of the deficits on the body. The left hemisphere is usually the dominant hemisphere; even left-handed people are left hemisphere dominant two-thirds of the time. Brain stem strokes often cause "crossed findings," i.e., deficits involving the left face and right side of the body. This is because almost all cranial nerves are ipsilateral, whereas the descending motor and sensory tracts are contralateral. For instance, a lesion in the left pons may cause left facial weakness (due to impairment of the left seventh cranial nerve) but right-sided weakness.

Table 1
Common Patterns of Neurologic Deficits in Ischemic Stroke

Left hemisphere (dominant hemisphere)
Aphasia
Right-sided weakness
Right-sided numbness
Right homonymous hemianopsia
Left gaze preference

Right hemisphere (Non-dominant Hemisphere)
Neglect or extinction
Left-sided weakness
Left-sided numbness
Left homonymous hemianopsia
Right gaze preference

Brain stem
Impaired consciousness
Ataxia/incoordination
Vertigo or dizziness
Double vision (diplopia)
Trouble swallowing (dysphagia)
Slurred speech (dysarthria)
Nystagmus

It is also important to differentiate ischemic stroke from common mimics. Processes that can mimic acute stroke symptoms include seizures, migraines, encephalopathy, positional vertigo, and hypo- or hyperglycemia. In the setting of aphasia, it can become particularly difficult to distinguish between focal language impairment and other causes of altered mental status, such as delirium. Often, the aphasic patient will be awake and alert, regarding the examiner but unable to follow commands, compared to the delirious patient, who often is agitated or somnolent/lethargic *(2)*. Headaches are uncommon in the setting of acute ischemic stroke because the brain itself is not sensitive to pain *(3)*.

The National Institutes of Health Stroke Scale (NIHSS) score (Table 2) is commonly employed by stroke neurologists to describe the deficits and determine the size of the stroke: the larger the stroke, the higher the NIHSS. The customary orientation questions are person and place. The routine commands are "Close your eyes" and "Show me two fingers." It is important for the examiner not to perform the tasks themselves and to prevent aphasic patients from mimicking. Technically, the NIHSS score should reflect the patient's total deficits, regardless of acuity. However, in clinical use, the NIHSS score is often scored to reflect the patient's new deficits. When used properly, the NIHSS serves to not only describe deficits, but also helps identify the occluded vessel and determine prognosis *(4)*. For example, a patient with an NIHSS of 20 likely has a carotid occlusion and poor prognosis.

The diagnosis of stroke can be made on the basis of history and clinical examination. Neuroimaging is critical to differentiate ischemic from hemorrhagic stroke *(5)*. The most commonly employed modality is computerized tomography (CT) scanning. A simple unenhanced CT scan of the head can consistently determine the presence of intracranial hemorrhage and diagnose some non-vascular causes such as malignancy *(6)*. CT scanning has important limitations. First, CT is relatively insensitive in detecting acute ischemic infarcts, as well as small cortical or subcortical strokes *(7)*. The inability of CT to determine acute infarcts is significant; therefore, the main utility of CT is to exclude hemorrhage and other causes. The diagnosis of acute ischemic stroke in the ED remains a largely clinical

Table 2
NIH Stroke Scale

1A. *Level of consciousness*
0 = Alert
1 = Arousable with minor stimulation
2 = Arousable with repeated stimulation
3 = Unresponsive or coma
1B. *Orientation questions (two questions)*
0 = Answers both correctly
1 = One question correct
2 = Neither question correct
1C. *Commands (two commands)*
0 = Follows both
1 = Follows one command
2 = Follows neither command

2. *Lateral Gaze*
0 = Normal horizontal eye movements
1 = Partial horizontal gaze palsy
2 = Complete gaze palsy or forced deviation

3. *Visual fields*
0 = Intact to confrontation
1 = Partial hemianopsia
2 = Complete hemianopsia
3 = Bilateral hemianopsia or blind

4. *Facial movement*
0 = Normal
1 = Minor facial weakness
2 = Paralysis of lower face or significant weakness
3 = Complete unilateral facial palsy

5. *Motor function in the arm (A=left, B=right)*
0 = Able to raise arm for 10 s without drift
1 = Arm drifts but does not touch bed
2 = Arm drifts down to bed before 10 s
3 = No movement against gravity, unable to raise
4 = No movement

6. *Motor function in the leg (A=left, B=right)*
0 = Able to raise for 5 s without drift
1 = Leg drifts but does not touch bed
2 = Leg drifts down to bed before 5 s
3 = No movement against gravity, unable to raise
4 = No movement

7. *Limb ataxia*
0 = No ataxia
1 = Ataxia in one limb
2 = Ataxia in two or more limbs

8. *Sensory*
0 = Normal
1 = Mild sensory loss
2 = Severe or total sensory loss

(Continued)

Table 2
(Continued)

9. *Language*
0 = Normal
1 = Mild aphasia, mild loss of fluency
2 = Severe aphasia, fragmented speech
3 = Mute of global aphasia

10. *Dysarthria*
0 = Normal
1 = Mild dysarthria but able to be understood
2 = Moderate dysarthria, unintelligible or mute

11. *Extinction or neglect*
0 = Absent
1 = Mild, extinction
2 = Severe neglect or inattention

diagnosis. Magnetic resonance imaging (MRI) is increasingly utilized in the ER as the initial neuroimaging modality and is discussed later.

- The diagnosis of stroke is based on the clinical exam and history.
- The CT scan is used to distinguish between ischemic and hemorrhagic stroke.
- The initial head CT may not detect an acute infract.

19.3. ACUTE THROMBOLYSIS AND TREATMENT

Thrombolysis has redefined the acute management of stroke. In 1995, the FDA approved recombinant tissue plasminogen activator (tPA) for use in the setting of an acute ischemic stroke based upon the results of the pivotal National Institute of Neurological Disorders and Stroke (NINDS) trial. In this study, 624 patients presenting within 3 h of symptom onset were randomized to treatment with intravenous (IV) tPA (0.9 mg/kg) or placebo. Patients treated with tPA were 30% more likely to have a favorable outcome at 3 months compared to placebo *(8)*. It is interesting to note that there was no significant decrease in the NIHSS scores at 24 h. So even if patients do not immediately improve, they are still more likely to have a favorable outcome at 3 months if treated with tPA. The most significant adverse effect of rtPA was intracerebral hemorrhage, which occurred in 6.4% of treated patients. The number of patients needed to treat with tPA to cause benefit is 3; whereas, the number needed to harm is 30 *(9)*. Proper selection of patients is critical. Criteria to select patients for treatment with tPA are summarized in Table 3 *(10)*. Deviations from published guidelines may increase the rate of intracranial hemorrhage *(11, 12)*.

Despite the approval of tPA for acute ischemic stroke, only a small percentage of patients nationwide receive the drug. The most common exclusion is presentation outside the 3 h window *(13)*. Most trials of tPA beyond 3 h have failed to show a benefit. However, a meta-analysis suggested a benefit to IV tPA beyond 3 h *(14)* and recently a large US trial showed a benefit of IV tPA up to 4.5 h after symptom onset *(15)*. At this time, treatment with IV tPA beyond 3 h should be done by experienced stroke physicians.

Another rapidly expanding area of acute stroke treatment is intra-arterial therapy (IAT). IAT is attractive because lytics can be administered directly into the clot, leading to higher recanalization

Table 3
Criteria for Treatment with tPA

Inclusion criteria
Clinical signs and symptoms consistent with ischemic stroke
Patient last seen normal in past 3 h
Significant neurologic deficit

Exclusion criteria
Any hemorrhage on neuroimaging
Symptoms suggestive of subarachnoid hemorrhage
Seizure at stroke onset that is thought to contribute to the neurologic deficit
Hypodensity in more than one-third of the cerebral hemisphere
SBP >185 mmHg or DBP >110 mmHg
Serum glucose <50 mg/dL
Platelet count <100 K/mm^3
INR >1.7
Elevated PTT
Any history of intracranial hemorrhage
Arterial puncture at non-compressible site in the past 7 days
Major surgery in the past 14 days
Gastrointestinal bleed or hematuria in the past 21 days
Ischemic stroke, myocardial infarction, or serious head trauma in the past 3 months

rates *(16)*. In addition to lytics, IAT has the added benefit of mechanical clot lysis via a plethora of specialized catheters and devices (Fig. 1). Problems with IAT include availability and time. Few centers have experienced neuro-interventionalists, and treatment requires activation of a specialized treatment team. IAT should be considered at experienced centers. Ideal patients may be those with moderate to severe strokes, who are otherwise not eligible for IV tPA. The availability of IAT should not preclude the use of IV tPA *(1)*. IAT should be performed after consultation with a stroke physician.

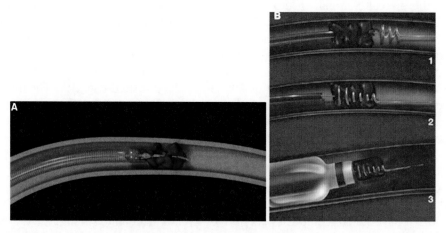

Fig. 1. Examples of intra-arterial catheters. (**a**) Penumbra Stroke System (Penumbra, Inc., Alameda, CA). The clot is broken up mechanically while continuous aspiration with the catheter prevents distal embolization. Image courtesy of Penumbra, Inc. (**b**) MERCI Retriever (Concentric Medical, Inc.). The microcatheter is advanced past the clot and the retriever deployed (*1*), then pulled back into the clot to ensnare it (*2*). Finally the device and microcatheter are withdrawn (*3*). Image courtesy of Concentric Medical.

- IV tPA is approved for ischemic stroke, if used within 3 h of symptom onset.
- IV tPA may be beneficial up to 4.5 h after symptom onset.
- Intra-arterial therapy is a promising field of reperfusion therapy.

19.4. IN-PATIENT GENERAL MEDICAL CARE

The in-patient care of stroke patients focuses on controlling risk factors and rehabilitation. Hypoxia can occur in patients with acute ischemic stroke, due to partial airway obstruction, hypoventilation, aspiration pneumonia, or atelectasis. Hypoxia should be treated to limit additional ischemic brain injury. Stroke patients with brain stem dysfunction or depressed consciousness are at particular risk of hypoxia due to impaired airway protective reflexes *(17)*. Many times stroke patients are routinely placed on supplemental oxygen, but benefit has not been proven *(18)*. The target blood oxygen saturation should be greater than or equal to 92% *(19)*. Endotracheal intubation should be performed if the airway is threatened. Hyperbaric oxygen has been studied in acute ischemic stroke; however, trials do not reveal improved outcomes *(20)*.

Fever is also associated with poor neurological outcomes after stroke. Possible mechanisms include increased metabolic demands, release of neurotransmitters, and free radical production *(21, 22)*. Treating fever may improve prognosis *(23)*. Fever may be secondary to a cause of stroke, such as endocarditis, or from a complication, such as deep venous thrombosis.

Hypothermia is a promising therapy for acute ischemic stroke. Hypothermia has already been shown to improve neurological outcomes after cardiac arrest *(24, 25)*. Small studies have evaluated the feasibility of hypothermia in acute ischemic stroke *(26–28)*. Patients can be cooled with external cooling devices, such as helmets, or internal catheters. Hypothermia is also being tested in combination with other potential neuroprotective agents, such as caffeinol (a combination of caffeine and alcohol) *(29)*. Although promising, hypothermia is associated with significant complications, such as hypotension, pneumonia, and cardiac arrhythmias *(30)*. Hypothermia in acute ischemic stroke is an active area of research, but at this time hypothermia is not recommended outside the setting of a clinical trial.

Cardiac arrhythmias and myocardial ischemia are potential complications of acute ischemic stroke *(31)*. Interestingly, strokes in the right hemisphere, particularly the insula, may have an increased risk of cardiac complications. The etiology is unknown, but thought to involve autonomic disturbances *(32, 33)*. In addition, stroke itself can cause ST segment depression, QT dispersion, inverted T waves, and prominent U waves *(34, 35)*. Cardiac monitoring is recommended for the first 24 h after admission. The most common arrhythmia in ischemic stroke patients is atrial fibrillation *(36)*.

The optimal management of blood pressure in ischemic stroke patients is controversial. Both hyper- and hypotension on admission are associated with increased mortality *(37)*. Theoretically, blood pressure lowering may reduce cerebral edema, lower the risk of hemorrhagic transformation, and prevent further vascular damage *(1)*. On the other hand, lowering blood pressure may also lead to neurologic worsening by decreasing cerebral perfusion *(38, 39)*. One randomized, controlled trial suggests that blood pressure can be acutely lowered safely, but further study is needed *(40, 41)*.

In the acute setting, elevated blood pressure is associated with an increased risk of hemorrhagic transformation after IV tPA *(42, 43)*. Therefore, the upper limit of BP is different in acute ischemic stroke patients treated with thrombolysis compared to those who are not. BP is generally not treated in the acute phase unless it exceeds the upper limits. Guidelines for acute BP management are summarized in Table 4 *(10)*. The general consensus is to allow "permissive hypertension" for the first few days of admission. This involves discontinuation of antihypertensive medications. Blood pressure is only treated if it exceeds the values in Table 4. The blood pressure is then gradually lowered by adding hypertensive medications during the in-patient stay.

Table 4
Blood Pressure Management Acute Ischemic Stroke

Blood pressure (mmHg)	Treatment
A. In patients not eligible for thrombolysis or other acute reperfusion therapies	
SBP ≤220 or DBP ≤120	Observation
SBP >220 or DBP 121–140	Enalapril (IV) or
	Hydralazine (IV) or
	Labetalol (IV) or
	Clonidine (IV or SC) or
	Nicardipine infusion (IV)
DBP >140	Nicardipine infusion (IV) or
	Nitroprusside infusion (IV)
B. In patients eligible for thrombolysis or other acute reperfusion therapies	
SBP ≤185 or DBP ≤110	Observation
SBP >185 or DBP >110	Labetalol (IV) or
	Hydralazine (IV) or
	Clonidine (IV or SC) or
	Nicardipine Infusion (IV)
DBP >140	Nicardipine infusion (IV) or
	Nitroprusside infusion (IV)

Hyperglycemia is often seen in ischemic stroke patients. The presence of hyperglycemia and diabetes is associated with worse outcomes and neurologic deterioration *(44–46)*. It is unclear if hyperglycemia causes worse outcomes or is merely a marker for more severe strokes. Treatment of blood glucose levels greater than 200 mg/dL is recommended *(1)*. Intensive glucose control does not seem to affect mortality and increases the incidence of hypoglycemia *(47, 48)*. Despite lack of good data to guide clinical decisions, it is generally agreed that hyperglycemia after stroke should be controlled *(49)*.

19.5. IN-PATIENT ISCHEMIC STROKE EVALUATION

The primary goals of the in-patient evaluation are to determine the etiology of the stroke, manage neurologic complications, and prevent future events. The first goal is to determine the size of the ischemic stroke and determine the etiology. Non-contrast CT scans can determine stroke size after the acute period has passed. Because the CT scan looks at brain structure, once 48 h have passed the infarct is much better defined on CT. The CT scan can also identify hemorrhagic transformation, which can affect the use of antiplatelet agents or anticoagulants. However, it is difficult to distinguish new from old areas of infarction on CT. In addition, small lacunar or brain stem strokes may be missed *(7)*.

Because of the limitations of CT, many centers employ MRI to evaluate stroke patients. The first important sequence is diffusion-weighted imaging (DWI), often called the "stroke sequence" (Fig. 2). Acute strokes will appear bright on DWI within an hour of ischemia and remain bright for approximately 2 weeks *(50)*. The companion image to the DWI is the ADC (Apparent Diffusion Coefficient); acute strokes appear dark on ADC and then normalize in 5–10 days *(51)*. After a few hours of ischemia, FLAIR (FLuid Attenuated Inversion Recovery) sequences identify areas of vasogenic edema, consistent with acute ischemic stroke *(51)*. FLAIR sequences also identify old areas of ischemia. Although CT reliably detects hemorrhage, GRE (GRadient Echo) images on MRI are much more sensitive for

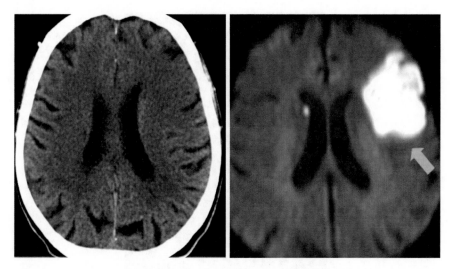

Fig. 2. DWI in ischemic stroke. In acute ischemic stroke the CT scan is often normal (**a**), but the stroke can easily be seen on DWI imaging (**b**).

areas of small petechial and old hemorrhages *(52, 53)*. Because of its many advantages over CT, MRI is the imaging modality of choice in stroke patients.

After determining the size and extent of the stroke, the next step is to determine the etiology of the vascular occlusion. Clots can be divided into two basic classes. A thrombus forms at the site of the occlusion, whereas an embolus forms in one place and then travels to occlude the artery. Because ischemic stroke can be due to either process, it is important to obtain vascular imaging to evaluate the arteries and cardiac imaging to evaluate for potential cardiac sources of emboli.

Carotid ultrasound (CUS) is a common technique to image the vessels of the neck. CUS is based on Doppler imaging of velocity in the carotid arteries. The advantages of CUS are that it is non-invasive, quick, and does not require contrast. As the diameter of the vessel decreases, the velocity must increase to maintain consistent flow. The degree of stenosis can be determined using velocity criteria *(54)*. The disadvantages of ultrasound are that it cannot image the entire length of the carotid or vertebral arteries and it provides no information about the intracranial vessels.

A technique to image the arterial circulation of the entire head and neck is CT angiography (CTA). This is done in the CT scanner. IV contrast is injected and allows for visualization of the vessel lumen. CTA of the neck can identify areas of stenosis or occlusion anywhere along the carotid or vertebral arteries *(55)*. CTA of the head can be performed at the same time and provides valuable information about the intracranial circulation. The main drawback of CTA is that it requires contrast, which is nephrotoxic, and must be used with caution in patients with renal insufficiency.

Because many stroke patients undergo an MRI while in the hospital, magnetic resonance angiography (MRA) has become a convenient non-invasive method of vascular imaging. MRA is based on flow of blood through the vessel *(56)*. An MRA of the head and neck will provide information similar to a CTA (Fig. 3).

The gold standard imaging technique remains invasive cerebral angiography. This is done in the angiography suite by direct arterial injection. Because of its invasive nature, the complications of angiography can be serious: arterial dissection, creation of emboli to cause further strokes, and even death. However, complication rates are low in the hands of experienced interventionalists *(56)*. Ultimately, the choice of vascular imaging is personal; different centers prefer different imaging modalities.

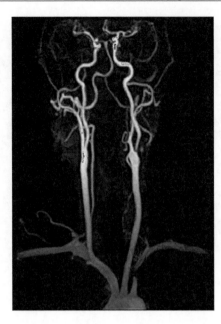

Fig. 3. MRA of the head and neck reveals a smooth narrowing of the left internal carotid artery *(arrow)*.

Since emboli leading to stroke are often cardiac in origin, echocardiography is done in almost every patient with ischemic stroke. Transthoracic echocardiography (TTE) provides information about the structure and function of the heart. Transesophageal echocardiography (TEE) provides better visualization of the atrial chambers and particularly the left atrial appendage, where many clots form. TEE also provides information about atherosclerotic disease in the arch, which may be an additional source of emboli. TEE is preferred over TTE *(57)*. Most centers routinely employ TTE, with selected patients undergoing TEE.

- Ischemic stroke patients should have vascular imaging to evaluate the vessels of the head and neck for areas of stenosis or occlusion.
- CT or MR angiography provides non-invasive imaging of the vasculature.
- Invasive cerebral angiography remains the gold standard vascular imaging technique.
- Echocardiography aids in the identification of causes of cardiogenic emboli.

19.6. IN-PATIENT MANAGEMENT OF NEUROLOGIC COMPLICATIONS

There are three significant acute neurological complications of ischemic stroke. First is cerebral edema, second is hemorrhagic transformation, and third is seizure. Consultation with a neurologist or a neurosurgeon is recommended for management of acute neurologic complications.

Signs of increased intracranial pressure due to cerebral edema include depressed consciousness or worsening neurological deficits. In some patients, cerebral edema can be severe enough to cause a shift of the intracranial structures. A particularly ominous sign is a fixed dilated pupil; this occurs with compression of the third cranial nerve.

Cerebral edema typically peaks about 4 days after stroke onset *(58)*. Although most strokes will have some degree of edema, relatively few have significant enough edema to warrant intervention *(59)*. Initial management of cerebral edema involves avoiding hypo-osmolar fluid (which theoretically may worsen edema). In addition, hypoxemia, hypercarbia, and hyperthermia may exacerbate swelling and should be managed appropriately. Antihypertensive agents should be avoided to maximize cerebral perfusion *(1)*.

Large middle cerebral artery strokes may cause significant intracranial shift. The definitive treatment is decompressive hemicraniectomy. This involves removing half the skull and cutting the dura on the side of the stroke, to allow room for the damaged brain to swell outward. The bone is saved and can be re-inserted later, after the edema has resolved. Decompressive hemicraniectomy has been a focus of significant research in the past few years. We now know that early hemicraniectomy (within 48 h of stroke onset) improves survival and outcomes, whereas delaying hemicraniectomy beyond 48 h improves survival but has little effect on outcomes *(60, 61)*. Hemicraniectomy should be considered in patients under the age of 60, with large hemispheric stroke involving more than two-thirds of the middle cerebral artery territory *(61)*. However, surviving patients often have significant neurological deficits, and quality of life after hemicraniectomy remains a topic of debate.

Management of hemorrhagic transformation depends upon the amount of bleeding and symptoms. Small petechial hemorrhages are usually asymptomatic. Large confluent hematomas can increase intracranial pressure and cause neurologic deterioration. Although hemorrhagic transformation is a well-known complication of ischemic stroke, optimal treatment strategies have not been defined. If a patient recently received tPA, the tPA should be reversed by administration of cryoprecipitate and platelets *(2)*. In late hemorrhagic transformation, antiplatelets and anticoagulants should be temporarily held.

Seizures are uncommon after ischemic stroke, occurring in about 5% of patients. They usually occur within 48 h of infarction. Most seizures are focal and do not generalize. Interestingly, seizures do not appear to be associated with worse outcome *(62)*. Little data exists about the management of seizures in ischemic stroke; therefore, management is similar to seizures in other neurological illnesses.

19.7. STROKE PREVENTION

The key component of stroke prevention is risk factor management. This section will begin by discussing risk factor management applicable to most ischemic stroke patients, such as hypertension, diabetes, and hypercholesterolemia. This is followed by a discussion of antiplatelet agents, indications for anticoagulation, and the treatment for other disease states that may be discovered during the inpatient evaluation, such as carotid artery disease and intracranial stenosis.

The association between blood pressure reduction and primary stroke prevention is well established *(63)*. Antihypertensives have also been shown to decrease recurrent stroke rates, regardless of whether the patient has hypertension or not *(64)*. Based on the current data, specific recommendations about choice of antihypertensive agents cannot be made, but antihypertensive therapy is recommended to prevent recurrent stroke and vascular events *(36)*.

As mentioned previously, hyperglycemia has been associated with worse outcomes in ischemic stroke patients. Glycemic control reduces the occurrence of microvascular complications *(65)*. Conventional reasoning would argue that glycemic control should, therefore, also prevent macrovascular complications and reduce vascular mortality in patients with diabetes. Interestingly, multiple studies now reveal that tight glycemic control in patients with type 2 diabetes does not reduce cardiovascular events and may actually increase mortality *(66–68)*. While glycemic control is probably still important in stroke prevention, aggressive glycemic control may not be the best strategy. The optimum blood glucose and hemoglobin A_{1c} concentrations to prevent recurrent strokes and cardiovascular events have not been established.

The association between hyperlipidemia and stroke risk has been a topic of much study and discussion. Prior studies have shown a weak correlation between lipid levels and stroke *(69)*. The pivotal study to prove that statin therapy reduced recurrent stroke in patients with stroke or TIA was the

SPARCL (Stroke Prevention by Aggressive Reduction in Cholesterol Levels) trial. This study proved that atorvastatin reduced the overall incidence of strokes and cardiovascular events *(70)*. Patients with stroke and elevated cholesterol should be treated according to the NCEP III guidelines with lifestyle modification, dietary guidelines, and medications *(71)*. The goal LDL in ischemic stroke patients is <100 and <70 mg/dL in very high-risk patients. Statins are suspected to have beneficial effects on the vascular endothelium, beyond cholesterol lowering. Therefore, patients with atherosclerotic ischemic stroke are reasonable candidates for statin therapy *(36)*.

In many patients, smoking cessation is the single most effective way to decrease the risk of recurrent vascular events. Smoking approximately doubles the risk of stroke compared to non-smokers *(72)*. In addition, second-hand smoke may also increase the risk of cardiovascular disease *(73–75)*. A combination of nicotine replacement therapy, social support, and skills training is the most effective approach to quitting smoking *(76)*. The increased risk of stroke disappears 5 years after smoking cessation *(77, 78)*.

Most studies suggest a J-shaped relationship between alcohol consumption and ischemic stroke. Consumption of 1 or 2 drinks/day appears to decrease the risk of stroke. Consumption of 0 or >5 drinks/day is associated with an increased stroke risk *(79)*. The current recommendations state that light to moderate levels of alcohol consumption (2 drinks/day for men, 1 drink/day for women who are not pregnant) may be beneficial *(1)*. Heavy drinkers should reduce their consumption *(36)*.

An increasing body mass index (BMI) increases stroke risk in men *(80)*, but the effect in women is unclear *(81)*. Although losing weight has not been shown to decrease stroke risk, losing weight improves blood pressure, glucose levels, and cholesterol *(82)*. The goal BMI is 18.5–24.9 kg/m^2 *(36)*.

Much attention is focused on the choice of antiplatelet agents to reduce recurrent stroke. At present there are three different agents that are commonly utilized—aspirin, dipyridamole+aspirin (Aggrenox), and clopidogrel (Plavix). Aspirin has been consistently shown to reduce the risk of recurrent stroke. The dose range varies from 50 to 1,300 mg/day. Both high- and low-dose aspirin have similar efficacy *(83, 84)*. However, higher doses of aspirin increase the risk of GI bleeding *(85)*. Clopidogrel is considered similar to aspirin for stroke prevention *(86)*. The combination of aspirin plus clopidogrel offers further benefit for stroke prevention, but this benefit is offset by an increased risk of intracranial hemorrhage in stroke patients *(87)*. Dipyridamole+aspirin has been shown superior to aspirin or dipyridamole alone *(88)*.

If dipyridamole+aspirin is superior to aspirin and clopidogrel is equivalent to aspirin; therefore dipyridamole+aspirin must be superior to both aspirin and clopidogrel. Based upon this logic, for years stroke neurologists considered dipyridamole+aspirin (Aggrenox) the antiplatelet of choice for secondary stroke prevention. Then in 2008, the results of a trial comparing dipyridamole+aspirin to clopidogrel (the largest stroke prevention trial to date) were released. Surprisingly, there was no significant difference *(89)*. The decision of which antiplatelet to use should be individualized. Patients who are unable to tolerate aspirin because of GI side effect may benefit from clopidogrel. Patients suffering headaches because of dipyridamole may benefit from aspirin or clopidogrel.

Many stroke patients presenting to the hospital are often already prescribed and taking an antiplatelet agent. A common practice is to change the antiplatelet prior to discharge, on the assumption that the current antiplatelet was ineffective. For example, if a patient has a stroke on aspirin, they are changed to clopidogrel on discharge, because they have "failed" aspirin therapy. If antiplatelet agents prevented 100% of recurrent strokes, then this would be acceptable. But just because a patient was taking aspirin and has a vascular event, this does not mean that the patient did not benefit from antiplatelet therapy. There is no data to support the common practice of changing antiplatelet therapy in patients presenting with ischemic stroke.

During the in-patient evaluation, extracranial carotid artery disease is frequently found in stroke patients. Atherosclerotic disease of the carotid artery tends to affect the internal carotid artery (ICA) near the bifurcation of the common carotid into the internal and external carotid arteries. The decision to intervene is based on the degree of stenosis and whether the lesion is symptomatic or asymptomatic.

A lesion is considered symptomatic if the stroke or TIA is on the ipsilateral hemisphere. If there is no stroke on the side of the stenosis, then the lesion is considered asymptomatic. If the ICA stenosis is less than 50%, there is no benefit to intervention. If the stenosis is greater than 50% and symptomatic, then carotid endarterectomy is recommended *(36)*. If the lesion is asymptomatic, then a stenosis of greater than 60% should be considered for intervention *(90)*. The current recommendations are that surgery be performed within 2 weeks of stroke or TIA *(36)*.

The intervention of choice in patients with ICA stenosis at the origin is carotid endarterectomy (CEA). This procedure is performed by making an incision in the neck exposing the ICA. The artery is then opened and the plaque cleaned out by hand. In recent years, carotid artery stenting (CAS) has become another available option. Studies comparing CEA to CAS so far have been inconclusive *(91–93)*. While CAS appears to be as effective as CEA for preventing stroke, CAS is associated with a higher peri-procedural stroke rate *(92)*. CEA remains the intervention of choice, with CAS being utilized in cases at a high risk of surgical complications or when CEA is technically difficult.

Intracranial atherosclerotic disease is also frequently encountered in ischemic stroke patients. Many physicians preferred anticoagulation in this setting to encourage blood flow through the stenosis and reduce the risk of occlusion or distal embolization. The Warfarin Aspirin Symptomatic Intracranial Disease (WASID) trial evaluated anticoagulation with warfarin versus aspirin. There was no significant difference between the two groups, and the study was stopped early due to increased mortality in the warfarin arm *(94)*. Patients with intracranial stenosis are usually managed medically. If the patient has recurrent events on best medical therapy, then endovascular therapy should be considered, but the benefit is uncertain *(36)*.

Occasionally, stroke patients admitted to the hospital are started on heparin to decrease the risk of neurological deterioration and recurrent stroke. Several studies have shown no benefit of routine anticoagulation *(2)*. Antiplatelet therapy remains preferred over anticoagulation to prevent recurrent stroke, except in certain circumstances.

The most common indication for anticoagulation in ischemic stroke patients is atrial fibrillation. Atrial fibrillation is the most common cardiac arrhythmia in the elderly *(36)*. Clinical trials have consistently shown a benefit to anticoagulation over placebo, aspirin and aspirin plus clopidogrel in ischemic stroke patients *(95–97)*. The goal INR is 2.0–3.0. In patients not eligible for warfarin, antiplatelet therapy still reduces stroke risk. Other indications for anticoagulation in ischemic stroke patients are acute MI with LV thrombus, rheumatic mitral valve disease, mechanical prosthetic heart valves, or bioprosthetic heart valves. Cardiac conditions in which anticoagulation or antiplatelet therapy is appropriate are dilated cardiomyopathy with a low EF and mitral regurgitation due to mitral annular calcification *(36)*. In addition, patients with arterial dissection are often placed on warfarin for 3–6 months, although data to support this practice are lacking *(36)*.

- Control of risk factors such as hypertension, hyperglycemia, hyperlipidemia, smoking, alcohol, and obesity is the most effect method to prevent recurrent stroke.
- Antiplatelet therapy is indicated in most patients with ischemic stroke.
- Carotid endarterectomy should be considered in patients with symptomatic stenosis >50% or asymptomatic stenosis >60%.
- Patient with intracranial atherosclerotic disease should be treated with antiplatelets.
- Indications for anticoagulation include atrial fibrillation and prosthetic heart valves.

19.8. SUMMARY

Ischemic stroke patients typically present with sudden onset of focal neurologic symptoms that follow a recognized neuro-anatomic pattern. Every patient should get neuroimaging in the ER, usually a non-contrast CT, mainly to exclude hemorrhage. Ischemic strokes will appear on CT a few hours after symptom onset.

In patients with acute ischemic stroke, the time of onset is critical. IV tPA is approved for acute ischemic stroke within 3 h of symptom onset, but likely has a benefit up to 4.5 h. Intra-arterial therapy is promising, but has not yet been shown to improve outcomes. IAT should be considered after consultation with a stroke physician.

The management of hypoxia, fever, and hyperglycemia is important and should not be overlooked. Permissive hypertension for the first few days may help optimize cerebral perfusion. Neuroimaging during the in-patient stay provides valuable information about stroke size and location. CT is often used. MRI has many advantages over CT, as it can distinguish acute from chronic infarcts and small strokes that are often missed by CT. Stroke patients should receive vascular imaging. Carotid ultrasound is a minimum, but CTA or MRA is preferred since these modalities allow for non-invasive imaging of the entire vasculature of the head and neck. The gold standard remains invasive cerebral angiography. Echocardiography is recommended to evaluate for cardiac sources of emboli.

Significant in-patient complications of ischemic stroke are cerebral edema, hemorrhagic transformation, and seizures. Decompressive hemicraniectomy improves morbidity and mortality when done within 48 h of large ischemic strokes.

Management of blood pressure, glucose, cholesterol, smoking, and obesity is much more effective than antiplatelet therapy for stroke prevention. Antiplatelets are generally indicated for ischemic stroke prevention. Anticoagulation should be reserved for patients with conditions such atrial fibrillation and mechanical heart valves. Carotid revascularization should be considered in symptomatic stenosis >50% or asymptomatic stenosis >60%. Carotid artery stenting is useful in patients at high risk of complications from CEA.

19.9. CASE STUDIES

19.9.1. Case Study 1

A 60-year-old Caucasian male presents to the emergency room with acute onset of left-sided weakness and numbness while at work at 9 a.m. He has a past medical history of diabetes and hypertension. Medications are aspirin, HCTZ, and metformin. Vital signs are unremarkable except a BP of 170/95. On examination he has a left facial droop and dysarthria. Cranial nerves are otherwise intact. He is able to raise his left arm and leg off the bed, but they drift to the bed in a few seconds. He has impaired sensation to all modalities on the left (NIHSS 7). CT of the head is normal. Laboratory studies are normal. You evaluate him at 11 a.m.

At this point he meets criteria for IV tPA, and he is treated at 11:30 a.m. His HCTZ and aspirin are held and he is admitted to the ICU for close monitoring and has no change in his symptoms overnight. The next day his aspirin is restarted. His total cholesterol is 180 mg/dL and LDL is 110 mg/dL. He has an MRI and an MRA, which reveal an acute infarct in the subcortical white matter of the right hemisphere and 60% stenosis of his right internal carotid artery. Transthoracic echocardiography reveals an EF of 55% and mild mitral regurgitation. During the next few days in the hospital, his sensation returns to normal and his strength improves to only subtle weakness on his left side. He is started on an ace inhibitor (diabetes and ischemic stroke) in addition to his HCTZ and a statin because his goal LDL is <70 mg/dL (diabetes and stroke).

Because the RICA stenosis meets criteria (>50% symptomatic stenosis), you consult a vascular surgeon, who feels he is a candidate for CEA. He undergoes the CEA next week without complications.

19.9.2. Case Study 2

A 55-year-old African-American male is found down by family at 7 p.m. He was last seen normal in the morning. His past medical history is hypertension, hyperlipidemia, and coronary artery disease. Medications are aspirin, clopidogrel, atorvastatin, and metoprolol. Upon examination his vital signs are normal except for BP 180/100. He has a left gaze deviation, right homonymous hemianopsia, and right facial droop. He is alert and follows commands but is unable to speak. He has no movement or response to pain on his right side (NIHSS 18). CT shows subtle hypodensity in the left hemisphere consistent with early ischemic stroke.

He does not meet criteria for tPA because he is outside the window for treatment (last seen normal in the morning). He is admitted to the hospital and his metoprolol held. Overnight telemetry shows paroxysmal atrial fibrillation. MRI and MRA the next day show a large infarct involving most of the left hemisphere and LICA occlusion.

You consult the neurosurgeon who performs a hemicraniectomy that night. During his hospital stay, his visual fields improve, and he is barely able to raise his right arm and leg off the bed. He requires PEG placement. Two weeks after the hemicraniectomy he is started on anticoagulation for his atrial fibrillation. He is discharged to in-patient rehabilitation.

You see him back in follow-up 3 months later. He has had a left cranioplasty and is back on anticoagulation. He has three-fifths strength on his right side. He mostly uses a wheelchair but is able to walk short distances. He is able to speak simple sentences. He is again able to swallow and his PEG has been removed.

You see him back 1 year after his stroke; he is walking with the use of a cane, and his aphasia has improved. He is doing well on anticoagulation.

REFERENCES

1. Adams HP Jr, del Zoppo G, Alberts MJ, et al. Guidelines for the early management of adults with ischemic stroke: a guideline from the American Heart Association/American Stroke Association Stroke Council, Clinical Cardiology Council, Cardiovascular Radiology and Intervention Council, and the Atherosclerotic Peripheral Vascular Disease and Quality of Care Outcomes in Research Interdisciplinary Working Groups: the American Academy of Neurology affirms the value of this guideline as an educational tool for neurologists. *Stroke.* 2007;38:1655–1711.
2. Khaja AM, Grotta JC. Established treatments for acute ischaemic stroke. *Lancet.* 2007;369:319–330.
3. Adams HP Jr, Adams RJ, Brott T, et al. Guidelines for the early management of patients with ischemic stroke: a scientific statement from the Stroke Council of the American Stroke Association. *Stroke.* 2003;34:1056–1083.
4. Frankel MR, Morgenstern LB, Kwiatkowski T, et al. Predicting prognosis after stroke: a placebo group analysis from the National Institute of Neurological Disorders and Stroke rt-PA Stroke Trial. *Neurology.* 2000;55:952–959.
5. Muir KW, Weir CJ, Murray GD, et al. Comparison of neurological scales and scoring systems for acute stroke prognosis. *Stroke.* 1996;27:1817–1820.
6. Jacobs L, Kinkel WR, Heffner RR Jr. Autopsy correlations of computerized tomography: experience with 6,000 CT scans. *Neurology.* 1976;26:1111–1118.
7. Mullins ME, Schaefer PW, Sorensen AG, et al. CT and conventional and diffusion-weighted MR imaging in acute stroke: study in 691 patients at presentation to the emergency department. *Radiology.* 2002;224:353–360.
8. The National Institute of Neurological Disorders and Stroke rt-PA Stroke Study Group. Tissue plasminogen activator for acute ischemic stroke. *N Engl J Med.* 1995;333:1581–1587.
9. Saver JL. Number needed to treat estimates incorporating effects over the entire range of clinical outcomes: novel derivation method and application to thrombolytic therapy for acute stroke. *Arch Neurol.* 2004;61:1066–1070.
10. Khaja AM. Acute ischemic stroke management: administration of thrombolytics, neuroprotectants, and general principles of medical management. *Neurol Clin.* 2008;26:943–961.
11. Katzan IL, Furlan AJ, Lloyd LE, et al. Use of tissue-type plasminogen activator for acute ischemic stroke: the Cleveland area experience. *JAMA.* 2000;283:1151–1158.
12. Katzan IL, Hammer MD, Furlan AJ, et al. Quality improvement and tissue-type plasminogen activator for acute ischemic stroke: a Cleveland update. *Stroke.* 2003;34:799–800.
13. Barber PA, Zhang J, Demchuk AM, et al. Why are stroke patients excluded from TPA therapy? An analysis of patient eligibility. *Neurology.* 2001;56:1015–1020.
14. Hacke W, Donnan G, Fieschi C, et al. Association of outcome with early stroke treatment: pooled analysis of ATLANTIS, ECASS, and NINDS rt-PA stroke trials. *Lancet.* 2004;363:768–774.
15. Hacke W, Kaste M, Bluhmki E, et al. Thrombolysis with alteplase 3–4.5 hours after acute ischemic stroke. *N Engl J Med.* 2008;359:1317–1329.

16. Qureshi AI. Endovascular treatment of cerebrovascular diseases and intracranial neoplasms. *Lancet.* 2004;363: 804–813.

17. Hacke W, Krieger D, Hirschberg M. General principles in the treatment of acute ishemic stroke. *Cerebrovasc Dis.* 1991;1(Suppl 1):93–99.

18. Ronning OM, Guldvog B. Should stroke victims routinely receive supplemental oxygen? A quasi-randomized controlled trial. *Stroke.* 1999;30:2033–2037.

19. American Heart Association guidelines for cardiopulmonary resuscitation and emergency cardiovascular care. *Circulation.* 2005;112(24 Suppl):IV1–IV203.

20. Oppel L. A review of the scientific evidence on the treatment of traumatic brain injuries and strokes with hyperbaric oxygen. *Brain Inj.* 2003;17:225–236.

21. Azzimondi G, Bassein L, Nonino F, et al. Fever in acute stroke worsens prognosis. A prospective study. *Stroke.* 1995;26:2040–2043.

22. Hajat C, Hajat S, Sharma P. Effects of poststroke pyrexia on stroke outcome: a meta-analysis of studies in patients. *Stroke.* 2000;31:410–414.

23. Jorgensen HS, Reith J, Nakayama H, et al. What determines good recovery in patients with the most severe strokes? The Copenhagen Stroke Study. *Stroke.* 1999;30:2008–2012.

24. The Hypothermia after Cardiac Arrest Study Group. Mild therapeutic hypothermia to improve the neurologic outcome after cardiac arrest. *N Engl J Med.* 2002;346:549–556.

25. Bernard SA, Gray TW, Buist MD, et al. Treatment of comatose survivors of out-of-hospital cardiac arrest with induced hypothermia. *N Engl J Med.* 2002;346:557–563.

26. Krieger DW, De Georgia MA, Abou-Chebl A, et al. Cooling for acute ischemic brain damage (cool aid): an open pilot study of induced hypothermia in acute ischemic stroke. *Stroke.* 2001;32:1847–1854.

27. Wang H, Olivero W, Lanzino G, et al. Rapid and selective cerebral hypothermia achieved using a cooling helmet. *J Neurosurg.* 2004;100:272–277.

28. Slotboom J, Kiefer C, Brekenfeld C, et al. Locally induced hypothermia for treatment of acute ischaemic stroke: a physical feasibility study. *Neuroradiology.* 2004;46:923–934.

29. Martin-Schild S, Hallevi H, Shaltoni H, et al. Combined neuroprotective modalities coupled with thrombolysis in acute ischemic stroke: a pilot study of caffeinol and mild hypothermia. *J Stroke Cerebrovasc Dis.* 2009;18:86–96.

30. Olsen TS, Weber UJ, Kammersgaard LP. Therapeutic hypothermia for acute stroke. *Lancet Neurol.* 2003;2:410–416.

31. Kocan MJ. Cardiovascular effects of acute stroke. *Prog Cardiovasc Nurs.* 1999;14:61–67.

32. Korpelainen JT, Sotaniemi KA, Huikuri HV, et al. Abnormal heart rate variability as a manifestation of autonomic dysfunction in hemispheric brain infarction. *Stroke.* 1996;27:2059–2063.

33. Orlandi G, Fanucchi S, Strata G, et al. Transient autonomic nervous system dysfunction during hyperacute stroke. *Acta Neurol Scand.* 2000;102:317–321.

34. Afsar N, Fak AS, Metzger JT, et al. Acute stroke increases QT dispersion in patients without known cardiac diseases. *Arch Neurol.* 2003;60:346–350.

35. McDermott MM, Lefevre F, Arron M, et al. ST segment depression detected by continuous electrocardiography in patients with acute ischemic stroke or transient ischemic attack. *Stroke.* 1994;25:1820–1824.

36. Sacco RL, Adams R, Albers G, et al. Guidelines for prevention of stroke in patients with ischemic stroke or transient ischemic attack: a statement for healthcare professionals from the American Heart Association/American Stroke Association Council on Stroke: co-sponsored by the Council on Cardiovascular Radiology and Intervention: the American Academy of Neurology affirms the value of this guideline. *Stroke.* 2006;37:577–617.

37. Vemmos KN, Tsivgoulis G, Spengos K, et al. U-shaped relationship between mortality and admission blood pressure in patients with acute stroke. *J Intern Med.* 2004;255:257–265.

38. Johnston KC, Mayer SA. Blood pressure reduction in ischemic stroke: a two-edged sword? *Neurology.* 2003;61: 1030–1031.

39. Goldstein LB. Blood pressure management in patients with acute ischemic stroke. *Hypertension.* 2004;43:137–141.

40. Martin-Schild S. Blood pressure in acute stroke: lower it or let the CHHIPS fall where they will. *Lancet Neurol.* 2009;8:23–24.

41. Potter JF, Robinson TG, Ford GA, et al. Controlling hypertension and hypotension immediately post-stroke (CHHIPS): a randomised, placebo-controlled, double-blind pilot trial. *Lancet Neurol.* 2009;8:48–56.

42. The NINDS t-PA Stroke Study Group. Intracerebral hemorrhage after intravenous t-PA therapy for ischemic stroke. *Stroke.* 1997;28:2109–2118.

43. Larrue V, von Kummer R, del Zoppo G, et al. Hemorrhagic transformation in acute ischemic stroke. Potential contributing factors in the European Cooperative Acute Stroke Study. *Stroke.* 1997;28:957–960.

44. Bruno A, Biller J, Adams HP Jr, et al. Acute blood glucose level and outcome from ischemic stroke. Trial of ORG 10172 in Acute Stroke Treatment (TOAST) Investigators. *Neurology.* 1999;52:280–284.

45. Lindsberg PJ, Roine RO. Hyperglycemia in acute stroke. *Stroke.* 2004;35:363–364.

46. Candelise L, Landi G, Orazio EN, et al. Prognostic significance of hyperglycemia in acute stroke. *Arch Neurol.* 1985;42:661–663.

47. Griesdale DE, de Souza RJ, van Dam RM, et al. Intensive insulin therapy and mortality among critically ill patients: a meta-analysis including NICE-SUGAR study data. *CMAJ.* 2009;180(8):821–827.

48. Finfer S, Heritier S. The NICE-SUGAR (Normoglycaemia in Intensive Care Evaluation and Survival Using Glucose Algorithm Regulation) Study: statistical analysis plan. *Crit Care Resusc.* 2009;11:46–57.

49. Levetan CS. Effect of hyperglycemia on stroke outcomes. *Endocr Pract.* 2004;10(Suppl 2):34–39.

50. Roberts TP, Rowley HA. Diffusion weighted magnetic resonance imaging in stroke. *Eur J Radiol.* 2003;45: 185–194.

51. Thulborn KR. MRI in the management of cerebrovascular disease to prevent stroke. *Neurol Clin.* 2008;26:897–921.

52. Atlas SW, Thulborn KR. MR detection of hyperacute parenchymal hemorrhage of the brain. *Am J Neuroradiol.* 1998;19:1471–1477.

53. Gomori JM, Grossman RI. Mechanisms responsible for the MR appearance and evolution of intracranial hemorrhage. *Radiographics.* 1988;8:427–440.

54. Grant EG, Benson CB, Moneta GL, et al. Carotid artery stenosis: gray-scale and Doppler US diagnosis—Society of Radiologists in Ultrasound Consensus Conference. *Radiology.* 2003;229:340–346.

55. Koelemay MJ, Nederkoorn PJ, Reitsma JB, et al. Systematic review of computed tomographic angiography for assessment of carotid artery disease. *Stroke.* 2004;35:2306–2312.

56. Jaff MR, Goldmakher GV, Lev MH, et al. Imaging of the carotid arteries: the role of duplex ultrasonography, magnetic resonance arteriography, and computerized tomographic arteriography. *Vasc Med.* 2008;13:281–292.

57. Homma S. Echocardiography in stroke patients (with emphasis on cryptogenic stroke). *Rinsho Shinkeigaku.* 2006;46:799–804.

58. Ropper AH, Shafran B. Brain edema after stroke. Clinical syndrome and intracranial pressure. *Arch Neurol.* 1984;41: 26–29.

59. Wijdicks EF, Diringer MN. Middle cerebral artery territory infarction and early brain swelling: progression and effect of age on outcome. *Mayo Clin Proc.* 1998;73:829–836.

60. Vahedi K, Hofmeijer J, Juettler E, et al. Early decompressive surgery in malignant infarction of the middle cerebral artery: a pooled analysis of three randomised controlled trials. *Lancet Neurol.* 2007;6:215–222.

61. Hofmeijer J, Kappelle LJ, Algra A, et al. Surgical decompression for space-occupying cerebral infarction (the Hemicraniectomy After Middle Cerebral Artery infarction with Life-threatening Edema Trial [HAMLET]): a multicentre, open, randomised trial. *Lancet Neurol.* 2009;8:326–333.

62. Kilpatrick CJ, Davis SM, Tress BM, et al. Epileptic seizures in acute stroke. *Arch Neurol.* 1990;47:157–160.

63. Lawes CM, Bennett DA, Feigin VL, et al. Blood pressure and stroke: an overview of published reviews. *Stroke.* 2004;35:776–785.

64. Rashid P, Leonardi-Bee J, Bath P. Blood pressure reduction and secondary prevention of stroke and other vascular events: a systematic review. *Stroke.* 2003;34:2741–2748.

65. Reichard P, Nilsson BY, Rosenqvist U. The effect of long-term intensified insulin treatment on the development of microvascular complications of diabetes mellitus. *N Engl J Med.* 1993;329:304–309.

66. Patel A, MacMahon S, Chalmers J, et al. Intensive blood glucose control and vascular outcomes in patients with type 2 diabetes. *N Engl J Med.* 2008;358:2560–2572.

67. Gerstein HC, Miller ME, Byington RP, et al. Effects of intensive glucose lowering in type 2 diabetes. *N Engl J Med.* 2008;358:2545–2559.

68. Duckworth W, Abraira C, Moritz T, et al. Glucose control and vascular complications in veterans with type 2 diabetes. *N Engl J Med.* 2009;360:129–139.

69. Gorelick PB. Stroke prevention therapy beyond antithrombotics: unifying mechanisms in ischemic stroke pathogenesis and implications for therapy: an invited review. *Stroke.* 2002;33:862–875.

70. Amarenco P, Bogousslavsky J, Callahan A 3rd, et al. High-dose atorvastatin after stroke or transient ischemic attack. *N Engl J Med.* 2006;355:549–559.

71. Expert Panel on Detection, Evaluation, and Treatment of High Blood Cholesterol in Adults. Executive summary of the third report of the National Cholesterol Education Program (NCEP) Expert Panel on Detection, Evaluation, and Treatment of High Blood Cholesterol in Adults (Adult Treatment Panel III). *JAMA.* 2001;285:2486–2497.

72. Shinton R, Beevers G. Meta-analysis of relation between cigarette smoking and stroke. *BMJ.* 1989;29:789–794.

73. He J, Vupputuri S, Allen K, et al. Passive smoking and the risk of coronary heart disease—a meta-analysis of epidemiologic studies. *N Engl J Med.* 1999;340:920–926.

74. You RX, Thrift AG, McNeil JJ, et al. Ischemic stroke risk and passive exposure to spouses' cigarette smoking. Melbourne Stroke Risk Factor Study (MERFS) Group. *Am J Public Health.* 1999;89:572–575.

75. Bonita R, Duncan J, Truelsen T, et al. Passive smoking as well as active smoking increases the risk of acute stroke. *Tob Control.* 1999;8:156–160.

76. Fiore MC. US public health service clinical practice guideline: treating tobacco use and dependence. *Respir Care.* 2000;45:1200–1262.

77. Wannamethee SG, Shaper AG, Whincup PH, et al. Smoking cessation and the risk of stroke in middle-aged men. *JAMA.* 1995;274:155–160.

78. Kawachi I, Colditz GA, Stampfer MJ, et al. Smoking cessation in relation to total mortality rates in women. A prospective cohort study. *Ann Intern Med.* 1993;119:992–1000.

79. Reynolds K, Lewis B, Nolen JD, et al. Alcohol consumption and risk of stroke: a meta-analysis. *JAMA.* 2003;289:579–588.

80. Kurth T, Gaziano JM, Berger K, et al. Body mass index and the risk of stroke in men. *Arch Intern Med.* 2002;162:2557–2562.

81. Lindenstrom E, Boysen G, Nyboe J. Lifestyle factors and risk of cerebrovascular disease in women. The Copenhagen City Heart Study. *Stroke.* 1993;24:1468–1472.

82. Anderson JW, Konz EC. Obesity and disease management: effects of weight loss on comorbid conditions. *Obes Res.* 2001;9(Suppl 4):326S–334S.

83. Antiplatelet Trialists' Collaboration. Collaborative overview of randomised trials of antiplatelet therapy—I: prevention of death, myocardial infarction, and stroke by prolonged antiplatelet therapy in various categories of patients. *BMJ.* 1994;308:81–106.

84. The Dutch TIA Study Group. The Dutch TIA trial: protective effects of low-dose aspirin and atenolol in patients with transient ischemic attacks or nondisabling stroke. *Stroke.* 1988;19:512–517.

85. Antithrombotic Trialists' Collaboration. Collaborative meta-analysis of randomised trials of antiplatelet therapy for prevention of death, myocardial infarction, and stroke in high risk patients. *BMJ.* 2002;324:71–86.

86. CAPRIE Steering Committee. A randomised, blinded, trial of clopidogrel versus aspirin in patients at risk of ischaemic events (CAPRIE). *Lancet.* 1996;348:1329–1339.

87. Diener HC, Bogousslavsky J, Brass LM, et al. Aspirin and clopidogrel compared with clopidogrel alone after recent ischaemic stroke or transient ischaemic attack in high-risk patients (MATCH): randomised, double-blind, placebo-controlled trial. *Lancet.* 2004;364:331–337.

88. Diener HC, Cunha L, Forbes C, et al. European Stroke Prevention Study. 2. Dipyridamole and acetylsalicylic acid in the secondary prevention of stroke. *J Neurol Sci.* 1996;143:1–13.

89. Sacco RL, Diener HC, Yusuf S, et al. Aspirin and extended-release dipyridamole versus clopidogrel for recurrent stroke. *N Engl J Med.* 2008;359:1238–1251.

90. Chaturvedi S, Bruno A, Feasby T, et al. Carotid endarterectomy—an evidence-based review: report of the Therapeutics and Technology Assessment Subcommittee of the American Academy of Neurology. *Neurology.* 2005;65:794–801.

91. Yadav JS, Wholey MH, Kuntz RE, et al. Protected carotid-artery stenting versus endarterectomy in high-risk patients. *N Engl J Med.* 2004;351:1493–1501.

92. Mas JL, Trinquart L, Leys D, et al. Endarterectomy versus angioplasty in patients with symptomatic severe carotid stenosis (EVA-3S) trial: results up to 4 years from a randomised, multicentre trial. *Lancet Neurol.* 2008;7:885–892.

93. Ricotta JJ 2nd, Malgor RD. A review of the trials comparing carotid endarterectomy and carotid angioplasty and stenting. *Perspect Vasc Surg Endovasc Ther.* 2008;20:299–308.

94. Chimowitz MI, Lynn MJ, Howlett-Smith H, et al. Comparison of warfarin and aspirin for symptomatic intracranial arterial stenosis. *N Engl J Med.* 2005;352:1305–1316.

95. Risk factors for stroke and efficacy of antithrombotic therapy in atrial fibrillation. Analysis of pooled data from five randomized controlled trials. *Arch Intern Med.* 1994;154:1449–1457.

96. Stroke Prevention in Atrial Fibrillation Investigators. Warfarin versus aspirin for prevention of thromboembolism in atrial fibrillation: Stroke Prevention in Atrial Fibrillation II Study. *Lancet.* 1994;343:687–691.

97. Healey JS, Hart RG, Pogue J, et al. Risks and benefits of oral anticoagulation compared with clopidogrel plus aspirin in patients with atrial fibrillation according to stroke risk: the atrial fibrillation clopidogrel trial with irbesartan for prevention of vascular events (ACTIVE-W). *Stroke.* 2008;39:1482–1486.

20 Aortic Aneurysms

Irfan Hameed, Eric M. Isselbacher,
and Kim A. Eagle

CONTENTS

Key Words: Abdominal aortic aneurysm; Endovascular stent-graft therapy; Matrix metalloproteinase; Thoracic aortic aneurysm.

KEY POINTS

Thoracic Aneurysms

- Thoracic aortic aneurysms are much less common than abdominal aortic aneurysms and occur most commonly in the sixth and seventh decades of life.
- Cystic medial degeneration is the major pathophysiology of thoracic aortic aneurysms and is common in Marfan syndrome, Ehlers–Danlos syndrome, familial aortic aneurismal disease clusters, and bicuspid aortic valve patients.
- The vast majority of thoracic aortic aneurysms is clinically silent and discovered incidentally. A minority of patients experience symptoms, and in rare instances acute aneurysm expansion, rupture, or dissection constitutes the initial presentation.
- Emergent surgery for thoracic aortic aneurysm is associated with substantial morbidity and mortality. The goal is to operate electively aorta reaches the critical size which increases the risk of rupture, i.e., 5.5 cm for the ascending aorta and 6 cm for the descending aorta.
- Surgical repair is the standard of care for symptomatic, large high risk or unstable aortic aneurysms. Asymptomatic patients are usually managed medically with aggressive blood pressure reduction, with beta-blocking agents, angiotensin receptor blockers (or angiotensin-converting enzyme inhibitors), reduction of cardiovascular risk factors, follow-up surveillance, and patient education.

From: *Contemporary Cardiology: Comprehensive Cardiovascular Medicine in the Primary Care Setting*
Edited by: Peter P. Toth, Christopher P. Cannon, DOI 10.1007/978-1-60327-963-5_20
© Springer Science+Business Media, LLC 2010

Abdominal Aortic Aneurysms

- Smoking is the strongest independent risk factor for abdominal aortic aneurysm, followed by male gender, age, hypertension, hyperlipidemia, and atherosclerosis.
- The triad of abdominal pain, pulsatile epigastric mass, and hypotension, although uncommon, suggests a leaking or ruptured AAA. Palpation of asymptomatic AAAs is safe and does not precipitate rupture.
- Ultrasound scanning is the preferred method for detecting and following AAAs; however, CTA and MRA are the "gold standards" in the preoperative and postoperative evaluation of AAAs.
- Currently, ultrasound screening for AAA is recommended in men 60 years of age or older who have a family history of AAA or men who are 65–75 years of age who have ever smoked (former or current). Screening of women is reserved for those who have a family history, a suggestive physical exam, and possibly those with established atherosclerosis beyond age 75 years.
- Baseline aortic aneurysm size and annual expansion rate are the most important predictors of aneurysm rupture, followed by smoking, hypertension, family history, and gender.
- Current guidelines recommended surgical repair of abdominal aortic aneurysms ≥5.5 cm in diameter in asymptomatic patients. AAAs measuring 4.0–5.4 cm in diameter should be monitored by ultrasound or CT scans every 6–12 months to detect expansion.
- Endovascular stent-graft therapy is a less invasive alternative to open repair with potentially fewer postoperative complications and lower morbidity.

20.1. INTRODUCTION

Aortic aneurysms are relatively common, and their management frequently involves cardiologists, primary care physicians, and surgeons. It is therefore important not only to understand the basic pathological mechanism and current treatment recommendations but also to recognize the different variants and their complications and to know the indications for aortic repair. This chapter will focus on the pathogenesis of aortic aneurysm, different types and classifications, prevalence and mortality associated with it, and current medical and surgical management guidelines.

20.2. AORTA

The aorta begins in the aortic annulus of the aortic valve and ends at the bifurcation into the common iliac arteries. Anatomically the aorta is divided into thoracic and abdominal components. The thoracic aorta is further divided into the ascending, arch, and descending segments, and the abdominal aorta into the suprarenal and infrarenal segments (Fig. 1) (1). The aortic arch gives rise to the brachiocephalic, left common carotid, and left subclavian arteries.

The aorta, the largest and strongest artery in the body, is composed of three layers: the intima (thin inner layer), media (thick middle layer), and adventia (thin outer layer). In adults, the aortic diameter is approximately 3 cm in the ascending portion, 2.5 cm in the descending portion, and 1.8–2 cm in the abdomen. The diameter of the normal aorta does increase slightly with age (2). Its diameter also varies with body size and gender.

20.3. AORTIC ANEURYSMS

Aortic aneurysms are the 13th leading cause of mortality in the United States (3). The term *aneurysm* refers to a pathological dilatation of one or more segments of a blood vessel. A *true aneurysm* involves all three layers of the vessel wall and is distinguished from a *pseudoaneurysm,* in which the dilated portion extends outside the aortic media (4). Dilatation is considered to be present with a diameter above the norm for age and body surface area. The term aneurysm has been defined as a 50% increase

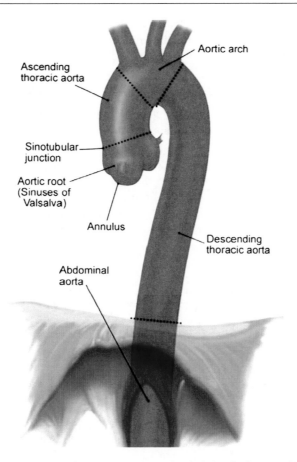

Fig. 1. Anatomy of thoracic and proximal abdominal aorta *(1)*.

above the expected normal diameter of that given arterial segment, but no definition is currently well enough accepted to define thoracic aortic aneurysms *(5)*. The reported incidence of aortic aneurysms is increasing with improvements in screening, as well as advances in imaging. Aneurysms are usually described in terms of their location, size, morphological appearance, and origin. The morphology of an aortic aneurysm is typically either *fusiform* (symmetrical dilatation involving the full circumference), or *saccular* (localized dilatation involving only one side). Aortic aneurysms are also classified according to location, i.e., abdominal versus thoracic. Aneurysms of the descending thoracic aorta are often contiguous with infradiaphragmatic aneurysms and are referred to as *thoracoabdominal aortic aneurysms.* The etiology, natural history, and treatment guidelines of aortic aneurysms differ according to the location (thoracic versus abdominal) and, consequently, they will be discussed separately.

20.4. THORACIC AORTIC ANEURYSM

Thoracic aortic aneurysms are much less common than abdominal aortic aneurysms; the incidence is estimated to be around 4.5 cases per 100,000 patient-years *(6)*. They are detected most commonly in the sixth and seventh decades of life; males are affected approximately two to four times more commonly than females *(7)*. In the case of aortic root aneurysms, patient are often younger (age 30–50 years), with a 1:1 sex ratio *(6)*. Thoracic aneurysms are classified by the segment of aorta involved: aortic root, ascending aorta, arch, or descending aorta (Fig. 1). In a recent series, the reported frequency of involvement of the thoracic aortic segment was 60% for the aortic root and/or ascending aorta, 40% for the descending aorta, 10% for the arch, and 10% for the thoracoabdominal aorta (with some involving >1 segment) *(1)*.

20.4.1. Etiology and Pathogenesis

Aortic aneurysms result from conditions that cause degradation or abnormal production of the aortic wall's structural components (elastin and collagen). The causes of aortic aneurysms may be broadly categorized as degenerative diseases, inherited or developmental diseases, infections, vasculitides, and trauma (Table 1) *(4)*. Aneurysms of the ascending thoracic aorta most often result from cystic medial degeneration, in which degeneration of elastic fiber and collagen appears histologically as empty spaces filled with mucoid material *(1)*. Medial degeneration leads to circumferential weakening and dilatation of the aortic wall, which in turn results in the development of fusiform aneurysms involving the ascending aorta and/or the aortic root. When such aneurysms involve the aortic root, the anatomy is often referred to as *annuloaortic ectasia (1)*.

Table 1
Etiology of Aortic Aneurysms *(1, 4)*

Causes	Remarks
Hereditary fibrillinopathies	
Marfan syndrome	Classic disorder with cystic medial degeneration due to mutations in the fibrillin-1 gene. Aortic aneurysms typically occur at the aortic root level but can occur in the entire aorta. Accounts for 6% of dissections
Ehlers–Danlos syndrome	Defects in type III collagen cause hyperelasticity; aortic root disease is uncommon
Familial TAA syndrome	Autosomal-dominant mode of inheritance, but marked variability in expression and penetrance; males present at a younger age
Hereditary vascular disease	
Bicuspid valve	Approximately 50% have a dilatation of the ascending aorta; cystic medial degeneration regarded as the main cause
Vascular inflammation	
Takayasu arteritis	Results in aortic dilatation in 15% of cases; occurs mostly in women
Syphilis	Spirochetal infection of the aortic media causes obliterative endarteritis of the vasa vasorum. Currently rare due to antibiotic treatment
Giant cell arteritis	Typically affects the temporal or cranial arteries, but can also produce thoracic aortic aneurysms (11%)
Ankylosing spondylitis	Associated with inflammation of fibrocartilage, potentially directed at tissues rich in fibrillin-1
Behçet disease	Leads more to local aneurysm formation and perforation than dissection
Kawasaki syndrome	Coronary artery aneurysms are typical, but also other arterial segments can be involved. More circumscript aneurysm formation
Deceleration trauma	
High speed accidents	Results in partial or complete transection of the aorta; usually occurs at the aortic isthmus

Cystic medial degeneration occurs normally to some extent with aging and the process is accelerated by hypertension *(8)*, but is particularly prevalent in patients with Marfan syndrome, Ehlers–Danlos syndrome type IV, congenital bicuspid aortic valves, and familial thoracic aortic aneurysm syndromes *(1)*. Marfan syndrome, the prototype of cystic medial degeneration, is an autosomal-dominant heritable disorder of connective tissue caused by mutations in the gene for fibrillin-1, a structural protein that is the major component of microfibrils of elastin. More than 100 mutations have been identified at one locus on the fibrillin gene *(2)*. There is also a strong association between bicuspid aortic valve and ascending thoracic aortic aneurysms, and cystic medial degeneration has been found to be the underlying cause of the aortic dilatation *(6)*.

20.4.2. Clinical Manifestations

Most thoracic aortic aneurysms are asymptomatic but are discovered incidentally on imaging studies (chest X-ray, CT scan, or echocardiogram) ordered for other indications *(9)*. Symptomatic thoracic aortic aneurysms may present either with a local mass effect or with a vascular consequence of the aneurysm. Vascular consequences include dilatation of the aortic root or ascending aorta, leading to aortic regurgitation and a diastolic murmur detectable on physical examination or, less often, progressing to congestive heart failure *(6)*. A local mass effect by aneurysms may cause symptoms of compression or erosion of adjacent tissue, such as compression of the trachea or mainstem bronchus (causing cough, dyspnea, wheezing, or recurrent pneumonitis), compression of the esophagus (causing dysphagia), or compression of the recurrent laryngeal nerve (causing hoarseness) *(1)*.

Rarely, chest or back pain may occur with non-dissecting aneurysms as a result of stretching of the aortic tissue, direct compression of other intrathoracic structures, or erosion into adjacent bone *(1)*. The most feared consequences of thoracic aortic aneurysms are aortic dissection or rupture, both of which are potentially lethal. Aortic dissection is typically accompanied by the sudden onset of severe thoracic pain, usually felt retrosternally in case of ascending aortic involvement or posteriorly, between the scapulae, when the descending aorta is involved. Acute aneurysm expansion, or subacute contained rupture, which may herald frank rupture, can cause similar pain *(4)*.

20.4.3. Diagnosis

A variety of noninvasive and invasive methods are useful for the diagnosis and evaluation of thoracic aortic aneurysms.

20.4.3.1. EKG

An EKG is an important test, especially in patients with chest pain, and may help differentiate pain from acute angina/myocardial infarction versus non-coronary pain.

20.4.3.2. CHEST X-RAY

A chest X-ray may be the first test to suggest the diagnosis of a thoracic aortic aneurysm. Most aneurysms are characterized by widening of the mediastinal silhouette, enlargement of the aortic knob, or tracheal deviation *(10)*. In the PA view, an enlarged ascending aorta may produce a convex contour of the right superior mediastinum (Fig. 2). In the lateral view, there may be a loss of the retrosternal air space. Aneurysms confined to the aortic root can be obscured by the cardiac silhouette and may not be evident on a chest radiograph *(6)*. Additionally, smaller aneurysms and even some large ones may not produce any abnormalities on chest X-ray, so this technique cannot be used to exclude the diagnosis of aortic aneurysm *(1)*. Similarly one cannot typically distinguish whether an enlarged aortic silhouette represents a tortuous aorta or the presence of an aneurysm. Consequently, an enlarged aortic silhouette on chest X-ray should prompt a further workup (e.g., CT scan or MRI) in the appropriate clinical setting *(1)*.

20.4.3.3. CT, MRA, AND AORTOGRAPHY

Contrast-enhanced computed tomography (CT), magnetic resonance angiography (MRA), and conventional invasive aortography are sensitive and specific tests for the assessment of aneurysms *(11)*.

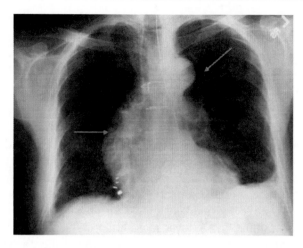

Fig. 2. Chest radiograph of a patient with a very large aneurysm of the ascending thoracic aorta *(4)*.

However, given the relative invasive nature of aortography, CT and MRA are preferred in most cases to define both aortic and branch vessel anatomy (Fig. 3). Among patients with known bicuspid aortic valves, the *2006 ACC/AHA Guidelines* recommend the use of MRA or CT when the morphology of the aortic root or ascending aorta cannot be accurately assessed by echocardiography *(12)*. Every patient with an aortic aneurysm detected by echocardiography or suspected based on chest X-ray should

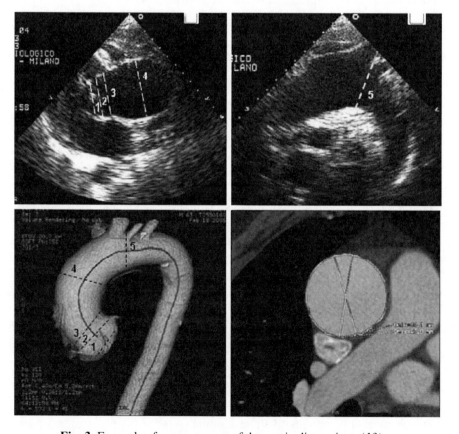

Fig. 3. Example of measurement of the aortic dimensions *(13)*.

undergo an initial CT or MRA examination of the entire aorta (thoracis and abdominal), because multiple aneurysms occur in 13% of patients diagnosed with a thoracic aneurysm *(4)*.

20.4.3.4. ECHOCARDIOGRAPHY

Transthoracic echocardiography (TTE) is effective for imaging the aortic root (Fig. 3), but it does not consistently visualize the mid or distal ascending aorta well, nor does it visualize the descending aorta well *(1, 11, 13)*. Therefore, after baseline CT or MRA, patients with Marfan syndrome and bicuspid aortic valve can then be followed by serial evaluation with TTE on a yearly basis with repeat CT or MRA less frequently if the CT/MRA shows normal aortic size and morphology beyond the aortic root *(1)*. Transesophageal echocardiography (TEE) can image almost the entire thoracic aorta quite well. However, given that TEE is a semi-invasive procedure, it is not favored for the routine imaging of those with stable (non-dissecting) thoracic aneurysms *(4)*.

20.4.4. Natural History

The natural history of thoracic aortic aneurysms is related to location and the etiology, which in turn predict the rate of growth and propensity for dissection or rupture. Therefore, it is appropriate to image aneurysms serially to document size and growth and perform surgery when aneurysms are large enough to be considered at significant risk for rupture and/or dissection *(1, 4)*. Studies focusing on the natural history of thoracic and thoracoabdominal aneurysms have found that the odds of rupture are increased by chronic obstructive pulmonary disease (COPD) (RR, 3.6), advanced age (RR, 2.6 per decade), and aneurysm-related pain (RR, 2.3) *(14)*.

Davies et al. reported a mean growth rate of 0.1 cm/year for the thoracic aortic aneurysms measuring 3.5 cm *(15)*. In this longitudinal study of more than 31 months, they found that the rate of growth was higher for aneurysms of the descending aorta versus ascending aorta, for dissected aneurysms versus non-dissected aortas, and for those with Marfan syndrome versus those without. In a multivariate logistic regression analysis, initial aneurysm diameter, Marfan syndrome, and female gender were found to be significant predictors of dissection or rupture. Initial aneurysm diameter is the single most important predictor of dissection, rupture, or death in several studies (Table 2) *(14–17)*. The critical point at which rupture or dissection occurred was at 6 cm for the ascending aorta and 7 cm for the descending aorta. Rupture and/or dissection occurs at smaller sizes in patients with Marfan syndrome *(16)*. Accordingly, it is important to intervene before aneurysm reaches this critical point (Table 2).

Table 2
Complications Based on Aortic Size *(16)*

Aortic size				
Yearly risk	>3.5 cm	>4 cm	>5 cm	>6 cm
Rupture (%)	0.0	0.3	1.7	3.6
Dissection (%)	2.2	1.5	2.5	3.7
Death (%)	5.9	4.6	4.8	10.8
Any of the above (%)	7.2	5.3	6.5	14.1

20.5. MANAGEMENT

20.5.1. Surgical Treatment

Symptomatic aortic aneurysms require surgery regardless of the size. Prophylactic surgical repair is often recommended to prevent the morbidity and mortality associated with aneurysm rupture (Table 3). However, the optimal timing of surgical repair of thoracic aortic aneurysms remains uncertain, particularly for aneurysms less than 5 cm in size. Significant risks are associated with thoracic

Table 3
Criteria for Resection of Thoracic Aortic Aneurysms (17)

Rupture
Acute aortic dissection
Ascending requires urgent operation
Descending requires complication—specific approach

Symptomatic states
Pain consistent with aortic origin and unexplained by other causes
Compression of adjacent organs especially trachea, esophagus, or left
  main bronchus
Significant aortic insufficiency in conjunction with ascending aortic
  aneurysm

Documented enlargement
Growth >1 cm/year or substantial growth and aneurysm is rapidly
  approaching absolute size criteria

Absolute size (cm)
  Marfan
  Ascending 5.0 cm
  Descending 6.0 cm
Non-Marfan
  Ascending 5.5 cm
  Descending 6.5 cm

Table 4
Risk Associated with Thoracic Aortic Surgery (4, 16)

	Mortality (%)	*Stroke (%)*	*Paraplegia (%)*
Ascending aorta/aortic arch	2.50	8.30	0
Descending aorta/thoracoabdominal aorta	8.20	4.10	2.00

aortic surgery, particularly in the arch and descending aorta (Table 4), which in many cases may outweigh the potential benefits of aortic repair, particularly in patients who have concomitant cardiovascular disease. Mortality rates in a recent case series are in the range of 5–9% for elective surgical repair and more than 50% in the setting of emergent or urgent surgical repair (15).

Therefore, the decision to operate is determined by the expected natural history of the aneurysm and the anticipated risk of the proposed surgical procedure. For most ascending thoracic aortic aneurysms of ≥5.5 cm in diameter and/or descending thoracic aortic aneurysms of 6 cm or greater, surgery is indicated (Table 3) (1, 2, 6, 15, 16). Among those with an increased operative risk (e.g., the elderly or those with significant comorbidities), the threshold for recommending surgery is raised (often by 1 cm) (17). Similarly, among patients who are at increased risk of aortic dissection or rupture (e.g., Marfan syndrome, bicuspid aortic valve, or a familial thoracic aortic aneurysm syndrome), aortic repair is recommended when the diameter reaches 5 cm.

20.5.1.1. Open Surgical Repair Versus Endovascular Stent-Graft

Choice of technique depends on the location of the aneurysm, the distal extent of aortic involvement, underlying pathology, comorbidities, life expectancy of the patient, and desired anticoagulation status. In general, patients requiring open surgical repair of an ascending thoracic aneurysm should undergo coronary angiography and echocardiography to evaluate the need for concomitant cardiac procedures as well as to assess the status of the aortic valve and root *(3)*. Thoracic aortic aneurysm repair requires cardiopulmonary bypass to support the circulation distal to the aneurysm. The aneurysmal segment is replaced with a prosthetic Dacron tube graft of appropriate size. Endovascular stent-graft implantation is an alternative approach for the repair of descending thoracic aneurysms in selected patients with favorable aortic anatomy. The role of catheter-based intraluminal stent grafting in thoracic aortic disease is undergoing active clinical investigation in both elective and emergency settings, and the indications for intervention remain to be fully defined. This technique has the advantage of being far less invasive than surgery with potentially fewer postoperative complications and lower morbidity *(1)*. Recently, the comparison of endovascular stent grafting with an open surgical repair cohort compiled for FDA analysis showed favorable early outcomes *(18)*. The devices were approved in 2005, and their use is rapidly growing *(4)*.

20.5.2. Medical Management

Asymptomatic patients with aneurysms below the size threshold for surgery are initially managed medically (Table 3), with risk factor reduction, control of hypertension, and smoking cessation, and serial imaging studies to monitor aortic growth and size. The goal systolic pressure is 105–120 mmHg if tolerated *(1)*. Currently, the choice of medical treatment to prevent the progression of aortic dilatation and reduce the risk of dissection or rupture is limited *(4)*. Reports of medical therapy in patients with Marfan syndrome have demonstrated that propranolol administration is associated with improvements in both aortic growth and 10-year survival *(19)*. Whether these benefits can truly be extrapolated to the non-Marfan population with thoracic aneurysms remains unknown.

In a non-randomized evaluation of angiotensin-converting enzyme inhibitors, Yetman and colleagues *(20)* noted a decrease in aortic growth for Marfan patients receiving enalapril compared with those receiving β(beta)-blockers. Recently, losartan, an angiotensin II type 1 receptor (AT1) blocker, was shown to prevent aortic aneurysm in a mouse model of Marfan syndrome, possibly secondary to its capacity to reduce transforming growth factor beta (TGF-β(beta)) expression and signaling *(21)*. There is some early experimental evidence that HMG–CoA reductase inhibitors (statins) may potentially have a protective effect, but further research and clinical validation is needed before any therapeutic implications can be drawn *(1, 22)*.

Associated cardiovascular risk factors should be aggressively controlled, and activities and lifestyle should be modified if needed. Patients should be informed about potential acute symptoms and instructed how to respond appropriately. Pregnancy is discouraged in patients with Marfan syndrome, especially if the aortic root diameter exceeds 40 mm. In the case of pregnancy in a female Marfan patient with an aortic root diameter of 40 mm or greater, close clinical and echocardiographic surveillance is necessary as well as treatment with beta-blocker therapy *(12)*.

The natural history of thoracic aortic aneurysm is generally that of inexorable expansion, so almost all patients require regular surveillance imaging. It is appropriate to obtain a first follow-up imaging study after 6 months and, if the aneurysm is stable, subsequent imaging studies on an annual basis in most cases. However, should there be a significant increase or rapid growth in aortic diameter, the interval between imaging studies should be decreased to 3 or 6 months *(1)*. One suggested protocol for surveillance is given in Table 5 *(3)*.

20.6. ABDOMINAL AORTIC ANEURYSM (AAA)

The abdominal aorta is the most common site of arterial aneurysm. Since the abdominal aorta tends to be about 2 cm in diameter, a true abdominal aortic aneurysm measures 3 cm or more *(5)*. Given the variation in normal aortic diameter, the diagnosis of abdominal aortic aneurysm should be adjusted for

Table 5
Suggested Imaging Surveillance for Patients with Thoracic Aortic Aneurysms (3)

Aortic pathology	Additional initial workup	First follow-up imaging	Subsequent imaging
Newly diagnosed TAA	Echocardiography to evaluate aortic valve structure and function	CT scan at 6 months	Annual CT scan if stable Annual echocardiography if initial study demonstrated moderate to severe aortic stenosis or insufficiency
Rapidly growing TAA	Echocardiography	CT scan at 3 months unless indication for operation exists	CT scan at 6 months if stable, then annually thereafter
	Right and left heart catheterization Carotid duplex Pulmonary function testing		CT scan every 3 months if growing further
Residual distal aortic dissection after repair of type A dissection	None	CT scan 3 months postoperatively	Annual CT scan if stable distal aortic dimension
Known TAA in setting of pregnancy	Echocardiography	6–8 weeks with repeat echocardiography	Echocardiography every 6–8 weeks including into first 3 postpartum months CT scan postpartum, then algorithm per rapidly growing TAA

age, gender, and body surface area (5). Hence, using the diameter ratio may be better, particularly in smaller people such as women and those of short stature (23). Similar to thoracic aortic aneurysms, abdominal aortic aneurysms are also classified according to their shape (fusiform or saccular) and the segment involved, as discussed above. Abdominal aortic aneurysms are much more common than thoracic aortic aneurysms and occur 5–10 times more frequently in males than in females. Age is an important risk factor (4). The incidence of abdominal aortic aneurysm rises rapidly after 55 years of age in males and 70 years of age in females (1); however, this may vary depending on the type of diagnostic imaging used, the diagnostic criteria applied, and the age and gender distribution of the population screened.

20.6.1. Etiology and Pathogenesis

Smoking is the strongest independent risk factor for abdominal aortic aneurysm, followed by older age, hypertension, hyperlipidemia, and atherosclerosis (24). Wilmink et al. reported that current smokers were 7.6 times more likely to have an abdominal aortic aneurysm than nonsmokers (23). Smoking increases not only the risks of aneurysm expansion and rupture but also the risk associated with aneurysm repair. Sex and genetics are the strongest non-modifiable risk factors. Males are 10 times more likely than females to have an abdominal aortic aneurysm of 4 cm or greater (1). However, females and those with a family history of abdominal aortic aneurysm have a higher risk of rupture *(4)*. Race also appears to influence the prevalence of AAAs. In the Veterans Affairs Study, abdominal aneurysms occurred approximately twice as frequently in whites compared to blacks *(25)*. Vasculitis (such as Takayasu arteritis, giant cell arteritis, spondyloarthropathies, rheumatoid arthritis) and infections disease (such as tuberculosis or mycotic aneurysms) are less commonly associated with abdominal aneurysms.

Classically, degenerative atherosclerotic disease has been considered the underlying cause of abdominal aortic aneurysms, but recent data suggest that many aneurysms form in response to altered expression patterns of tissue matrix metalloproteinases that diminish the integrity of the arterial wall *(5)*. Matrix metalloproteinases are enzymes that are produced by smooth muscle and inflammatory cells, can degrade elastin and collagen, and may participate in abdominal aortic aneurysm formation. There is growing evidence that atherosclerotic and inflammatory abdominal aortic aneurysms share a common underlying pathophysiology *(8)*. The wall of the infrarenal abdominal aorta is thinner, has fewer adventitial vasa vasora than the thoracic aorta, is more prone to atherosclerosis, and therefore is the most common site of abdominal aneurysm formation *(23)*.

20.6.2. Clinical Manifestations

In most cases, abdominal aortic aneurysms are asymptomatic, expand silently, and are discovered incidentally on routine physical examination or on imaging studies ordered for other indications *(1, 4)*. Up to 50% of abdominal aneurysms can be recognized on plain roentgenograms as a calcified aneurysmal wall *(23)*. Younger patients are more likely to be symptomatic at the time of diagnosis *(4)*. In symptomatic abdominal aneurysms, pain is the typical complaint and is usually located in the hypogastrium or lower back. The usual description is steady and gnawing in nature, lasting hours to days *(1, 4)*.

Sudden worsening of pain or development of new pain may herald expansion or impending rupture of an aneurysm, whereas frank rupture is associated with abrupt onset of back pain along with abdominal pain and tenderness *(4)*. Most patients have a palpable, pulsatile abdominal mass, unless they are hypotensive because of blood loss. The classic pathognomic triad of abdominal/back pain, a pulsatile abdominal mass, and hypotension is seen in only few cases *(5)*. Hemorrhagic shock and its complications may ensue rapidly in cases of rupture.

20.6.3. Physical Examination

The sensitivity of physical examination to detect a pulsatile mass varies and increases with the size of the aneurysm; 29–61% for abdominal aneurysms 3.0–3.9 cm in diameter and 76–82% for aneurysms 5.0 cm or larger *(26)*. Generally, it is easier to detect a pulsatile mass in thin individuals who do not have a tense abdomen and more difficult to detect in overweight or obese patients *(26)*. Contrary to a once popular belief, gentle palpation of AAAs is safe and does not precipitate rupture *(23)*.

20.6.4. Diagnosis and Sizing

A number of diagnostic imaging modalities are available for detecting and serially monitoring abdominal aortic aneurysms.

20.6.4.1. PLAIN FILM

Fifteen to 85% of abdominal aneurysms are discovered because of curvilinear aortic wall calcification that represents an incidental finding on a plain abdominal film that was obtained for other purposes *(5)*. However, it is not the current standard of care to use plain radiographic studies for screening or surveillance of aneurysms.

20.6.4.2. ULTRASONOGRAPHY

B-mode or real-time abdominal ultrasonography is perhaps the most practical way to screen, assess, and follow abdominal aneurysms because it is relatively inexpensive, noninvasive, and does not require the use of a contrast agent (Fig. 4) *(1)*. Multiple studies have suggested that ultrasound is a reliable method of imaging to determine the presence or absence of an infrarenal aortic aneurysm compared to suprarenal aortic aneurysm *(5)*. Diagnostic specificity for the presence of an infrarenal aortic aneurysm is nearly 100%, with sensitivity ranging from 92 to 99% *(5)*. Given the limited ability to visualize the extent of disease (cephalic and/or pelvic) and define the anatomy of mesenteric and renal arteries, ultrasound is insufficient for planning operative repair *(4)*.

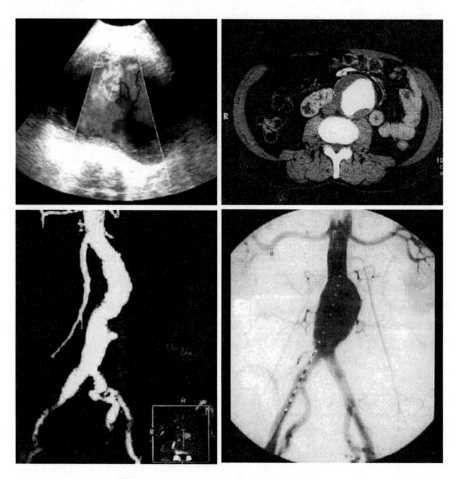

Fig. 4. Abdominal aortic aneurysm *(34)*.

20.6.4.3. CONTRAST-ENHANCED COMPUTED TOMOGRAPHIC (CT) SCANNING AND MAGNETIC RESONANCE ANGIOGRAPHY (MRA)

Contrast CT and MRA provide detailed information about the site, size, shape, extent, and local anatomic relationships of the aneurysm and are therefore valuable when planning abdominal aneurysm repair (Fig. 4) *(4)*. They are also better than ultrasonography in imaging suprarenal aortic aneurysms. Their cost, use of ionizing radiation (CT scan), intravenous contrast media (CT scan and MRA), and inconsistent availability (MRA) are major disadvantages that make these tests less practical for screening. Nevertheless, their high accuracy in sizing aneurysms makes them excellent modality(ies) for serially monitoring changes in aneurysm size *(1)*. Because of improved techniques, their relatively noninvasive nature, and relative cost advantage over transcatheter angiography, CTA and MRA have emerged as current "gold standards" in the preoperative and postoperative evaluation of abdominal aneurysms *(27)*.

20.6.5. Screening

Aortic diameter can be measured accurately by ultrasound imaging in more than 97% of subjects, and screening by this method has the potential to reduce the incidence of aortic rupture *(5)*. The effectiveness of population-based ultrasound screening has been evaluated in several studies, with specific targeting of high-risk groups, such as those with hypertension, coronary disease, or tobacco use. In a population-based screening of men aged 65–74 years by Multicenter Aneurysm Screening Study Group, patients with abdominal aortic aneurysms of 3 cm or greater were followed up with serial ultrasound scans for a mean of 4 years *(28)*. There were 113 aneurysm-related deaths in the control group versus 65 in the screening group, yielding an estimated risk reduction of 42%. Another study addressed the potential usefulness of repeated screening for abdominal aneurysms and reported that a normal ultrasonogram at age 65 effectively excludes the risk of a clinically significant aneurysm for life *(29)*. A recent consensus statement from the Society of Vascular Surgery, the American Association of Vascular Surgery, and the Society of Vascular Medicine and Biology recommended that all men age 60–85 years be screened for abdominal aneurysms, as should women age 60–85 years with cardiovascular risk factors, and men and women older than 50 years with a family history of abdominal aneurysm *(30)*. More recently, based on a meta-analysis of the currently published international data, the US Preventive Services Task Force (USPSTF) recommends one-time screening for abdominal aneurysms by ultrasonography in men age 65–75 years who have ever smoked *(31)*.

20.6.6. Natural History

The natural history of abdominal aortic aneurysms is distinguished by gradual and/or sporadic expansion in diameter and by the accumulation of mural thrombus. The major risk posed by an expanding abdominal aortic aneurysm is rupture and its associated mortality risk *(1)*. Among the participants in the United Kingdom Small Aneurysm Trial who suffered a ruptured abdominal aneurysm, 79 out of 103 died without abdominal aneurysm repair (25% died before reaching a hospital and 51% died at the hospital without undergoing surgery), and of those who had surgery, the operative mortality was 46%, yielding an overall 30-day survival of 11% *(32)*. Therefore, the goal is to prevent rupture by having patients undergoing elective aortic repair (with a mortality of only 4–6%) when aneurysms are considered to be at significant risk of rupture *(1)*.

In a classic report, Szilagyi et al. noted that the risk for spontaneous rupture was a direct function of aneurysm size *(33)*. Additional factors also may influence the rupture rate, such as hypertension, COPD and/or tobacco abuse, female gender, and a family history of aortic aneurysms (particularly when a woman with an aortic aneurysm is present in the proband *(5)*). Nevertheless, baseline aneurysm size remains the single most important predictor of aneurysm growth rate and rupture, and the risk of rupture increases with aneurysm size, with larger aneurysms expanding more rapidly than small ones (Fig. 5) *(34)*. The mean rate of expansion within a population is extremely variable, and, according to one study, the mean expansion rate of ruptured versus non-ruptured aneurysms was 0.82 and 0.42 cm/year, respectively *(35)*. Thus, a small AAA that expands ≥0.5 cm over 6 months of follow-up is considered at high risk for rupture *(5)*.

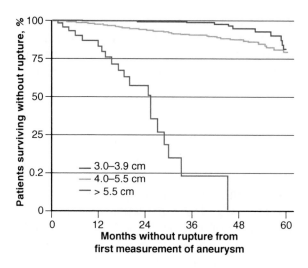

Fig. 5. Risk of rupture of aneurysm according to the first measured aortic diameter *(34)*.

20.7. MANAGEMENT

20.7.1. Surgical Treatment

Operative mortality for elective aneurysm repair is 4–6% overall and as low as 2% in low-risk patients *(1)*. However, operative mortality rises to 19% for urgent aortic repair and reaches 50% for repair of a ruptured aneurysm. The decision to operate must weigh the expected natural history of the aneurysm and life expectancy of the patient against the anticipated morbidity and mortality of the proposed surgical procedure. Aneurysm size is the primary indicator for repair of asymptomatic aneurysms and according to the recently published set of guidelines, the Joint Council of the American Association for Vascular Surgery and Society for Vascular Surgery agreed with the 5.5 cm threshold for the "average" male patient, but recommended that women should undergo elective repair at a smaller aortic diameter of 4.5–5 cm *(36)*. The *2005 ACC/AHA Guidelines* recommended surgical repair of abdominal aortic aneurysms ≥5.5 cm in diameter in asymptomatic patients *(5)*.

20.7.1.1. OPEN AORTIC ANEURYSM REPAIR VERSUS ENDOVASCULAR AORTIC ANEURYSM REPAIR (EVAR)

The choice of endovascular repair versus open surgery depends on the patient's condition, preference, life expectancy, urgency of the procedure, and the surgeon's experience *(23)*. Procedural mortality of endovascular repair is lower than with open surgical repair, but the long-term outcome of endovascular stent-graft repair versus open surgical repair remains uncertain.

Open aortic aneurysm repair is performed by a midline transabdominal approach (or an extraperitoneal incision in the left flank), whereas endovascular abdominal aneurysm repair can be performed under regional or even local anesthesia and can avoid a major transabdominal procedure. Thus, the minimally invasive technique clearly represents a major advancement in the management of high-risk patients with aneurysms who have severe cardiopulmonary disease or advanced age *(5)*. However, endovascular repair also has been offered at many centers to low- or average-risk patients who have no particular contraindications to open surgical repair *(5)*. According to available data, the rate of successful stent-graft implantation ranges from 78 to 99%, with several recent large series reporting rates of 98% *(1, 4)*. Despite these encouraging results, only 30–60% of patients have suitable anatomy for endovascular repair *(4)*. A number of recent trials demonstrated a clear early mortality advantage for endovascular repair but offer no clear late advantage over open repair among those who are good candidates for either procedure. Therefore, the endovascular repair has generally been limited to a subset of patients, typically older patients or those at high risk for open surgical repair *(4)*.

20.7.2. Preoperative Risk Assessment

Because atherosclerosis is a common finding in patients with abdominal aneurysms, the likelihood of concomitant coronary artery disease (CAD) increases significantly *(4)*. Thus, patients undergoing major vascular surgery, such as open surgical repair in the presence of concomitant CAD, are at high risk of perioperative cardiac events. Indeed, one-half of all perioperative deaths from aneurysm repair result from myocardial infarction *(1, 4)*. Recently, however, studies on prophylactic coronary revascularization in stable CAD and high-risk patients (with preoperative extensive stress-induced ischemia) undergoing vascular surgery were not associated with an improved outcomes *(37, 38)*. The *ACC/AHA 2007 Guidelines* do not recommend (indeed discourage) the routine use of prophylactic coronary revascularization in stable CAD before noncardiac surgery *(39)*. However, the *ACC/AHA 2007 Guidelines* recommend that patients with active cardiac conditions such as unstable coronary syndromes, decompensated heart failure, significant arrhythmias, or severe valvular disease should undergo evaluation and treatment before noncardiac surgery *(39)*. Treatment for patients requiring percutaneous coronary intervention (for MI or ACS) who need subsequent surgery should be based on the urgency of procedure and risk of bleeding *(39)*.

Current data does not support indiscriminate use of beta-blockers in patients undergoing vascular surgery because several recent randomized trials have not confirmed the efficacy of these agents in contrast to the earlier studies that appeared to demonstrate efficacy *(39)*. The ACC/AHA recommends the use of perioperative beta-blockers in patients undergoing vascular surgery who are at high cardiac risk owing to the finding of ischemia on preoperative testing and encourage beta-blocker use in whom preoperative assessment identifies coronary heart disease or more than one clinical risk factor. The agent should be initiated preoperatively and titrated carefully to avoid severe bradycardia and/or hypotension. There is also a protective effect of perioperative statin use during noncardiac surgery, especially vascular surgery *(39)*. In a meta-analysis of 15 studies evaluating the overall effect of preoperative statin therapy, a 44% reduction in mortality was observed *(39)*.

20.7.3. Medical Management

Medical management involves early detection, surveillance, and risk factor modification. It is widely recognized that patients with abdominal aneurysms have significantly more cardiovascular risk factors such as smoking, hypertension, hypercholesterolemia, and atherosclerosis of other vessels than do age- and gender-matched controls *(5)*. Therefore, finding an abdominal aneurysm is an opportunity to start risk factor modification and should be fundamental in the medical management of abdominal aortic aneurysms. Smoking cessation and management of hypertension are the mainstays of medical therapy. Given the increased risk of aneurysm rupture among active smokers and hypertensive patients, cigarette smoking must be discontinued and hypertension should be controlled *(23)*.

Beta-blockers have long been considered an important therapy for reducing the risk of aneurysm expansion and rupture and have numerous benefits in patients with cardiovascular disease *(4)*. In animal model, propranolol delays the development of aneurysms prone to spontaneous aortic rupture. In humans, the data are mixed. Three randomized trials reported that beta-blockers did not slow the growth rate of most small aneurysms. However, slower growth rates were noted in a beta-blocker subgroup that had aneurysms larger than 3.9 cm at enrollment, suggesting that the beta-blocker had a small effect *(23, 40)*. Therefore, beta-blockers should be recommended for patients with larger aneurysms or in hypertensive aneurysm patients who are managed medically. In the absence of other indications for beta-blockers, there is insufficient evidence to recommend using them routinely for the sole purpose of slowing aneurysm growth *(23)*. Treatment with statins, although not proven to affect aneurysm expansion or rupture, may prolong survival by their effect on low-density lipoprotein (LDL) and cardiac and cerebrovascular disease. Given the strong association of abdominal aortic aneurysm with coronary artery disease in epidemiological studies, the National Cholesterol Education Program (NCEP) defines aortic abdominal aneurysms as a CHD equivalent *(41)*. Therefore, the goal of the treatment should be the same as for patients with coronary artery disease, i.e., <100 for LDL and <130 for non-HDL cholesterol *(41)*.

Follow-up surveillance to monitor the size of aortic aneurysms (either rapid expansion >0.5 cm/year or an increase in size to 5.5 cm or larger) is a critical part of management in patients not treated surgically; however, the optimal surveillance schedule has not been clearly defined. The *2005 ACC/AHA Guidelines* recommended that patients with abdominal aneurysms measuring 4.0–5.4 cm in diameter should be monitored by ultrasound or CT scans every 6–12 months, whereas abdominal aneurysms <4.0 cm in diameter, monitoring by ultrasound examination every 2–3 years is reasonable *(23)*.

20.8. CASE STUDIES

20.8.1. Case Study 1: Thoracic Aortic Aneurysms

A 32-year-old man with Marfan syndrome and a strong family history of aneurysmal disease was referred to our center for a newly discovered cardiac murmur. Initial examination revealed a tall, lean man with long arm span. His fingers were long and slender and had a spider-like appearance (arachnodactyly). He had reduced vision because of dislocations of lenses (ectopia lentis). Vitals sign were stable except heart rate was 55 beats/minute. Cardiac auscultation revealed a midsystolic click followed by a late systolic murmur. Standing and Valsalva maneuver made the click and murmur louder and earlier in systole. Two-dimensional echocardiography not only confirmed the clinical impression of MVP with regurgitation but also revealed aortic root dilation. The patient subsequently underwent magnetic resonance angiography (MRA) which showed a thoracic aortic aneurysm involving the aortic root and ascending thoracic aorta (4.4 cm at root/sinuses and 4.1 cm at ascending). He was started on angiotensin receptor blocker and had a repeat imaging (MRA) at 6 months which did not a show significant change in the size of aneurysm. Later he continued to follow-up with yearly imaging. The above case illustrates the importance of the initial examination and appropriate surveillance studies to look for both valvular and aortic effects of Marfan syndrome.

20.8.2. Case Study 2: Abdominal Aortic Aneurysms

A 70-year-old male with a past medical history of COPD, HTN, dyslipidemia, and colon cancer was referred for the management of rapidly increasing abdominal aortic aneurysm. The aneurysm was diagnosed 3 years ago when a computed tomography (CT) scan was done for another reason (colon cancer). At that time, the size of the aneurysm was only 4 cm in diameter. After the colon surgery the patient was lost to follow-up. He was recently admitted for new onset back pain, along with abdominal pain and tenderness.

He has continued to smoke (2 packs/day, duration 50 years) and was non-compliant with his antihypertensive and statin medications in the past 2 years. On examination his vitals were stable; however, there was tender pulsatile abdominal mass. Ultrasonography showed an infrarenal abdominal aortic aneurysm of 5.8 cm, which was subsequently confirmed with CT scan. The patient underwent urgent endovascular aortic aneurysm repair (EVAR). The above case illustrates that aneurysms can rapidly increase in size especially in patients with risk factors for atherosclerosis (especially smoking) and can present acutely with rupture or impending rupture.

20.9. CONCLUSIONS

Aortic aneurysms are the 13th leading cause of mortality in the United States. The incidence of aortic aneurysms is increasing with improvements in screening as well as advances in imaging. Care of aortic aneurysm patients often involves physicians from different specialties such as primary care, hospitalists, cardiologists, emergency physicians, and, ultimately, surgeons. Knowledge of the etiology, natural history, and prognosis help determine optimal management, e.g., medical versus surgical treatment, and the frequency of surveillance, ultrasound versus computed tomography scan, and family education about the expected outcomes and screening of other family members. It is well known that most aortic aneurysms are clinically silent and discovered incidentally, but occasionally the aorta undergoes expansion, rupture, or dissection, and such presentations of aortic aneurysms are potentially lethal. Emergent surgery for aortic aneurysm is associated with a substantial morbidity and mortality and so the goal is to operate electively before reaching the critical points of rupture/dissection. The current paradigm of surgical management is switching from open repair to endovascular repair and its use is increasing in the younger patient population whereas previously it was used primarily in an older and sicker patient.

REFERENCES

1. Isselbacher EM. Thoracic and abdominal aortic aneurysms. *Circulation.* 2005;111:816–828.
2. Erbel R, Eggebrecht H. Aortic dimensions and the risk of dissection. *Heart.* 2006;92:137–142.
3. Patel HJ, Deeb GM. Ascending and arch aorta: pathology, natural history, and treatment. *Circulation.* 2008;118:188–195.
4. Isselbacher EM. Diseases of the aorta. In: Libby P, ed. *Braunwald's Heart Disease: A Textbook of Cardiovascular Medicine.* 8th ed. Philadelphia, PA: WB Saunders; 2008:1457–1467.
5. Hirsch AT, Haskal ZJ, Hertzer NR, et al. ACC/AHA 2005 practice guidelines for the management of patients with peripheral arterial disease (lower extremity, renal, mesenteric, and abdominal aortic): a collaborative report from the American Association for Vascular Surgery/Society for Vascular Surgery, Society for Cardiovascular Angiography and Interventions, Society for Vascular Medicine and Biology, Society of Interventional Radiology, and the ACC/AHA Task Force on Practice Guidelines (Writing Committee to Develop Guidelines for the Management of Patients With Peripheral Arterial Disease): Endorsed by the American Association of Cardiovascular and Pulmonary Rehabilitation; National Heart, Lung, and Blood Institute; Society for Vascular Nursing; Trans Atlantic Inter-Society Consensus; and Vascular Disease Foundation. *Circulation.* 2006;113:e463–e654.
6. Nataf P, Lansac E. Dilation of the thoracic aorta: medical and surgical management. *Heart.* 2006;92:1345–1352.
7. Frydman G, Walker PJ, Summers K, et al. The value of screening in siblings of patients with abdominal aortic aneurysm. *Eur J Vasc Endovasc Surg.* 2003;26:396–400.
8. Guo DC, Papke CL, He R, Milewicz DM. Pathogenesis of thoracic and abdominal aortic aneurysms. *Ann N Y Acad Sci.* 2006;1085:339–352.
9. Pressler V, McNamara JJ. Aneurysm of the thoracic aorta. Review of 260 cases. *J Thorac Cardiovasc Surg.* 1985;89:50–54.
10. von Kodolitsch Y, Nienaber CA, Dieckmann C, et al. Chest radiography for the diagnosis of acute aortic syndrome. *Am J Med.* 2004;116:73–77.
11. Hartnell GG. Imaging of aortic aneurysms and dissection: CT and MRI. *J Thorac Imaging.* 2001;16:35–46.
12. Bonow RO, Carabello BA, Kanu C, et al. ACC/AHA 2006 guidelines for the management of patients with valvular heart disease: a report of the American College of Cardiology/American Heart Association Task Force on Practice Guidelines (Writing Committee to Revise the 1998 Guidelines for the Management of Patients with Valvular Heart Disease): developed in collaboration with the Society of Cardiovascular Anesthesiologists: endorsed by the Society for Cardiovascular Angiography and Interventions and the Society of Thoracic Surgeons. *Circulation.* 2006;114:e84–e231.
13. Tamborini G, Galli CA, Maltagliati A, et al. Comparison of feasibility and accuracy of transthoracic echocardiography versus computed tomography in patients with known ascending aortic aneurysm. *Am J Cardiol.* 2006;98:966–969.
14. Griepp RB, Ergin MA, Galla JD, et al. Natural history of descending thoracic and thoracoabdominal aneurysms. *Ann Thorac Surg.* 1999;67:1927–1930; discussion 53–58.
15. Davies RR, Goldstein LJ, Coady MA, et al. Yearly rupture or dissection rates for thoracic aortic aneurysms: simple prediction based on size. *Ann Thorac Surg.* 2002;73:17–27; discussion 8.

16. Elefteriades JA. Natural history of thoracic aortic aneurysms: indications for surgery, and surgical versus nonsurgical risks. *Ann Thorac Surg.* 2002;74:S1877–S1880; discussion S92–S98.

17. Elefteriades JA. Thoracic aortic aneurysm: reading the enemy's playbook. *Curr Probl Cardiol.* 2008;33:203–277.

18. Bavaria JE, Appoo JJ, Makaroun MS, Verter J, Yu ZF, Mitchell RS. Endovascular stent grafting versus open surgical repair of descending thoracic aortic aneurysms in low-risk patients: a multicenter comparative trial. *J Thorac Cardiovasc Surg.* 2007;133:369–377.

19. Shores J, Berger KR, Murphy EA, Pyeritz RE. Progression of aortic dilatation and the benefit of long-term beta-adrenergic blockade in Marfan's syndrome. *N Engl J Med.* 1994;330:1335–1341.

20. Yetman AT, Bornemeier RA, McCrindle BW. Usefulness of enalapril versus propranolol or atenolol for prevention of aortic dilation in patients with the Marfan syndrome. *Am J Cardiol.* 2005;95:1125–1127.

21. Habashi JP, Judge DP, Holm TM, et al. Losartan, an AT1 antagonist, prevents aortic aneurysm in a mouse model of Marfan syndrome. *Science.* 2006;312:117–121.

22. Ejiri J, Inoue N, Tsukube T, et al. Oxidative stress in the pathogenesis of thoracic aortic aneurysm: protective role of statin and angiotensin II type 1 receptor blocker. *Cardiovasc Res.* 2003;59:988–996.

23. Almahameed A, Latif AA, Graham LM. Managing abdominal aortic aneurysms: treat the aneurysm and the risk factors. *Cleve Clin J Med.* 2005;72:877–888.

24. Lederle FA, Johnson GR, Wilson SE, et al. Prevalence and associations of abdominal aortic aneurysm detected through screening. Aneurysm Detection and Management (ADAM) Veterans Affairs Cooperative Study Group. *Ann Intern Med.* 1997;126:441–449.

25. Lederle FA, Johnson GR, Wilson SE, et al. The aneurysm detection and management study screening program: validation cohort and final results. Aneurysm Detection and Management Veterans Affairs Cooperative Study Investigators. *Arch Intern Med.* 2000;160:1425–1430.

26. Fink HA, Lederle FA, Roth CS, Bowles CA, Nelson DB, Haas MA. The accuracy of physical examination to detect abdominal aortic aneurysm. *Arch Intern Med.* 2000;160:833–836.

27. Rubin GD, Armerding MD, Dake MD, Napel S. Cost identification of abdominal aortic aneurysm imaging by using time and motion analyses. *Radiology.* 2000;215:63–70.

28. Multicentre aneurysm screening study (MASS) Group. Multicentre aneurysm screening study (MASS): cost effectiveness analysis of screening for abdominal aortic aneurysms based on four year results from randomised controlled trial. *BMJ.* 2002;325:1135.

29. Crow P, Shaw E, Earnshaw JJ, Poskitt KR, Whyman MR, Heather BP. A single normal ultrasonographic scan at age 65 years rules out significant aneurysm disease for life in men. *Br J Surg.* 2001;88:941–944.

30. Kent KC, Zwolak RM, Jaff MR, et al. Screening for abdominal aortic aneurysm: a consensus statement. *J Vasc Surg.* 2004;39:267–269.

31. U.S. Preventive Services Task Force. Screening for abdominal aortic aneurysm: recommendation statement. *Ann Intern Med.* 2005;142:198–202.

32. Brown LC, Powell JT. Risk factors for aneurysm rupture in patients kept under ultrasound surveillance. UK Small Aneurysm Trial Participants. *Ann Surg.* 1999;230:289–296; discussion 96–97.

33. Szilagyi DE, Smith RF, DeRusso FJ, Elliott JP, Sherrin FW. Contribution of abdominal aortic aneurysmectomy to prolongation of life. *Ann Surg.* 1966;164:678–699.

34. Powell JT, Greenhalgh RM. Clinical practice. Small abdominal aortic aneurysms. *N Engl J Med.* 2003;348:1895–1901.

35. Gadowski GR, Pilcher DB, Ricci MA. Abdominal aortic aneurysm expansion rate: effect of size and beta–adrenergic blockade. *J Vasc Surg.* 1994;19:727–731.

36. Brewster DC, Cronenwett JL, Hallett JW Jr, Johnston KW, Krupski WC, Matsumura JS. Guidelines for the treatment of abdominal aortic aneurysms. Report of a subcommittee of the Joint Council of the American Association for Vascular Surgery and Society for Vascular Surgery. *J Vasc Surg.* 2003;37:1106–1117.

37. McFalls EO, Ward HB, Moritz TE, et al. Coronary artery revascularization before elective major vascular surgery. *N Engl J Med.* 2004;351:2795–2804.

38. Poldermans D, Schouten O, Vidakovic R, et al. A clinical randomized trial to evaluate the safety of a noninvasive approach in high-risk patients undergoing major vascular surgery: the DECREASE–V Pilot Study. *J Am Coll Cardiol.* 2007;49:1763–1769.

39. Fleisher LA, Beckman JA, Brown KA, et al. ACC/AHA 2007 guidelines on perioperative cardiovascular evaluation and care for noncardiac surgery: executive summary: a report of the American College of Cardiology/American Heart Association Task Force on Practice Guidelines (Writing Committee to Revise the 2002 Guidelines on Perioperative Cardiovascular Evaluation for Noncardiac Surgery). Developed in Collaboration with the American Society of Echocardiography, American Society of Nuclear Cardiology, Heart Rhythm Society, Society of Cardiovascular Anesthesiologists, Society for Cardiovascular Angiography and Interventions, Society for Vascular Medicine and Biology, and Society for Vascular Surgery. *J Am Coll Cardiol.* 2007;50:1707–1732.

40. Propanolol Aneurysm Trial Investigators. Propranolol for small abdominal aortic aneurysms: results of a randomized trial. *J Vasc Surg.* 2002;35:72–79.

41. National Cholesterol Education Program (NCEP) Expert Panel on Detection, Evaluation, and Treatment of High Blood Cholesterol in Adults (Adult Treatment Panel III). Third report of the National Cholesterol Education Program (NCEP) Expert Panel on Detection, Evaluation, and Treatment of High Blood Cholesterol in Adults (Adult Treatment Panel III) final report. *Circulation.* 2002;106:3143–3421.

21 Erectile Dysfunction

Thorsten Reffelmann and Robert A. Kloner

Contents

Key Words: Vardenafil; Erectile dysfunction; Tadalafil; Phosphodiesterase-5 inhibitor; Sildenafil.

KEY POINTS

- The majority of cases of erectile dysfunction are associated with a general vascular process including endothelial dysfunction and may be classified as vascular-type erectile dysfunction.
- Cardiovascular risk factors, such as smoking, dyslipidemia, diabetes mellitus, arterial hypertension, are very common among patients with erectile dysfunction.
- Erectile dysfunction might be an (early) harbinger of other vascular disease such as silent myocardial ischemia or cerebrovascular and peripheral arterial disease. Erectile dysfunction should initiate a cardiovascular work-up including a complete history and physical exam, an ECG, and in many cases also an exercise test. Referral to a cardiologist might be appropriate in certain patients.
- Reduction of cardiovascular risk factors, be it lifestyle change or medical intervention, should be the first step for treatment of erectile dysfunction due to vascular dysfunction.

From: *Contemporary Cardiology: Comprehensive Cardiovascular Medicine in the Primary Care Setting*
Edited by: Peter P. Toth, Christopher P. Cannon, DOI 10.1007/978-1-60327-963-5_21
© Springer Science+Business Media, LLC 2010

- When cardiovascular medications, in particular antihypertensives, are prescribed, careful selection of appropriate drugs is prudent because many, in particular thiazide diuretics and β-blockers, may worsen erectile function.
- Before an appropriate treatment option is considered, patients, especially those with preexisting cardiovascular disease, should be evaluated for the issue of whether sexual intercourse can be safely recommended or whether further stabilization of the medical condition is mandatory.
- For evaluation of cardiovascular patients, recommendations of the first and second Princeton Consensus Conference may be applied.
- Oral treatment with inhibitors of phosphodiesterase-5, such as sildenafil, vardenafil, and tadalafil, is highly effective in a broad spectrum of patients presenting with erectile dysfunction.
- The use of drugs serving as nitric oxide donors, such as nitrates, is an absolute contraindication for the use of phosphodiesterase-5 inhibitors.
- A stable blood pressure (at least >90/60 mmHg) is a prerequisite for the use of phosphodiesterase-5 inhibitors. In general, concomitant use of antihypertensive therapy is well tolerated. Special caution is advisable when α(alpha)-receptor—antagonists are used simultaneously.
- Other treatment strategies, for instance testosterone replacement in hypogonadism or psychotherapy and antidepressants in major depression, are restricted to special indications and may in certain cases be combined with phosphodiesterase-5 inhibitors. Non-oral treatment strategies for erectile dysfunction, such as vacuum pumps, intracavernosal self-injection, or intraurethral application of alprostadil or penile prostheses, have become second- or third-line therapies.
- Dopamine agonists, such as sublingual apomorphine (available in Europe, but not FDA approved in the United States), are less effective than phosphodiesterase-5 inhibitors, but may be useful, in particular when contraindications do not allow use of phosphodiesterase-5 inhibitors.

21.1. DEFINITION, PREVALENCE, AND CAUSES OF ERECTILE DYSFUNCTION

Erectile dysfunction is commonly defined as the inability to attain or maintain a penile erection sufficient for satisfactory sexual intercourse. The prevalence, as estimated in a cross-sectional national probability survey in the United States of America (men aged 40 years and more, May 2001–January 2002), was 22% with significant increase with aging *(1)*. A similar prevalence of 19.2% was found in an urban area in Germany (30–80 years of age), with an increase from 2% among the youngest group to 53% in the oldest group *(2)*. Twenty-six new cases per 1,000 men were the estimated annual incidence of erectile dysfunction determined in the Massachusetts Male Aging Study (40- to 69-year-old men) *(3)*.

There are numerous causes of erectile dysfunction that should be considered when a patient first presents with this problem. Apart from neurologic and anatomic disorders and conditions following spinal cord injury, many medical diseases are commonly associated with some degree of erectile dysfunction. For example, endocrine disorders associated with erectile dysfunction do not merely comprise hypogonadism, thyroid disorders, or hyperprolactinemia, but also diabetes mellitus, which, as a cardiovascular risk factor, may also be classified as vascular-type erectile dysfunction. Table 1 presents an overview, compiled from various references *(4–15)*, of associated disorders and conditions to be considered for a patient suffering from erectile dysfunction. Of note, also various drugs frequently used in clinical practice may be associated with some degree of erectile dysfunction.

21.2. CARDIOVASCULAR RISK FACTORS IN ERECTILE DYSFUNCTION

Why should erectile dysfunction, a disorder at first sight belonging to the medical discipline of urology, be discussed in a book dealing with cardiovascular medicine? As early as 1985, this question was asked in a modified fashion in an article published in Lancet entitled "Is Impotence an Arterial

Table 1
Conditions and Disorders to be Considered in Patients with Erectile Dysfunction *(4–15)*

	Associated conditions
Vascular-type erectile dysfunction	1. Cardiovascular risk factors: Arterial hypertension Smoking Diabetes mellitus Dyslipidemia, hypercholesterolemia Obesity sedentary lifestyle 2. Endothelial dysfunction, atherosclerosis
Medical disorders	1. Renal failure, dialysis, hepatic failure, sickle cell disease, leukemia 2. Endocrine disorders: Hypogonadism Hyperprolactinemia Thyroid disease Diabetes mellitus
Neurological conditions	1. Spinal cord injury, nerve damage due to prostate surgery, cerebrovascular insult, multiple sclerosis 2. Neuropathy (e.g., diabetic)
Anatomical disorders	1. Peyronie's disease, trauma, priapism
Psychogenic/psychiatric disease	1. Depression, anxiety disorder, etc.
Drugs (selection)	1. Thiazide diuretics, spironolactone, digoxin, antidepressants, β-blockers, centrally acting antihypertensives, fibrates, phenothiazines, histamine-2-receptor antagonists, allopurinol, indomethacin, tranquilizer, chemotherapeutics, etc. 2. Alcohol

Disorder?" *(16)*. The paper reported the prevalence of atherogenic risk factors in 440 men suffering from erectile dysfunction. Smoking (64%), diabetes mellitus (30%), and hyperlipidemia (34%) were significantly more common in patients with erectile dysfunction in comparison with a male population of similar age.

In the Massachusetts Male Aging Study, the incidence of erectile dysfunction increased markedly with each decade of age, and clearly, heart disease, diabetes, and hypertension were identified as major risk factors in this prospective analysis *(3)*. An investigation of 154 patients suffering from erectile dysfunction in the United States reported a prevalence of 44% for hypertension, 23% for diabetes mellitus, 16% for tobacco use, 79% for obesity, and 74% for elevated low-density lipoprotein cholesterol levels (>120 mg/dL) *(17)*.

Endothelial dysfunction might be the common denominator of erectile dysfunction and atherosclerotic risk factors. A generalized vascular process involving atherosclerosis and endothelial dysfunction appears to be the basis for many forms of erectile dysfunction. Endothelial dysfunction, measured as flow-dependent and flow-independent vasodilation of the brachial artery, was strongly associated with first symptoms of erectile dysfunction prior to manifestation of atherosclerotic disease in a cohort of 30 patients in comparison with age-matched controls *(18)*. In some cases, erectile dysfunction may be a warning sign of silent cardiac disease before symptoms of heart disease are present *(19)*. Among patients with diabetes mellitus type 2, erectile dysfunction was identified as a predictor of silent coronary artery disease apart from traditional risk factors *(20)*. In general, endothelial dysfunction is supposed to precede the morphologic development of atherosclerotic lesions *(21)*. As a consequence, the association with erectile dysfunction might suggest that the presence of erectile dysfunction can predict the development of atherosclerotic disease in an early stage. Notably, a retrospective analysis, including more than 24,000 men with and without erectile dysfunction, demonstrated a twofold increased risk for acute myocardial infarction among men with erectile dysfunction in comparison to men without erectile dysfunction after adjustment for age, smoking, obesity, and medication *(22)*. Thus, detecting the underlying cardiovascular disease in men with erectile dysfunction and then treating the underlying risk factors may help to prevent future clinical manifestations of atherosclerotic disease.

21.3. BRIEF OVERVIEW: PHYSIOLOGY AND PATHOPHYSIOLOGY OF ERECTILE FUNCTION

The process of penile erection involves the sequence of tumescence and detumescence regulated by a complex neurophysiological process involving coordinated relaxation and contraction of smooth muscle cells within the corpora cavernosa of the penis. Increasing blood flow toward the corpus cavernosum while simultaneously reducing the outflow results in a penile erection.

Release of nitric oxide from non-adrenergic, non-cholinergic nerves and endothelial cells as a result of sexual stimulation enhances the activity of the enzyme guanylate cyclase of penile artery smooth muscle cells. This enzyme catalyzes the formation of $3'5'$-cyclic guanosine monophosphate (cGMP), which serves as a second messenger leading to reduced intracellular Ca^{2+}-activity and relaxation of the penile arteries, arterioles, and sinusoids. Total blood volume within the rigid tunica albuginea increases as draining venules are compressed by the rigid tunica albuginea. This results in a penile erection. The breakdown of cGMP is catalyzed by isoform 5 of the enzyme phosphodiesterase-5. Thus, when cGMP formation via guanylate cyclase decreases, falling concentrations of intracellular cGMP are accompanied by penile detumescence.

While alteration of various steps within this physiological model might conceivably worsen erectile function, the availability of nitric oxide appears to be crucial for initiation and maintenance of an erection. As a reduced availability of nitric oxide and, consequently, compromised endothelial-dependent vasodilation is a central characteristic of endothelial dysfunction, one might easily imagine that endothelial dysfunction may be the pathophysiological link to compromised erectile function.

21.4. EVALUATION OF A PATIENT PRESENTING WITH ERECTILE DYSFUNCTION

Even if various diseases are to be considered as a potential cause of erectile dysfunction (Table 1), erectile dysfunction associated with a generalized vascular process will play a prominent role in the patient population in the primary care setting. Of note, during routine outpatient cardiology visits, a prevalence of erectile dysfunction of 75% among patients with chronic stable coronary artery disease, as evaluated by a standardized questionnaire, was estimated *(23)*. Most of these patients had never discussed issues related to sexual function with their doctor. It appears to be important that the primary care physician or cardiologist should give patients at risk for erectile dysfunction, in particular cardiovascular patients, the opportunity to discuss potential problems regarding sexual functioning, depending on the patient's readiness to discuss these issues.

On the other hand, patients complaining of erectile dysfunction should be thoroughly evaluated regarding cardiovascular risk factors and potential silent cardiovascular disease. A detailed medical history, including sexual and psychosocial history, and evaluation of a potential genetic predisposition to cardiovascular disease, as well as a complete list of drugs the patient takes, are necessary.

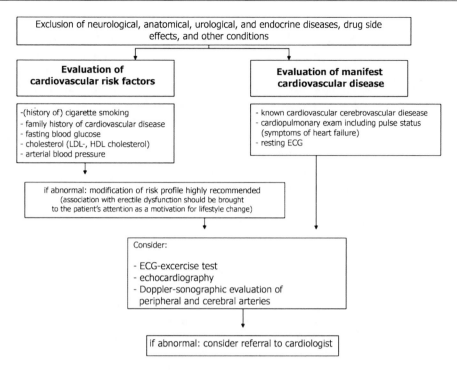

Fig. 1. Algorithm for the evaluation of a patient presenting with erectile dysfunction.

A history of hypertension, dyslipidemia, smoking, diabetes mellitus, obesity, and lack of physical activity are crucial to elicit during the work-up. Exertional dyspnea or anginal symptoms should be investigated. A careful clinical exam, including genitourinary examination, and also a complete cardiovascular (including blood pressure, heart rate measurement and assessment of peripheral pulses, complete pulse status), pulmonary, and neurologic exam are indispensable. If special medical diseases as a cause for erectile dysfunction (Table 1) are suspected, laboratory tests or further technical work-up may be required. If no obvious cause, such as neurologic, endocrine, or anatomic disorders, can be detected, a detailed cardiovascular work-up is worthwhile in order to see whether the classification as vascular-type erectile dysfunction is plausible and whether cardiovascular risk factors or manifest cardiovascular disease are also present. In Fig. 1, we propose a practical approach to the patient. In particular, an ECG-exercise test may be helpful in detecting silent coronary artery disease, abnormal blood pressure regulation, and overall physical fitness. In some cases, referral to a cardiologist, either for further diagnostic testing or for stabilization of the medical condition, might be necessary.

21.5. TREATMENT OF CARDIOVASCULAR RISK FACTORS—THERAPY FOR ERECTILE DYSFUNCTION?

The statistical association between cardiovascular risk factors and erectile dysfunction as well as pathophysiological concepts suggests that reducing modifiable cardiovascular risk factors may also improve erectile function. Even if this is not undoubtedly proven for the majority of risk factors, the association between risk factors and erectile dysfunction might be a relative concrete motivation for the patient to modify his risk profile, change lifestyle, and, in some cases, also initiate medical interventions. The following facts could help when discussing these issues with a patient.

Smoking cigarettes can lead to endothelial dysfunction, which provides a link to the close relation with erectile dysfunction in smokers. The risk for erectile dysfunction appears to be approximately twofold increased in smokers in comparison with non-smokers *(24, 25)*. One can conjecture that cessation of tobacco use could reverse erectile dysfunction, as in one study (in contrast to others) the prevalence of erectile dysfunction in former smokers was not different from individuals that had never smoked *(24, 26, 27)*.

Increasing physical activity, among other *lifestyle changes,* can significantly reduce the risk of developing erectile dysfunction, as reported in a prospective cohort study in men aged 40–70 years *(28)*. It is interesting that the same investigation reported that weight loss, reduction of alcohol consumption, and also smoking cessation had little beneficial effects on erectile dysfunction when initiated at higher age. Presumably, lifestyle change, once atherosclerosis has already developed, may be too late to reverse erectile dysfunction, but it might prevent its progression. Therefore, change of lifestyle should be strongly encouraged as early as possible.

For diabetic patients, a strong association between glycemic control and the prevalence of erectile dysfunction seems to be well established, even if there are no prospective trials showing reversal of erectile dysfunction after intensified treatment of diabetes *(29)*.

Treatment of hyperlipidemia, as either primary or secondary prophylaxis, should be recommended for any patients with dyslipidemia. Dietary measures should be the first step to correct the altered lipid balance. While fibrates can also induce erectile dysfunction as a drug-specific side effect, information regarding the effect of statins on erectile function is controversial. In general, statins seem to have positive effects on endothelial function *(30)*. In a similar manner, small studies also reported a positive effect on erectile function, in particular in conjunction with phosphodiesterase-5 inhibitors *(31)*. Case series from Spain and France, however, also demonstrated a low, but significant incidence of erectile dysfunction probably related to statin therapy *(32)*. Thus, even if treatment of high cholesterol levels is strongly recommended in this risk population, a positive effect on erectile function is not undoubtedly proven *(33–35)*.

Arterial hypertension should consequently be treated to achieve adequate target levels of blood pressure, because it is closely related to endothelial dysfunction. However, there is no scientific proof that this has the potential to reverse erectile dysfunction. To the contrary, some antihypertensive drugs, in particular thiazide diuretics and slightly less frequently β-blockers, may worsen erectile function as a side effect (compare Table 1). Nonetheless, with the currently available spectrum of antihypertensive drugs, it should be possible to find an effective combination without these side effects. Angiotensin-converting enzyme inhibitors appear to be neutral, while angiotensin-receptor blockers were actually reported to slightly improve erectile function *(36–38)*. Calcium antagonists have a low risk of deteriorating erectile function, but sometimes they increase prolactin levels which could have negative effects.

21.6. THE CARDIOVASCULAR PATIENT PRESENTING WITH ERECTILE DYSFUNCTION

In patients with manifest cardiovascular disease, erectile dysfunction is quite common. A healthy sexual life significantly contributes to quality of life, which is particularly true for the cardiovascular patient. Nonetheless, there is substantial uncertainty among patients and doctors whether a patient, e.g., after a myocardial infarction, may engage in sexual activity without increased cardiovascular risk. Furthermore, patients asking for treatment of erectile dysfunction may long have abstained from sexual activity, and it may not be evident whether physical activity during sexual intercourse is adequate for their cardiovascular status. Therefore, patients asking for medical treatment for erectile dysfunction should not only be checked for potential drug interactions and contraindications when prescribing oral treatment but also be evaluated to determine whether they can safely expend the physical activity needed for sexual activity.

The level of physical exertion during sexual intercourse may vary depending on several factors; in healthy males a peak heart rate of 110–127 per min was measured during intercourse with their usual female partner in a laboratory setting *(39)*. As a rule of thumb, historically, the stair-climbing test was introduced to simulate the level of physical activity during intercourse by Larson et al., who demonstrated an increased heart rate of 115 ± 7 per min and a systolic blood pressure of 164 ± 7 mmHg during sexual intercourse, and a heart rate of 118 ± 6 per min and a systolic blood pressure of 144 ± 6 mmHg with stair-climbing in patients with coronary artery disease *(40)*. In these investigations, 10 min of brisk walking was followed by climbing two flights of stairs, which approximates 5–6 METs, and may provide a general impression of the level of energy expenditure during sexual intercourse.

To quantify the level of physical exertion, the metabolic equivalent of energy expenditure at the resting state (MET, approximately 3.5 mL/kg/min oxygen consumption) is usually used for various physical activities (e.g., climbing two flights of stairs equals approximately 3 METs and digging in the garden 5 METs). Bohlen et al. found that 2.5–3.3 METs are attained during sexual stimulation and orgasm (maximum 5.4 METs) *(39)*.

Therefore, an exercise test might approximate the potential cardiac stress during sexual activity. A patient achieving 3–5 METs on exercise testing without signs of ischemia or arrhythmias is most likely not at risk for developing ischemia during intercourse.

21.7. RISK STRATIFICATION (FIRST AND SECOND PRINCETON CONSENSUS PANEL)

A cardiovascular patient asking for treatment options for erectile dysfunction should first be given a realistic estimate of a potential risk of sexual intercourse depending on his cardiovascular condition. For most patients, the risk of a cardiac event will be very low. The recommendations from the first and second Princeton Consensus Conference *(41, 42)* may be applied because they provide an approach that is useful in daily practice. Cardiovascular patients are categorized into three groups (Table 2): the low-risk, high-risk, and indeterminate-risk group. In the indeterminate-risk group, further diagnostic testing or therapeutic stabilization of the cardiovascular condition is required before the patient can be re-evaluated and categorized into either low-risk group or high-risk group. For most of these patients, referral to a cardiologist is appropriate to clarify the cardiovascular disease by further diagnostic testing (echocardiography, exercise testing, for some patients cardiac catheterization) and to plan treatment options including revascularization and adequate medical treatment.

Patients in the low-risk group, e.g., those with medically controlled arterial hypertension, or less than three cardiovascular risk factors, can be assured of a very low risk of a cardiovascular event during sexual intercourse, and treatment for erectile dysfunction can be safely prescribed. Patients with mild angina pectoris should undergo non-invasive evaluation including exercise-ECG. If angina pectoris occurs only at very high levels of exertion, the risk appears to be low. Nonetheless, in some patients the antianginal drug regimen may need to be modified to accommodate drug therapy for erectile dysfunction (e.g., no nitrates when a phosphodiesterase-5 inhibitor is prescribed). In patients with successful revascularization, i.e., percutaneous coronary interventions or bypass grafting, an exercise test should be used to document that there is no remaining ischemia. Traditionally, it has been recommended that sexual activity be avoided for 6–8 weeks after an acute myocardial infarction. In those who have undergone successful revascularization with no remaining exercise-induced ischemia, this period may be reduced to 3–4 weeks. Of note, exercise training (cardiac rehabilitation program) after myocardial infarction and also β-blockers may reduce the risk of a cardiac event during sexual activity.

Table 2
Categorization of Cardiovascular Patients (Modified Recommendations According to the First and Second Princeton Consensus Panel (38, 39))

Low-risk group	Indeterminate-risk group	High-risk group
≤ 2 atherogenic risk factors,	≥ 3 atherogenic risk factors	Unstable angina/refractory angina
Controlled hypertension	Moderate, stable angina	Uncontrolled arterial hypertension
Mild, stable angina (consider exercise test)	Myocardial infarction (2–6 weeks after the acute event)	Congestive heart failure (NYHA III–IV)
After successful coronary revascularization (either percutaneous coronary interventions or bypass surgery, without remaining ischemia)	Congestive heart failure NYHA II	Myocardial infarction (within the last 2 weeks)
	Stroke, peripheral vascular disease	
After uncomplicated myocardial infarction (>6–8 weeks)		Recent stroke
Mild valvular disease		Moderate to severe valvular heart disease or hypertrophic obstructive cardiomyopathy
Congestive heart failure NYHA I		
		High-risk arrhythmia

Within the table, connecting arrows: "Further diagnostic testing, interventional or medical treatment" ← "Further diagnostic testing" →

For high-risk patients, adequate treatment must be initiated before sexual activity may be recommended. Revascularization is required for unstable angina and medical treatment for uncontrolled hypertension and congestive heart failure. Cardiac valve disease may require heart valve replacement, and for malignant ventricular arrhythmia an implanted cardioverter/defibrillator may be adequate. In any case, stabilization of the cardiovascular condition is necessary before any treatment for erectile dysfunction is prescribed.

21.8. TREATMENT OF ERECTILE DYSFUNCTION

Phosphodiesterase-5 inhibitors, such as sildenafil, vardenafil, and tadalafil, have become first-line treatments for many patients with different degrees and etiologies of erectile dysfunction. Efficacy has been demonstrated in a broad spectrum of causes, including diabetes and hypertension.

Phosphodiesterase-5 inhibitors have become first-line treatment options for erectile dysfunction in a broad spectrum of patients. By inhibiting isoform 5 of the enzyme phosphodiesterase, which is abundant in penile smooth muscle cells, vasodilation, and thereby blood flow into the corpus cavernosum, is enhanced and prolonged, which in turn explains their positive effect in erectile dysfunction.

The most important contraindication to the use of phosphodiesterase-5 inhibitors is the concurrent medication of a nitric oxide donor, e.g., nitroglycerine as an antianginal drug. The combination of both drugs may result in life-threatening hypotension due to generalized vasodilation. Any patient on a phosphodiesterase-5 inhibitor must be informed about this absolute contraindication.

Sildenafil has a half-life of about 4 h, and 6 half-lives (24 h) were recommended as an interval before any nitrate may be given. Vardenafil has a similar half-life; therefore, a 24-h interval between vardenafil intake and application of nitrates may be sufficient. For tadalafil with 17.5 h half-life, the interval should be at least 48 h.

In general, combination of phosphodiesterase-5 inhibitors with a broad spectrum of antihypertensive agents is well tolerated (43–45). Blood pressure lowering effects of phosphodiesterase-5 inhibitors are small. Zusman et al. reported a non-dose-dependent reduction of systolic and diastolic arterial blood pressure after sildenafil of 7–10 mmHg *(46)*. Combination with calcium channel blockers, β-blockers, angiotensin-converting enzyme inhibitors, and other antihypertensive drugs are well tolerated in hypertensive patients. A resting blood pressure of 90/60 mmHg is the prerequisite for initiation of a phosphodiesterase-5 inhibitor. Caution is mandatory when phosphodiesterase-5 inhibitors are combined with α(alpha)-blockers, as hypotensive effects might be stronger than expected.

For some patients, sublingual apomorphine (dopamine agonist) may be an alternative, in particular when the patient is on nitrates. Sublingual apomorphine is not yet available in the United States but is available in parts of Europe. Even if the efficacy rate is slightly lower, the therapeutic potential was demonstrated in a broad spectrum of patients, including cardiovascular patients and diabetics. Baseline hypotension, however, is an absolute contraindication. As vagal tone (sometimes leading to nausea) might be increased by sublingual apomorphine, caution is advisable in patients with baseline bradycardia and atrioventricular conduction disturbances.

Other therapies, such as intracavernosal self-injection and intraurethral alprostadil, or vacuum pumps and penile protheses are second- or third-line treatment options for the majority of patients.

21.9. SUMMARY

Atherogenic risk factors are extremely common in the patient population suffering from erectile dysfunction. Many forms of erectile dysfunction may be classified as vascular-type erectile dysfunction and are closely related to endothelial dysfunction. Therefore, patients with erectile dysfunction should be encouraged to minimize their risk profile by lifestyle changes and in some cases by medical therapy. It is worthwhile initiating a cardiovascular diagnostic work-up when a patient presents with erectile dysfunction, as cardiovascular risk factors or manifest cardiovascular disease, such as silent myocardial ischemia, can be detected in a substantial percentage of patients. Any cardiovascular patient asking for treatment of erectile dysfunction should be closely evaluated before any treatment is prescribed. Recommendations of the Princeton Consensus Conference are useful in daily practice. An exercise test may be required in some patients to see whether the patient is able to tolerate physical exercise at a level usually performed during sexual intercourse without evidence for ischemia or arrhythmia. Phosphodiesterase-5 inhibitors and for some patients sublingual apomorphine are effective treatment options. Phosphodiesterase-5 inhibitors must not be combined with any nitric oxide donor as this may lead to potentially life-threatening hypotension.

21.10. CASE STUDIES

21.10.1. Case Study 1

A 56-year-old man asks his family doctor for some pills for treatment of erectile dysfunction. The problem had developed over the last 3 years. He is in a stable relationship with his wife, and both partners discussed whether treatment with these tablets could improve their sex life. He is apparently healthy, has no history of cardiovascular diseases, and is not on any medical treatment. He stopped smoking 3 years ago (30 pack years). The clinical exam (height 5.8 ft/178 cm, weight 199 pounds/90 kg), including cardiopulmonary exam and pulse status, is unremarkable except for blood pressure.

The cardiovascular risk profile is further characterized: fasting glucose, 5.0 mmol/L; blood pressure, 165/100 mmHg; LDL-cholesterol, 4.6 mmol/L; HDL-cholesterol, 1.1 mmol/L; triglycerides, 1.5 mmol/L; no family history of vascular disease; resting ECG, normal.

The patient is asked to return to the outpatient office to re-evaluate his blood pressure, and after two more measurements, the diagnosis of arterial hypertension was confirmed. The association of vascular risk factors with his primary problem, erectile dysfunction, is discussed with the patient. He is encouraged to reduce weight, start a low-cholesterol diet, and increase physical activity. Furthermore, the use of statins to lower LDL cholesterol, as a primary prophylactic measure, is discussed. Because he has multiple risk factors and is physically inactive, the patient is referred to a cardiologist for further evaluation of potential secondary causes of his arterial hypertension and for an exercise test to determine whether he can achieve 3–5 METs (metabolic equivalent of energy expenditure) needed for sexual activity.

An exercise-ECG does not provide evidence for myocardial ischemia, no secondary causes of arterial hypertension are found, and an echocardiogram is normal. Blood pressure treatment is initiated using an angiotensin-receptor blocker, and a statin is added. The patient increased his physical activity and tried to lose weight, which seemed to improve his general well-being.

A phosphodiesterase-5 inhibitor, prescribed for the treatment of erectile dysfunction, worked well, as reported at the next follow-up visit.

21.10.2. Case Study 2

A 62-year-old man with a medical history of myocardial infarction and subsequent coronary bypass grafting 6 years ago asks his family doctor for some treatment for erectile dysfunction. The patient is in a stable cardiovascular condition. His daily medication includes aspirin, a β(beta)-blocker, angiotensin-converting-enzyme inhibitor, and a statin. Sometimes during very heavy exercise and emotional stress he develops angina, which is promptly relieved by sublingual nitroglycerine.

The doctor tells the patient that phosphodiesterase-5 inhibitors, which nowadays are commonly prescribed for the treatment of erectile dysfunction, cannot be used, as the patient sometimes uses nitroglycerine. The concomitant use of phosphodiesterase-5 inhibitors and a nitrate may lead to a life-threatening blood pressure drop.

However, the doctor recommends further cardiological work-up to see whether there are further treatment options for his stable angina. A scintigraphic investigation demonstrates myocardial ischemia at a higher level of exertion. Cardiac catheterization reveals a high-grade graft stenosis. Stent implantation was successful. Thereafter the patient feels well and does not suffer from further angina even at relative high levels of exertion. The patient does not use nitroglycerine any more. After 4 weeks, the patient returns to the office. He reports about his improved cardiac condition and asks what treatment options for his erectile dysfunction might be considered. As the patient is stable without further use of nitrates, the prescription of nitroglycerine is stopped and a phosphodiesterase-5 inhibitor is prescribed for treatment of erectile dysfunction, which worked well.

REFERENCES

1. Laumann EO, West S, Glasser D, Carson C, Rosen R, Kang JH. Prevalence and correlates of erectile dysfunction by race and ethnicity among men aged 40 or older in the United States: from the male attitudes regarding sexual health survey. *J Sex Med*. 2007;4:57–65.
2. Braun M, Wassmer G, Klotz T, Reifenrath B, Mathers M, Engelmann U. Epidemiology of erectile dysfunction: results of the "Cologne Male Survey". *Int J Impot Res*. 2000;12:305–311.
3. Johannes CB, Araujo AB, Feldman HA, Derby CA, Kleinman KP, McKinlay JB. Incidence of erectile dysfunction in men 40–69 years old: longitudinal results from the Massachusetts Male Aging Study. *J Urol*. 2000;163:460–463.
4. Levine LA. Diagnosis and treatment of erectile dysfunction. *Am J Med*. 2000;109:3S–12S.
5. Benet AE, Melman A. The epidemiology of erectile dysfunction. *Urol Clin North Am*. 1995;22:699–709.
6. Greiner KA, Weigel JW. Erectile dysfunction. *Am Fam Physician*. 1996;54:1675–1682.
7. Nicolosi A, Moreira E, Shirai M, Bin Mohd Tambi MI, Glasser DB. Epidemiology of erectile dysfunction in four countries: cross-national study of the prevalence and correlates of erectile dysfunction. *Urology*. 2003;61:201–206.
8. NIH Consensus Development Panel on Impotence. Impotence. *JAMA*. 1993;270:83–90.
9. Nusbaum MR. Erectile dysfunction: prevalence, etiology, and major risk factors. *J Am Osteopath Assoc*. 2002;102: S1–S6.

10. McVary KT, Carrier S, Wessells H. Subcommittee on Smoking and Erectile Dysfunction Socioeconomic Committee, Sexual Medicine Society of North America. Smoking and erectile dysfunction: evidence based analysis. *J Urol.* 2001;166:1624–1632.

11. Brock GB, Lue TF. Drug-induced male sexual dysfunction. An update. *Drug Saf.* 1993;8:414–446.

12. Keene LC, Davies PH. Drug-related erectile dysfunction. *Adverse Drug React Toxicol Rev.* 1999;18:5–24.

13. Nurnberg HG, Hensley PL, Gelenberg AJ, Fava M, Lauriello J, Paine S. Treatment of antidepressant-associated sexual dysfunction with sildenafil: a randomized controlled trial. *JAMA.* 2003;289:56–64.

14. Roth A, Kalter-Leibovici O, Kerbis Y, et al. Prevalence and risk factors for erectile dysfunction in men with diabetes, hypertension, or both diseases: a community survey among 1,412 Israeli men. *Clin Cardiol.* 2003;26:25–30.

15. Moulik PK, Hardy KJ. Hypertension, anti-hypertensive drug therapy and erectile dysfunction in diabetes. *Diabet Med.* 2003;20:290–293.

16. Virag R, Bouilly P, Frydman D. Is impotence an arterial disorder? A study of arterial risk factors in 440 impotent men. *Lance.* 1985;1:181–184.

17. Walczak MK, Lokhandwala N, Hodge MB, Guay AT. Prevalence of cardiovascular risk factors in erectile dysfunction. *J Gend Specif Med.* 2002;6:19–24.

18. Kaiser DR, Billups K, Mason C, Wetterling R, Lundberg JL, Bank AJ. Impaired brachial artery endothelium-dependent and -independent vasodilation in men with erectile dysfunction and no other clinical cardiovascular disease. *J Am Coll Cardiol.* 2004;43:179–184.

19. O'Kane PD, Jackson G. Erectile dysfunction: is there silent obstructive coronary artery disease? *Int J Clin Pract.* 2001;55:219–220.

20. Gazzaruso C, Giordanetti S, De Amici E, et al. Relationship between erectile dysfunction and silent myocardial ischemia in apparently uncomplicated type 2 diabetic patients. *Circulation.* 2004;110:22–26.

21. Billups KL. Endothelial dysfunction as a common link between erectile dysfunction and cardiovascular disease. *Curr Sex Health Rep.* 2004;1:137–141.

22. Blumentals WA, Gomez-Caminero A, Joo S, Vannappagari V. Should erectile dysfunction be considered as a marker for acute myocardial infarction? Results from a retrospective cohort study. *Int J Impot Res.* 2004;16:350–353.

23. Kloner RA, Mullin SH, Shook T, et al. Erectile dysfunction in the cardiac patient: how common and should we treat? *J Urol.* 2003;170:S46–S50.

24. McVary KT, Carrier S, Wessells H. Subcommittee on Smoking and Erectile Dysfunction Socioeconomic Committee, Sexual Medicine Society of North America: smoking and erectile dysfunction: evidence based analysis. *J Urol.* 2001;166:1624–1632.

25. Dorey G. Is smoking a cause of erectile dysfunction? A literature review. *Br J Nurs.* 2001;10:455–465.

26. Jeremy JY, Mikhailidis DP. Cigarette smoking and erectile dysfunction. *J R Soc Health.* 1998;118:151–155.

27. Mirone V, Imhimbo C, Bortolotti A, et al. Cigarette smoking as risk factor for erectile dysfunction: results from an Italian epidemiological study. *Eur Urol.* 2002;41:294–297.

28. Derby CA, Mohr BA, Goldstein I, Feldman HA, Johannes CB, McKinlay JB. Modifiable risk factors and erectile dysfunction: can lifestyle changes modify risk? *Urology.* 2000;56:302–306.

29. Romeo JH, Seftel AD, Madhum ZT, Aron DC. Sexual function in men with diabetes type 2: association with glycemic control. *J Urol.* 2000;163:788–791.

30. Wassmann S, Laufs U, Bäumer AT, et al. HMG-CoA reductase inhibitors improve endothelial dysfunction in normocholesterolemic hypertension via reduced production of reactive oxygen species. *Hypertension.* 2001;37:1450–1457.

31. Herrmann HC, Levine LA, Macaluso J, et al. Can atorvastatin improve the response to sildenafil in men with erectile dysfunction not initially responsive to sildenafil? Hypothesis and pilot trial results. *J Sex Med.* 2006;3:303–308.

32. Carvajal A, Macias D, Sáinz M, et al. HMG CoA reductase inhibitors and impotence: two case series from the Spanish and French drug monitoring systems. *Drug Saf.* 2006;29:143–149.

33. Ralph D, McNicholas T. Erectile Dysfunction Alliance. UK management guidelines for erectile dysfunction. *BMJ.* 2000;321:499–503.

34. Rizvi K, Hampson JP, Harvey JN. Do lipid-lowering drugs cause erectile dysfunction? A system review. *Fam Pract.* 2002;19:95–98.

35. Schachter M. Erectile dysfunction and lipid disorders. *Curr Med Res Opin.* 2000;16:S9–S12.

36. Carvajal A, Lérida MT, Sánchez A, Martín LH, de Diego IM. ACE inhibitors and impotence: a case series from the Spanish drug monitoring system. *Drug Saf.* 1995;13:130–131.

37. Llisterri JL, Lozano Vidal JV, Aznar Vicente J, et al. Sexual dysfunction in hypertensive patients treated with lorsatan. *Am J Med Sci.* 2001;321:336–341.

38. Reffelmann T, Kloner RA. Sexual function in hypertensive patients receiving treatment. *Vasc Health Risk Manag.* 2006;2:447–455.

39. Bohlen JG, Held JP, Sanderson MO, Patterson RP. Heart rate, rate–pressure product and oxygen uptake during four sexual activities. *Arch Intern Med.* 1984;144:1745–1748.

40. Larson JL, McNaughton MW, Kennedy JW, Mansfield LW. Heart rate and blood pressure response to sexual activity and a stair-climbing test. *Heart Lung*. 1980;9:1025–1030.

41. DeBusk R, Drory Y, Goldstein I, et al. Management of sexual dysfunction in patients with cardiovascular disease: recommendations of the Princeton Consensus Panel. *Am J Cardiol*. 2000;86:175–181.

42. Kostis JB, Jackson G, Rosen R, et al. Sexual dysfunction and cardiac risk (the second Princeton consensus conference). *Am J Cardiol*. 2005;96:313–321.

43. Reffelmann T, Kloner RA. Cardiovascular effects of phosphodiesterase 5 inhibitors. *Curr Pharm Des*. 2006;12: 3485–3494.

44. Reffelmann T, Kloner RA. Vardenafil: a selective inhibitor of phosphodiesterase-5 for the treatment of erectile dysfunction. *Expert Opin Pharmacother*. 2007;8:965–974.

45. Reffelmann T, Kloner RA. The cardiovascular safety of tadalafil. *Expert Opin Drug Saf*. 2008;7:43–52.

46. Zusman RM, Morales A, Glasser DB, Osterloh IH. Overall cardiovascular profile of sildenafil citrate. *Am J Cardiol*. 1999;83:35C–44C.

IV CARDIAC DISEASE

22 Valvular Heart Disease

Garrick C. Stewart and Patrick T. O'Gara

CONTENTS

Keywords: Aortic stenosis; Endocarditis; Mitral regurgitation; Mitral stenosis; Murmur.

KEY POINTS

- Once valvular heart disease is identified, the clinical history and examination as well as serial echocardiography are the crucial elements in ensuring timely referral for valve surgery.
- Compensatory remodeling often allows chronic severe valvular heart disease to have a long latent phase, but onset of clinical symptoms is a turning point marking cardiac decompensation.
- Severe aortic stenosis accompanied by symptoms of angina, syncope, dyspnea, or frank heart failure has a poor prognosis without valve replacement surgery. There is no strict age limit for aortic valve replacement.
- Congenitally bicuspid aortic valve predisposes to early aortic stenosis, aortic regurgitation, and/or aortic root dilatation.
- Aortic regurgitation may be caused by either aortic valve (infective endocarditis, rheumatic disease, bicuspid aortic valve) or aortic root pathology (Marfan syndrome, connective tissue disease, or syphylitic aortitis).
- Mitral regurgitation begets mitral regurgitation and may result from disease affecting any part of the mitral valve apparatus—from the valve leaflets, annulus, and chordae tendinae to the papillary muscles and subadjacent ventricle.
- Though mitral valve prolapse has a generally benign course, it is the most common cause of severe MR requiring surgical treatment in North America.

From: *Contemporary Cardiology: Comprehensive Cardiovascular Medicine in the Primary Care Setting*
Edited by: Peter P. Toth, Christopher P. Cannon, DOI 10.1007/978-1-60327-963-5_22
© Springer Science+Business Media, LLC 2010

- Percutaneous balloon mitral valvotomy is now the treatment of choice for appropriate anatomic candidates with rheumatic mitral stenosis.
- The choice between mechanical and bioprosthetic heart valve weighs valve durability against the risks of anticoagulation.
- Antibiotic prophylaxis against infective endocarditis is recommended only for those patients at greatest risk for complications from endocarditis—patients with a prosthetic valve, previous endocarditis, complex congenital heart disease, or cardiac transplantation.

22.1. INTRODUCTION

Primary valvular heart disease remains a source of significant morbidity and mortality. Over 5 million Americans are living with valvular heart disease and nearly 100,000 undergo valve surgery each year *(1)*. Valvular heart disease is often first identified after a murmur is appreciated during a primary care visit and subsequently characterized by echocardiography (Fig. 1) *(2)*. Optimal management of valvular heart disease requires close collaboration among primary care physicians, cardiologists, and cardiac surgeons. With timely recognition and appropriate referral to cardiac specialists, in most instances patients with valvular heart disease can lead a normal life span.

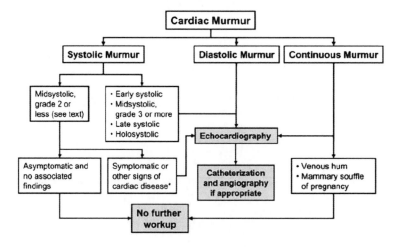

Fig. 1. Strategy for evaluation of heart murmurs *(9)*.

22.2. AORTIC STENOSIS

22.2.1. Etiology

Aortic stenosis (AS) accounts for one-quarter of all chronic valvular heart disease; approximately 80% of symptomatic cases in adults occur in males. Common etiologies of valvular AS include age-related calcific degeneration, stenosis of a congenitally bicuspid valve, or rheumatic heart disease. Age-related degenerative calcific AS is the most common cause of AS among adults in the United States. Over 30% of adults >65 years of age exhibit aortic valve sclerosis, while 2% have more severe valvular stenosis. Aortic sclerosis involves thickened or calcified valve cusps, often with a systolic ejection murmur, without significant outflow obstruction. On histology these valves appear thickened, inflamed, and calcified, similar to atherosclerosis. Interestingly, age, male sex, smoking, diabetes mellitus, hypertension, chronic kidney disease, and hypercholesterolemia are all risk factors for calcific AS. Both calcific AS and aortic sclerosis appear to be a marker for coronary heart disease events *(3)*. Recent studies suggest calcific AS is the end-result of an active disease process rather than the inevitable consequence of aging *(4)*.

Congenitally bicuspid aortic valves are present in 1–2% of the population without serious narrowing of the aortic orifice in childhood. The abnormal valve architecture makes the leaflets susceptible to ordinary hemodynamic stresses, ultimately leading to thickened, calcified leaflets, and narrowing of the orifice *(5)*. AS develops earlier in bicuspid valves, usually in the fifth or sixth decades, compared to trileaflet aortic valves, where degenerative calcific AS rarely develops before the sixth or seventh decade of life. Bicuspid aortic valves are also associated with aortic regurgitation, aortic root dilatation, and aortic coarctation.

Rheumatic disease may affect the aortic leaflets leading to commissural fusion, fibrosis, and calcification, with narrowing of the valve orifice. Rheumatic AS is almost always accompanied by involvement of the mitral valve or concomitant aortic regurgitation. By the time AS becomes severe, superimposed calcification may make it difficult to determine underlying valve architecture and the precise etiology of AS. In addition to valvular AS, other causes of left ventricular (LV) outflow obstruction include hypertrophic obstructive cardiomyopathy, a congenitally unicuspid aortic valve, discrete congenital subvalvular AS resulting from a fibromuscular membrane, and supravalvular AS. The various causes of LV outflow obstruction can be differentiated by careful physical examination and transthoracic echocardiography.

22.2.2. Pathophysiology

Obstruction to LV outflow produces a pressure gradient between the ventricle and the aorta. The ventricle responds to this pressure overload by concentric hypertrophy, which is initially adaptive because it reduces wall stress. This hypertrophy may accommodate a large pressure gradient for years before it becomes maladaptive and LV function declines, with chamber dilatation and reduced cardiac output. A mean gradient >40 mmHg or an effective aortic valve orifice of <1 cm^2 is considered as severe AS. Cardiac output, while normal at rest, may fail to rise appropriately with exercise. Coronary flow reserve may be reduced because of the increased oxygen demand of the thick-walled LV, increased transmural pressure gradient, and the longer distance blood must travel to reach the subendocardial surface. This may result in subendocardial ischemia even in the absence of epicardial coronary artery disease. The loss of appropriately timed atrial contraction, such as occurs with atrial fibrillation, may cause rapid progression of symptoms because of the reliance on atrial systole to fill a stiff and hypertrophied LV.

22.2.3. Symptoms

Most patients with AS have gradually increasing LV obstruction over many years with a long latent phase and no symptoms. Even with severe AS, the hypertrophied LV can produce the elevated pressures necessary to maintain an adequate stroke volume. Symptoms from AS are rare until the valve orifice has narrowed to approximately 1 cm^2 or less. The onset of symptoms usually indicates severe AS and often heralds the need for surgical evaluation and treatment because of the markedly reduced survival in symptomatic severe AS *(6)*.

Exertional dyspnea, angina pectoris, and syncope are the cardinal symptoms of AS. Oftentimes an insidious history of fatigue and dyspnea may be present, accompanied by a reduction in activity. Dyspnea primarily results from the elevated LV filling pressures necessary to fill the non-compliant, hypertrophied LV during diastole. Angina typically occurs later because of a mismatch between myocardial oxygen supply and demand from the thickened LV, even in the absence of obstructive epicardial coronary disease. Exertional syncope may result from an inability to augment cardiac output through the stenotic aortic valve orifice or from a sudden fall in output produced by an arrhythmia. Because of variable rates of AS progression, all patients with known AS should report any changes in symptoms to their physician *(7)*.

Symptoms of frank LV failure, such as orthopnea, paroxysmal nocturnal dyspnea, and pulmonary edema, are not present until the advanced stages of AS with LV systolic dysfunction. Signs of low cardiac output, such as marked fatigue, cyanosis, and cachexia, are not present until AS reaches the end stage, as are severe pulmonary hypertension, RV failure, and systemic venous congestion leading to hepatomegaly. In patients with severe, symptomatic AS, sudden cardiac death may occur in the setting of hypotension or arrhythmia due to ischemia, LV hypertrophy, or impaired LV function.

22.2.4. Physical Findings

The hallmark of AS is a carotid arterial pulse that rises slowly to a delayed and sustained peak (pulsus parvus et tardus). In the elderly, stiffened arterial walls may mask this finding, while patients with concomitant aortic regurgitation may have preservation of arterial pulsation due to elevated stroke volumes. The LV apical impulse may be displaced laterally and sustained due to LV hypertrophy and prolonged systolic ejection in the face of valve obstruction.

The murmur of AS is a systolic ejection murmur commencing shortly after S1, rising in intensity with a peak in mid-ejection and ending just before aortic valve closure. It is characteristically low-pitched, harsh, or rasping in character and best heard at the base of the heart in the second right intercostal space. It is transmitted upward along the carotid arteries, though may sometimes be transmitted downward to the apex where it may be confused with the murmur of MR (Gallavardin effect). The intensity of the murmur does not necessarily correspond to the severity of AS. The murmur of AS is diminished with Valsalva maneuver and standing, in contrast to the murmur of LV outflow tract obstruction in hypertrophic cardiomyopathy, which gets louder with these maneuvers.

When AS becomes more severe, the aortic component of S2 diminishes and may even disappear. Often S2 becomes paradoxically split in severe AS because of prolonged LV ejection across the stenotic valve. An S4 is audible at the apex and reflects LV hypertrophy with an elevated LV end-diastolic pressure. An S3 generally occurs late in the course of AS when LV dilatation is present. The best predictors of AS severity on physical exam are a late peak to the systolic murmur, a single S2 (absent aortic valve closure sound), and a pulsus parvus et tardus.

22.2.5. Diagnostic Testing

22.2.5.1. ECG

Most patients with AS have evidence of LV hypertrophy. In advanced cases there may be ST depression and T-wave inversion in the lateral leads. There is no correlation between ECG findings and severity of obstruction. The absence of LV hypertrophy does not exclude severe obstruction.

22.2.5.2. CHEST X-RAY

The chest radiograph usually shows a normal heart size. There may be post-stenotic dilation of the ascending aorta or a widened mediastinum if aneurysmal dilatation is present in patients with a bicuspid aortic valve. Aortic valve calcification may be identified on the lateral film. In the later stages of AS, the LV dilates leading to a widened cardiac silhouette, often accompanied by pulmonary congestion.

22.2.5.3. ECHOCARDIOGRAPHY

Key findings include LV hypertrophy and, in patients with valvular calcification (most adults with symptomatic AS), bright, thick echoes on the aortic valve. Eccentric valve cusps are characteristic of congenitally bicuspid aortic valves. Valve gradient and area are estimated by Doppler measurement of transaortic velocity (Fig. 2). Severe AS is defined as a valve area <1 cm^2, moderate as 1.0–1.5 cm^2, and mild AS as 1.5–2.0 cm^2. Echocardiography is useful for identifying coexisting valvular disease and differentiating valvular AS from other forms of LV outflow tract obstruction. There may also be

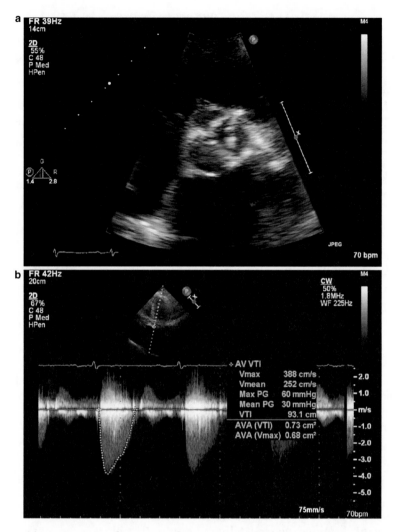

Fig. 2. Echocardiographic appearance of severe aortic stenosis. (**a**) Parasternal short-axis view at the level of the aortic valve during systole showing thickened, calcified aortic valve cusps with reduced excursion and a stenotic orifice. (**b**) Continuous wave Doppler interrogation of flow across the aortic valve with a peak velocity (*V*max) of 3.9 m/s. This produces an estimated peak gradient (Max PG) of 60 mmHg and a mean gradient (Mean PG) of 30 mmHg, with an approximate aortic valve area (AVA) of 0.7 cm^2.

aneurysmal enlargement of the aortic root or ascending aorta in up to 20–30% of patients with bicuspid aortic valves. Dobutamine stress echocardiography may be useful for the evaluation of patients with severe AS and reduced LV function (EF<35%).

22.2.5.4. CARDIAC CATHETERIZATION

Non-invasive assessment with echocardiography is now standard, but catheterization may be helpful as there is a discrepancy between the clinical and echocardiographic findings. Concerns have been raised about the risk of cerebral embolization during attempts to cross the aortic valve to directly measure the transaortic gradient. Coronary angiography is indicated to detect coronary artery disease in patients >45 years old who are being considered for operative treatment of severe AS. Coronary CT angiography is likely to be performed more often for this indication.

22.2.6. Natural History

In the era before widespread surgical treatment, average time to death after onset of AS symptoms was angina pectoris, 3 years; syncope, 3 years; dyspnea, 2 years; congestive heart failure, 1–2 years (Fig. 3). Sudden death is very uncommon (<1% per year) in asymptomatic adult patients with severe AS. Obstructive calcific AS is a progressive disease with an average annual reduction in valve area of approximately 0.1 cm^2. Death in patients with severe AS most commonly occurs in the seventh and eighth decades. Asymptomatic patients with severe calcific AS should be followed carefully for the development of symptoms and by serial echocardiograms for evidence of deteriorating LV function.

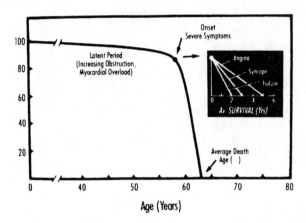

Fig. 3. Natural history of aortic stenosis. There is a long, latent period during which survival is similar to patients without aortic stenosis. Once symptoms develop, survival declines dramatically. Half of the patients do not survive 5 years after angina onset, 3 years after syncope, and only 2 years after heart failure develops in the absence of aortic valve replacement surgery *(6)*.

22.2.7. Treatment

22.2.7.1. MEDICAL TREATMENT

In patients with severe AS, strenuous physical activity should be avoided even in the asymptomatic phase. Hypertension medications such as ACE inhibitors or beta blockers are generally safe for asymptomatic patients. Nitroglycerin may be helpful in relieving angina pectoris in patients with known CAD, though should be used with caution for fear of hypotension with severe AS. If congestive heart failure is present, diuretic therapy may be helpful to regulate fluid retention. There has been enthusiasm for use of HMG-CoA reductase inhibitors (statins) to reduce the rate of progression of calcific degenerative AS, though prospective studies have thus far not shown benefit. In patients with mild-to-moderate asymptomatic AS, intensive lipid-lowering therapy with combination simvastatin and ezetimibe failed to reduce aortic valve events, a combined endpoint that included aortic valve replacement, congestive heart failure due to AS, and cardiovascular death *(8)*. Ultimately, medical therapy alone is ineffective treatment for severe symptomatic AS.

22.2.7.2. SURGICAL TREATMENT

Surgery is indicated in patients with symptomatic severe AS (<1.0 cm^2), in those patients have LV dysfunction (EF<50%), and in those patients with AS and an aneurysmal or expanding aortic root (>4.5 cm or increase in size >0.5 cm/year), even if they are asymptomatic (Fig. 4) *(9)*. Surgery may be postponed in patients with severe, asymptomatic AS and normal LV function because they may do well for years *(10)*. The risk of surgery exceeds that of sudden death in asymptomatic patients. In patients without heart failure, the overall operative mortality for aortic valve replacement (AVR) is

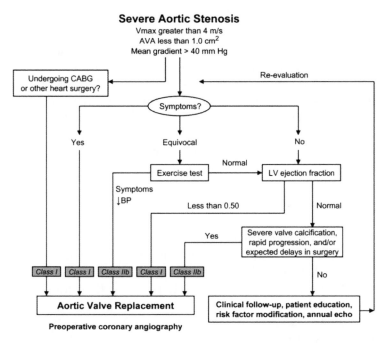

Fig. 4. Management strategy for patients with severe aortic stenosis *(9, 35)*. AVA = aortic valve area, BP = blood pressure, CABG = coronary artery bypass graft surgery, Echo = echocardiography, LV = left ventricle, Vmax = maximal velocity across aortic valve by Doppler echocardiography.

approximately 3% *(7)*. AVR may also be performed in patients with moderate AS undergoing coronary artery bypass grafting. AVR should be carried out before LV failure develops. At this late stage with a low EF and stroke volume, the transaortic gradient may be reduced. The operative mortality may exceed 15–20% in such patients and LV dysfunction may persist after AVR. Operative mortality depends to a substantial extent on pre-operative clinical and hemodynamic status. Because many patients with calcific degenerative AS are elderly, attention to pulmonary, renal, and hepatic function is required before AVR. Age alone is not a contraindication to AVR. The overall 10-year survival for patients with AVR is approximately 60%.

22.2.7.3. Percutaneous Aortic Balloon Valvotomy (PABV)

This procedure is often used instead of an operation in children and young adults with congenital, non-calcific AS. It is not widely used in adults with severe calcific AS because of high restenosis rates, embolic complications, and the development of AR after PABV. Given these risks, it is seldom used even in a palliative setting. In rare cases, it may be used as a bridge to AVR in patients with severe LV dysfunction and shock who are too ill to tolerate surgery without a period of metabolic recovery. Clinical trials are under way to develop new techniques for percutaneous aortic valve replacement and early results are very promising *(11)*.

22.3. AORTIC REGURGITATION

Chronic aortic regurgitation (AR) may be caused by disorders of either the aortic valve leaflets or aortic root *(12)*. The most common causes of primary valvular AR include rheumatic heart disease, bicuspid aortic valve, and infective endocarditis. Significant valvular AS may coexist with AR due to stiff, retracted leaflets, particularly in rheumatic disease, and in some patients with calcific degeneration. In patients with primary valvular AR, the aortic annulus may dilate secondarily, further worsening AR. Primary aortic root disease without involvement of the valve leaflets may also cause AR. Common etiologies of aortic root enlargement with AR include Marfan syndrome with associated cystic medial degeneration, connective tissue diseases, syphilitic aortitis, or aortic dissection.

The total volume of blood ejected by the heart is increased in AR. There is, however, significant regurgitation back into the LV due to aortic valve incompetence leading to a decrease in effective forward stroke volume. Over time, the LV dilates and thickens to accommodate the increased regurgitant volume, maintaining forward flow at a reduced wall tension. Eventually, these adaptive measures fail and the ejection fraction and forward stroke volume decline. Deterioration of LV function often precedes symptom development. At autopsy, the hearts of patients with severe AR are among the largest encountered.

22.3.1. Symptoms

Chronic severe AR may have a long latent period with patients remaining asymptomatic for as long as 10–15 years *(13)*. Some patients may have an uncomfortable awareness of their heartbeat, particularly when lying down, or head pounding due to the increased stroke volume. Exertional dyspnea from reduced cardiac reserve is usually the first symptom, followed by orthopnea, paroxysms of nocturnal dyspnea, and excessive diaphoresis. Angina, particularly at night, may also be present even in the absence of coronary artery disease. Systemic congestion with ankle edema and hepatomegaly may be present late in the disease course.

22.3.2. Physical Findings

Physical examination in chronic severe AR centers on signs of an increased stroke volume and detection of conditions predisposing to AR. The arterial pulse rises rapidly and collapses suddenly. Capillary pulsations in the nail bed may be appreciated when pressure is applied to the nail tip (Quinke's pulse). A "pistol-shot" sound can be heard over the femoral artery and a to-and-fro murmur may be audible when the femoral artery is lightly compressed with the stethoscope. The arterial pulse pressure is widened and often accompanied by an elevated systolic pressure. Palpation of the heart in chronic severe AR reveals a heaving, laterally displaced LV impulse. Both an apical diastolic thrill and systolic thrill at the base of the neck may be present. In some patients with severe AR, the carotid pulse may be bisferiens with two systolic waves separated by a trough.

In patients with severe AR, the aortic valve closure sound (A2) may be absent. The murmur of AR is a high-pitched, blowing decrescendo murmur. It is often loudest along the left sternal border, though may be heard along the right sternal border in patients with aortic root disease. The murmur of AR is often best appreciated with the patient leaning forward and after a breath hold following forced expiration. A mid-systolic flow murmur may also be heard at the base from increased stroke volume. A low-pitched mid-diastolic rumble, known as the Austin Flint murmur, may be produced in severe AR from displacement of the anterior mitral valve leaflet. Vigorous handgrip, which increases systemic resistance, augments the murmur of aortic regurgitation.

22.3.3. Diagnostic Testing

With chronic AR, the ECG will often have LV hypertrophy, left atrial abnormality, and a left axis deviation. With acute AR, the ECG may only have sinus tachycardia. Chest radiography often reveals cardiomegaly in chronic AR because of significant eccentric hypertrophy. Echocardiography is helpful in evaluating valve morphology and aortic root abnormalities. Doppler interrogation of the aortic valve and descending aorta helps quantify AR severity. Most importantly, echocardiography can identify LV enlargement and reduced systolic function, which may trigger operative intervention even before the onset of frank symptoms in chronic severe AR.

22.3.4. Treatment

Early symptoms of dyspnea and exercise intolerance often respond to treatment with diuretics and vasodilators such as dihydropyridine calcium channel blockers, ACE inhibitors, or hydralazine. The use of vasodilators to prolong the asymptomatic phase of chronic severe AR is controversial. Vasodilators, however, are an important means of controlling hypertension in this population (goal systolic blood pressure <140 mmHg). Nitrates may be used to control angina from AR, but are less effective than in coronary artery disease. Patients with severe AR should avoid isometric exercises.

Management of chronic severe AR often hinges on the timing of operation. In most cases of AR, valve replacement instead of repair is required, in contrast to MR. Patients with chronic severe AR usually do not become symptomatic until after LV dysfunction develops (14). In deciding when to operate on asymptomatic patients, the risks of the operation and prosthesis must be weighed against the risks of delaying surgery. Operation should be carried out in patients with LV ejection fraction of <50%, an LV end-systolic dimension of >55 mmHg, or an end-diastolic dimension of >75 mmHg. Patients with severe AR without indication for operation should be followed by serial echocardiography every 3–12 months to ensure operation before irreversible LV dysfunction develops. If a patient becomes symptomatic from severe AR, then valve replacement is indicated. The presence of new onset heart failure indicates cardiac decompensation, irrespective of echocardiographic evidence of LV dysfunction (15). When delayed too long (>1 year after symptom onset or echocardiographic evidence of LV dysfunction), surgical therapy may not restore LV function.

Surgical therapy for severe AR has evolved considerably in recent decades. Operations for isolated valvular AR involve prosthetic valve replacement. Primary aortic root disease without valvular involvement may respond to aortic root replacement with a native valve sparing method. As in other valve abnormalities, mortality after surgery depends in large part on the stage of disease and ventricular function at the time of operation. The overall mortality for isolated AVR is 3%. However, in patients with an enlarged or dysfunction LV at surgical referral, operative mortality is 10% and late mortality is 5% per year because of LV failure. Because prognosis is poor with medical management alone, even patients with LV failure should be considered for operation.

22.3.5. Acute Aortic Regurgitation

With acute aortic regurgitation, patients appear gravely ill and have tachycardia, significant dyspnea, and often hypotension. It is a medical emergency requiring rapid stabilization and surgery and is rarely encountered in the primary care setting. Most cases of acute severe AR are caused by infective endocarditis, but other causes include aortic dissection and trauma. Because compensatory eccentric hypertrophy has not had time to develop, a wide pulse pressure from increased stroke volume may not be present, and there may only be a short diastolic murmur. Once acute AR is suspected, prompt echocardiography and transfer to a center with cardiac surgical capabilities are imperative. Hemodynamic monitoring and therapy with intravenous vasodilators may be required to stabilize patients before surgery. Prompt surgical treatment may be life saving in acute severe AR.

22.4. MITRAL REGURGITATION

22.4.1. Etiology

Mitral regurgitation (MR) may arise from disorders affecting any part of the mitral valve apparatus. The mitral valve apparatus is composed of the anterior and posterior mitral valve leaflets, the annulus, chordae tendinae, papillary muscle, and the subadjacent left ventricular myocardium. Primary MR refers to defects of any element of the mitral valve apparatus above the level of the ventricle. Functional or secondary MR usually refers to a disorder of the left ventricle itself (16).

Similarly, MR can be separated into acute or chronic causes. Acute MR can occur in the setting of acute myocardial infarction with papillary muscle dysfunction or rupture, after blunt chest wall trauma, or in the course of infective endocarditis. Transient acute MR may result from papillary muscle ischemia, often presenting with angina accompanied by significant shortness of breath or pulmonary edema. Chronic MR may result from rheumatic disease, mitral valve prolapse, mitral annular calcification, hypertrophic obstructive cardiomyopathy, and dilated cardiomyopathy. Chronic MR may also result from geometric changes in the left ventricular after infarction, including remodeling that leads to leaflet tethering and fibrosis of the papillary muscles *(17)*. This same process can lead to MR in non-ischemic forms of dilated cardiomyopathy with an enlarged ventricular chamber and stretching of the annulus. Chronic severe MR is often progressive with atrial and ventricular remodeling leading to further leaflet displacement, greater regurgitation, and a vicious cycle. Mitral regurgitation begets mitral regurgitation.

22.4.2. Pathophysiology

With chronic mitral regurgitation, resistance to LV emptying is reduced because blood can eject into a compliant, enlarged low-pressure left atrium. Both LV filling and stroke volume are augmented because there is a greater return of blood from the atrium so that forward LV output is preserved. As LV volume increases over time, contractile function begins to deteriorate. Since ejection fraction rises in chronic severe MR in the presence of normal LV function, even a modest reduction (<60%) reflects significant dysfunction. In acute MR, the LV ejects blood into a small, non-compliant left atrium leading to a rapid rise in left atrial pressure during systole. This, in turn, increases pulmonary venous pressures and can lead to pulmonary edema. The difference in left atrial compliance and size explains why chronic MR (increased compliance) can be well tolerated and why acute MR (reduced compliance) is not.

22.4.3. Symptoms

Patients with MR in the compensated phase of their disease are typically asymptomatic and can tolerate even relatively strenuous exercise *(18)*. With acute onset MR or in the late stages of chronic MR, symptoms of left-sided heart failure predominate, including exertional dyspnea, orthopnea, paroxysmal nocturnal dyspnea, and fatigue. Palpitations are common and may signify the onset of atrial fibrillation. In severe chronic MR and pulmonary hypertension, symptoms of right heart failure may also be present.

22.4.4. Physical Findings

In patients with chronic severe MR, the LV is hyperdynamic with a brisk systolic impulse that may be laterally displaced and accompanied by an S3 gallop. In acute MR, signs of pulmonary congestion predominate and the pulse pressure may be narrowed due to reduced forward stroke volume. Chronic MR is marked by a blowing holosystolic murmur with a reduced S1, which may be obscured by murmur onset. This systolic murmur may sometimes be accompanied by a rumbling mid-diastolic murmur from the large volume of blood filling the LV. The murmur of severe chronic MR is usually at least III/VI in intensity and loudest at the apex with radiation to the axilla. In patients with ruptured chordae, the systolic murmur often radiates away from the leaflet that prolapses or is flail. If the posterior leaflet is affected, the murmur radiates to the base, whereas anterior leaflet involvement will produce a regurgitant jet directed posteriorly and, thus, a murmur transmitted to the back. The murmur of chronic MR is increased with isometric exercise (hand grip) and reduced during the strain phase of the Valsalva maneuver. MR may be distinguished from tricuspid regurgitation. Tricuspid regurgitation usually produces a less intense murmur heard at the left lower sternal border, which varies in intensity with inspiration and is accompanied by large "v" waves in the jugular venous pulsation. A ventricular septal defect also produces a holosystolic murmur, which varies inversely in intensity with defect size, is usually accompanied by a palpable thrill, and also does not vary with inspiration.

22.4.5. Diagnostic Testing

ECG often reveals left atrial enlargement, but right atrial enlargement may be present when pulmonary hypertension is severe. Chronic severe MR is associated with atrial fibrillation. There may also be signs of LV hypertrophy. Chest x-ray may reveal an enlarged cardiac silhouette in the late stages of chronic MR because of massive LV and left atrial dilation. Calcification of the mitral annulus may be visualized, particularly on lateral views. In acute severe MR, patients may have evidence of pulmonary edema, which may be asymmetric because the regurgitant jet may be directed to one set of pulmonary veins. Transthoracic echocardiography with Doppler is indicated to assess the etiology and severity of MR (Fig. 5). Serial assessment of global LV function and size are of particular importance in following patients with chronic severe MR *(19)*.

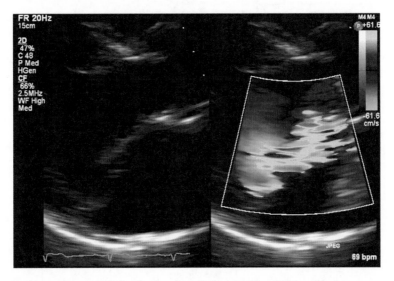

Fig. 5. Echocardiographic appearance of mitral valve prolapse. The *left panel* shows severe prolapse of the posterior mitral valve leaflet due to myxomatous degeneration. When color flow Doppler is applied, there is an anteriorly directed jet of severe mitral regurgitation associated with leaflet prolapse during systole.

22.4.6. Treatment

22.4.6.1. MEDICAL

In patients with acute severe MR, stabilization and preparation for surgery often involves the use of intravenous diuretics, vasodilators, and even intra-aortic balloon counterpulsation. In contrast, the use of vasodilators for treatment of chronic severe MR is only indicated in the presence of systemic hypertension. MR in the setting of heart failure with reduced ejection fraction may be improved by evidence-based treatments such as ACE inhibitors, beta blockers, diuretics, and cardiac resynchronization therapy. Asymptomatic patients with severe MR and normal LV size and function should avoid isometric exercise.

22.4.6.2. SURGICAL

In selecting patients for surgery for chronic severe MR, the slowly progressive nature of the disease must be weighed against the immediate and long-term risks of operation *(20)*. The risks are substantially lower for valve repair compared to replacement. Repair involves valve reconstruction using a variety of valvuloplasty techniques and insertion of an annuloplasty ring. In addition to reducing the need for anticoagulation and the risk of late prosthetic valve failure, valve repair preserves the integrity of the subvalvular apparatus, which maintains LV function to a greater degree.

Surgery for chronic severe MR is indicated once symptoms occur, especially if repair is feasible (Fig. 6). Other indications for early repair include recent onset of atrial fibrillation or pulmonary hypertension (>50 mmHg at rest, >60 mmHg with exercise). Surgery is also indicated in asymptomatic patients with LV ejection fraction <60% or end-systolic cavity dimension >40 mmHg. The aggressive indications for surgery are expanding given the outstanding results of mitral valve repair. In patients

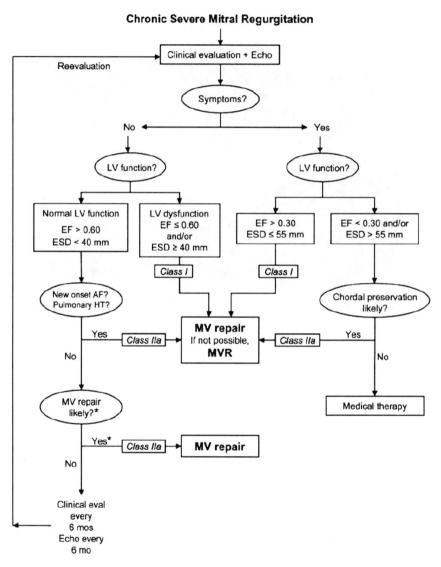

Fig. 6. Management strategy for patients with chronic severe mitral regurgitation. Mitral valve repair may be performed in asymptomatic patients with normal left ventricular (LV) function if performed by an experienced surgical team and if the likelihood of successful MV repair is >90% *(9)*. AF = atrial fibrillation, echo = echocardiography, EF = ejection fraction, ESD = end-systolic dimension, eval = evaluation, HT = hypertension, MVR = mitral valve replacement.

<75 years old with normal LV function and no coronary disease, there is <1% perioperative mortality with primary valvuloplasty with reoperation rates ~1% per year for 10 years after surgery *(21)*. The risk of surgery rises in patients with reduced LV function, particularly in those with LV ejection fraction <30%, because of persistence or worsening of LV dysfunction. When surgery is contemplated, cardiac catheterization may be helpful in delineating discrepancies between echocardiography and clinical exam, along with identifying patients who may also require coronary revascularization.

22.5. MITRAL VALVE PROLAPSE

Mitral valve prolapse (MVP) is a common (2.4% of population), highly variable clinical syndrome resulting from one of several disorders of the mitral valve apparatus *(22, 23)*. Among these are excessive or redundant mitral leaflet tissue associated with myxomatous degeneration, which may be related to disorders of collagen formation, or heritable connective tissue disorders such as Marfan and Ehler–Danlos syndromes. In most patients with MVP, the underlying cause is unknown. Myxomatous degeneration of the heart valves is often confined to the mitral valve, most commonly the posterior leaflet. In many patients elongated, redundant chordae may contribute to regurgitation. MVP may lead to stress on the papillary muscle and result in papillary dysfunction from ischemia. Ruptured chordae tendinae and annular dilation also contribute to regurgitation, further stressing the diseased valve apparatus, creating a vicious cycle.

MVP is more prevalent in females, most commonly between ages 15 and 30. Their clinical course is typically benign *(24)*. MVP has also been observed in patients >50 years old who are predominantly males and in whom MR is more severe and often requires surgery. MVP encompasses a broad spectrum of severities, ranging from a systolic click and murmur and mild prolapse of the posterior leaflet to severe MR with massive bileaflet prolapse. Most patients are asymptomatic and remain so for their entire lives. However, in North America, MVP is now the most common cause of severe MR requiring surgical treatment. MVP may be associated with arrhythmias such as premature ventricular contractions, paroxysmal supraventricular tachycardia, and ventricular tachycardia which may lead to palpitations, lightheadedness, or syncope. Sudden death is a rare complication, usually occurring only with severe MR and LV dysfunction. Many patients have a difficult-to-evaluate chest pain syndrome that is often substernal and unrelated to exertion. MVP may also have an association with migraine headaches.

On physical examination, the most important finding is a mid-systolic to late-systolic click thought to be produced by the sudden tensing of slack, elongated chordae tendineae, or the prolapsing mitral leaflet reaching its maximum excursion. Systolic clicks may be followed by a late-systolic crescendo–decrescendo murmur, which is occasionally "whooping" or "honking" and best heard at the apex. Any maneuver that reduces LV volume, such as standing or the Valsalva maneuver, will exaggerate the propensity of the mitral valve to prolapse and move the click and murmur earlier during systole. Squatting or isometric exercises, in contrast, will cause an increase in LV volume, reduce prolapse, and move the click and murmur later in systole. Some patients will have either a click or murmur, but not both together.

MVP is defined on echocardiography by systolic displacement of the mitral valve leaflets >2 mm into the left atrium above the plane of the mitral annulus (Fig. 5). Color flow and Doppler are useful in quantifying the degree of mitral regurgitation. Predictors of adverse outcome with MVP include older age, severe MR, thickened valve leaflets, and a dilated LV or left atrium. If the MR is only mild or moderate, patients can be provided with reassurance and have serial echocardiography every 3–5 years. Screening echocardiography is recommended for first-degree relatives of patients with MVP. Infective endocarditis prophylaxis is only indicated for patients with a prior history of endocarditis. Beta blockers may be helpful in relieving symptoms of chest pain or palpitations.

22.6. MITRAL STENOSIS

Rheumatic fever is the leading cause of mitral stenosis (MS). Widespread use of programs for the detection and treatment of Group A streptococcal pharyngitis have reduced the incidence of rheumatic fever in the developed world. As a result, the incidence of rheumatic MS has declined considerably in recent decades. Rheumatic heart disease remains the dominant cause of valvular disease in developing countries *(25)*. In patients with rheumatic heart disease, 28% have pure MS, 40% have mixed MS/MR, and 28% have mixed valve disease. Two-thirds of patients with MS are female. Rheumatic fever leads to inflammation and scarring of the mitral valve with fusion of the valve commissures and subvalvular apparatus. Although the initial insult is rheumatic, altered flow patterns may lead to calcification and further valve deformity. Taken together, these changes lead to a narrowing at the apex of a funnel-shaped ("fish-mouth") valve (Fig. 7).

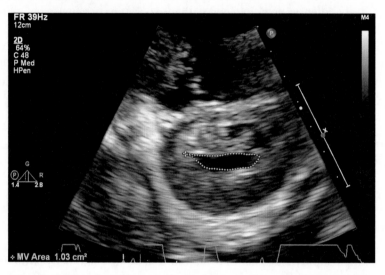

Fig. 7. Severe rheumatic mitral stenosis. This parasternal short-axis image at the level of the mitral valve leaflet tips shows that classic "fish-mouth" appearance of rheumatic mitral stenosis. Direct planimetry shows the effective mitral valve orifice to be 1 cm^2, consistent with severe mitral stenosis.

In normal adults, the mitral valve orifice is 4–6 cm^2, and MS develops when the area is reduced to <2 cm^2 and an elevated left atrioventricular pressure gradient is required to propel blood across the mitral valve. Severe MS is present when the valve area is <1 cm^2. The elevated left atrial pressures lead to pulmonary hypertension, exercise intolerance, and eventually right-sided heart failure. Adequate transit time is required to allow blood to flow across the stenotic mitral valve during diastole. As a consequence, the first symptoms are often precipitated by conditions resulting in tachycardia, such as fevers, anemia, hyperthyroidism, pregnancy, sexual intercourse, infection, or atrial fibrillation (AF). Chronically elevated left atrial pressures in MS contribute to the development of AF, which may in turn put patients at risk for thrombus formation and arterial embolization.

MS is a slowly progressive disease with a latent period of up to two decades between the episode of rheumatic carditis and symptom onset. The disease led to death within 2–5 years in the era before the development of mitral valvotomy *(26)*. As symptoms progress, lesser stresses precipitate symptoms and the patient becomes limited in her daily activities; orthopnea and paroxysmal nocturnal dyspnea develop. Development of permanent atrial fibrillation marks a turning point in the patient's course with an accelerated rate of symptom progression. Systemic embolization may be the first clue to the presence of MS, both from atrial fibrillation and the calcified mitral valve itself, with up to 20% of embolic events occurring during normal sinus rhythm. Patients may also suffer from hemoptysis due to shunting between the bronchial and pulmonary veins, leading to rupture. Rarely patients with MS may present with hoarseness because of compression of the recurrent laryngeal nerve due to severe left atrial enlargement (Ortner's syndrome).

22.6.1. Physical Findings

Patients with MS may have signs of heart failure, including pulmonary rales or pleural effusion, peripheral edema, ascites, an elevated jugular venous pressure, and congestive hepatomegaly. In severe mitral stenosis, patients may also have a malar flush with pinched and blue facies. The first heart sound (S1) is usually accentuated and slightly delayed. The opening snap (OS) of MS is best appreciated in early diastole during expiration with the diaphragm near the cardiac apex. The time interval between aortic valve closure (A2) and OS varies inversely with the severity of MS and the height of the left atrial pressures. The OS is followed by a low-pitched rumbling diastolic murmur best heard at the apex with the patient in the left lateral decubitus position. It is accentuated by mild exercise (e.g., a few sit-ups) performed just before auscultation. In general, the duration of the murmur corresponds to the severity of stenosis. Associated valvular lesions including the murmurs of pulmonic valve regurgitation and tricuspid regurgitation may be present along with a loud P2 from pulmonary hypertension.

The murmur of MS must be distinguished from several other conditions. A diastolic flow murmur may be present in severe MR, but commences later than the murmur of MS and is associated with signs of LV enlargement. Similarly, the apical diastolic murmur of severe AR (Austin Flint murmur) may be mistaken for MS but can be differentiated because it is not intensified following atrial presystole in patients in sinus rhythm. The murmur of an atrial septal defect or that of a left atrial myxoma may also be confused with MS. An ASD, however, usually is associated with fixed splitting of S2. Patients with left atrial myxoma often have signs of systemic illness, such as weight loss, and marked change in their exam based on body position. If there is doubt, echocardiography is invaluable in distinguishing amongst these conditions.

22.6.2. Diagnostic Testing

In patients with MS in sinus rhythm, left atrial enlargement is present. The QRS complex is usually normal. In severe pulmonary hypertension from MS, there may be right axis deviation and right ventricular (RV) hypertrophy. Chest x-ray may reveal signs of left atrial enlargement including upward displacement of the left main bronchus. Kerley B lines along the periphery of the middle and low lung fields may be present. Echocardiography with both two-dimensional imaging and color flow Doppler can estimate transmitral gradients and orifice size. Echocardiography is important for determining the presence and severity of accompanying MR, along with rheumatic involvement of the other valves and the degree of pulmonary hypertension. If there is a discrepancy between the clinical findings and echocardiography, either cardiac catheterization or cardiac magnetic resonance imaging may be indicated. All patients should be referred for further evaluation if the estimated mitral valve area is <1.5 cm^2, if they are symptomatic or develop atrial fibrillation, or if there is evidence of pulmonary hypertension on clinical exam or Doppler interrogation.

22.6.3. Treatment

22.6.3.1. MEDICAL THERAPY

Preventing management are prevention of recurrent rheumatic carditis, treating the consequences of MS, and monitoring for its progression. Appropriate patients with MS should receive penicillin prophylaxis against recurrent Group A beta-hemolytic streptococcal infections (27). No treatment is required for asymptomatic patients in sinus rhythm. Diuretic therapy along with dietary salt restriction is the mainstay for treating symptoms of pulmonary congestion. If AF develops, rate control with digoxin, beta blockers, or non-dihydropyridine calcium channel blockers (e.g., diltiazem or verapamil) is crucial because a rapid heart rate reduces mitral inflow time, thereby increasing left atrial pressure and reducing cardiac output. Warfarin to an INR of 2–3 should be administered to all patients with MS with either AF or history of thromboembolism. Once the ventricular rate has been slowed in AF, chemical or electrical cardioversion is indicated to restore sinus rhythm once the patient has been therapeutically anticoagulated for 4 weeks. If more urgent cardioversion is required, transesophageal echocardiography may be required to exclude left atrial thrombus. Patients with MS should be followed by clinical examination and echocardiography until symptoms limit lifestyle, atrial fibrillation develops or pulmonary hypertension becomes severe (>50 mmHg), at which time they should be referred for mechanical correction of the stenosis.

22.6.3.2. MITRAL VALVOTOMY AND REPLACEMENT

In the absence of any contraindication, mitral valvotomy is indicated in symptomatic (New York Heart Association Class II–IV) patients with isolated severe MS (valve area is <1 cm^2). Unlike PABV, percutaneous mitral balloon valvotomy (PMBV) has achieved durable results *(28)*. PMBV is performed by transseptal puncture, passing a guidewire across the mitral valve, and inflating a balloon (Inoue balloon) across the mitral orifice to split the commissures and widen the stenotic valve. Ideal patients for PMBV are younger (<45 years old) and have pliable mitral leaflets with little calcification, no left atrial thrombus and no more than mild MR *(29)*. Favorable PMBV candidates can be identified by careful echocardiographic study *(30)*. Such patients have excellent event-free survival after PMBV with rates of 80–90% over 3–7 years when performed by a skilled operator in a high-volume center. Successful PMBV doubles the mitral valve area, reduces transmitral gradient, and improves symptoms. If anatomy is unfavorable for PMBV due to thickening and heavy calcification of the mitral apparatus or significant concomitant MR, or if the initial PMBV is unsuccessful, then surgical commissurotomy may be performed, which requires thoracotomy and cardiopulmonary bypass *(31)*. Persistence of symptoms after commissurotomy suggests that it induced MR or that underlying LV dysfunction or associated subvalvular disease was present. There is a significant rate of restenosis after both percutaneous and surgical commissurotomy with most patients requiring a repeat procedure within 10–15 years.

Mitral valve replacement (MVR) is necessary in patients with MS and significant MR and those in whom valve anatomy is too distorted for commissurotomy alone. MVR is performed with preservation of the chordal attachments to preserve LV geometry and function. Given the long-term complications of MVR, it should be considered only in those patients with a valve area <1 cm^2 and NYHA III–IV symptoms. The average operative risk for MVR is 5%, with an overall 10-year survival in surgical survivors of 70%. Long-term prognosis is influenced by patient age, comorbid conditions, and the presence of concomitant pulmonary hypertension and RV dysfunction.

22.7. TRICUSPID REGURGITATION

Tricuspid regurgitation (TR) is most commonly functional and related to marked dilatation of the tricuspid annulus due to RV infarction, severe pulmonary hypertension, or dilated cardiomyopathy. The most important causes of primary valvular tricuspid regurgitation are trauma and infective endocarditis, particularly in patients who abuse injected intravenous drugs. Carcinoid is another cause, as is Ebstein's anomaly, a congenital heart defect in which the annulus of the tricuspid valve is displaced apically into the right ventricle. TR is often first identified in patients with evidence of a holosystolic murmur along the left sternal border. When severe, TR may contribute to symptoms of right heart failure, including fatigue, edema, and ascites. The murmur of TR usually increases in intensity with inspiration (Carvallo's sign) since inspiration augments RV filling. Examination of the neck veins reveals large V-waves. A pulsatile liver edge may also be felt in the right upper quadrant.

ECG often reveals right axis deviation and RV hypertrophy. Chest radiography may show an enlarged right heart border and obliteration of the retrosternal window. Echocardiography is valuable for identifying the cause of TR and estimating its severity. Primary valvular disease, such as vegetations with endocarditis, may be noticed and pulmonary pressures can be estimated to determine if underlying pulmonary hypertension is present. There is almost universal right ventricular and atrial enlargement. Severe TR may be accompanied by hepatic vein systolic flow reversal.

Despite the significant volume load with severe TR, in general the RV tolerates TR remarkably well and operation is rarely indicated. Therapy for TR is targeted as the underlying disease process. For example, if there is left ventricular failure, appropriate management with dieresis and afterload reduction may reduce the degree of functional TR. Similarly treatment of pulmonary hypertension may reduce the degree of TR. In severe TR, chronic diuretics are the mainstay of therapy to reduce symptoms RV volume overload and systemic venous hypertension. Tricuspid annuloplasty or replacement may be required for severe TR with primary involvement of the valve causing refractory symptoms of right heart failure or worsening RV systolic dysfunction.

22.8. PROSTHETIC HEART VALVES

Valve replacement surgery has been a major breakthrough allowing patients with severe cardiac valvular disease to have better quality and length of life *(32)*. Successful valve replacement surgery is dependent on the patient's myocardial function and general medical condition, as well as careful intraoperative and postoperative care. Durability and anticoagulation are the two most important long-term considerations. All valve prostheses have drawbacks, including the risk of thromboembolism, infective endocarditis, and mechanical failure *(33)*. As a consequence, there has been an increasing emphasis on valve repair rather than replacement in recent years, particularly for mitral regurgitation.

Prosthetic valves may be either mechanical or bioprosthetic. Bioprosthetic valves are usually xenografts (porcine aortic valves or cryopreserved, mounted bovine pericardium), but homografts from human cadavers may be used in complicated aortic valve endocarditis. In choosing an appropriate valve prosthesis, the need for anticoagulation, hemodynamic profile, durability, and patient preference must all be considered. In general, considerations for choice of valve are similar for the aortic and mitral positions.

Mechanical valves have excellent durability and hemodynamic performance. However, all patients who have undergone valve replacement with a mechanical prosthesis are at risk for thromboembolic complications and must be maintained on systemic anticoagulation with warfarin, which in turn increases the risk of bleeding *(33)*. The target INR level for a mechanical valve in the mitral position is higher (2.5–3.5) than the aortic position (2.0–3.0). Patients with a mechanical valve at high risk for thrombotic events, including those with atrial fibrillation, left ventricular dysfunction, previous thromboembolic event or hypercoagulable state, should have a target INR of 2.5–3.5. High-risk patients with a bioprosthetic valve should have INR targets of 2.0–3.0. Low-dose aspirin therapy is recommended for all patients with a prosthetic valve *(9)*.

The principal advantage of bioprosthetic valves is the virtual absence of thrombotic complication after 3 months, except when there are risk factors such as a hypercoagulable state or chronic atrial fibrillation with atrial enlargement *(34)*. Bioprostheses are at increased risk for structural deterioration. This deterioration requires repeat valve surgery in up to 30% of patients by 10 years and in 50% by 15 years. Bioprosthetic valves remain the preferred choice for patients >65 years old. They are also indicated for women who expect to become pregnant, as well as in others who have a contraindication to or refuse to take anticoagulation. In patients without contraindication to anticoagulation who are <65 years old, a mechanical prosthesis is reasonable. There has been a trend to using bioprosthetic valves in younger patients given the increased durability of the new generation bioprosthetic valves, decreased risk at reoperation, and aggregate risks of long-term anticoagulation, with full knowledge that reoperation will be likely over time.

22.9. PREVENTING INFECTIVE ENDOCARDITIS

Emerging data on the lifetime risk of infective endocarditis, as well as trends in antibiotic resistance and antibiotic-associated adverse events, have led to changes in guideline recommendations for antibiotic prophylaxis *(27)*. Infective endocarditis is much more likely to occur from frequent exposure to random bacteremias associated with daily activities than with medical or dental procedures. Antibiotic prophylaxis for infective endocarditis should only be provided to patients at greatest risk for complication from endocarditis. This includes patients with prosthetic valves, previous endocarditis, complex congenital heart disease, or cardiac transplantation. Routine antibiotic prophylaxis for mitral valve prolapse is no longer recommended. Prophylaxis in these high-risk populations is recommended for all dental procedures involving manipulation of gingival tissue or perforation of oral mucosa. Antibiotic prophylaxis may also be reasonable for procedures involving the respiratory tract, infected skin, or the musculoskeletal system. Antibiotic therapy solely to prevent endocarditis is no longer recommended for genitourinary or gastrointestinal procedures. Antibiotic prophylaxis is targeted to gram-positive oral and skin flora. Standard prophylaxis regimens in adults include amoxicillin (2 g 1 h before procedure), or if penicillin-allergic then clindamycin (600 mg 1 h before procedure) or azithromycin (500 mg 1 h before procedure).

22.10. CASE STUDIES

22.10.1. Case Study 1

Mrs. C.H. is a 77-year-old woman with a history of controlled hypertension, type 2 diabetes mellitus, and hypercholesterolemia who was noted to have a 2/6 systolic ejection murmur after hospitalization for total hip arthoplasty 5 years previously. She had no difficulty rehabilitating from her surgery and resumed her normal activities, including walking the two flights of stairs in her house and doing her own grocery shopping. She returns to the clinic for her semi-annual check-up and is now noted to have a late-peaking 3/6 systolic ejection murmur loudest at the base and radiating to the carotids with a diminished aortic component of the second heart sound. She has an apical S4 gallop, clear lungs, and no ankle edema. ECG reveals sinus rhythm and left ventricular hypertrophy. Echocardiography reveals a thickened and calcified aortic valve with reduced leaflet excursion. Her ejection fraction is 60% and her peak transaortic velocity is 3.9 m/s with a peak gradient of 60 mmHg and an aortic valve area of 0.7 cm^2, findings consistent with severe aortic stenosis (Fig. 2). She is referred to a cardiologist for further evaluation.

Age-related calcific degeneration of the aortic valve with stenosis is associated with traditional coronary risk factors, including hypertension, diabetes mellitus, and dyslipidemia. Calcific AS is a progressive disease, though may have a long latent phase during which mortality may be similar to that of similar patients without AS. Because of the importance of symptoms in determining the timing of referral for aortic valve surgery, Mrs. C.H. is told to seek medical attention immediately if she develops chest pain, shortness of breath, lightheadedness, or any reduction in exercise capacity (Fig. 4). Given her severe AS, serial echocardiography and clinical follow-up every 6 months is arranged to monitor left ventricular function and progression of her already severe valve disease. In the meantime, she will be maintained on an anti-hypertensive regimen featuring an ACE inhibitor for hypertension, insulin therapy for diabetes, as well as HMG-CoA reductase inhibitor (statin) therapy for her hypercholesterolemia.

22.10.2. Case Study 2

Mr. C.D. is a 49-year-old man who was found to have a systolic ejection click and murmur 13 years ago during a routine health maintenance physical. He underwent echocardiography, which revealed myxomatous degeneration of the mitral valve with prolapse of the posterior mitral valve leaflet and moderate, anteriorly directed mitral regurgitation. He remained asymptomatic working as an investment banker. While walking to work 1 day, he developed palpitations and visited his primary care physician. Physical examination revealed a regular rhythm, with a 3/6 holosystolic murmur radiating throughout the precordium, accompanied by an enlarged, laterally displaced point of maximal impulse. He was referred to a cardiologist for further evaluation given his mitral regurgitation with palpitations and evidence of left ventricular enlargement on exam.

Resting ECG showed normal sinus rhythm with left atrial enlargement, and holter monitoring revealed paroxysms of atrial tachycardia. Echocardiography demonstrated mitral valve prolapse with severe mitral regurgitation, moderate left atrial enlargement, and a left ventricular ejection fraction of 65% (Fig. 5). Given the absence of myocardial dysfunction, he was provided reassurance that asymptomatic severe mitral regurgitation can be well tolerated for many years. However, he has been carefully followed every 6 months with serial echocardiography and clinical evaluations to determine when mitral valve repair would be indicated (Fig. 6).

Mr. C.D. continues to work and has no exertional dyspnea in his daily activities or with light aerobic exercise, but has been counseled against performing strenuous isometric exercise such as weight lifting. He does not require routine antibiotic prophylaxis for dental procedures since he is not at high risk for complication from endocarditis. He has been told to seek medical attention if develops symptoms of exertional dyspnea, orthopnea, paroxysmal nocturnal dyspnea, and fatigue, at which point mitral valve repair will be recommended. Mitral valve prolapse is the most common cause of severe mitral regurgitation in North America requiring surgical therapy.

REFERENCES

1. Rosamond W, Flegal K, Furie K, et al. Heart disease and stroke statistics—2008 update: a report from the American Heart Association Statistics Committee and Stroke Statistics Subcommittee. *Circulation.* 2008;117:e25–e146.
2. O'Gara PT, Braunwald E. Approach to the patient with a heart murmur. In: Braunwald E, Fauci AS, Kasper DL, Hauser SL, Longo DL, Jameson JL, eds. *Harrison's Principles of Internal Medicine.* 15th ed. New York, NY: McGraw-Hill; 2001:207–211.
3. Otto CM, Lind BK, Kitzman DW, Gersh BJ, Siscovick DS. Association of aortic-valve sclerosis with cardiovascular mortality and morbidity in the elderly. *N Engl J Med.* 1999;341:142–147.
4. Freeman RV, Otto CM. Spectrum of calcific aortic valve disease: pathogenesis, disease progression, and treatment strategies. *Circulation.* 2005;111:3316–3326.
5. Fedak PW, Verma S, David TE, Leask RL, Weisel RD, Butany J. Clinical and pathophysiological implications of a bicuspid aortic valve. *Circulation.* 2002;106:900–904.
6. Ross J Jr. Braunwald E. Aortic stenosis. *Circulation.* 1968;38(1 Suppl):61–67.
7. Carabello BA. Clinical practice. Aortic stenosis. *N Engl J Med.* 2002;346:677–682.
8. Rossebo AB, Pedersen TR, Boman K, et al. Intensive lipid lowering with simvastatin and ezetimibe in aortic stenosis. *N Engl J Med.* 2008;359:1343–1356.
9. Bonow RO, Carabello BA, Kanu C, et al. ACC/AHA 2006 guidelines for the management of patients with valvular heart disease: a report of the American College of Cardiology/American Heart Association Task Force on Practice Guidelines (Writing Committee to Revise the 1998 Guidelines for the Management of Patients with Valvular Heart Disease): developed in collaboration with the Society of Cardiovascular Anesthesiologists: endorsed by the Society for Cardiovascular Angiography and Interventions and the Society of Thoracic Surgeons. *Circulation.* 2006;114:e84–e231.
10. Pellikka PA, Sarano ME, Nishimura RA, et al. Outcome of 622 adults with asymptomatic, hemodynamically significant aortic stenosis during prolonged follow-up. *Circulation.* 2005;111:3290–3295.
11. Coats L, Bonhoeffer P. New percutaneous treatments for valve disease. *Heart (British Cardiac Society).* 2007 May;93(5):639–644.
12. Enriquez-Sarano M, Tajik AJ. Clinical practice. Aortic regurgitation. *N Engl J Med.* 2004;351:1539–1546.

13. Bonow RO, Lakatos E, Maron BJ, Epstein SE. Serial long-term assessment of the natural history of asymptomatic patients with chronic aortic regurgitation and normal left ventricular systolic function. *Circulation*. 1991;84:1625–1635.
14. Dujardin KS, Enriquez-Sarano M, Schaff HV, Bailey KR, Seward JB, Tajik AJ. Mortality and morbidity of aortic regurgitation in clinical practice. A long-term follow-up study. *Circulation*. 1999;99:1851–1857.
15. Klodas E, Enriquez-Sarano M, Tajik AJ, Mullany CJ, Bailey KR, Seward JB. Optimizing timing of surgical correction in patients with severe aortic regurgitation: role of symptoms. *J Am Coll Cardiol*. 1997;30:746–752.
16. Otto CM. Clinical practice. Evaluation and management of chronic mitral regurgitation. *N Engl J Med*. 2001;345: 740–746.
17. Carabello BA. Ischemic mitral regurgitation and ventricular remodeling. *J Am Coll Cardiol*. 2004;43:384–385.
18. Rosenhek R, Rader F, Klaar U, et al. Outcome of watchful waiting in asymptomatic severe mitral regurgitation. *Circulation*. 2006;113:2238–2244.
19. Etchells E, Bell C, Robb K. Does this patient have an abnormal systolic murmur? *JAMA*. 1997;277:564–571.
20. Carabello BA. The current therapy for mitral regurgitation. *J Am Coll Cardiol*. 2008;52:319–326.
21. STS Adult Cardiovascular National Surgery Database—STS national database risk calculator. Available online at http://www.sts.org/sections/stsnationaldatabase/riskcalculator/
22. Freed LA, Levy D, Levine RA, et al. Prevalence and clinical outcome of mitral-valve prolapse. *N Engl J Med*. 1999;341:1–7.
23. O'Rourke RA, Crawford MH. The systolic click-murmur syndrome: clinical recognition and management. *Curr Probl Cardiol*. 1976;1:1–60.
24. Avierinos JF, Gersh BJ, Melton LJ 3rd, Bailey KR, Shub C, Nishimura RA, et al. Natural history of asymptomatic mitral valve prolapse in the community. *Circulation*. 2002;106:1355–1361.
25. Nkomo VT, Gardin JM, Skelton TN, Gottdiener JS, Scott CG, Enriquez-Sarano M. Burden of valvular heart diseases: a population-based study. *Lancet*. 2006;368:1005–1011.
26. Horstkotte D, Niehues R, Strauer BE. Pathomorphological aspects, aetiology and natural history of acquired mitral valve stenosis. *Euro Heart J*. 1991;12(Suppl B):55–60.
27. Wilson W, Taubert KA, Gewitz M, et al. Prevention of infective endocarditis: guidelines from the American Heart Association: a guideline from the American Heart Association Rheumatic Fever, Endocarditis, and Kawasaki Disease Committee, Council on Cardiovascular Disease in the Young, and the Council on Clinical Cardiology, Council on Cardiovascular Surgery and Anesthesia, and the Quality of Care and Outcomes Research Interdisciplinary Working Group. *Circulation*. 2007;116:1736–1754.
28. Reyes VP, Raju BS, Wynne J, et al. Percutaneous balloon valvuloplasty compared with open surgical commissurotomy for mitral stenosis. *N Engl J Med*. 1994;331:961–967.
29. Palacios IF, Sanchez PL, Harrell LC, Weyman AE, Block PC. Which patients benefit from percutaneous mitral balloon valvuloplasty? Prevalvuloplasty and postvalvuloplasty variables that predict long-term outcome. *Circulation*. 2002;105:1465–1471.
30. Wilkins GT, Weyman AE, Abascal VM, Block PC, Palacios IF. Percutaneous balloon dilatation of the mitral valve: an analysis of echocardiographic variables related to outcome and the mechanism of dilatation. *British Heart J*. 1988;60:299–308.
31. Ben Farhat M, Ayari M, Maatouk F, et al. Percutaneous balloon versus surgical closed and open mitral commissurotomy: seven-year follow-up results of a randomized trial. *Circulation*. 1998;97:245–250.
32. Vongpatanasin W, Hillis LD, Lange RA. Prosthetic heart valves. *N Engl J Med*. 1996;335:407–416.
33. Goldsmith I, Turpie AG, Lip GY. Valvar heart disease and prosthetic heart valves. *BMJ*. 2002;325:1228–1231 (Clinical research ed.).
34. Cannegieter SC, Rosendaal FR, Wintzen AR, van der Meer FJ, Vandenbroucke JP, Briet E. Optimal oral anticoagulant therapy in patients with mechanical heart valves. *N Engl J Med*. 1995;333:11–17.
35. Otto CM. Valvular aortic stenosis: disease severity and timing of intervention. *J Am Coll Cardiol*. 2006;47:2141–2151.

23 Pericardial Diseases

Fidencio Saldana and Leonard S. Lilly

CONTENTS

KEY POINTS
INTRODUCTION
ANATOMY/PHYSIOLOGY
ACUTE PERICARDITIS
RECURRENT PERICARDITIS
PERICARDIAL EFFUSION
PULSUS PARADOXUS
CONSTRICTIVE PERICARDITIS
REFERENCES

Key Words: Dressler's syndrome; Pericarditis; Pericardial effusion; Cardiac tamponade; Friction rub.

KEY POINTS

- The pericardium is a two-layered sac that anchors the heart in the mediastinum. It normally contains a small amount of pericardial fluid that is thought to provide a lubrication function.
- Acute pericarditis is characterized by pleuritic, positional chest pain, a pericardial friction rub, and specific ECG abnormalities. It is most commonly post-viral or "idiopathic" in origin.
- Non-steroidal anti-inflammatory drugs and colchicine are the main treatments for acute viral/idiopathic pericarditis.
- Recurrent episodes of pericarditis occur in up to 30% of patients. Initial treatment of acute pericarditis with corticosteroids poses a risk for disease recurrence.
- The most common etiologies of large pericardial effusions are "idiopathic," neoplastic, and uremic.
- A small non-hemodynamically significant pericardial effusion can be medically managed. An effusion that results in hemodynamic compromise (cardiac tamponade) requires referral for urgent evacuation.
- Constrictive pericarditis is an insidious condition manifested by abnormal pericardial rigidity that impairs filling of the ventricles. Right-sided heart failure and decreased cardiac output are common findings. Advanced cases require surgical resection of the pericardium.

23.1. INTRODUCTION

Pericardial disease may present as an isolated condition or as a manifestation of systemic illness. Recognition of the clinical signs and symptoms of such conditions in the primary care setting is critical for appropriate, and potentially lifesaving, triage and management. This chapter considers

From: *Contemporary Cardiology: Comprehensive Cardiovascular Medicine in the Primary Care Setting*
Edited by: Peter P. Toth, Christopher P. Cannon, DOI 10.1007/978-1-60327-963-5_23
© Springer Science+Business Media, LLC 2010

acute pericarditis and its potential complications relevant to the primary care provider: recurrent pericarditis, pericardial effusion, and constrictive pericarditis.

23.2. ANATOMY/PHYSIOLOGY

The pericardium is a fibro-serous sac that consists of two layers. The outer fibrous layer (the *parietal pericardium*) is largely acellular and is composed of collagen and elastic fibers, which allow it to gradually expand if subjected to chronic stretch. The internal portion of the fibrous pericardium is composed of a serous layer, which reflects onto the epicardial surface of the heart, forming the *visceral pericardium (1)*. The space between the parietal and visceral layers normally contains 15–35 mL of serous fluid, providing lubrication to the heart's movements. The pericardium is well innervated with nerve afferents so that acute inflammation produces pain and vagal reflexes *(2)*.

The pericardium attaches to the diaphragm, sternum, and other neighboring structures in the anterior mediastinum and, in this manner, serves to anchor the heart within the thorax. Additionally, the pericardium is thought to limit acute dilatation of the heart *(3, 4)*. The ability to restrain myocardial expansion is likely one of the most important functions of the pericardium. Despite these presumed actions, the complete absence of the pericardium (e.g., congenitally) is generally without clinical consequence *(5, 6)*.

The fibrous pericardium has the tensile strength of rubber *(7)*. As such, a sudden increase in volume within the pericardial space results in an equal external pressure against each of the cardiac chambers, which can lead to hemodynamic instability, as described below. Conversely, a slow increase in volume, over weeks to months, allows gradual stretching and accommodation of greater volume before such chamber compression occurs.

23.3. ACUTE PERICARDITIS

23.3.1. Case Study 1

A 51-year-old woman with a history of Hodgkin's lymphoma presents to the outpatient office with the gradual onset of left anterior pleuritic chest pain and mild dyspnea. The chest pain is non-radiating, dull, worse with chest and arm movements, and is relieved by sitting forward. She also

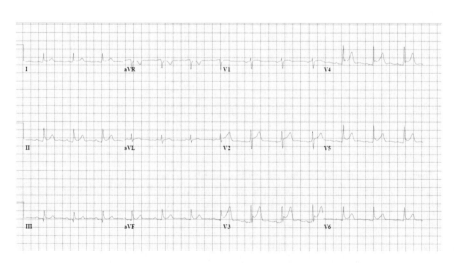

Fig. 1. Twelve-lead electrocardiogram of acute pericarditis, Stage 1. Diffuse concave-upward ST-segment elevation is present.

reports 2 weeks of malaise and fatigue accompanied by low-grade fever. On physical examination, she appears uncomfortable and anxious. The temperature is 98°F, pulse rate 120 bpm, blood pressure 125/70 mmHg, with pulsus paradoxus of 6 mmHg. The jugular venous pressure is 7 cm water. Her chest is clear to percussion and auscultation. On cardiac examination there is no retrosternal dullness. No murmurs, gallops, or rubs are auscultated. The electrocardiogram (Fig. 1) demonstrates diffuse ST-segment elevations in most of the ECG leads. A transthoracic echocardiogram (Fig. 2) obtained at the outpatient center reveals a small circumferential pericardial effusion with no signs of cardiac tamponade physiology.

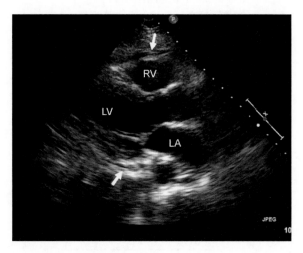

Fig. 2. Case Study 1. Two-dimensional echocardiogram, parasternal long-axis view, demonstrating a small pericardial effusion (*black arrows*). LA = left atrium, LV = left ventricle, RV = right ventricle.

23.3.1.1. EPIDEMIOLOGY AND ETIOLOGY

Case Study 1 depicts the classic presentation of acute pericarditis, an inflammatory condition of the pericardial sac, the differential diagnosis of which is broad (Table 1). As many as 90% of cases of acute pericarditis are considered to be post-viral or of unknown ("idiopathic") origin *(7)*. The majority of idiopathic cases are actually likely due to undetected viral infection, with agents such as Coxsackie and Echovirus species *(8)*. Less common viral causes of acute pericarditis include CMV, mumps, Ebstein–Barr virus, Varicella, Rubella, Parvovirus, and HIV. Acute pericarditis can also result from non-viral infections, autoimmune disorders, malignancy (most commonly lung or breast carcinoma or lymphoma), uremia, following transmural myocardial infraction, cardiac surgery or chest irradiation therapy, and as a result of specific medications such as isoniazid and hydralazine *(7, 9, 10)*.

Tuberculosis (TB) is only rarely encountered as a cause of pericarditis in industrialized countries. However, it is an important etiology in immunocompromised patients and in less developed regions of the world. In Africa, TB is the most common source of pericardial disease in patients with HIV infection.

Pericardial involvement is common in autoimmune disorders. Up to 25% of patients with rheumatoid arthritis, 40% of those with systemic lupus erythematosus, and 10% of individuals with progressive systemic sclerosis experience clinical manifestations of acute pericarditis in the course of their systemic disease.

The form of post-MI pericarditis most likely to be encountered in the primary care office is *Dressler's syndrome,* which can arise weeks or months following an acute myocardial infarction and is thought to be of autoimmune origin, resulting from exposure to antigens released from necrotic

Table 1
Causes of Acute Pericarditis

Infectious
Viral
Bacterial and mycobacterial
Fungal and protozoal

Autoimmune disorders
Systemic lupus erythematosus
Rheumatoid arthritis
Scleroderma

Malignancy
Breast and lung carcinoma
Lymphoma

Metabolic disorders
Uremia
Hypothyroidism

Drugs
Hydralazine
Procainamide
Diphenylhydantoin
Isoniazid

Following mediastinal irradiation
Following cardiothoracic surgery
Following myocardial infarction

myocardial cells. A similar syndrome, *post-pericardiotomy pericarditis,* may present weeks following cardiac surgical procedures.

23.3.1.2. Clinical Presentation

Patients with acute pericarditis typically present with chest discomfort that may mimic more serious conditions such as myocardial infarction or pulmonary embolism *(11).* However, the pain is typically pleuritic and positional in nature, worsening with recumbency and improving when the patient sits and leans forward. The discomfort can radiate widely, however localization to the trapezius ridge is highly suggestive of pericardial irritation, as the phrenic nerve innervates both the pericardium and the trapezius muscle *(2).* It tends to be rapid in onset and can then last for hours to days *(9).*

Symptoms of a viral syndrome, including low-grade fever and malaise, may precede post-viral pericarditis. In cases of pericarditis that develop more gradually (e.g., uremia, collagen vascular conditions, tuberculosis, neoplastic disease), the patient may not describe any chest pain at all. *High fever* and more severe symptomatology are typical of bacterial (purulent) pericarditis.

A thorough review of systems and past history can help identify specific etiologies of acute pericarditis. For example, drug-induced pericarditis should be considered in a patient taking isoniazid, diphenylhydantoin, or hydralazine. A history of HIV or mycobacterium infection should lead to consideration of those pathogens or associated complications. A prior malignancy may raise the concern of recurrence manifesting as pericardial involvement.

23.3.1.3. Physical Examination

The majority of patients with acute pericarditis demonstrate a pericardial friction rub *(12).* It is best auscultated over the left mid-to-lower sternal border while the patient leans forward *(13).* The character of the rub can be scratchy, leathery, or the crunchy sound of walking in snow and can be distinguished from a pleural rub by a breath hold, which extinguishes the latter *(9, 13, 14)*. It is most often triphasic, representing the phases of rapidly changing cardiac volumes: ventricular ejection, rapid ventricular filling in early diastole, and atrial systole *(7, 11, 13)*. The mechanism that produces the rub may not solely be the interaction between the inflamed pericardial layers as the finding can be detected even in patients with large pericardial effusions, in whom the layers are widely separated from one another *(13)*. In any patient with acute pericarditis, it is important to inspect for potential signs of cardiac tamponade described in more detail below: hypotension, distended neck veins, and distant heart sounds.

23.3.1.4. ELECTROCARDIOGRAM

The electrocardiogram can help distinguish pericarditis from other forms of chest discomfort. There are usually diffuse ST-segment elevations in the limb and precordial leads, typically with the exception of lead aVR *(9)*. This is accompanied by PR-segment deviation opposite to the direction of the P-wave. These findings reflect epicardial irritation of both the ventricles and the atria *(15)*. The electrocardiographic abnormalities typically evolve in four stages *(2, 16, 17)*:

Stage 1—Diffuse ST-segment elevations and possible PR-segment deviations (see Fig. 1)
Stage 2—Normalization of the ST- and PR-segments
Stage 3—Diffuse T-wave inversions (often weeks later)
Stage 4—Complete resolution

More than 80% of patients with acute pericarditis present with Stage 1 electrocardiographic findings. Anti-inflammatory treatment has been shown to prevent further progression of the ECG abnormalities *(8, 18)*.

There are several characteristics that distinguish the ECG findings of pericarditis from those of acute myocardial infarction. In patients with acute ST-segment elevation myocardial infarction (STEMI), the ST-segment elevation is localized to the region of the involved myocardium and is accompanied by ST depression in the opposite leads *(9)*. The direction of the ST-segment elevation is typically concave upward in pericarditis, but convex upward in STEMI. In addition, in infarction, T-wave inversions develop while the ST-segments are still elevated, whereas this occurs days later in pericarditis, after the ST-segments have returned to baseline (Stage 3). Finally, acute myocardial infarction does not cause deviations of the PR-segment.

Individuals with the common ECG variant known as *early repolarization* display baseline ST elevations that can mimic Stage 1 pericarditis. However, in distinction to those with early repolarization, the height of the ST-segment in acute pericarditis tends to be >25% of the height of the T-wave.

23.3.1.5. CHEST X-RAY

The chest radiograph may be normal in uncomplicated pericarditis. However, the presence of a large effusion (>250 mL) is manifest as a symmetrically enlarged cardiac silhouette *(11, 14)*.

23.3.1.6. BLOOD STUDIES

Measurement of acute and convalescent serum viral titres is not of practical value in the diagnosis of pericarditis as most patients will have recovered before such results are available. And while indicators of systemic inflammation are often elevated in acute pericarditis, there is no consensus on the utility of measuring markers, such as C-reactive protein or erythrocyte sedimentation rate (ESR), in establishing the diagnosis or following the course of disease *(11)*. In general, a modestly elevated ESR is consistent with idiopathic or post-viral pericarditis, while higher levels are suggestive of more active inflammatory states such as rheumatoid arthritis, systemic lupus erythematosus, or tuberculosis *(9)*. Similarly, a mild leukocytosis is typical of viral or idiopathic pericarditis, whereas a markedly elevated white blood cell count is more consistent with purulent pericarditis *(11)*. In 35–50% of patients with pericarditis, troponin levels are increased due to extension of inflammation to the adjacent myocardium *(8, 19, 20)*. However, elevation of cardiac-specific troponins is not a negative prognostic marker in acute pericarditis *(21–23)*.

23.3.1.7. ECHOCARDIOGRAM

Current guidelines recommend that a transthoracic echocardiogram be obtained in patients with suspected pericardial disease to assess for effusion, contributing pathology, and for evidence of impending hemodynamic compromise *(24)*. In patients with uncomplicated pericarditis the echocardiogram may be completely normal. If a pericardial effusion has formed, it is visualized as an echo-free space external to the cardiac chambers, as in Fig. 2 *(9)*. The smallest effusions appear posterior to the left ventricle because of the effect of gravity. Larger effusions wrap around the sides of the heart and, if more than approximately 250 mL has accumulated, appear anterior to the right ventricle as well.

23.3.1.8. TREATMENT

Idiopathic or post-viral pericarditis is a self-limited condition that tends to improve spontaneously within 1–3 weeks. Drug therapies are employed for earlier symptomatic relief. While there is little in the way of randomized trials to guide the treatment of acute pericardial disease, the European Society of Cardiology has published guidelines with management strategies *(25)*. The mainstay of acute treatment is oral non-steroidal anti-inflammatory agent therapy (NSAIAs) such as aspirin (2–4 g daily), ibuprofen (1,600–3,200 mg daily), or indomethacin (75–225 mg daily) *(11)*. No one NSAIA appears to be more effective than others; however, certain circumstances may favor the use of a particular agent *(26)*. Ibuprofen is used frequently because of its general tolerability *(9)*. Indomethacin has been shown to reduce epicardial coronary flow and the European guidelines suggest that it should be avoided in elderly patients *(25)*. For individuals who have sustained a recent myocardial infarction, aspirin is the drug of choice given a concern of impairment of healing of infarcted tissue by other NSAIAs in animal models *(11)*. In addition to oral NSAIAs, parenteral keterolac has been shown to be effective at resolving symptomatic acute pericarditis *(27)*.

Recently, colchicine has entered the armamentarium for the treatment of pericarditis *(9)*. The COlchicine for acute PEricarditis (COPE) Trial demonstrated that colchicine (1 mg po bid on first day, then 0.5 mg bid for 3 months), in conjunction with aspirin, reduced the rate of recurrent pericarditis in patients with a first episode from 32.3% to 10.7% *(28)*. Conversely, corticosteroids are not recommended as first line agents in uncomplicated pericarditis as their use predisposes to relapse after they are tapered *(8, 25, 28)*. Recurrences have been identified in up to 86.7% of patients treated initially with corticosteroids alone *(28)*.

Symptoms typically resolve within days of treatment, often after the first few doses. NSAIAs are usually continued for 7–14 days followed by gradual reduction in dosage over 1–2 weeks for a total treatment time of 3–4 weeks. If colchicine is used it should be continued for 3 months as was the protocol in the COPE trial. Acute pericarditis is not an absolute contraindication to concurrent warfarin therapy in patients for whom anticoagulation is indicated (e.g., atrial fibrillation, intracardiac thrombus). However, the risks and benefits of continued anticoagulation must be evaluated on a patient-by-patient basis.

23.3.1.9. TRIAGE

Identification of high-risk features is important in the triage of patients with acute pericarditis. Findings that warrant hospitalization and close observation include a large circumferential pericardial effusion, cardiac tamponade findings, patients who are on anticoagulation therapy, a high fever, an underlying immunosuppressed state, evidence of accompanying myocarditis, or trauma-associated pericarditis (Fig. 3) *(11, 22, 29)*. There is no consensus on triage of patients who do not exhibit such

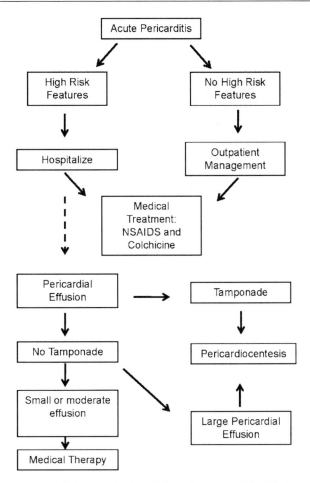

Fig. 3. Approach to the management of acute pericarditis and pericardial effusion. NSAIDS = non-steroidal anti-inflammatory drugs.

high-risk features. The European Society of Cardiology recommends hospitalization for most patients with acute pericarditis to facilitate work up and observe the effectiveness of treatment *(25)*. Others have shown that uncomplicated idiopathic/post-viral pericarditis can be safely treated in a day-hospital setting where the patient can be observed for several hours, have an echocardiogram performed, and if stable, return home *(22)*.

23.4. RECURRENT PERICARDITIS

Between 15% and 30% of patients treated for acute pericarditis experience relapses *(9)*. Symptoms are similar to the initial episode, characterized by fever, pleuritic chest pain, a pericardial rub, and elevation of inflammatory makers *(30)*. Recurrent pericarditis may occur as anti-inflammatory therapy is tapered (*incessant* pericarditis) at varying intervals following the cessation of treatment (*intermittent* pericarditis). Recurrences may or relate to an immune-mediated reaction following the initial episode or may be the manifestation of a previously undiagnosed and ongoing inflammatory condition such as an autoimmune disorder *(9, 11)*.

Relapses can be challenging to suppress. The first defense is prevention of recurrent episodes by optimizing treatment of the index presentation. As noted above, the COPE trial demonstrated a decreased recurrence rate in patients with acute pericarditis treated with aspirin plus colchicine compared with aspirin alone *(28)*. Once a recurrence develops, symptoms often respond to renewed therapy with an NSAIA agent with the addition of colchicine. In the prospective Colchicine for Recurrent Pericarditis (CORE) Trial, 84 patients with a first bout of recurrent pericarditis were randomized to aspirin alone (800 mg daily every 6 or 8 h for 7–10 days, then tapered over 3–4 weeks) versus aspirin in addition to colchicine (1.0–2.0 mg on the first day, then 0.5–1.0 mg daily for 6 months). Compared with aspirin alone, the combination reduced further recurrences by 50%, and symptom persistence at 72 h fell by approximately 33% *(30)*. Recurrent episodes with refractory symptoms may require the use of a corticosteroid *(25)*. In such cases, the *European Society of Cardiology Guidelines* recommends a regimen of prednisone 1–1.5 mg/kg for 1 month, then a gradual taper over 3 months, as an NSAIA or colchicine is then reintroduced. However, a recent retrospective review of 100 patients with recurrent pericarditis concluded that lower steroid doses (prednisone 0.2–0.5 mg/kg/day) were better tolerated and were associated with fewer subsequent recurrences *(31)*. Patients with persistent symptoms or recurrent episodes that fail to cease with these measures should be referred to a specialist for consideration of more extreme approaches, such as pericardiectomy *(9)*.

23.5. PERICARDIAL EFFUSION

23.5.1. Case Study 2

The 51-year-old woman from Case Study 1 returns to her primary care doctor 2 weeks after her initial presentation. Her symptoms had responded initially to a course of ibuprofen plus colchicine. The colchicine was discontinued after a few days due to diarrhea. Her current symptoms are increasing dyspnea on exertion and chest fullness when she leans toward her left side. She denies fevers, sweats, or chills.

On physical examination the temperature is 98°F, heart rate 115 bpm, blood pressure 112/70 mmHg with a pulsus paradoxus of 15 mmHg. The jugular venous pressure is 12 cm water. The chest is clear to auscultation. On cardiac exam, there is retrosternal dullness and a pericardial friction rub is auscultated. There is no abdominal distension, hepatomegaly, or peripheral edema. The patient undergoes an urgent echocardiogram (Fig. 4), which demonstrates a large circumferential pericardial effusion with right atrial and right ventricular diastolic collapse.

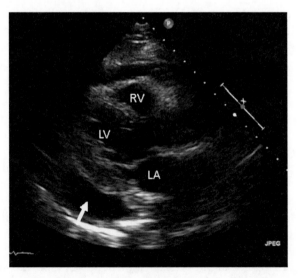

Fig. 4. Case Study 2. Echocardiogram demonstrating a large pericardial effusion (*white arrow*). LA = left atrium; LV = left ventricle; RV = right ventricle.

23.5.1.1. ETIOLOGY

A pericardial effusion results from the accumulation of fluid within the potential space between the visceral and parietal pericardial layers *(32)*. Fluid accumulation can result from an inflammatory reaction, direct trauma, or obstruction of lymphatic drainage *(9)*. The etiologies of acute pericardial disease in Table 1 are all potential causes of pericardial effusion accumulation. Large effusions are most commonly idiopathic, neoplastic, or uremic in origin *(33, 34)*. As many as 15% of patients with idiopathic pericarditis and 60% of patients with purulent or malignant present with an effusion *(10, 35)*.

Effusions that are most likely to progress to tamponade are those caused by trauma, non-viral infections (bacterial, fungal), and malignancy *(9)*. It is unusual for idiopathic/post-viral pericarditis to lead to tamponade.

23.5.1.2. PATHOPHYSIOLOGY

The pericardium has only a limited potential for expansion. A sudden increase in pericardial volume can lead to hemodynamic instability due to external compression of the cardiac chambers, resulting in diminished cardiac output and possible cardiogenic shock. Conversely, a slowly accumulating effusion (over weeks or months) can stretch the pericardium and attain a much larger volume (e.g., > 1 L) before tamponade physiology develops *(7)*.

23.5.1.3. CLINICAL PRESENTATION

In the primary care setting, a pericardial effusion may come to light in the setting of known pericarditis, as an incidental finding on an imaging study, or in an individual who presents with symptoms of tamponade *(2, 9, 36)*. In the absence of tamponade physiology, a patient with a pericardial effusion may not have symptoms attributable to it. Conversely, patients with tamponade typically manifest dyspnea, chest discomfort, cough, and evidence of decreased cardiac output *(36)*.

23.5.1.4. PHYSICAL EXAMINATION

Patients with a small pericardial effusion may not have any abnormal findings on exam. The only clue to its presence may be distant heart sounds on auscultation and retrosternal dullness to percussion. A pericardial rub may be present *(13)*. Conversely, in patients who have developed tamponade, the triad of hypotension, distant heart sounds, and elevated jugular venous pressure is expected *(37)*. Furthermore, tamponade physiology produces pulsus paradoxus, an abnormal decline in blood pressure with normal inspiration (see Section 23.6) *(2, 38)*. A recent review analyzed five features observed in patients with tamponade: dyspnea, tachycardia, pulsus paradoxus, elevated jugular venous pressure, and cardiomegaly on chest radiography. Of these features a pulsus paradoxus >10 mmHg identified the presence of tamponade with a sensitivity of 98% and specificity of 70% *(37, 39)*. Of note, pulsus paradoxus may not appear in tamponade when coexisting conditions impede respiratory alterations in left ventricular filling, including left ventricular dysfunction, aortic regurgitation, and atrial septal defects. Conversely, conditions that cause large alterations in intrathoracic pressure (e.g., advanced obstructive airways disease or pulmonary embolism) can produce pulsus paradoxus in the absence of tamponade.

23.6. PULSUS PARADOXUS

Measurement of pulsus paradoxus at the bedside is of great value in assessing the hemodynamic significance of a pericardial effusion. During the respiratory cycle in healthy patients, inspiration draws blood from the systemic veins into the thorax and the right side of the heart, causing the interventricular septum to bow toward the left, which transiently reduces LV filling. As a result, LV stroke volume declines and systolic blood pressure normally falls slightly (< 10 mmHg) with inspiration. In tamponade, this mechanism is exaggerated by the presence of high pressure pericardial effusion compressing the cardiac chambers. The more marked inspiratory decline in LV filling in tamponade reduces the LV stroke volume to a greater extent, and the systolic blood pressure falls >10 mmHg.

23.6.1. Procedure to Measure Pulsus Paradoxus

The arm sphygmomanometer is inflated to a level greater than the systolic pressure. As the cuff is slowly deflated, note the pressure at which the first Korotkoff sound is heard. Next listen as the Korotkoff sound at that level disappears with inspiration. Then continue to deflate the cuff slowly until the Korotkoff sounds stop drifting in and out, i.e., they are heard during both inspiration and expiration. The difference in pressure between the first Korotkoff sound and when the Korotkoff sounds are heard during both inspiration and expiration is the pulsus paradoxus.

23.6.2. Electrocardiogram

A large pericardial effusion decreases transmission of electrical forces from the myocardium resulting in decreased voltage on the ECG *(37)*. In addition, a sufficiently large effusion allows the heart to swing back and forth within the pericardial sac. This is manifest as beat to beat variation in the axis of the QRS complex on the ECG, causing *electrical alternans* (Fig. 5) *(40)*.

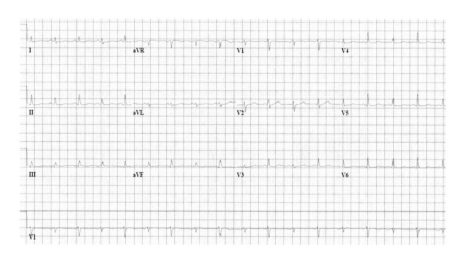

Fig. 5. Twelve-lead electrocardiogram and V1 rhythm strip demonstrating electrical alternans.

23.6.3. Chest X-Ray

If a pericardial effusion is greater than ~250 mL in volume, the cardiac silhouette enlarges, typically in a symmetrical fashion.

23.6.4. Echocardiogram

The echocardiogram is the most useful non-invasive modality in the diagnosis of pericardial effusion and cardiac tamponade *(41)*. The location and size of the pericardial effusion as well as its hemodynamic impact can be readily assessed. Important signs of tamponade include diastolic collapse of the right ventricle and the right atrium, distention of the inferior vena cava, and exaggerated reciprocal respiratory variations in mitral and tricuspid diastolic Doppler velocities *(42)*. Magnetic resonance imaging and computed tomography can also help localize and characterize pericardial effusions, but rarely add to the clinical information afforded by echocardiography in the evaluation of tamponade physiology.

23.6.5. Treatment of Pericardial Effusion with Cardiac Tamponade

Cardiac tamponade is a medical emergency requiring rapid recognition and management. Patients who present in the primary care setting with findings consistent with this diagnosis should be immediately triaged to the hospital for consideration of urgent pericardiocentesis. When performed, pericardial fluid analysis for diagnostic purposes should include blood counts and cytology, and bacterial, fungal, and mycobacterial cultures *(9, 43)*. However, the diagnostic yield of pericardial fluid culture for M. tuberculosis is low. If TB is suspected, a more rapid diagnosis from the pericardial fluid can be accomplished by polymerase chain reaction (where available) or by the finding of an elevated level of adenosine deaminase (>30 U/L in tuberculosis).

23.6.6. Management of Pericardial Effusion Without Tamponade

Asymptomatic patients with small- to moderate-sized effusions can be followed with serial echocardiograms to ensure ultimate resolution. Pharmacologic treatment aimed at decreasing pericardial inflammation should be initiated (e.g., NSAIA and/or colchicine, see Section 23.3) *(25)*. When the cause of effusion is not clear from the clinical presentation, testing for specific etiologies should be considered, such as PPD skin testing for tuberculosis, serologic testing (e.g., antinuclear antibodies) for collagen vascular diseases, mammography, and chest CT for screening of breast and lung cancers, respectively, and in the appropriate clinical contexts, testing for Lyme disease or hypothyroidism.

Patients with asymptomatic large chronic pericardial effusions who are being followed in the outpatient setting may occasionally develop tamponade unexpectedly *(44)*. Reassuringly, in one series of 45 patients with large pericardial effusions managed conservatively, no progression to tamponade was demonstrated *(43)*.

23.7. CONSTRICTIVE PERICARDITIS

23.7.1. Etiology and Pathophysiology

Constrictive pericarditis is characterized by a thickened and scarred pericardium with abnormal rigidity that impairs filling of the cardiac chambers *(9, 25)*. Any of the etiologies of acute pericarditis listed in Table 1 can result in constrictive pericarditis. The most common causes are idiopathic pericarditis, post-cardiac surgery, and prior mediastinal radiation therapy *(45, 46)*. Tuberculous pericarditis, previously a common cause of constrictive pericarditis in the developed world, remains an important etiology in developing countries *(9)*.

In constriction, pericardial compliance becomes the limiting factor of ventricular filling leading to elevation and equalization of diastolic intracardiac pressures *(7)*. In early diastole (just after the mitral and tricuspid valves open), the ventricles actually begin to fill quite briskly because atrial pressures are typically elevated. However, as soon as the ventricles fill to the limit imposed on them by the surrounding rigid pericardium, filling abruptly ceases. Venous congestion results from the elevated diastolic pressures, and the reduced LV filling impairs ventricular stroke volume and forward cardiac output.

23.7.2. Clinical Presentation

Clinical findings in constrictive pericarditis develop insidiously over a period of months to years. Patients typically present with systemic congestion out of proportion to pulmonary congestion. Symptoms of right-sided heart failure in constriction include elevated jugular venous pressure, hepatic congestion, early satiety, ascites, and peripheral edema. Dyspnea in the absence of pulmonary congestion is also common *(25)*. Late in the disease, signs of reduced cardiac output become manifest including cachexia and muscle wasting *(7)*.

23.7.3. Physical Exam

The jugular venous pressure is markedly elevated with two prominent descents during each cardiac cycle (*x* and *y* descents), creating a distinctive filling and collapsing pattern that is often evident from across the room. In distinction to normal individuals the degree of jugular venous distention fails to decrease, or may increase further, with inspiration (*Kussmaul sign*). In normal individuals, inspiration decreases intrathoracic pressure resulting in increased venous return to the heart and a decline in jugular venous pressure. Conversely, in pericardial constriction the inspiratory decrease in intrathoracic pressure is not transmitted through the rigid pericardium to the cardiac chambers, resulting in the increased jugular venous pressure instead *(7)*. On cardiac auscultation there may be a *pericardial knock*. This is a high-pitch sound that is best heard at the left sternal border or the apex in early diastole. It corresponds to the abrupt cessation of ventricular filling in early diastole *(9)*. Additional physical findings include abdominal distension, ascites, and peripheral edema.

23.7.4. Laboratory Studies

There are no specific findings of constrictive pericarditis on the electrocardiogram, usually simply nonspecific ST- and T-wave abnormalities. However, atrial arrhythmias such as atrial fibrillation are common and about one-third of patients manifest low QRS voltage *(46)*. The chest radiograph may show a rim of pericardial calcification, particularly in those with chronic tuberculous pericarditis, best observed at the right heart border on a lateral projection. Echocardiography may demonstrate a thickened pericardium, but this is often difficult to visualize by a standard transthoracic study.

Table 2
Findings that Differentiate Constrictive Pericarditis from Restrictive Cardiomyopathy

	Constrictive pericarditis	*Restrictive cardiomyopathy*
Physical examination		
Kussmaul's sign	Common	Absent
Pericardial knock	May be present	Absent
Chest X-ray		
Pericardial calcification	May be present	Absent
Echocardiography		
Thickened pericardium	Present	Absent
Thickened myocardium	Absent	Present (may be "speckled" in infiltrative disease)
Exaggerated variation in transvalvular velocities	Present	Absent
Doppler tissue imaging at mitral annulus (represents LV relaxation rate at earliest phase of diastole)	Normal (>8 cm/s)	Reduced (<8 cm/s)
CT or MRI		
Thickened pericardium	Usually	Absent
Cardiac catheterization		
Equalized RV and LV diastolic pressures	Yes	LV often > RV by more than 3–5 mmHg
Endomyocardial biopsy	Normal	Usually abnormal (e.g., amyloid)

LV = left ventricle, PA = pulmonary artery, RV = right ventricle.

Doppler analysis reveals a characteristic pattern that can be differentiated from other causes of diastolic dysfunction such as restrictive cardiomyopathy (see Table 2). Cardiac magnetic resonance imaging and computed tomography are superior to echocardiography in visualizing pericardial anatomy. Pericardial thickness is usually increased at >2 mm in patients with constrictive pericarditis, though a minority of patients with proven constriction have normal thickness *(9)*. Cardiac catheterization demonstrates elevation and equalization of right and left ventricular diastolic pressures with unimpeded early diastolic filling followed by abrupt cessation of filling as ventricular volumes reach the limit imposed by the constricting pericardium.

23.7.5. Treatment

Complete surgical pericardiectomy is the mainstay of treatment in patients with advanced constrictive pericarditis *(46)*. Pericardiectomy results in symptomatic improvement rapidly in many patients, but recovery may be more gradual in those with associated myocardial stiffness or fibrosis. Patients with constriction due to viral/idiopathic pericarditis have the best outcomes after surgery, while results are less favorable in those with radiation-associated constriction *(45)*.

23.7.6. Constrictive Pericarditis Versus Restrictive Cardiomyopathy

The clinical findings of constrictive pericarditis can closely resemble those of restrictive cardiomyopathy (e.g., cardiac amyloidosis). Both of these pathologies result in impaired diastolic ventricular filling. The distinction is important as constrictive pericarditis is treatable with surgical resection, while options for restrictive cardiomyopathies are much more limited. Table 2 lists common features that cardiologists consider in differentiating these entities.

REFERENCES

1. Moore K, Dalley A. *Clinically Oriented Anatomy.* 5th ed. Philadelphia, PA: Lippincott Williams & Wilkins; 2005: 137–141.
2. Spodick DH. *The Pericardium: A Comprehensive Textbook.* New York, NY: Marcel Dekker, Inc; 1997:7.
3. Applegate RJ, Johnston WE, Vinten-Johansen J, Klopfenstein HS, Little WC. Restraining effect of intact pericardium during acute volume loading. *Am J Physiol.* 1992;262:H1725–H1733.
4. Freeman GL, LeWinter MM. Pericardial adaptations during chronic cardiac dilation in dogs. *Circ Res.* 1984;54: 294–300.
5. Kansal S, Roitman D, Sheffield LT. Two-dimensional echocardiography of congenital absence of pericardium. *Am Heart J.* 1985;109:912–915.
6. Abbas AE, Appleton CP, Liu PT, Sweeney JP. Congenital absence of the pericardium: case presentation and review of literature. *Int J Cardiol.* 2005;98:21–25.
7. Little WC, Freeman GL. Pericardial disease. *Circulation.* 2006;113:1622–1632.
8. Spodick DH. Acute pericarditis: current concepts and practice. *JAMA.* 2003;289:1150–1153.
9. LeWinter MM. Pericardial diseases. In: Libby P, Bonow R, Mann D, Zipes D, eds. *Braunwald's Heart Disease.* 8th ed. Philadelphia, PA: Sauders Elsevier; 2008:1829–1853.
10. Permanyer-Miralda G, Sagrista-Sauleda J, Soler-Soler J. Primary acute pericardial disease: a prospective series of 231 consecutive patients. *Am J Cardiol.* 1985;56:623–630.
11. Lange RA, Hillis LD. Clinical practice. Acute pericarditis. *N Engl J Med.* 2004;351:2195–2202.
12. Zayas R, Anguita M, Torres F, et al. Incidence of specific etiology and role of methods for specific etiologic diagnosis of primary acute pericarditis. *Am J Cardiol.* 1995;75:378–382.
13. Spodick DH. Pericardial rub. Prospective, multiple observer investigation of pericardial friction in 100 patients. *Am J Cardiol.* 1975;35:357–362.
14. Troughton RW, Asher CR, Klein AL. Pericarditis. *Lancet.* 2004;363:717–727.
15. Wang K, Asinger RW, Marriott HJ. ST-segment elevation in conditions other than acute myocardial infarction. *N Engl J Med.* 2003;349:2128–2135.
16. Spodick DH. Diagnostic electrocardiographic sequences in acute pericarditis. Significance of PR segment and PR vector changes. *Circulation.* 1973;48:575–580.

17. Spodick DH. Electrocardiogram in acute pericarditis. Distributions of morphologic and axial changes by stages. *Am J Cardiol*. 1974;33:470–474.

18. Ginzton LE, Laks MM. The differential diagnosis of acute pericarditis from the normal variant: new electrocardiographic criteria. *Circulation*. 1982;65:1004–1009.

19. Bonnefoy E, Godon P, Kirkorian G, Fatemi M, Chevalier P, Touboul P. Serum cardiac troponin I and ST-segment elevation in patients with acute pericarditis. *Eur Heart J*. 2000;21:832–836.

20. Brandt RR, Filzmaier K, Hanrath P. Circulating cardiac troponin I in acute pericarditis. *Am J Cardiol*. 2001;87: 1326–1328.

21. Imazio M, Demichelis B, Cecchi E, et al. Cardiac troponin I in acute pericarditis. *J Am Coll Cardiol*. 2003;42: 2144–2148.

22. Imazio M, Demichelis B, Parrini I, et al. Day-hospital treatment of acute pericarditis: a management program for outpatient therapy. *J Am Coll Cardiol*. 2004;43:1042–1046.

23. Spodick DH. Risk prediction in pericarditis: who to keep in hospital? *Heart*. 2008;94:398–399.

24. Cheitlin MD, Armstrong WF, Aurigemma GP, et al. ACC/AHA/ASE 2003 guideline update for the clinical application of echocardiography: summary article: a report of the American College of Cardiology/American Heart Association Task Force on Practice Guidelines (ACC/AHA/ASE Committee to Update the 1997 Guidelines for the Clinical Application of Echocardiography). *Circulation*. 2003;108:1146–1162.

25. Maisch B, Seferovic PM, Ristic AD, et al. Guidelines on the diagnosis and management of pericardial diseases executive summary; the task force on the diagnosis and management of pericardial diseases of the European Society of Cardiology. *Eur Heart J*. 2004;25:587–610.

26. Berman J, Haffajee CI, Alpert JS. Therapy of symptomatic pericarditis after myocardial infarction: retrospective and prospective studies of aspirin, indomethacin, prednisone, and spontaneous resolution. *Am Heart J*. 1981;101:750–753.

27. Arunasalam S, Siegel RJ. Rapid resolution of symptomatic acute pericarditis with ketorolac tromethamine: a parenteral nonsteroidal antiinflammatory agent. *Am Heart J*. 1993;125:1455–1458.

28. Imazio M, Bobbio M, Cecchi E, et al. Colchicine in addition to conventional therapy for acute pericarditis: results of the COlchicine for acute PEricarditis (COPE) trial. *Circulation*. 2005;112:2012–2016.

29. Imazio M, Cecchi E, Demichelis B, et al. Indicators of poor prognosis of acute pericarditis. *Circulation*. 2007;115: 2739–2744.

30. Imazio M, Bobbio M, Cecchi E, et al. Colchicine as first-choice therapy for recurrent pericarditis: results of the CORE (COlchicine for REcurrent pericarditis) trial. *Arch Intern Med*. 2005;165:1987–1991.

31. Imazio M, Brucato A, Cumetti D, et al. Corticosteroids for recurrent pericarditis: high versus low doses: a nonrandomized observation. *Circulation*. 2008;118:667–671.

32. Braunwald E. Pericardial disease. In: Fauci A, Braunwald E, Kasper D, et al., eds. *Harrison's Principles of Internal Medicine*. New York, NY: McGraw Hill; 2008: 1488–1495.

33. Sagrista-Sauleda J, Merce J, Permanyer-Miralda G, Soler-Soler J. Clinical clues to the causes of large pericardial effusions. *Am J Med*. 2000;109:95–101.

34. Ben-Horin S, Bank I, Guetta V, Livneh A. Large symptomatic pericardial effusion as the presentation of unrecognized cancer: a study in 173 consecutive patients undergoing pericardiocentesis. *Medicine*. 2006;85:49–53.

35. Permanyer-Miralda G. Acute pericardial disease: approach to the aetiologic diagnosis. *Heart*. 2004;90:252–254.

36. Spodick DH. Acute cardiac tamponade. *N Engl J Med*. 2003;349:684–690.

37. Roy CL, Minor MA, Brookhart MA, Choudhry NK. Does this patient with a pericardial effusion have cardiac tamponade? *JAMA*. 2007;297:1810–1818.

38. Shabetai R. Pericardial and cardiac pressure. *Circulation*. 1988;77:1–5.

39. Curtiss EI, Reddy PS, Uretsky BF, Cecchetti AA. Pulsus paradoxus: definition and relation to the severity of cardiac tamponade. *Am Heart J*. 1988;115:391–398.

40. Spodick DH, Usher BW. Electrical alternans. *Am Heart J*. 1972;84:574–575.

41. Pande AN, Lilly LS. Pericardial disease. In: Solomon SD, ed. *Essential Echocardiography*. Totowa, NJ: Humana Press; 2007: 191–208.

42. Oh JK, Seward JB, Tajik AB. *The Echo Manual*. 3rd ed. Philadelphia, PA: Lippincott Williams & Wilkins; 2007: 289–309.

43. Merce J, Sagrista-Sauleda J, Permanyer-Miralda G, Soler-Soler J. Should pericardial drainage be performed routinely in patients who have a large pericardial effusion without tamponade? *Am J Med*. 1998;105:106–109.

44. Sagrista-Sauleda J, Angel J, Permanyer-Miralda G, Soler-Soler J. Long-term follow-up of idiopathic chronic pericardial effusion. *N Engl J Med*. 1999;341:2054–2059.

45. Bertog SC, Thambidorai SK, Parakh K, et al. Constrictive pericarditis: etiology and cause-specific survival after pericardiectomy. *J Am Coll Cardiol*. 2004;43:1445–1452.

46. Ling LH, Oh JK, Schaff HV, et al. Constrictive pericarditis in the modern era: evolving clinical spectrum and impact on outcome after pericardiectomy. *Circulation*. 1999;100:1380–1386.

24

Common Atrial and Ventricular Arrhythmias

Blair Foreman

CONTENTS

Key Words: Arrhythmia ablation; Antiarrhythmic drugs; Atrial fibrillation; Atrial flutter; Ventricular tachycardia; Sick sinus syndrome.

KEY POINTS

- Appropriate history taking facilitates arrhythmia diagnosis.
- A systematic approach to ECG interpretation helps avoid diagnostic pitfalls.
- Many clinical syndromes are due to a continuum of cardiovascular disease.
- Atrial fibrillation and atrial flutter are often grouped together but comprise distinct clinical entities.
- Genetic cardiac diseases and their evaluation are growing in today's clinical practice.
- Guidelines have been published on the evaluation and treatment of a myriad of cardiac arrhythmic syndromes.
- Antiarrhythmic drug therapy is often giving way to aggressive therapy with pacemaker, implantable cardioverter–defibrillators, and invasive arrhythmia ablation.

24.1. INTRODUCTION

Cardiac arrhythmias and their clinical correlates form the basis for some of the most intriguing aspects of cardiac care. During training, however, emphasis is often placed on care related to congestive heart failure, myocardial infarction, and the treatment of dyslipidemias. Unfortunately, patient complaints related to cardiac arrhythmias are often a common reason for a patient's presentation to emergency rooms, for office visits, and for referrals to subspecialists.

One must develop a basic understanding of cardiac anatomy, cardiac pharmacology, and basic electrocardiogram (ECG) interpretation to accurately evaluate and treat cardiac arrhythmias. Combining the patient's history with knowledge of expected arrhythmias associated with a variety of disease

From: *Contemporary Cardiology: Comprehensive Cardiovascular Medicine in the Primary Care Setting*
Edited by: Peter P. Toth, Christopher P. Cannon, DOI 10.1007/978-1-60327-963-5_24
© Springer Science+Business Media, LLC 2010

states, the ECG can then be used as a tool to verify a patient's specific arrhythmic complaint. In certain circumstances, while the clinical complaints suggest an arrhythmic component, one may often find through thorough evaluation that indeed no arrhythmia exists. Only through a systematic approach to evaluation can one make the correct diagnosis.

Clinical manifestations of cardiac arrhythmias include symptoms of irregular heart beating or awareness of heart beating (palpitations), altered consciousness, light headedness, chest fullness, chest pain, heart failure, syncope, and may include sudden cardiac death. Recurrent symptoms may also be a clue to the arrhythmia.

Inherent in the identification of common and less common arrhythmias is the importance of timing in evaluation and treatment. Multiple guidelines and consensus statements have been published over the last several years to help guide the evaluation and treatment of arrhythmic abnormalities. Throughout the chapter, use of these guidelines that may aid in the prompt diagnosis of the majority of the arrhythmias will be presented. Treatment strategies will also be discussed.

The surface ECG is a culmination of cardiac cellular depolarization and repolarization within the atria and ventricles. Changes in the normal pattern of cellular electrophysiologic events result in pattern changes at the macroscopic level. To better understand cardiac arrhythmias, a basic understanding of these events is helpful. Due to special conduction tissue within the heart, sinus node and atrioventricular (AV) node tissue are distinctly different than atrial tissue, Purkinje tissue, or ventricular myocardium. In Fig. 1, generalized cellular activation is shown for both tissue groups. Features of the sinus and AV node tissue include a calcium-dependent upstroke of phase 0 of the action potential and prolonged action potential duration and refractory period at more rapid rates. This results in slower propagation through the tissue at faster intrinsic heart rates. At faster rates, early-coupled extra-systoles are less likely to be propagated.

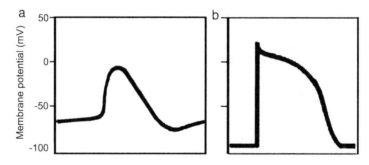

Fig. 1. Stylized representation of the action potential in predominantly calcium-dependent cardiac tissues and sodium-dependent cardiac tissues. (**a**) Sinoatrial node and AV node tissue rely on a slower, calcium dependent phase 0 depolarization. (**b**) Non-specialized atrial and ventricular tissue, typical accessory pathways, and His-Purkinje tissue rely on rapid phase 0 depolarization.

In contrast, atrial, His-Purkinje, and ventricular tissue have a rapid, sodium-dependent upstroke in phase 0. At faster rates, action potential duration shortens resulting in a shorter refractory period, and conduction rates through tissue are unchanged or slightly improved (1). Early coupled extra-systoles are, thus, more likely to be propagated at faster baseline heart rates.

The surface ECG is a culmination of multiple cellular events throughout the cardiac chambers. As shown in Fig. 2, normal cardiac activation arises from the sinus node complex located in the superior-medial aspect of the right atrium. Atrial activation proceeds across the right atrium and into the left atrium and from a superior to inferior direction resulting in the normal P-wave on the surface ECG (2). Atrial activation typically takes less than 100 ms. Atrial enlargement or atrial disease processes may significantly increase the magnitude or duration of the P-wave on the ECG. As the wavefront enters into the AV node, additional delay is encountered prior to activation of the His-Purkinje system. The

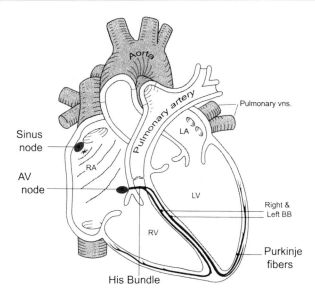

Fig. 2. Schematic representation of cardiac activation originating in the sinus node and penetrating the AV node. Conduction delay occurs in the AV node and then rapidly traverses the His bundle and into the right and left bundle branches to depolarize ventricular myocardium. RA = right atrium, RV = right ventricle, LA = left atrium, LV = left ventricle, AV = atrioventricular, vns. = veins.

resultant PR interval is considered normal if its duration is between 120 and 200 ms. Rapid activation of the myocardium through the Purkinje network results in a QRS complex duration between 80 and 120 ms in normal myocardium. Delay through the right bundle or the left bundle fascicles results in prolongation of the QRS. Activation of the myocardium without utilizing the His-Purkinje tissue (via a premature ventricular contraction, a paced complex, or an accessory pathway) also results in abnormally slow activation of the ventricles and, thus, prolonged QRS duration. As the ventricular myocardium repolarizes, the QT interval occurs *(3)*. Repolarization of atrial tissue also occurs after the P-wave, but it is not detectable on the surface ECG due to its small magnitude and frequency compared to ventricular activation occurring simultaneously.

Drugs, aging, ischemia, and metabolic derangements can affect myocardial cells. These changes can lead to alterations in excitability resulting in increased or decreased automaticity. Additionally, spontaneous or drug-associated atrial or ventricular activation may occur due to triggered activity. The resultant atrial or ventricular ectopy or sustained arrhythmia would be the surface ECG correlate. Alterations in conduction due to changes at the level of the sinus node or AV node can result in sinus exit block, sinus pauses, AV node Wenckebach, or higher grade AV block. Changes in conduction at the Purkinje level can lead to left or right bundle branch block and even re-entrant ventricular arrhythmias. Alterations in myocardial propagation, often in the setting of scar, can lead to functional or anatomic block resulting in re-entrant atrial or ventricular arrhythmias *(4)*.

24.2. CLINICAL ARRHYTHMIAS

One can organize arrhythmias based on their mechanism, origin, or clinical scenario with which they are associated. In daily practice, utilizing a clinical approach based on arrhythmia origin is often useful. The approach outlined here is anatomy-based, beginning with the atrium and progressing through the AV or accessory pathway and then into the His-Purkinje system and onward into the ventricle. Additional delineation based on a bradycardic or tachycardic rhythm or isolated event versus sustained arrhythmia is also proposed.

24.2.1. Supraventricular Arrhythmias

24.2.1.1. ATRIAL-BASED ARRHYTHMIAS

24.2.1.1.1. Sinus Arrhythmia. Under normal physiologic conditions, the sinus rate at rest is considered normal between the rates of 60 and 100 beats/min (bpm). During regular rhythm, variations in rate occur, usually in a rhythmic pattern. Under autonomic control, sinus rhythm is influenced by variations in sympathetic and parasympathetic input *(5–8)*. Usually varying by only a few beats per minute under normal circumstances and nearly imperceptible, sinus arrhythmia can be more pronounced, at other times. More noticeable changes often occur during sleep when the influences of vagal tone may dominate *(9)*. Variations in sinus rate and the concomitant sinus arrhythmia are normal (Fig. 3). No therapy is needed or recommended. Absence of some degree of heart rate (HR) variation over the course of evaluation would be considered abnormal and may occur in some dysautonomias, most commonly advanced diabetes and heart failure *(10–13)*. Excessive variation and noticeable pauses during sleep may suggest medical conditions such as central or obstructive sleep apnea that may require treatment of the underlying condition *(14)*.

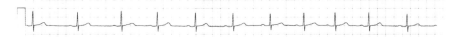

Fig. 3. Sinus arrhythmia. Rhythmic variation in the sinus rate is noted across the rhythm strip. P-wave morphology and PR intervals remain essentially unchanged.

24.2.1.2. BRADYARRHYTHMIAS

24.2.1.2.1. Sinus Bradycardia, the Sinus Pause, and Sinus Arrest. Sinus bradycardia is by definition a regular atrial rhythm less than 60 bpm with a P-wave morphology similar to that of normal sinus rhythm (Fig. 4). In today's world of polypharmacy and increase in the average age of patients, drugs are a common cause of sinus bradycardia not associated with sleep. Most beta-blockers and calcium channel blockers have a direct effect on sinus rates. Even agents once thought to exhibit little sinus slowing, such as angiotensin-converting enzyme inhibitors or angiotensin receptor blockers, have slowing effects in vitro and in vivo *(15)*. Not all sinus bradycardia should be considered abnormal. Some individuals will exhibit sinus bradycardia due to rigorous physical aerobic training or may have a more unusual finding of familial bradycardia *(16, 17)*. Unfortunately, no widely accepted pharmacologic therapy for symptomatic sinus bradycardia exists despite data to suggest some benefit. Theophylline compounds have been studied and are occasionally tolerated and may be effective in patients with sinus node dysfunction *(18)*. There are unfortunately, no safe, long-term beta-agonists available in oral form. Acute increases in heart rate may be accomplished with direct or indirect beta-agonists such as isuprel, dopamine, and dobutamine. Parasympathetic blockade with atropine may also be helpful acutely in certain cases *(19, 20)*.

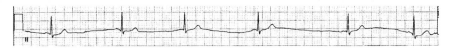

Fig. 4. Marked sinus bradycardia at a rate of approximately 30–40 bpm. Competing junctional beats are noted in the third and fourth beats with a PR interval shorter than expected.

Patients with asymptomatic awake heart rates above 40 bpm do not usually require additional therapy, most notably atrial pacing. Symptomatic patients and minimally symptomatic patients with resting bradycardia less than 40 bpm may benefit from pacing *(21)*. Consideration of dual chamber pacing in certain patients should be considered given the tendency to go on to symptomatic AV block in a notable proportion. Again, evaluation for an underlying cause should be considered as hypertension, coronary disease, sleep apnea, and infiltrative diseases such as sarcoidosis, hemosiderosis, or amyloidosis may cause sinus bradycardia.

As atrial disease progresses, sinus node automaticity may decline erratically resulting in pauses that may become more symptomatic *(22)*. This is often due to simple aging, the use of drug therapy, or advancing cardiopulmonary disease. While variations in heart rate are certainly common, and vagally mediated slowing is noticed frequently at night, pauses in excess of second are abnormal (Fig. 5). In the absence of other reversible causes, pauses in excess of 5 s suggest significant sinus node disease and may warrant pacing to prevent symptomatic postural events that may result in injury *(21)*. Vagally mediated pauses of greater than 20–30 s are not uncommon during tilt table tests or with carotid sinus massage in susceptible patients. Again, drug therapy is often insufficient, and pacing may be required in certain circumstances *(23)*.

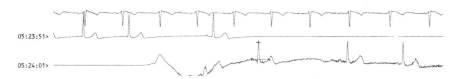

Fig. 5. Sinus slowing and sinus arrest. Early morning monitoring reveals a sudden slowing and then a nearly 10-s episode of sinus arrest. Return rate is slow initially and then increases.

24.2.1.3. Wandering Atrial Pacemaker, Premature Atrial Contractions, and Ectopic Atrial Rhythm

Related to sinus arrhythmia and resulting in heart rate variation at physiologic rates, a wandering atrial pacemaker rhythm represents a change in the origin of the atrial activation periodically outside the normal sinus complex and into adjacent atrial tissue and sometimes into AV junctional tissue *(24)*. The morphology of the P-wave changes shape and often direction, and the changes in rate are typically more abrupt than with sinus arrhythmia. Due to changes in atrial origin, the resultant atrial conduction time to the AV node and changes in the degree of prematurity, changes in the PR interval are often seen *(25)*. As the changes become even more noticeable and less regular, sinus rhythm with premature atrial contractions (PACs) becomes the rhythm designation. Wandering atrial pacemaker rhythm is a less commonly used term but typically reflects a physiologic rhythm. This is found more commonly in the setting of normal hearts but altered autonomic tone may influence arrhythmogenesis in the setting of atrial disease and intrinsic sinus node disease.

Premature atrial contractions arise from abrupt, early activation of the atria and may arise from either the right or the left atrium. Newer evidence suggests atrial ectopy may frequently arise from electrically active tissue within the pulmonary veins and may be the trigger for atrial fibrillation *(26)*. Usually a benign rhythm, PACs may be quite bothersome with symptoms of palpitations or tachypalpitations. Premature atrial contractions may reflect underlying atrial disease either intrinsic in nature or associated with a pulmonary process, hypertension, valvular heart disease, ischemic cardiac disease, or even infiltrative heart disease *(27)*. Consideration of patient age, associated medical problems, and underlying cardiac disease should be made when determining the clinical ramifications of symptomatic or asymptomatic PACs (Fig. 6).

A regular, persistent atrial rhythm originating outside the sinus node gives rise to a P-wave morphology distinct from the typical sinus P-wave. Termed ectopic atrial rhythm, patients are usually asymptomatic, and the rhythm is benign (Fig. 7). An ectopic atrial rhythm is not infrequently seen in the setting of concurrent medical or metabolic derangement such as acute or chronic pulmonary

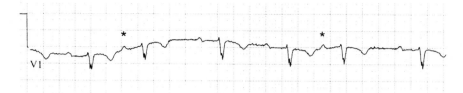

Fig. 6. Sinus rhythm with first-degree AV block and occasional premature atrial complexes. Noted on the second and fifth beat (∗), early atrial complexes with a different morphology are noted giving rises to an irregular rhythm.

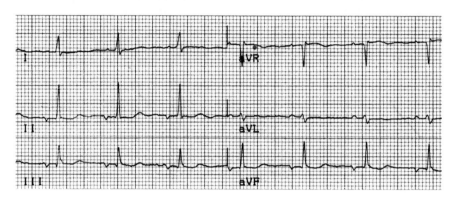

Fig. 7. Ectopic atrial rhythm. An regular rhythm at approximately 85 beats is noted with inverted P-waves in the inferior leads and upright in aVR suggesting an origin in the low septal right or left atrium.

disease or alcohol excess or ischemia. These slower rhythms may also be a clinical sign of advancing sinus node or atrial tissue disease *(4)*.

The clinical term sick sinus syndrome (SSS) is applied when a variety of atrial bradycardias and tachycardias are noted. It encompasses clinical palpitations associated with sinus pauses, sinus brady-cardia, premature atrial complexes, a variety of atrial dysrhythmias, atrial fibrillation, and atrial flutter *(28, 29)*. Sick sinus syndrome is reflective of advanced sinus node and atrial disease and is typically progressive. Treatment to reduce rapidly conducted atrial tachycardias is complicated by intrinsic sinus node dysfunction often giving rise to excessive resting bradycardia and frequently concurrent therapy with pacing is required *(21)*.

24.2.1.4. Tachyarrhythmias

24.2.1.4.1. Sinus Tachycardia. As atrial rates increase, additional rhythm disorders come into play. The simplest tachyarrhythmia arising from the atria is sinus tachycardia. While one could dis-miss this as just a normal sinus mechanism at a faster rate, one has to remember that sinus tachycardia occurring in patients that are supine, resting in an office, or in a hospital bed is usually inappropriate and may point to conditions that may have been overlooked. Metabolic derangements may manifest early as sinus tachycardia. Thyroid toxicosis, sepsis syndrome, shock, hypovolemia, pheochromocy-toma, diabetes-associated autonomic dysfunction, substance abuse, malignant hyperthermia, myocar-dial infarction, drug toxicity, and pain are just a few clinical scenarios that may predispose a patient to sinus tachycardia *(30)*. Additionally, clinical tachyarrhythmias may also arise in or around the sinus node unrelated to clinical or metabolic disorders and are discussed below.

24.2.1.4.2. Ectopic Atrial Tachycardia.   Atrial tachyarrhythmias arising from a single region also include ectopic atrial tachycardias (EAT). These arrhythmias often have abrupt onset of a regular tachycardia with P-waves that are distinctly different from the typical sinus P-wave (Fig. 8) *(31)*. Abrupt onset and offset often occur but a mild warm-up at initiation and a mild slowing prior to termination also suggest a certain degree of autonomic modulation. Additionally, the arrhythmia rates appear to be under the control of autonomic input as assessed by heart rate variability obtained by time- and frequency-domain methods. However, short R–R changes may result from an intrinsic abnormality of the ectopic rhythm or possibly from a specific autonomic difference *(32)*.

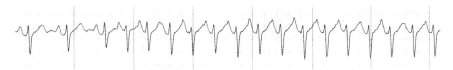

Fig. 8. Ectopic atrial tachycardia. Sinus rhythm with peaked P-waves suggestive of atrial overload is replaced by a sudden onset of regular atrial tachycardia at a rate of 160 bpm. The new P-wave morphology is noticeably different beginning with the first early beat (fourth P-wave).

Most atrial tachycardias are non-sustained and asymptomatic found during routine ambulatory monitoring. However, they can become incessant resulting in a rate-related cardiomyopathy *(33)*. The origin of the ectopic atrial arrhythmia may be throughout either the right or left atria. Hot spots within atrial appendages, along the cristae terminalis, and around the pulmonary veins have been described *(34–38)*. Drug therapy in patients with atrial tachyarrhythmias such as ectopic atrial tachycardia may include beta-blockers, calcium channel blockers, and Vaughan Williams class Ic and III drugs *(30)*. Radiofrequency ablation has been used in patients with symptomatic ectopic atrial rhythms in which type Ic or III agents fail or are not preferred. Unfortunately, many of these arrhythmias are often difficult to initiate with programmed stimulation in the electrophysiology lab *(38)*.

24.2.1.4.3. Multifocal Atrial Tachycardia.   An atrial tachyarrhythmia warranting mention is multifocal atrial tachycardia (MAT). Characterized by heart rates greater than 100 bpm and an irregular rhythm with greater than two atrial P-wave morphologies, MAT often arises in the setting of metabolic or respiratory distress. Treatment of the underlying medical illness is the treatment of choice. Verapamil has been shown to help to a limited degree. Digoxin use is discouraged due to limited value and concerns over digoxin toxicity-associated atrial tachycardia with block going unrecognized in the setting of MAT. There is no role for direct current cardioversion (DCC), ablation, or antiarrhythmic drugs *(30)*.

24.2.1.4.4. Sinus Node Re-entry Tachycardia, Positional Orthostatic Tachycardia Syndrome, Inappropriate Sinus Tachycardia, and Neurocardiogenic Syncope.   Similar to the ectopic atrial tachycardias, atrial tachycardias associated with or originating in the sinus node may occur. Sinus node re-entrant tachycardia (SNRT) arises from the sinus node complex and is associated with an abrupt change in heart rate with a P-wave morphology similar to the sinus P-wave. The re-entrant mechanism may be entirely within the sinus node or involve nearby transitional atrial myocardium. Treatment of SNRT involves similar drug therapy to EAT *(39)*. However, due to extensive autonomic innervation of the sinus node complex, treatment may be more difficult to manage. Ablation therapy may be appropriate in many cases *(40)*. Sinus node re-entry may occur as an isolated finding or may be associated with occult or overt cardiac disease. Automatic or triggered atrial tachycardias can also arise within the sinus node complex and may be treated similarly.

Additional clinical syndromes may also result in sinus tachycardia. Patients suffering from postural orthostatic tachycardia syndrome (POTS) will manifest abrupt increases in heart rate, usually sustained, with upright posture. Volume expansion and re-evaluation to exclude hypovolemia as a cause of tachycardia is necessary. Clinical elimination of other dysautonomic syndromes is also necessary to make the diagnosis. POTS likely involves a cardiac sympathetic dysautonomia mediated by increased norepinephrine release from intact cardiac sympathetic nerves. This is not associated with fixed abnormalities in cell activity or sympathetic innervation density *(41)*. Treatment with a beta-blocker may control postural changes in heart rate, often with good success *(42–45)*.

Over a decade ago, Lee and colleagues described a group of patients with inappropriate sinus tachycardia (IST) *(46)*. Inappropriate sinus tachycardia is a syndrome affecting young women almost exclusively. Patients have consistently higher heart rates for a given activity or even at rest. P-wave morphology is identical or similar to sinus rhythm, and there is not another identifiable cause for the sinus tachycardia. It has a gradual onset and offset in contrast to paroxysmal atrial tachycardias. In these patients, symptoms of palpitations and heart racing are difficult to control with beta-blockers, calcium channel blockers, volume expansion, or antiarrhythmic drugs. In one series, patients were treated with invasive ablation of their sinus node complex resulting in resting bradycardia *(46)*. Extensive destruction of the sinus node may result in bradycardia severe enough to warrant pacing to restore appropriate quality of life. Interestingly, many of the patients in this study were health-care personnel. Additional studies have since demonstrated efficacy of ablation in the management of this disorder *(47–49)*.

Vasovagal syncope (VVS) or neurocardiogenic syncope (NCS) may also be preceded by dramatic increases in heart rate just prior to abrupt decline in heart rate and vasodilation resulting in loss of consciousness. Situational events such as public speaking, a sudden frightening event, external or internal painful stimuli, and hypovolemia may be the precipitating factor for the initial increase in heart rate. Studies have demonstrated that both sympathetic activation just prior to syncope and sympathetic withdrawal may occur, resulting in initial tachycardia *(50–52)*.

24.2.1.4.5. Atrial Fibrillation and Atrial Flutter. No other arrhythmias have been more thoroughly studied, evaluated, and written about than atrial fibrillation (AF) and atrial flutter (AFL). Despite this, atrial fibrillation remains the number one cause for hospital admissions among arrhythmias. Atrial fibrillation affects nearly 2.2 million people in America and 4.5 million people in the European Union. The incidence of AF continues to grow due to the aging population, obesity, hypertension, and better screening techniques. By the year 2050, atrial fibrillation is expected to affect nearly 5.6 million individuals in the United States *(53)*.

Atrial fibrillation and atrial flutter are often grouped together as a single entity. This tendency by practitioners occurs due to nearly identical symptoms, treatment, and clinical outcomes with respect to stroke and stroke prevention. However, mechanistically, atrial fibrillation and flutter are distinct entities and should be understood as such.

Atrial fibrillation is characterized by the absence of organized atrial electrical activity resulting in the loss of mechanical function. On the surface ECG, no discernable P-waves are seen but are replaced by multiform oscillations in the baseline. The ventricular response is typically irregular and rapid, as disorganized atrial activity is conducted through the AV node. The ventricular response in patients with normal AV node physiology is usually rapid. Heart block with a junctional or ventricular escape rhythm may also be seen. This is most common in older patients, those with advanced AV node disease, or individuals undergoing pharmacologic treatment with beta-blockers, calcium channel antagonists, or digoxin (Fig. 9) *(54)*.

In contrast, typical atrial flutter is a macro-re-entrant arrhythmia occupying nearly the entire right atrium. Impulses travel up the interatrial septum, across the roof of the atrium superior and laterally, and traverse inferiorly along the lateral wall along the crista. Propagation progresses medially along the cavotricuspid isthmus and then back up the interatrial septum. Left atrial activation occurs with each rotation while conduction down to the ventricle typically occurs in a 2:1, 3:1 or 4:1 atrial to ventricular

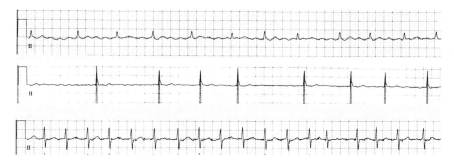

Fig. 9. Variably conducted atrial fibrillation. In panel **1**, coarse atrial fibrillation is conducted at a normal, variable rate between 55 and 80 bpm. In panel **2**, AF is conducted slowly at a rate of between 32 and 70 bpm. In panel **3**, AF is conducted rapidly at around 120 bpm. In each case R–R intervals are variable demonstrating absence of heart block.

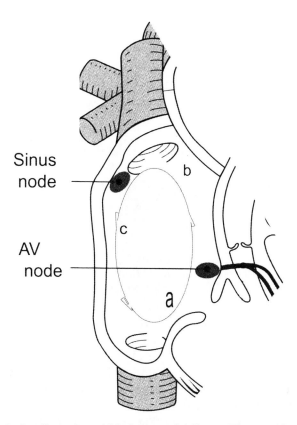

Fig. 10. Typical counterclockwise Cavotricuspid isthmus atrial flutter. The wavefront at (**a**) moves laterally to medial across the isthmus between the inferior vena cava and the tricuspid annulus. It propagates superiorly up the interatrial septum (**b**) and traverses the roof medial to lateral and down the lateral wall along the cristae (**c**) to propagate another cycle. Typical conduction slowing is often found along the isthmus.

activation pattern (Fig. 10). Cavotricuspid isthmus atrial flutter has a rate around 240–300 bpm with conducted ventricular rates an integer of that or around 150, 100, 75, or 60 bpm. Typical AFL on the surface ECG is seen as a regular sawtooth pattern of atrial activity most easily discerned in the inferior leads with negative flutter waves and a positive flutter wave in V1 *(37, 55)*. The majority of atrial flutter is of a counterclockwise rotation. Ten percent of the time this atrial flutter wave rotates clockwise, and in some patients, both can be seen at different times (Fig. 11). Macro-re-entrant left-sided atrial flutter or macro-re-entrant atypical atrial flutter around the right atrial cristae are beyond the scope of this chapter. However, evaluation and possible treatment considerations are similar as described below.

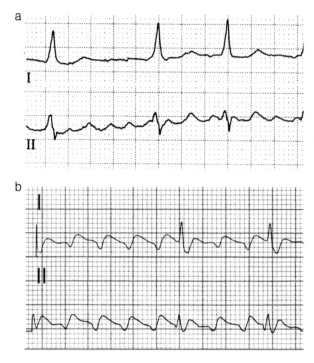

Fig. 11. Typical clockwise (**a**) and counterclockwise (**b**) atrial flutter with variable conduction to the ventricle.

Atrial fibrillation is now classified in a scheme that provides a framework for appropriate evaluation and treatment regimens. The ACC/AHA/ESC 2006 Practice Guidelines on Atrial Fibrillation outline the current system. First-detected atrial fibrillation is simply when AF is originally diagnosed, recognizing that prior asymptomatic or symptomatic episodes may have already occurred. When two or more episodes have occurred, AF is considered recurrent. Episodes of self-terminating AF of less than 7 days are considered paroxysmal, while those lasting greater than 7 days are considered persistent. Persistent atrial fibrillation also includes long-standing AF (very long duration), which usually results in permanent AF. Permanent AF also includes atrial fibrillation in which pharmacologic or electrical cardioversion has not been tried or has failed *(55)*.

Risk factors for the development of atrial fibrillation include progressive myocardial fibrosis, surgical manipulation, pressure and volume overload with atrial stretch and enlargement, genetic predisposition related to sodium and potassium channelopathies, and possible abnormalities in intercellular gap junctions, alterations in the renin–angiotensin–aldosterone system, and inflammatory and infiltrative changes. Clinical syndromes of valvular heart disease, obesity, hypertension, sleep apnea, thyroid disease, acute pulmonary embolism or pneumonia, heart failure, and ischemic heart disease are associated with increased rates of atrial fibrillation *(56–69)*. When a patient presents with atrial fibrillation, one should consider these disease states in their evaluation as a potential treatment mechanism both to prevent future AF breakthrough and to affect the long-term outcome of a patient's non-arrhythmic health.

The clinical symptoms of AF are often protean with little or no symptoms in some individuals while others may suffer an advanced heart failure exacerbation, severe palpitations, chest pain, syncope, or even catastrophic stroke. An individual may have a clinical course that varies depending on volume status, age, heart rate, and changes in underlying health status *(70–74)*. In patients with paroxysmal AF of short duration, the diagnosis is often delayed. Patients presenting to the office or emergency room for evaluation are often in sinus rhythm on evaluation, delaying the correct diagnosis. Symptoms may also predominantly occur with resolution of AF, culminating in long pauses and syncope with ECG evaluation at follow-up being normal (Fig. 12) *(75)*. Ambulatory short-term (24–48 h) or long-term (30 day) monitoring may demonstrate episodes of asymptomatic AF or symptomatic aspects of associated tachycardia or bradycardia *(76)*. Associated signs of sinus node or atrial disease, such as moderate frequency atrial ectopy, bursts of ectopic atrial tachycardia, or asymptomatic pauses, may also raise the suspicion of AF for a patient's tachypalpitations.

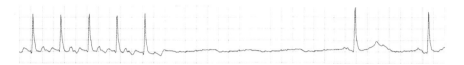

Fig. 12. Pause associated with termination of atrial flutter with restoration of sinus bradycardia in a patient with episodes of intermittent transient light headedness and syncope.

Advancements in the treatment strategies for atrial fibrillation are ongoing. In the past, most clinicians concentrated on restoring sinus rhythm as the primary therapy for atrial fibrillation. Short-term anticoagulation drug therapy with AV nodal blocking agents and antiarrhythmic drugs were utilized and cardioversion is performed. More recently a paradigm shift has occurred as a result of two large trials that looked at event rates in warfarin anticoagulated patients who were randomized to either rate control or maintenance of sinus rhythm. The AFFIRM trial studied patients that were an average age of 69 years old with a high incidence of hypertension and coronary artery disease. Structural heart disease with left atrial enlargement was noted in 67% and left ventricular (LV) dysfunction in 26%. Patients were followed for 5 years. This large trial of 4,060 patients demonstrated that restoration of sinus rhythm offered no survival advantage over the rate-control strategy. In addition, it affirmed the continued role of warfarin even after restoration of sinus rhythm in prevention of stroke *(77)*. This trial and earlier smaller trials *(78–81)* have led to appropriate chronic anticoagulation and rate control as first-line therapy in many patients with AF. Considerable debate has been raised with respect to the advanced age in the patient populations studied, the moderate crossover from rate to rhythm control arms, low beta-blocker use in the rhythm strategy arm, and a lower incidence of heart failure in both groups *(82)*. Despite these shortcomings, evidence suggests that many typical AF patients can be treated with simple rate-control and chronic warfarin anticoagulation.

In a second major trial reported in 2008, the AF-CHF trial studied patients with atrial fibrillation and a history of left ventricular ejection fraction of 35% or less and symptoms of heart failure. Time to death from cardiovascular causes was the primary endpoint. In this trial of 1,376 patients followed for a mean of 37 months, no difference in CV death rate was seen (27% versus 25% for the rhythm-control versus rate-control group). Secondary endpoints were also similar including all-cause mortality, stroke, worsening heart failure, and composites of the same. In summary, even in patients with depressed LV function and heart failure, AF may be reasonably treated with a rate-control and anticoagulation strategy *(82)*.

To achieve clinical results with a rate-control and anticoagulation strategy, appropriate use of pharmacotherapy and patient follow-up is needed. Anticoagulation with either aspirin or warfarin should be initiated in the appropriate patients *(83)*. Warfarin dosing is recommended to be followed at weekly intervals until a stable International Normalized Ratio value (INR) is reached. At a minimum, monthly INR evaluation should be obtained in stable patients thereafter *(55)*. Unfortunately, many drugs may interfere with warfarin, and more frequent evaluation may be warranted in those circumstances *(84, 85)*.

In many trials, beta-blockers were utilized as the primary AV node blocking agent. Concurrent digoxin and non-dihydropyridine agents may also be useful. Long-acting metoprolol succinate or twice daily metoprolol tartrate are often used due to ease of use and being beta-1adrenergic receptor selective. In addition, these drugs have a positive mortality benefit in patients with depressed LV systolic function and heart failure symptoms *(86)*. Other beta-blockers may also be used to affect AV node blockade. When additional rate control is needed, the addition of digoxin to this regimen after up-titration of the beta-blocker to maximal tolerated dose can prove useful. In patients with normal LV systolic function or isolated diastolic dysfunction, diltiazem or verapamil may be added to control the rate (Table 1). In some individuals, rate control may require polypharmacy and may still not

Table 1
Common Drugs, Drug Dosing, and Route for Rate Control in Atrial Fibrillation

Drug	Dose	Frequency	Route	Comments
Digoxin	0.125–0.25 mg	Daily	i.v. or p.o	0.25–1.0 mg load, drug levels available (inc. mortality above 1.0 in HF) usually inadequate as a single agent
Beta-Blockers *Non-selective*				
Inderal	10–30 mg	t.i.d.	p.o.	Non-selective beta-blocker (parent compound)
Inderal LA	30–60 mg	Daily–b.i.d.	p.o.	Long acting
Pindolol	5–30 mg	b.i.d.	p.o.	Intrinsic sympathomimetic action
Beta-1 selective				
Acebutolol	200–600 mg	b.i.d.	p.o.	Lower doses may be effective once daily
Bisoprolol	2.5–20 mg	Daily	p.o.	Mild intrinsic sympathomimetic action
Esmolol	500 mcg/kg over 1 min	Load	i.v.	Ultra short acting, acute onset
	50–200 mcg/kg	Continuous	i.v.	
Metoprolol tartrate	5 mg	b.i.d.–q.i.d.	i.v.	Short onset, medium duration
	25–100 mg	b.i.d–t.i.d	p.o.	
Metoprolol succinate	25–100 mg	Daily–b.i.d	p.o.	Slow onset, long acting
Mixed alpha/beta				
Labetalol	100–400 mg	b.i.d.	p.o.	Predominantly used for hypertension
Carvedilol	3.125–50 mg	b.i.d.	p.o.	Used extensively in heart failure therapy
Calcium channel blockers				
Diltiazem	5–15 mg/h		i.v.	(0.25–0.35 mg/kg initial bolus)
Diltiazem	30–120 mg	t.i.d.	p.o.	Quick onset, short duration
Diltiazem extended	120–540 mg daily	Daily	p.o.	
Verapamil	2.5–10 mg	Bolus	i.v.	Short acting, acute onset
Verapamil	40–12 mg	t.i.d.	p.o.	Potent AV node blocker, negative inotropic effect in HF
Verapamil extended	180–480 mg	Daily	p.o.	

be achieved. More invasive methods may be required such as AV junctional ablation and pacing in these patients *(55)*. AV junction ablation and biventricular pacing has been proposed to potentially reduce the risk of pacing associated cardiomyopathy. This approach has not been fully validated in a prospective, randomized clinical trial.

The evaluation of heart rate control is not solely based on the resting pulse or ECG. Heart rate may appear controlled at rest yet inappropriately increase with even minimal activity. In the AFFIRM trial, a resting HR of less than 80 bpm was required as well as an average heart rate of less than 100 bpm over 18 h of ambulatory monitoring. Heart rates could not exceed the 100% age-predicted maximum heart rate during rest or activity *(77)*. In common practice, hourly average heart rates of less than 100 bpm are expected. Variability in the conducted HR also provides some insight into the status of autonomic control and may have some prognostic implications *(87–90)*.

While rate control as an alternative to rhythm control has gained popularity, electrophysiologists continue to find ways to restore sinus rhythm. Two major strategies for rhythm control include antiarrhythmic drug use or invasive techniques of either pulmonary vein isolation or surgical atrial reduction and isolation. Antiarrhythmic drug use since the mid-1980s has been relegated mostly to cardiologists and electrophysiologists due to the recognition of potentially significant proarrhythmic properties of some drugs and increased risk for mortality associated with their use. However, identification of patients at low risk for iatrogenic arrhythmogenesis can be undertaken, and antiarrhythmic drugs initiated in a monitored setting appropriately by nearly all practitioners.

In patients considered for antiarrhythmic drug use, identification of structural heart disease through echocardiography, electrocardiography, and evaluation of ischemic heart disease through history, exercise testing, or angiography should be performed. In addition, evaluation of renal function, hepatic function, and pulmonary and thyroid function may be necessary in certain cases. Evaluation of patient compliance and dosing schedules are also important.

In the 2006 ACC/AHA/ESC Guidelines for the Treatment of Atrial Fibrillation, high-risk features for proarrhythmia for class Ia, Ic, and III drugs are presented. In patients being considered for class Ia or III agents, underlying prolonged QT or concurrent use of agents that can prolong the QT interval, female gender, bradycardia, structural heart disease, high dose or rapid increase in dosing, as well as renal dysfunction and depressed LV function all increase the chance of proarrhythmia. In patients being considered for type Ic drugs, a prolonged QRS duration, structural heart disease with or without LV dysfunction, rapid heart rates, and high drug dose or rapid dose acceleration can all increase proarrhythmia *(55)*.

For acute conversion of atrial fibrillation, the class Ic agents propafenone and flecainide can be used in patients without significant structural heart disease *(91–95)*. The class III, short acting i.v. ibutilide can also be used with high efficacy *(96–98)*. In patients with structural heart disease such as left ventricular hypertrophy (LVH) or with coronary artery disease with preserved ejection fraction, the class III agents dofetilide *(99–103)* and amiodarone can be used *(91, 104–106)*. These agents may also be helpful in patients with normal hearts in which earlier agents have been ineffective. Finally, in patients with heart failure or LV dysfunction, dofetilide and amiodarone may be used *(105, 106)*. Again, consideration of drug clearance and other factors that may affect drug choice should be made *(55)*.

Other antiarrhythmic drugs may also be efficacious but are being replaced. For acute conversion of atrial fibrillation, quinidine, procainamide, and disopyramide have fallen out of favor due to lack of efficacy compared to other agents or increased risk for adverse effects. Digoxin and verapamil or diltiazem may be helpful in slowing conducted atrial rates, but are not effective in converting AF to sinus rhythm *(55)*.

Compared to acute conversion of AF to sinus, the maintenance of sinus rhythm in patients is very similar. The major difference is that sotalol plays a role in patients with normal hearts as well as in patients with hypertension without left ventricular hypertrophy (LVH), and patients with revascularized coronary artery disease with preserved ejection fraction. Beta-blockers and disopyramide also may play a role in selected patient groups *(107–111)*. In addition, amiodarone has taken on a large role due to the safety and efficacy of outpatient initiation and reduction in recurrence rate and duration of atrial fibrillation in relation to other antiarrhythmic drugs *(112–116)*.

Restoration of sinus rhythm by pharmacologic therapy alone is often not enough. Direct current cardioversion is often necessary either with or without the use of antiarrhythmic treatment. In patients with highly symptomatic paroxysmal or persistent AF or permanent AF, an appropriate anticoagulation regimen is utilized and cardioversion can be effective with a low risk for thromboembolism. Efficacy of direct current cardioversion utilizing a biphasic rectilinear waveform defibrillator was greater than 99% in 1,877 procedures *(117)*. Atrial fibrillation of prolonged duration (greater than 1 year) has a significantly lower rate of conversion and maintenance of sinus rhythm.

More recently completed trials and registries have looked at the role of various forms of invasive treatment of atrial fibrillation. Pioneering surgical therapies in which surgical cutting and re-sewing the atrium into multiple sections to effectively produce conduction block and atrial size reduction accomplished the elimination of atrial fibrillation through a surgical technique *(118–124)*. Swartz and associates demonstrated AF could be eliminated through endocardial radiofrequency ablation using similar ablation lines *(125)*. Over the next one and one-half decades, various techniques have been advanced to reduce procedure times, decrease complications, and still yield effective therapy.

Limited single center and multicenter trials and surveys form the bulk of literature to assess the efficacy of AF suppression after radiofrequency ablation, quality of life, and the morphologic changes in atrial and ventricular myocardium. In the 2007 Consensus Statement on Catheter and Surgical Ablation of Atrial Fibrillation, indications for ablation, anticoagulation, surgical approaches, and outcomes were summarized. Patients were considered appropriate candidates for AF ablation if they continue to have highly symptomatic atrial fibrillation despite at least one antiarrhythmic drug trial in the setting of appropriate rate control and anticoagulation. Individuals that were younger in age, had smaller atria, absence of significant valvular disease, and preserved LV function were considered more ideal candidates. Currently, a patient's desire alone to eliminate anticoagulation should not be considered an appropriate indication for AF ablation, as long-term stroke risk after successful ablation of anticoagulation has not been studied *(126)*.

Table 2 outlines the results of non-randomized and randomized trials as well as that of a large ablation survey including 9,000 patients. Generalization of the trials suggests success rates are higher for patients with paroxysmal rather than persistent AF and multiple procedures are required to affect a success with or without suppressive antiarrhythmic drugs. In addition, major complications of ablation in the survey were relatively high at 6%.

The impetus to pursue maintenance of sinus rhythm without pharmacotherapy continues as several trials have demonstrated significant improvements in objective cardiac parameters including a reduction in left atrial size and function and improvements in LV ejection fraction *(133–140)*. Quality of life indicators have also been shown to improve in many trials. However, many were unblinded or non-randomized, and the role of a placebo effect may be difficult to exclude *(98, 99)*.

Supporting the growing role of AF ablation, a recent trial by Khan and colleagues randomized patients with heart failure and an ejection fraction of 40% or less to either a pulmonary vein isolation ablation procedure or to AV junctional ablation and biventricular pacing for rate control. The composite score of ejection fraction, distance on 6-min walk test, and Minnesota Living with Heart Failure (MLWHF) score was the primary endpoint. In this small trial, success rates for freedom from AF in the ablation arm were 88% with or without antiarrhythmic drug use. Quality of life, improvement in LV systolic function, and 6-min walk test all statistically improved. In patients randomized to AV junctional ablation and biventricular ablation, ejection fraction remained unchanged, and quality of life and 6-min walk test improved only modestly. Of note, 30% of patients in the pacing arm had progression

Table 2
Summary of Clinical Trials Evaluating the Role of Radiofrequency Ablation and Drugs on the Treatment of
Atrial Fibrillation. Recurrence Rates for Isolated and Multiple Procedures Are Summarized for the
Non-randomized Trials. In the Survey, Results Are Grouped

Non-randomized clinical trials		
	Single procedure success	*Multiple procedure success*
Paroxysmal AF	38–78% (most >60%)	54–80% (most >70%)
Persistent AF	22–45% (most <30%)	37–88% (most >50%)
Mixed AF	16–84%	30–81%
Randomized clinical trials		
	Recurrence	*Comments*
Wazni et al. *(127)* (*n* = 70)	Drug: 63% ≥1	(Paroxysmal AF, flecainide or sotalol, 1 year f/u)
	RFA: 13% ≥1	
Oral et al. *(128)* (*n* = 168)	DCC: 42%	(Persistent AF, DCC vs. RFA 1 year f/u)
	RFA: 26%	
Stabile et al. *(129)* (*n* = 137)	Drug: 91%	(PAF and persistent AF, drug vs. RFA)
	RFA: 44%	
Pappone et al. *(130)* (*n* = 199)	Drug: 78%	(Paroxysmal AF, drug vs. RFA)
	RFA: 14%	
Jais et al. *(131)* (*n* = 53)	Drug: 93%	(Drug vs. RFA)
	RFA: 25%	
Survey *(132)* (*n* = 9,000)	RFA: 48%	(Includes single and multiple procedures and paroxysmal and persistent AF)
	RFA + Drug: 24%	

of their atrial fibrillation. Larger trials are needed to validate these findings. A standard rate-control arm may also help elucidate the functional changes in myocardial structure and function *(141)*.

Additional ongoing trials are likely to further demonstrate the importance of atrial fibrillation ablation procedures in selected groups. However, the economic impact of the procedure and the potential complications should not be understated *(126)*. In addition, standard surgical and minimally invasive surgical techniques have also been developed over the last 20 years, and procedure rates are growing in specialty centers with good results *(142–148)*. Clearly the future of atrial fibrillation management is a moving target. A proposed algorithm for the treatment of atrial fibrillation is shown in Fig. 13.

In contrast to atrial fibrillation, typical cavotricuspid isthmus-dependent atrial flutter ablation has a high success rate and is less complex to perform. Linear lesions, typically utilizing radiofrequency current or cryoablation, are delivered between the tricuspid annulus toward the inferior vena cava. This isthmus is a critical portion of the macro-re-entrant rhythm of atrial flutter. As the wavefront collides into the ablation line, the atrial flutter terminates and sinus rhythm is restored (Fig. 14). Following ablation, pacing the right atrium from the coronary sinus activates the atrium superiorly and also infero-laterally along the isthmus. Wavefront collision with the ablation line laterally in the isthmus results in activation of the lateral wall in a superior to inferior direction. This is in contrast to the activation pattern prior to ablation where lateral wall activation from coronary sinus pacing typically occurs in an inferior to superior manner (Fig. 15). Success rates are often as high as 90% with very low complication rates, making cure through ablation the treatment of choice for many individuals *(149, 150)*. Unfortunately, patients may have intermittent atrial fibrillation and long-term anticoagulation may need to be continued.

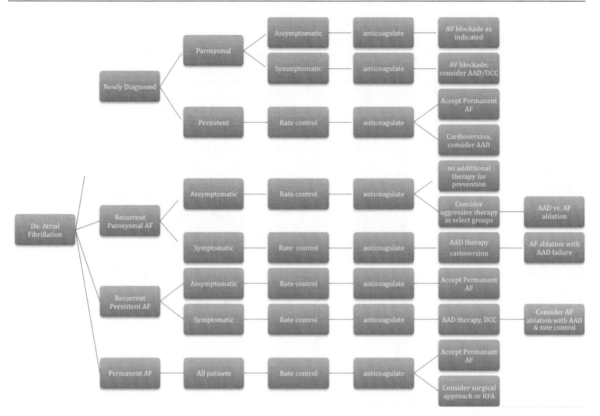

Fig. 13. Algorithm for the treatment of newly diagnosed AF, recurrent paroxysmal AF, recurrent persistent AF, and permanent AF. Treatment with warfarin is generally indicated in most groups unless specifically contraindicated. AAD = antiarrhythmic drug, DCC = direct current cardioversion.

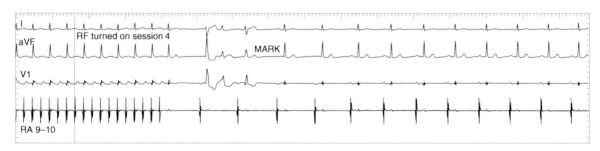

Fig. 14. Termination of atrial flutter during radiofrequency ablation along the venocaval–tricuspid isthmus. Rapid intracardiac depolarizations during atrial flutter are replaced by slower sinus depolarizations noted in lead RA 9–10. Surface leads II, aVF, V1, and intracardiac atrial recording from the high right atrium (RA 9–10) are shown.

24.2.2. Atrioventricular Chamber-Associated Arrhythmias

24.2.2.1. BRADYCARDIC ARRHYTHMIAS

24.2.2.1.1. Atrioventricular Block. Changes in atrioventricular (AV) node and His-Purkinje physiology over time or as a consequence of drugs or disease states are common. Progressive AV block is demonstrated in Fig. 16. The simplest form of abnormal AV association is first-degree AV block and is seen as a prolongation of the AV interval over 200 ms (Fig. 16a). It is usually not a clinically important ECG finding and rarely progresses to complete heart block *(151)*. Conduction delay

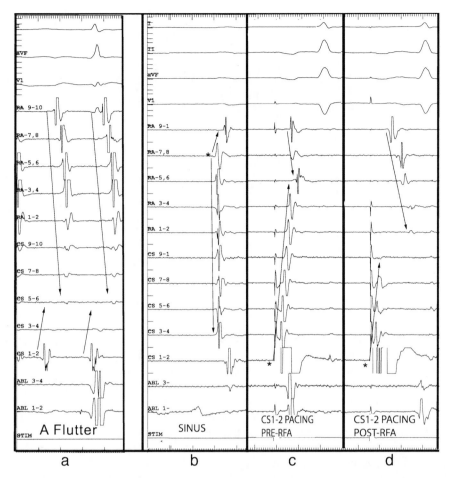

Fig. 15. Intracardiac recordings of atrial flutter during AFL, sinus rhythm, and during coronary sinus pacing prior to ablation and following isthmus ablation demonstrating medial to lateral block along the cavotricuspid isthmus at intracardiac recording (CS 9–10). (**a**) The AFL wavefront travels counterclockwise from RA 9–10 laterally along the cristae eventually reaching csv5–6. Conduction delay is noted to CS 3–4 and CS 1–2 and then rapidly ascends up the interatrial septum back to RA 9–10. (**b**) During sinus, RA 7–8 near the sinus node is earliest with activation down the crista and superior medially toward RA 9–10. CS 1–2 representing low LA activation is also late. (**c**) Pacing in the CS (at CS 1–2) propagates laterally along the isthmus and then up the lateral wall toward RA 3–4. A simultaneous wavefront reaches the superior-medial electrode at CS 9–10 and then laterally toward the opposing wavefront to collide at or near RA 3–4. Finally, in (**d**) following isthmus ablation, pacing from the CS (at CS 1–2) results in propagation across only part of the isthmus with termination of the wavefront at CS 9–10. A simultaneous wavefront from the CS 1–2 pacing propagates up the interatrial septum to the RA 9–10 electrode and then laterally along the crista toward the RA 1–2 electrode.

in first-degree AV block is usually at the AV node level, but in rare circumstances can also occur in His-Purkinje tissue *(152, 153)*. An electrophysiology study is necessary to confirm the level of conduction delay and is rarely indicated for first-degree AV block. However, very long AV intervals in which atrial activation occurs prior to opening of the tricuspid and mitral valve from the prior ventricular depolarization can give rise to atrial stretch and loss of effective atrial contribution to cardiac output and resultant symptoms.

As AV conduction becomes more affected, Type I second-degree AV block can be seen. With this, there is progressive prolongation of conduction time of each atrial depolarization through the AV node and His-Purkinje tissue with PR prolongation until conduction fails and no intrinsic QRS is seen. The

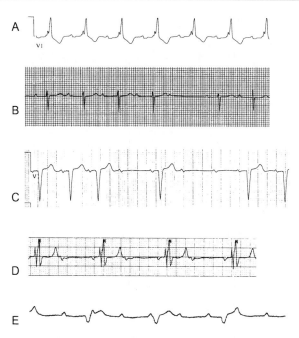

Fig. 16. Varying degrees of AV block. (**a**) Sinus rhythm with first-degree AV block with prolonged PR interval. (**b**) Type I, second-degree AV block (Wenckebach) with progressive PR prolongation followed by non-conducted P-wave and then a shorter PR interval on the next conducted P-wave. (**c**) Type II second degree and higher grade AV block. The third QRS complex is followed by a non-conducted P-wave without PR prolongation. The fourth QRS is followed by two consecutive non-conducted P-waves followed by two normally conducted beats. (**d**) 2:1 AV block is noted with every other P-wave being conducted. (**e**) Complete heart block with wide QRS escape rhythm. Atrial and ventricular depolarizations are independent.

PR interval on the first conducted beat after the dropped QRS is shorter than the last conducted PR interval prior to the dropped beat, confirming the diagnosis (Fig. 16b) *(154)*.

Asymptomatic Type I AV block is commonly seen during sleep and in trained athletes *(155)*. In patients without structural heart disease, Type I AV block is usually benign. However, in patients with structural heart disease, its importance is dictated by the severity of the underlying heart disease and symptoms *(156)*. Like first-degree AV block, Type I AV block is usually a product of AV nodal tissue delay but can occur in the His-Purkinje tissue and is usually seen in patients with significant bundle branch block on surface ECG as well *(157, 158)*.

As AV association becomes even more strained, Type II second-degree AV block is noted during regular sinus rhythm with a fixed AV interval followed by failure to conduct to the ventricle with a dropped QRS (Fig. 16c). The PR interval on the return beat is the same as that just prior to the dropped beat. Higher degrees of AV block are seen such as 2:1 AV block where every other QRS is dropped (Fig. 16c, d). Type II AV block is usually associated with underlying bundle branch block and delay within or below the His bundle *(159, 160)*. Pacing is typically indicated, as it is not uncommon for patients with underlying bundle branch block to progress to paroxysmal heart block or suffer Stokes–Adams type syncopal spells *(132, 161, 162)*.

Complete heart block is seen when no atrial conduction to the ventricle occurs. Non-conducted P-waves are seen with a junctional or ventricular escape rhythm eventually seen (Fig. 16e). Complete heart block may also occur as a congenital disorder with treatment concentrating on pacing in brady-cardic patients with low cardiac output and those with a wide QRS escape rhythm where heart block is presumed to occur below the level of the His bundle *(163)*.

In general, acquired heart block is usually associated with drugs, ischemic heart disease, or degenerative processes. Beta-blockers, non-dihydropyridine calcium antagonists, and membrane active antiarrhythmic drugs such as amiodarone, procainamide, propafenone, and flecainide are just a few drugs responsible for alterations in AV conduction at the level of the AV node or His-Purkinje system. Degenerative diseases such as Lenegre or Lev's disease or infectious etiologies such as rheumatic fever, Chagas disease, and rheumatic diseases including ankylosing spondylitis and rheumatoid arthritis, and infiltrative processes (amyloidosis, sarcoid, or Hodgkin's disease) are less common *(4)*.

24.2.2.2. TACHYARRHYTHMIAS

24.2.2.2.1. Junctional Rhythm, AV Nodal Re-entrant Tachycardia, and AV Reciprocating Tachycardia.
Junctional rhythm occurs when the automaticity of the AV node is faster than that of the sinus node and typically a regular narrow QRS rhythm is noted. Retrograde activation of the atrium may result in an inverted P-wave immediately following the QRS or there may be ventriculoatrial dissociation. Occasionally, antegrade conduction from a spontaneous atrial depolarization through the AVN may occur, advancing the next QRS and confirming the absence of complete heart block. At rates greater than 60 beats/min, junctional rhythm is considered to be abnormal and termed accelerated junctional rhythm. Junctional rhythm often occurs during times of heightened vagal tone such as sleep or rest but may also be seen with digoxin toxicity *(164, 165)*. Junctional and accelerated junctional rhythm may also be seen frequently after valvular surgery or after major cardiac surgery where sinus node function may be transiently impaired or the AV node is mechanically irritated.

Atrioventricular nodal (junctional) re-entrant tachycardia (AVNRT) is the most common form of sustained supraventricular tachycardia excluding atrial fibrillation and flutter *(166, 167)*. In this arrhythmia, the AV node has functionally two pathways termed slow and fast pathways. Re-entrant tachycardia occurs when an impulse travels down one of the pathways and back up the other. Perpetuation of the tachycardia occurs when the impulse again travels down the initial pathway and around again. Retrograde activation of the atrium occurs and inverted P-waves are often seen in the terminal portion of the QRS in the most common form (Figs. 17 and 18). Due to autonomic input into the AV node, maneuvers to enhance vagal tone such as valsalva maneuvers or carotid sinus massage can often terminate the arrhythmia *(166, 168)*. Drugs affecting the AV node including beta-blockers, nondihydropyridine calcium antagonists, and digoxin are used to suppress recurrence. Adenosine injected rapidly intravenously is often used to terminate the arrhythmias in emergency rooms with high success rates *(169–171)*.

An important tachycardia that should not be missed by the practicing physician is a bypass tract-mediated tachycardia. Commonly referred to as Wolf-Parkinson-White syndrome, clinical tachypalpitations and the presence of a delta wave in sinus rhythm are clues to the possible mechanism of a patient's clinical arrhythmia. In the setting of manifest or overt preexcitation during sinus rhythm, a narrow QRS tachycardia with retrograde P-waves distinct from the terminal portion of the QRS strongly suggests orthodromic atrioventricular tachycardia. The arrhythmia in this setting utilizes the AV node, His-Purkinje tissue, and ventricle in an antegrade limb. The ventricular myocardium is thus activated normally and results in a narrow QRS. Retrograde atrial activation occurs when the bypass tract is activated from ventricular depolarization. Atrial activation then perpetuates antegrade ventricular activation and the circuit perpetuates (Fig. 19).

In antidromic AV re-entrant tachycardia (AVRT) or circus movement tachycardia, the bypass tract is utilized antegrade and the tachycardia is a wide complex tachycardia as a result of slower cell-to-cell ventricular myocardial activation, not His-Purkinje based activation (Fig. 20) *(1)*. Retrograde activation of the atrium occurs usually through the His-Purkinje–AV node axis but may rarely utilize a second bypass tract in the retrograde direction. Antidromic AV reciprocating tachycardia may mimic ventricular tachycardia and is suggested when preexcitation of the QRS is noted after restoration of sinus rhythm. Agents such as verapamil or diltiazem that may enhance antegrade AV conduction over the bypass tract in the setting of atrial fibrillation may result in ventricular fibrillation and are contraindicated.

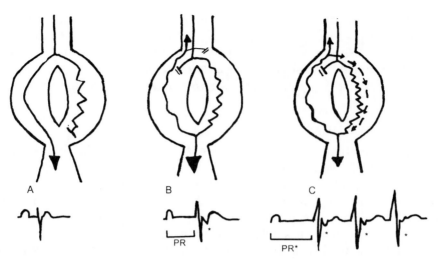

Fig. 17. Initiation of typical AV nodal re-entry tachycardia (AVNRT). (**a**) Normal activation sequence. An impulse travels through the AV node then travels down two simultaneous pathways. Ventricular activation under normal circumstances occurs rapidly through the fast pathway and results in a normal PR interval. Conduction block occurs in the slower pathway as the impulse collides with the depolarized shared tissue. (**b**) Isolated re-entry echo beat. An atrial impulse or premature beat initially travels down the faster pathway but encounters block. Conduction then travels along the slower pathway activating the ventricle resulting in a longer PR interval. The impulse then travels retrograde up the fast pathway that either has not been depolarized or is no longer refractory and activates the atrium (*). The slow pathway is refractory to activation and antegrade conduction is blocked. (**c**) Initiation and perpetuation of tachycardia. An atrial beat or premature atrial beat again blocks in the fast pathway. Activation proceeds along the slow pathway giving rise to an even longer PR interval. Retrograde fast pathway activation occurs, and the atrium is activated giving rise to the inverted P-wave (*). Due to the additional recovery time, the previously refractory antegrade slow pathway is now excitable and the wavefront progresses to activate the ventricle. The circuit repeats giving rise to the tachycardia.

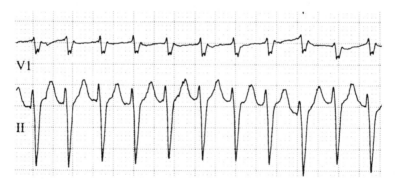

Fig. 18. Typical atrioventricular tachycardia (AVNRT). Lead V1 and lead II show a narrow complex tachycardia with no discernible retrograde P-waves during the tachycardia.

24.2.2.3. VENTRICULAR ORIGIN ASSOCIATED ARRHYTHMIAS

24.2.2.3.1. Premature Ventricular Contractions. The most common type of ventricular arrhythmia is that of the simple premature ventricular contraction (PVC). An early ventricular depolarization occurs prior to the normal antegrade activation from the atrium or the normal AV node–His-Purkinje axis. Occurring in normal and abnormal myocardium, PVCs may be asymptomatic but also may give rise to the sensation of palpitations and on occasion light headedness. In very high frequency, ventric-

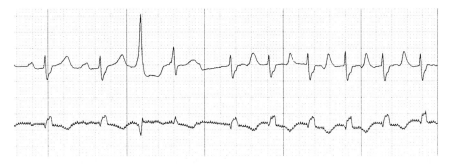

Fig. 19. Initiation of orthodromic AV reciprocating tachycardia. A P-wave arrives early resulting in a prolonged PR interval. Normal ventricular activation occurs through the AV node. Retrograde atrial activation occurs over the bypass tract giving rise to a long VA time. Perpetuation of re-entry then occurs.

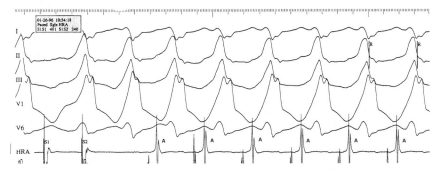

Fig. 20. Imitation and perpetuation of antidromic AV reciprocating tachycardia. An atrial premature is delivered (S2) during antegrade pacing with manifest preexcitation (wide QRS and short AV time). Retrograde atrial activation is noted in the HRA channel followed by a regular wide complex tachycardia with a right bundle branch block/right axis tachycardia consistent with a left lateral bypass tract.

ular ectopy may be entirely asymptomatic but may also give rise to decreased cardiac output states in patients with both normal and abnormal systolic function. The morphology of the PVCs and sequential PVCs can give clues to their ventricular location and may suggest a certain type of pathophysiology or syndrome *(172, 173)*.

Premature ventricular contractions that are of a single morphology are termed monomorphic or uniform and those that have multiple morphologies, polymorphic or polyform *(174)*. In the setting of no significant structural heart disease, monomorphic PVCs with a left bundle branch block, normal axis frequently arises from the pulmonary outflow tract region and are usually thought to be benign (Fig. 21a) *(175)*. Termed RV outflow tract PVCs (RVOT PVCs), these beats may be suppressed with beta-blockers, calcium antagonists, and Vaughan Williams class I and class III drugs. In the asymptomatic patient, no therapy is generally needed. In cases of drug failure or intolerance in the symptomatic patient, or in individuals with greater than 20% ectopy with decreased LV systolic function, ablation therapy is utilized with typically good success *(175–177)*. In making the diagnosis of benign RVOT PVCs, one first needs to confirm the absence of ischemia, as anterior wall distribution ischemia may also give rise to frequent asymptomatic and symptomatic PVCs.

Right bundle branch block (RBBB) superior axis monomorphic PVCs suggest an inferior origin of the left ventricle (Fig. 21b). Careful inspection of the resting ECG may reveal a prior inferior infarct suggesting that the ventricular ectopy is arising in the setting of myocardial scar or ischemia and may not be benign *(178–182)*. Patients with left ventricular dysfunction (ejection fraction less than 40%), prior myocardial infarction, and high frequency ventricular ectopy have a high incidence of sudden

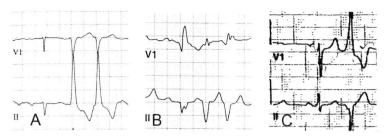

Fig. 21. Premature ventricular contraction (PVC) variability. (**a**) Left bundle/normal axis PVCs arising from the right ventricular outflow tract. (**b**) Right bundle branch/superior axis PVC arising from left ventricular inferior scar. (**c**) A right bundle branch/superior axis PVC with a narrower QRS consistent with fascicular PVCs arising from the left posterior fascicle.

cardiac death *(183–187)*. These individuals have been the subject of many drug and device trials over the last two decades as well as those with non-sustained ventricular tachycardia *(188–191)*.

In other patients, uniform ectopy arising from the inferior base of the left ventricle may also appear as RBBB, superior axis PVCs in the absence of structural heart disease (Fig. 21c). These may arise from the posterior fascicles of the left bundle and may be associated with a typically benign form of normal heart ectopy or ventricular tachycardia, albeit often symptomatic *(192)*. The PVC and ventricular tachycardia-associated QRS morphology is often subtlety narrower than scar-related or ischemia-related ventricular tachycardia and may help in the diagnosis *(193–196)*. This verapamil or adenosine sensitive rhythm is typically benign, but may require treatment in symptomatic patients.

When reviewing an ECG or rhythm strip, attention to the variable morphologies of ventricular ectopy is equally important. Individuals with polyform ventricular ectopy with left bundle branch block (LBBB)/superior axis and LBBB/normal axis or moderate variability of the LBBB-type QRS morphology in the setting of normal, non-ischemic left ventricular function may be found to have arrhythmogenic right ventricular cardiomyopathy (ARVC). This is a progressive disease of the right ventricular myocardium with premature cellular apoptosis and replacement with fatty tissue *(197)*. Associated with palpitations, syncope and sudden cardiac death thought secondary to malignant ventricular tachycardia or ventricular fibrillation, ARVC may be detected with ECG-gated computed tomography, MRI, or occasionally with endomyocardial biopsy *(198–201)*. The high suspicion and early referral to a specialist is often necessary to prevent untoward events. Drug therapies with sotalol, beta-blockers, and implantable defibrillators have been used. Ablation therapy may be used to reduce episodes of sustained ventricular tachycardia (VT). New origins for VT arise as the disease progresses, however, making ventricular tachycardia ablation alone less reliable *(202)*.

Multiform or polyform PVCs also occur in the setting of ongoing or prior ischemic heart disease. Symptoms of heart failure exacerbation, new chest pain, or prior infarct increases suspicion that the ventricular ectopy is an indicator of unstable myocardium. Evaluation of left ventricular function and noninvasive or invasive ischemic evaluation is warranted *(202)*. Depressed LV systolic function coupled with a high level of ventricular ectopy foreshadows a poor prognosis. In the GISSI-2 study, patients with normal and depressed left ventricular function and with varying degrees of ventricular ectopy were evaluated. Patients with depressed LV function and high degrees of ventricular ectopy had significantly higher mortality than those with low frequency ectopy and normal LV function *(203)*.

24.2.2.3.2. Non-ischemic Ventricular Tachycardia. Ventricular ectopy associated with non-ischemic entities such as right ventricular outflow tract PVCs, arrhythmogenic right ventricular cardiomyopathy, and verapamil sensitive tachycardia may all be associated with sustained ventricular tachycardia. Management and treatment of these arrhythmias is similar to treatment of the asymptomatic patient with PVCs alone. In symptomatic patients, however, specific drug therapy, ablation therapy, and implantable defibrillator placement may take on a greater role.

An additional ventricular tachycardia associated with non-ischemic cardiomyopathy is bundle branch re-entry tachycardia. In this tachycardia, the re-entrant circuit involves antegrade conduction down the right bundle branch and retrograde conduction up the left bundle branch, turning around at the His bundle. The tachycardia has a LBBB normal axis morphology and should be considered in patients with non-ischemic cardiomyopathy. Elimination of the tachycardia is accomplished through ablation at the right bundle *(204)*. Unfortunately, many patients may have additional ventricular tachyarrhythmias in the setting of non-ischemic cardiomyopathy and may still warrant treatment with implantable defibrillators.

Ventricular tachycardia may occur in the setting of surgical scar, sarcoidosis, scleroderma, Chagas disease, and after treatment of complex congenital heart disease repair. Long-term follow-up of many of these entities is limited with respect to ablation therapy. The role of implantable cardioverter–defibrillators (ICDs) has expanded to include many of these disease states as pacing indications are also met. Ventricular tachycardia ablation may be used to reduce the frequency of VT and ICD discharge in these patients *(205, 206)*.

24.2.2.3.3. Ischemic Ventricular Tachycardia.

As ventricular ectopy becomes more frequent and runs or short salvos of non-sustained ventricular tachycardia occur, risk of sudden cardiac death (SCD) increases *(179–182, 184–186)*. Greater than three consecutive beats at a rate of more than 100 bpm is termed non-sustained ventricular tachycardia (NSVT). Greater than 30 s of VT would be considered sustained VT even if it terminates spontaneously *(202)*. A regular slower ventricular rhythm less than 100 bpm is termed accelerated idioventricular rhythm (AIVR). While abnormal, this rhythm has not been used as a criterion for SCD risk management in modern day trials.

Several large trials of high-risk patients with prior cardiac arrest or who are thought to be at high risk for sudden cardiac death have utilized ventricular tachycardia, either spontaneous or induced as a risk stratifier, for evaluation and treatment. In the secondary prevention AVID trial *(207)*, patients with prior cardiac arrest without reversible cause, unexplained syncope with inducible ventricular tachycardia in the setting of LV dysfunction, and individuals with sustained, symptomatic ventricular tachycardia were evaluated and treated either with drug therapy (predominantly amiodarone) or implantable cardioverter–defibrillator (ICD) therapy. This trial and others have demonstrated the superior effectiveness of device therapy to drug therapy for the secondary prevention of SCD in high-risk patients *(208, 209)*.

Patients with underlying ischemic heart disease with prior infarct and non-sustained VT by ambulatory holter monitoring were evaluated by invasive electrophysiology study in the MADIT and MUSST trials *(210, 211)*. Individuals with inducible ventricular tachycardia through programmed stimulation that was not suppressible with drug therapy were deemed to be at high risk and were treated with conventional antiarrhythmic drug therapy or implantable defibrillators. In these landmark trials, implantable defibrillators were shown to be superior to drug therapy in this high-risk group for the primary prevention of SCD. In addition, antiarrhythmic drug use was associated with event rates greater than that of patients treated with placebo *(211)*. Over the last 10 years, several additional trials have been completed that emphasize the importance of left ventricular ejection fraction as an independent risk factor for SCD and the importance of standard drug therapy for the treatment of left ventricular dysfunction and device therapy in the reduction of premature death *(212, 213)*.

24.2.2.4. Special Considerations in Evaluation of Arrhythmias

24.2.2.4.1. Ventricular Tachycardia—Identification by Surface ECG.

A difficult problem that often occurs in clinical practice is distinguishing ventricular tachycardia from supraventricular tachycardia with aberrancy or pacing. At rapid rates or in the setting of an abnormal QRS during intrinsic ventricular activation, QRS morphology can become wide and resemble ventricular tachycardia. Several papers have been written over the last 30 years to help the clinician distinguish between these two entities. Important in the evaluation of the rhythm strip or ECG is the baseline QRS and clinical history of prior infarct and drug therapy. As with most tests, clinical information can greatly enhance the specificity of test findings (214).

Inherent in the evaluation of the wide complex rhythm are certain features of the QRS complex including duration, axis, precordial concordance, and Q-wave morphology. Additional information including AV dissociation, presence of fusion beats, and QRS alternans can be used. In 1978, Wellens and colleagues characterized QRS morphology and duration in RBBB wide complex tachycardias as well as presence of AV dissociation to distinguish ventricular tachycardia and supraventricular tachycardia (215). In 1988, Josephson and colleagues characterized QRS morphologies in LBBB wide complex tachycardias (216). Separate papers published in 1991 characterized most wide complex tachycardias based on a hierarchical evaluation of the QRS morphology and AV association (217, 218). In 1997, additional evaluation of patients with intraventricular conduction disease was reported (219). Newer criteria by Vereckei and associates utilized additional criteria of the QRS complex during tachycardia to improve specificity over prior algorithms. While potentially useful, these criteria too have shortcomings in certain patient populations including patients with prior infarction, preexcited tachycardias, and those on medications (220). Inherent in all the algorithms is the importance of the patients' clinical history. Patients with prior myocardial infarction with or without left ventricular dysfunction are much more likely to have ventricular tachycardia compared to aberrant supraventricular tachycardia (SVT) as the correct diagnosis during wide complex tachycardias (221). Detailed evaluation of these algorithms is beyond the scope of this text and the reader is referred to the cited articles.

24.2.2.4.2. Arrhythmias Associated with Genetic Disorders.   Abnormalities of cardiac depolarization and repolarization occur in patients with genetic disorders typically involving sodium and potassium channels. Table 3 lists common and some uncommon arrhythmic syndromes and their presumed genetic mutations (222–224). In many circumstances, genetic miscoding is not readily apparent on surface ECG and provocative measures may be required to elucidate them. In patients with familial hypertrophic cardiomyopathy, the electrocardiogram may be normal despite the fact that this mutation can result in adverse clinical events (225, 226).

Abnormalities in sodium and potassium channels and their subunits as well as regulatory proteins have been implicated in Brugadas syndrome and long QT syndrome. In the Brugada syndrome, an atypical RBBB with persistent ST elevation and frequently associated T-wave inversion is noted on the surface ECG and is most notable in leads V1–3 (Fig. 22). Subsequent evaluation has linked this syndrome to *SCN5A*, the gene responsible for the alpha subunit of the sodium channel and is inherited in an autosomal-dominant pattern with variable penetrance. Electrical abnormalities of right ventricular epicardium appear to be responsible for the abnormal ECG pattern (227–229).

Genetic polymorphisms in the sodium and potassium channels and their subunits have been demonstrated for a variety of individuals with long QT syndrome. Prolongation of ventricular myocardial repolarization due to genetic errors or drugs is manifested on the ECG by a long QT interval. A table of normal values for men and women is shown (Table 4) (230). Individuals with prolongation of the QT interval with unexplained syncope, light headedness, or a family history of sudden cardiac death warrant further evaluation. Asymptomatic patients may also warrant further evaluation, as sudden cardiac death may be the first presenting sign of patients at risk.

Polymorphous ventricular tachycardia with acquired long QT in the setting of drugs or pause-dependent QT prolongation may be seen. In Fig. 23, frequent PVCs result in bradycardia-dependent QT prolongation and a second PVC produces an R-on-T phenomenon resulting in non-sustained polymorphous ventricular tachycardia that appears to twist about a point termed torsades de pointes. Temporary pacing, isuprel infusion to increase intrinsic heart rate, beta-blockers, and lidocaine may be useful in reducing these events. Removing offending QT prolonging drugs is necessary.

Table 3
Gene, Gene Locus, Protein, Physiologic Effect, and Associated Clinical Syndromes Associated with Several Common and Less Common Cardiac Arrhythmias

Gene	Locus	Protein	Effect	Syndrome
SCN5A	3p24–p21	Sodium channel (hH1)	Repolarization (I_{Na} current)	Long QT 3, Brugada syndrome, progressive cardiac conduction disease, AV block, atrial standstill
SCN4B	11q23	Sodium channel subunit Navβ4	Repolarization	Long QT 10
CAV3	3p25	Caveolin-3 protein	Repolarization (alters sodium channel current)	Long QT 9
KCNQI	11p15.5	Potassium channel-alpha subunit (K_vLQT1)	Repolarization (I_{Ks} current)	Long QT 1, short QT syndrome, chronic AF, sudden infant death
KCNH2 (HERG)	7q35–q36	Potassium channel-alpha subunit	Repolarization (I_{Kr} current)	Long QT 2, Short QT syndrome, AF
KCNE1	21q22	Potassium channel-beta subunit (mink)	Repolarization (I_{Ks} current)	Long QT 5
KCNE2	21q22	Potassium channel-beta subunit (MirP)	Repolarization (I_{Kr} current)	Long QT 6, paroxysmal AF
KCNJ2	17q23	Potassium channel	Resting membrane potential maintenance (I_{Kr} current)	Long QT 7
CACNA1c	12p13.3	Calcium channel Cav1.2		Long QT 8, congenital heart disease, Brugadas syndrome-3
AnkB	4q25–q27	Anchoring protein	Altered Ca^{2+}, cellular disruption/organization, reduced protein levels	Long QT 4, AF
Ryr2	1q42.1–q43	Cardiac ryanodine receptor	Ca^{2+} release channel of endoplasmic reticulum (ER)	Catecholaminergic polymorphic ventricular tachycardia
CASQ2	1p13–p11	Calsequestrin	Ca^{2+} storage of ER	Catecholaminergic polymorphic ventricular tachycardia
HCN4	15q24–q25	Cation channel	Spontaneous diastolic depolarization (I_f current)	Sinus bradycardia
PRKAG2	7q36	cAMP-activated protein kinase	Glycogen metabolism	WPW, hypertrophic cardiomyopathy (HCM)
CSX	5q34	Transcription factor	Heart chamber growth/formation	AV block, congenital heart disease
TNNT2	1q32	Troponin T	Sarcomere contractile protein	Idiopathic ventricular tachycardia, HCM
GJA5	1q21.1	Connexin-40	Cell signaling-gap junctions	AF
Unknown	10q22–24	Possible alpha-, beta, receptor, or G-protein receptor kinase	Unknown	Familial paroxysmal and chronic AF
Unknown	6q14–16	Unknown	Unknown	Familial PAF progressing to chronic AF
Unknown	5p13	Unknown	Unknown	Chronic AF young associated with neonatal death, VF

AV = atrioventricular, AF = atrial fibrillation, WPW = Wolf-Parkinson-White.

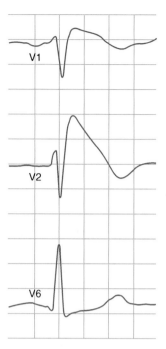

Fig. 22. Atypical right bundle branch block. QRS activation is noted in precordial leads V1, V2, and V6. The slurred, downsloping ST segment is most notable in V2 in this example.

Table 4
Normal QT Intervals for Individuals Under the Age of 15 and for Adult Men and Women

Rating	1–15 years (ms)	Adult male (ms)	Adult female (ms)>
Normal	<440	<430	<450
Borderline	440–460	430–450	450–470
Prolonged	>460	>450	>470

ms = milliseconds

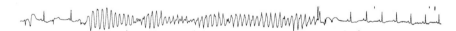

Fig. 23. Initiation and spontaneous termination of polymorphous ventricular tachycardia (PMVT). Variation in the RR interval results in pause-dependent QT prolongation. A PVC then initiates a PMVT that appears to twist about a point termed torsades de pointes. The arrhythmia terminates and sinus rhythm results.

Ventricular fibrillation may also occur in the setting of inherited channelopathies and in familial and sporadic hypertrophic cardiomyopathies *(222, 223, 225)*. Ventricular fibrillation is also frequently seen associated with acute ischemic events and may follow prolonged sustained monomorphic ventricular tachycardia as the myocardial substrate changes. Prompt treatment with advanced cardiopulmonary resuscitation and direct current cardioversion is required.

24.2.2.4.3. Paced Rhythms. An important rhythm seen commonly during ambulatory ECG monitoring and routine ECG is the paced atrial and ventricular complex. Many modern day pacemakers and pacemaker defibrillators are designed not only to sense normal intrinsic atrial and ventricular depolarization but also to distinguish the onset and offset of various atrial and ventricular arrhythmias. In certain modes, devices may be programmed to identify the rhythm and attempt to pace faster than the tachycardia in an effort to terminate it. Implantable cardioverter–defibrillators are designed to also deliver a high-voltage shock to terminate the arrhythmia automatically (Fig. 24). Complex algorithms within the device's program help prevent unwarranted shocks for rapidly conducted atrial fibrillation or sustained supraventricular tachycardia.

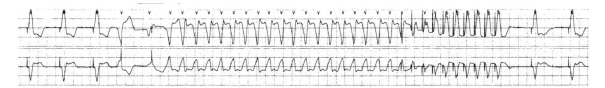

Fig. 24. Pace Termination of ventricular tachycardia (VT). A paced rhythm is followed by a premature ventricular contraction and rapid VT. Ten rapid pulses delivered from an implantable defibrillator are delivered automatically and terminates the tachycardia.

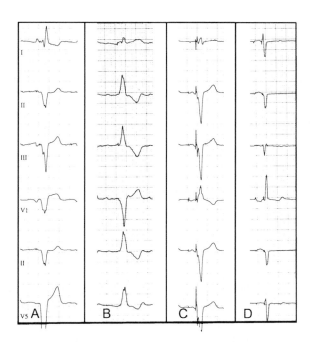

Fig. 25. QRS morphology is dependent on ventricular lead placement. (**a**) Pacing in the right ventricular apex gives rise to a right bundle branch block (LBBB) superior axis. (**b**) Right ventricular outflow tract pacing gives rise to a normal axis LBBB pattern. (**c**) Left ventricular apical pacing results in a superior axis, right bundle branch block (RBBB) pattern. (**d**) Simultaneous right and left ventricular activation results in a narrow, RBBB pattern with a superior axis.

Basic components of the pacemaker include the pace generator, the battery and computer, and the lead. The pacing wire is typically placed endovascularly and traverses the subclavian vein, into the superior vena cava, and is delivered to the right atrium, right ventricle, or, in certain circumstances, within the coronary sinus. These soft, flexible wires are design to affix to the endomyocardium in a variety of techniques, including passive adherence and screws. The pacing wire is able to carry electrical signals from the heart to the pacemaker generator where timing circuits analyze whether an impulse is to be delivered to the myocardium. As indicated impulse travels from the generator to the myocardium via the lead, activating the endomyocardium directly and initiates a wavefront across the affected chamber.

Inherently slower than specialized atrial tissue or the Purkinje system of the ventricular myocardium, activation is typically prolonged resulting in prolonged P-wave duration when pacing in the atrium or a bundle branch block appearance of the QRS during ventricular stimulation. Activation of the right ventricle with pacing results in a left bundle branch block pattern, while activation of the left ventricle results in a RBBB pattern. Apical activation results in a superior axis while right ventricular outflow position results in a normal axis. Pacing in the coronary sinus typically results in a right bundle branch block pattern (Fig. 25). However, inadvertent delivery of a lead across a patent foramen ovale, ventricular septal defect, or perforation of the right ventricle with pacing of the left ventricular epicardium can also occur. Knowledge of the lead delivery technique in patients with RBBB paced QRS configuration is important in avoiding embolic phenomenon from left ventricular endocardial placement or other serious complications such as tamponade from erroneous lead perforation.

24.3. CONCLUSION

Through careful attention to the clinical history, association of atrial and ventricular impulses and morphology of atrial and ventricular depolarization on the surface ECG, most common clinical arrhythmias can be accurately diagnosed. In many instances, treatment of an arrhythmia can be straightforward and handled without referral or consultation. However, new and expanding treatment options including device therapy and ablation as well as specific antiarrhythmic drug management may often require additional expertise. Cardiac arrhythmias associated with genetic mutations are becoming more recognized. While gene therapy is not currently available, genetic identification of many disorders is available and characterization in certain groups may aid in diagnosis of asymptomatic or high-risk patients and lead to pharmacologic or invasive procedures.

24.4. CASE STUDIES

24.4.1. Case Study 1

GB was a 52-year-old professional truck driver that presented to the emergency room following a single vehicle accident while driving across the state. The patient does not recall the accident and had eaten lunch about an hour earlier. He is diabetic, obese; he smokes one and a half packs of cigarettes per day; and he has a history of dyslipidemia. He takes a diuretic for mild hypertension but frequently does not use it due to his occupation. His wife reports he snores. He reports frequent morning headaches and when not working complains of fatigue, lack of energy, and falls asleep easily while watching TV. He reports occasional heart racing that usually lasts only a few minutes but can last up to an hour. He denies angina, orthopnea or paroxysmal nocturnal dyspnea, stroke-like symptoms, episodes of hypoglycemia or syncope. His HgbA1c is 9.0%.

Initial evaluation demonstrates a 5'10" male with a BMI of 42.3. Blood pressure was 148/84 and his serum glucose in the office is 186 mg/dL. Oxygen saturation was 94%. Potassium was 3.8, blood urea nitrogen 31, and creatinine 1.3 with a bicarbonate of 31. His cardiac exam is normal except for jugular venous distention, decreased heart sounds, and moderate lower extremity edema.

24.4.1.1. CLINICAL TESTING

Initial ECG demonstrated sinus arrhythmia with an incomplete right bundle branch block. Chest X-ray reveals moderate changes consistent with chronic obstructive lung disease. Cardiac size was upper limits of normal. Hemoglobin was 17.2 mg/dL. A head CT demonstrated no hemorrhage or mass.

24.4.1.2. DISCUSSION

The differential diagnosis for this patient is large. He has had a presumed syncopal event while operating a motor vehicle. Altered consciousness secondary to metabolic derangement, rapid atrial or ventricular arrhythmias, or heart block should be entertained due to the patients' history of palpitations and an abnormal ECG. There are symptoms to also suggest significant pulmonary disease and the history is concerning for sleep apnea.

The patient was hospitalized. Overnight telemetry demonstrated sinus arrhythmia and nocturnal pauses of 4.2 s. Heavy snoring while sleeping was noted by nursing staff. Bedside oximetry revealed frequent desaturation to 78% during apnea events. An echocardiogram revealed mild left ventricular hypertrophy with normal left ventricular function. Bi-atrial enlargement and right ventricular enlargement with an estimated systolic pulmonary pressure of 47 mmHg was noted. An exercise stress test was abnormal. Subsequent coronary angiography revealed mild, non-occlusive coronary disease.

The tentative diagnosis of sleep apnea was made. However, symptoms of palpitations suggested associated atrial fibrillation and underlying incomplete bundle branch block made heart block a possibility. Electrophysiology testing for evaluation of heart block revealed normal baseline intracardiac intervals and no evidence to suggest block within or inferior to the bundle of His. The patient was instructed to not drive until outpatient evaluation was complete. Formal sleep apnea testing was performed revealing severe sleep apnea. Continuous positive airway pressure therapy was initiated. In follow-up, additional ambulatory testing was performed revealing paroxysmal atrial fibrillation with rapid ventricular response. The patient was anticoagulated with warfarin given the presence of multiple risk factors for stroke. He was also given verapamil for hypertension and rate control during recurrent atrial fibrillation events. In follow-up, he has lost 55 pounds, has not had a recurrence of syncope, and his quality of life appears to have improved.

24.4.2. Case Study 2

TF is a 46-year-old electrician. He presented to the emergency room following cardiac arrest. His event was witnessed. Cardiopulmonary resuscitation (CPR) was initiated and he was promptly defibrillated at his workplace by a trained bystander using a new Automated External Defibrillator (AED). Paramedics transferred the patient to the ER. He was on nasal cannula and complained of chest pain. He reports feeling fine prior to the event and remembers his colleague at his side after defibrillation.

Initial evaluation revealed a normally developed 6'2" male. Blood pressure was 128/68, respirations 18 and unlabored, and his pulse was 110. Oxygen saturation was 99%. Exam also revealed a prominent, sustained cardiac PMI. A systolic murmur was noted in the aortic outflow position. Arterial pulses in the upper and extremity were normal.

24.4.2.1. CLINICAL TESTING

Initial ECG demonstrated sinus tachycardia. Left ventricular hypertrophy with moderate repolarization changes was seen. No evidence for acute or prior myocardial infarction was noted. Chest X-ray demonstrated cardiac enlargement. Routine serum chemistries and blood cell counts were normal. Cardiac enzymes were normal.

24.4.2.2. DISCUSSION

Ventricular fibrillation may result from metabolic abnormalities, acute or chronic ischemia, genetic arrhythmic disorders, inherited cardiomyopathies, or be associated with mechanical events such as acute pulmonary embolism or severe valvular heart disease. Further clinical history revealed a paternal uncle and grandfather that died suddenly in their early fifties. Autopsies were not performed. No documented family history of premature atherosclerosis was known.

Concentrating on the additional history, cardiac echo revealed severe left ventricular hypertrophy with an interventricular septum measuring 4.2 cm. Near cavitary obliteration with systole is noted. Flow velocities beneath and across the aortic valve are increased but did not demonstrate subvalvular or valvular stenosis. A tentative diagnosis of familial hypertrophic cardiomyopathy was made. Coronary angiography was performed to exclude occult coronary disease. Given high-risk features for sudden cardiac death (interventricular septum greater than 3 cm and prior ventricular arrest), an implantable defibrillator was placed. Beta-blockers at high doses were initiated to limit rapidly conducted atrial arrhythmias and to reduce recurrent ventricular fibrillation.

In follow-up over the next 2 years the patient developed progressive dyspnea. No recurrent ventricular fibrillation events occurred. Pulmonary pressures assessed by echocardiogram were increased at 52 mmHg and left atrial enlargement noted. Clinical systolic heart failure secondary to left ventricular hypertrophy was made and after failure of additional oral negative inotrope use to improve symptoms, the patient was referred for surgical myomectomy. Following successful surgery, the patient has returned to work and is with minimal symptoms. Recurrent ventricular events have subsequently been appropriately treated by his implantable defibrillator and sotalol was initiated to reduce recurrent arrhythmic events.

REFERENCES

1. Josephson ME. Preexcitation syndromes. *Clinical Cardiac Electrophysiology: Techniques and Interpretations*. 3rd ed. Philadelphia, PA: Lippincott Williams & Wilkins; 2002:322–424.
2. Boyett MR, Honjo H, Kodama I. Review: the sinoatrial node, a heterogeneous pacemaker structure. *Cardiovas Res*. 2000;47:658–687.
3. Marriott HJL. Chamber enlargement. *Practical Electrocardiography*. 7th ed. Baltimore, MD: Williams and Wilkins; 1983:58–59.
4. Daviddnko JM. Spiral waves in the heart: experimental demonstration of a theory. In: Zipes DP, Jalife J, eds. *Cardiac Electrophysiology—From Cell to Bedside*. 2nd ed. Philadelphia, PA: W.B. Saunders Co.; 1995:478–487.
5. Desai JM, Scheinman MM, Strauss HC, et al. Electrophysiologic effects of combined autonomic blockade in patients with sinus node disease. *Circulation*. 1981;63:953–960.
6. Boineau JP, Canavan TE, Schuessler RB, et al. Demonstration of a widely distributed atrial pacemaker complex in the human heart *Circulation*. . 1988;77:1221–1237.
7. Boineau JP, Schuessler RB, Roeske WR, et al. Quantitative relation between sites of atrial muscle origin and cycle length. *Am J Physiol*. 1983;245:H781–H789.
8. Mackeray AJC, Opthof T, Leeker WK, Jongsma HJ, Bouman LN. Interaction of adrenaline and acetylcholine on sinus node function. In: Bouman LN, Jongsma HJ, eds. *Cardinal Rate and Rhythm*. The Hague: Marinus Nijhoff; 1982: 507–523.
9. Zwillich C, Deulin T, White D, et al. Bradycardia during sleep apnea. Characteristics and mechanisms. *J Clin Invest*. 1982;69(6):1286–1292.
10. Frenneaux MP. Autonomic changes in patients with heart failure and in post myocardial infarction patients. *Heart*. 2004;90:1248–1255.
11. Madsen B, Rasmussen V, Hansen J. Predictors of sudden death and death from pump failure in congestive heart failure are different. Analysis of 24 h Holter monitoring, clinical variables, blood chemistry, exercise test and radionuclide angiography. *Int J Cardiol*. 1997;58:1561–1562.
12. Guzzetti S, La Rovere MT, Pinna G, et al. Different spectral components of 24 h heart rate variability are related to different modes of death in chronic heart failure. *Eur Heart J*. 2005;26:357–362.
13. Galinier M, Pathak A, Fourcade J, et al. Depressed low frequency power of heart rate variability as an independent predictor of sudden death in chronic heart failure. *Eur Heart J*. 2000;21:475–482.
14. Grimm W, Hoffmann J, Menz V, et al. Electrophysiologic evaluation of sinus node function and atrioventricular conduction in patients with prolonged ventricular asystole during obstructive sleep apnea. *Am J Cardiol*. 1996;77(15):1310–1314.
15. Ribuot C, Godin D, Couture R, Regoli D, Nadeau R. In vivo B2-receptor-mediated negative chronotropic effect of bradykinin in canine sinus node. *Am J Physiol Heart Circ Physiol*. 1993;265:H876–H879.
16. Srein R, Medeiros CM, Rosito GA, et al. Intrinsic sinus and atrioventricular node electrophysiologic adaptations in endurance athletes. *J Am Coll Cardiol*. 2002;39(6):1033–1038.

17. Milanesi R, Baroscotti M, Gnecchi-Ruscone T, DiFrancesco D. Familial sinus bradycardia associated with a mutation in the cardiac pacemaker channel. *N Engl J Med.* 2006;354:151–157.
18. Alboni P, Menozzi C, Brignole M, Paparella N, et al. Effects of permanent pacemaker and oral theophylline in sick sinus syndrome. The THEOPACE study: a randomized controlled trial. *Circulation.* 1997;96:260–266.
19. Scheinman MM, Thorburn D, Abbott JA. Use of atropine in patients with acute myocardial infarction and sinus bradycardia. *Circulation.* 1975;52:627–633.
20. Spiridoula Vavetsi S, Nikolaou N, Tsarouhas K, et al. Consecutive administration of atropine and isoproterenol for the evaluation of asymptomatic sinus bradycardia. *Europace.* 2008;10(10):1176–1181.
21. Epstein AE, DiMarco JP, Ellenbogen KA, et al. ACC/AHA/HRS 2008 guidelines for device-based therapy of cardiac rhythm abnormalities: a report of the American College of Cardiology/American Heart Association Task Force on Practice Guidelines (Writing Committee to Revise the ACC/AHA/NASPE 2002 Guideline Update for Implantation of Cardiac Pacemakers and Antiarrhythmia Devices). *J Am Coll Cardiol.* 2008;51:e1–e62.
22. Kistler PM, Sanders P, Fynn SP, Stevenson IH, et al. Electrophysiologic and electroanatomic changes in the human atrium associated with age. *J Am Coll Cardiol.* 2004;44:109–116.
23. Barón-Esquivias G, Pedrote A, Cayuela A, Valle JI, Fernández JM, et al. Long-term outcome of patients with asystole induced by head-up tilt test. *Eur Heart J.* 2002;23:483–489.
24. Goldman MJ. *Principles of Clinical Electrocardiography.* 12th ed. Los Altos, CA: Lange Medical Publications; 1986:224.
25. Batsford WP, Akhtar M, Caracta AR, et al. Effect of atrial stimulation site on electrophysiological properties of atrioventricular node in man. *Circulation.* 1974;50:283–292.
26. Haissaguerre M, Jais P, Shah DC, et al. Spontaneous initiation of atrial fibrillation by ectopic beats originating in the pulmonary veins. *N Engl J Med.* 1998;339:659–666.
27. Steinbeck G, Hoffmann E. "True" atrial tachycardia. *Eur Heart J.* 1998;19(Suppl E):E10–E19.
28. Ferrer MJ. The sick sinus syndrome in atrial disease. *JAMA.* 1968;206:645–646.
29. Rubenstein JJ, Schulman CL, Yurchck PM, DeSanctis RW. Clinical spectrum of the sick sinus syndrome. *Circulation.* 1972;46:5–13.
30. Blomström-Lundqvist C, Scheinman MM, Aliot EM, et al. ACC/AHA/ESC guidelines for the management of patients with supraventricular arrhythmias—executive summary: a report of the American College of Cardiology/American Heart Association Task Force on Practice Guidelines, and the European Society of Cardiology Committee for Practice Guidelines (Writing Committee to Develop Guidelines for the Management of Patients With Supraventricular Arrhythmias). *J Am Coll Cardiol.* 2003;42:1493–1531.
31. Saoudi N, Cosio F, Waldo A, et al. A classification of atrial flutter and regular atrial tachycardia according to electrophysiological mechanisms and anatomical bases; a statement from a joint expert group from The Working Group of Arrhythmias of the European Society of Cardiology and the North American Society of Pacing and Electrophysiology. *Eur Heart J.* 2001;22:1162–1182.
32. Huikuri HV, Poutiainen AM, Ma¨kikallio TH, et al. Dynamic behavior and autonomic regulation of ectopic atrial pacemakers. *Circulation.* 1999;100:1416–1422.
33. Poutiainen AM, Koistinen MJ, Airaksinen KE, et al. Prevalence and natural course of ectopic atrial tachycardia. *Eur Heart J.* 1999;20:694–700.
34. Kalman JM, Olgin JE, Karch MR, et al. . "Cristal tachycardias:" origin of right atrial tachycardias from the crista terminalis identified by intracardiac echocardiography. *J Am Coll Cardiol.* 1998;31:451–459.
35. Tada H, Nogami A, Naito S, et al. Simple electrocardiographic criteria for identifying the site of origin of focal right atrial tachycardia. *Pacing Clin Electrophysiol.* 1998;21:2431–2439.
36. Hoffmann E, Reithmann C, Nimmermann P, et al. Clinical experience with electroanatomic mapping of ectopic atrial tachycardia. *Pacing Clin Electrophysiol.* 2002;25:49–56.
37. Sippen Groenewegen A, Lesh MD, Rothinger FX, et al. Body surface mapping of counterclockwise and clockwise typical atrial flutter: a comparative analysis with endocardial activation sequence mapping. *J Am Coll Cardiol.* 2000;35:1276–1287.
38. Walsh EP, Saul JP, Hulse JE, et al. Transcatheter ablation of ectopic atrial tachycardia in young patients using radiofrequency current. *Circulation.* 1992;86:1138–1146.
39. Cossu SF, Steinberg JS. Supraventricular tachyarrhythmias involving the sinus node: clinical and electrophysiologic characteristics. *Prog Cardiovasc Dis.* 1998;41:51–63.
40. Goya M, Lesaka Y, Takahashi A, et al. Radiofrequency catheter ablation for sinoatrial node re-entrant tachycardia: electrophysiologic features of ablation sites. *Jpn Circ J.* 1999;63:177–183.
41. Goldenstein DS, Holmes C, Frabj SM, et al. Cardiac sympathetic dysautonomia in chronic orthostatic intolerance syndromes. *Circulation.* 2002;106:2358–2365.
42. Romano SM, Lazzeri C, Chiostri M, Gensini GF. Beat-to-beat analysis of pressure wave morphology for presymptomatic detection of orthostatic intolerance during head-up tilt. *J Am Coll Cardiol.* 2004;44:1891–1897.

43. Low PA, Opfer-Gehrking TL, Textor SC, et al. Postural tachycardia syndrome (POTS). *Neurology.* 1995;45 (Suppl 5):S19–S25.

44. Grubb BP, Kosinski DJ, Boehm K, Kip K. The postural orthostatic tachycardia syndrome: a neurocardiogenic variant identified during heart-up tilt table testing. *Pacing Clin Electrophysiol.* 1997;20:2205–2212.

45. Bush VE, Wight VL, Brown CM, Hainsworth R. Vascular responses to orthostatic stress in patients with postural tachycardia syndrome (POTS) in patients with low orthostatic tolerance, and in asymptomatic controls. *Clin Auton Res.* 2000;10:279–284.

46. Lee RJ, Kalman JM, Fitzpatrick AP, et al. Radiofrequency catheter modification of the sinus node for "inappropriate" sinus tachycardia. *Circulation.* 1995;92:2919–2928.

47. Mischke K, Stellbrink C, Hanrath P. Evidence of sinoatrial block as a curative mechanism in radiofrequency current ablation of inappropriate sinus tachycardia. *J Cardiovasc Electrophysiol.* 2001;12:264–267.

48. Man KC, Knight B, Tse HF, et al. Radiofrequency catheter ablation of inappropriate sinus tachycardia guided by activation mapping. *J Am Coll Cardiol.* 2000;35:451–457.

49. Sato T, Mitamura H, Murata M, et al. Electrophysiologic findings of a patient with inappropriate sinus tachycardia cured by selective radiofrequency catheter ablation. *J Electrocardiol.* 2000;33:381–386.

50. Van Lieshout JJ, Wieling W, Karemaker JM, Eckberg DL. The vasovagal response. *Clin Sci.* 1991;81:575–586.

51. Sander-Jensen K, Secher NH, Astrup A, et al. Hypotension induced by passive head-up tilt: endocrine and circulatory mechanisms. *Am J Physiol.* 1986;251:R742–R748.

52. Morillo CA, Eckberg DL, Ellenbogen KA, et al. Vagal and sympathetic mechanisms in patients with orthostatic vaso-vagal syncope. *Circulation.* 1997;96:2509–2513.

53. Go AS, Hylek EM, Phillips KA, et al. Prevalence of diagnosed atrial fibrillation in adults. National implications for rhythm management and stroke prevention: the anticoagulation and Risk Factors In Atrial Fibrillation (ATRIA) study. *JAMA.* 2001;285:2370–2375.

54. Prystowsky EN, Katz AM. Atrial fibrillation. In: Topol EJ, ed. *Textbook of Cardiovascular Medicine.* Philadelphia, PA: Lippincott-Raven; 1998:1661.

55. Fuster V, Rydén LE, Cannom DS, et al. ACC/AHA/ESC 2006 guidelines for the management of patients with atrial fibrillation: a report of the American College of Cardiology/American Heart Association Task Force on Practice Guidelines and the European Society of Cardiology Committee for Practice Guidelines (Writing Committee to Revise the 2001 Guidelines for the Management of Patients with Atrial Fibrillation). *J Am Coll Cardio.* 2006;48:e149–e246.

56. Polontchouk L, Haefliger JA, Ebelt B, et al. Effects of chronic atrial fibrillation on gap junction distribution in human and rat atria. *J Am Coll Cardiol.* 2001;38:883–891.

57. Pokharel S, van Geel PP, Sharma UC, et al. Increased myocardial collagen content in transgenic rats overexpressing cardiac angiotensin converting enzyme is related to enhanced breakdown of N-acetyl-Ser-Asp-Lys-Pro and increased phosphorylation of Smad2/3. *Circulation.* 2004;110:3129–3135.

58. Sharma OP, Maheshwari A, Thaker K. Myocardial sarcoidosis. *Chest.* 1993;103:253–258.

59. Maixent JM, Paganelli F, Scaglione J, et al. Antibodies against myosin in sera of patients with idiopathic paroxysmal atrial fibrillation. *J Cardiovasc Electrophysiol.* 1998;9:612–617.

60. Tsai CF, Tai CT, Hsieh MH, et al. Initiation of atrial fibrillation by ectopic beats originating from the superior vena cava: electrophysiological characteristics and results of radiofrequency ablation. *Circulation.* 2000;102:67–74.

61. White CW, Kerber RE, Weiss HR, et al. The effects of atrial fibrillation on atrial pressure-volume and flow relationships. *Circ Res.* 1982;51:205–215.

62. Kamkin A, Kiseleva I, Wagner KD, et al. Mechanically induced potentials in atrial fibroblasts from rat hearts are sensitive to hypoxia/reoxygenation. *Pflugers Arch.* 2003;446:169–174.

63. Schauerte P, Scherlag BJ, Pitha J, et al. Catheter ablation of cardiac autonomic nerves for prevention of vagal atrial fibrillation. *Circulation.* 2000;102:2774–2780.

64. Pappone C, Santinelli V, Manguso F, et al. Pulmonary vein denervation enhances long-term benefit after circumferential ablation for paroxysmal atrial fibrillation. *Circulation.* 2004;109:327–334.

65. Gami AS, Pressman G, Caples SM, et al. Association of atrial fibrillation and obstructive sleep apnea. *Circulation.* 2004;110:364–367.

66. Tsai CT, Lai LP, Hwang JJ, et al. Molecular genetics of atrial fibrillation. *J Am Coll Cardiol.* 2008;52:241–250.

67. Tsang TS, Gersh BJ, Appleton CP, et al. Left ventricular diastolic dysfunction as a predictor of the first diagnosed nonvalvular atrial fibrillation in 840 elderly men and women. *J Am Coll Cardiol.* 2002;40:1636–1644.

68. Wang TJ, Parise H, Levy D, et al. Obesity and the risk of new-onset atrial fibrillation. *JAMA.* 2004;292:2471–2477.

69. Coromilas J. Obesity and atrial fibrillation: is one epidemic feeding the other? *JAMA.* 2004;292:2519–2520.

70. Fetsch T, Bauer P, Engberding R, et al. Prevention of atrial fibrillation after cardioversion: results of the PAFAC trial. *Eur Heart J.* 2004;25:1385–1394.

71. Israel CW, Gronefeld G, Ehrlich JR, et al. Long-term risk of recurrent atrial fibrillation as documented by an implantable monitoring device: implications for optimal patient care. *J Am Coll Cardiol.* 2004;43:47–52.

72. Page R, Wilkinson WE, Clair WK, et al. Asymptomatic arrhythmias in patients with symptomatic paroxysmal atrial fibrillation and paroxysmal supraventricular tachycardia. *Circulation.* 1994;89:224–227.

73. Page RL, Tilsch TW, Connolly SJ, et al. Asymptomatic or "silent" atrial fibrillation: frequency in untreated patients and patients receiving azimilide. *Circulation.* 2003;107:1141–1145.

74. Kerr CR, Boone J, Connolly SJ, et al. The Canadian Registry of Atrial Fibrillation: a noninterventional follow-up of patients after the first diagnosis of atrial fibrillation. *Am J Cardiol.* 1998;82:82N–85N.

75. Olson JA, Fouts AM, Padanilam BJ, Prystowsky EN. Utility of mobile cardiac outpatient telemetry for the diagnosis of palpitations, presyncope, syncope, and the assessment of therapy efficacy. *J Cardiovasc Electrophysiol.* 2007;18(5):473–477.

76. Vasamreddy CR, Dalal D, Dong J, et al. Symptomatic and asymptomatic atrial fibrillation in patients undergoing radiofrequency catheter ablation. *J Cardiovasc Electrophysiol.* 2006;17(2):134–139.

77. AFFIRM I. A comparison of rate control and rhythm control in patients with atrial fibrillation. *N Engl J Med.* 2002;347:1825–1833.

78. Hagens VE, Ranchor AV, Van Sonderen E. Bosker et al. Effect of rate or rhythm control on quality of life in persistent atrial fibrillation. Results from the Rate Control Versus Electrical Cardioversion (RACE) Study. *Am Coll Cardiol.* 2004;43(2):241–247.

79. Van Gelder I, Hagens VE, Bosker HA, Kingma H, et al. A comparison of rate control and rhythm control in patients with recurrent persistent atrial fibrillation. *N Engl J Med.* 2002;347:1834–1840.

80. Opolski G, Torbicki A, Kosior DA, et al. Rate control vs. rhythm control in patients with nonvalvular persistent atrial fibrillation: the results of the Polish How to Treat Chronic Atrial Fibrillation (HOT CAFE) Study. *Chest.* 2004;26:476–486.

81. Hohnloser SH, Kuck KH, Lilienthal J. Rhythm or rate control in atrial fibrillation—Pharmacological Intervention in Atrial Fibrillation (PIAF): a randomized trial. *Lancet.* 2000;356:1789–1794.

82. Roy DR, Nattel S, Wyse G, et al. Rhythm control versus rate control for atrial fibrillation and heart failure. *N Engl J Med.* 2008;358:2667–2677.

83. Gage BF, Waterman AD, Shannon W, Boechler M, Rich MW, Radford MJ. Validation of clinical classification schemes for predicting stroke. Results from the National Registry of Atrial Fibrillation. *JAMA.* 2001;285:2864–2870.

84. Ebell MH. A systematic approach to managing warfarin doses. *Fam Pract Manag.* 2005;5:77–83.

85. O'Reilly RA. Anticoagulant, antithrombotic, and thrombolytic drugs. In: Gilman AG, Goodman LS, Rall TW, Murad F, eds. *Goodman and Gilman's: The Pharmacological Basis of Therapeutics.* 7th ed. New York, NY: MacMillan Publishing Co; 1985:1344–1352.

86. Willenheimer R, Lechat P. New concepts in managing patients with chronic heart failure: the evolving importance of beta-blockade. *Eur Heart J Supp.* 2006;8(Supp C):c.

87. Stein KM, Borer JS, Hochreiter C, et al. Variability of the ventricular response in atrial fibrillation and prognosis in chronic nonischemic mitral regurgitation. *Am J Cardiol.* 1994;74:906–911.

88. Frey B, Heinz G, Binder T, et al. Diurnal variation of ventricular response to atrial fibrillation in patients with advanced heart failure. *Am Heart J.* 1995;129:58–65.

89. Atwood JE, Myers J, Sandhu S, et al. Optimal sampling interval to estimate heart rate at rest and during exercise in atrial fibrillation. *Am J Cardiol.* 1989;63:45–48.

90. Olshansky B, Rosenfeld LE, Warner AL, et al. The Atrial Fibrillation Follow-up Investigation of Rhythm Management (AFFIRM) study: approaches to control rate in atrial fibrillation. *J Am Coll Cardiol.* 2004;43:1201–1208.

91. Donovan KD, Power BM, Hockings BE, et al. Intravenous flecainide versus amiodarone for recent-onset atrial fibrillation. *Am J Cardiol.* 1995;75:693–697.

92. Suttorp MJ, Kingma JH, Jessurun ER, et al. The value of class IC antiarrhythmic drugs for acute conversion of paroxysmal atrial fibrillation or flutter to sinus rhythm. *J Am Coll Cardiol.* 1990;16:1722–1727.

93. Botto GL, Capucci A, Bonini W, et al. Conversion of recent onset atrial fibrillation to sinus rhythm using a single oral loading dose of propafenone: comparison of two regimens. *Int J Cardiol.* 1997;58:55– 61.

94. Donovan KD, Dobb GJ, Coombs LJ, et al. Reversion of recent-onset atrial fibrillation to sinus rhythm by intravenous flecainide. *Am J Cardiol.* 1991;67:137–141.

95. Bertini G, Conti A, Fradella G, et al. Propafenone versus amiodarone in field treatment of primary atrial tachydysrhythmias. *J Emerg Med.* 1990;8:15–20.

96. Stambler BS, Wood MA, Ellenbogen KA. Antiarrhythmic actions of intravenous ibutilide compared with procainamide during human atrial flutter and fibrillation: electrophysiological determinants of enhanced conversion efficacy. *Circulation.* 1997;96:4298–4306.

97. Guo GB, Ellenbogen KA, Wood MA, et al. Conversion of atrial flutter by ibutilide is associated with increased atrial cycle length variability. *J Am Coll Cardiol.* 1996;27:1083–1089.

98. Ellenbogen KA, Stambler BS, Wood MA, et al. Efficacy of intravenous ibutilide for rapid termination of atrial fibrillation and atrial flutter: a dose-response study. *J Am Coll Cardiol.* 1996;28:130–136.

99. Falk RH, Pollak A, Singh SN, Friedrich T. Intravenous dofetilide, a class III antiarrhythmic agent, for the termination of sustained atrial fibrillation or flutter. Intravenous Dofetilide Investigators. *J Am Coll Cardiol.* 1997;29:385–390.

100. Norgaard BL, Wachtell K, Christensen PD, et al. Efficacy and safety of intravenously administered dofetilide in acute termination of atrial fibrillation and flutter: a multicenter, randomized, double-blind, placebo controlled trial. Danish Dofetilide in Atrial Fibrillation and Flutter Study Group. *Am Heart J.* 1999;137:1062–1069.

101. Sedgwick ML, Lip G, Rae AP, et al. Chemical cardioversion of atrial fibrillation with intravenous dofetilide. *Int J Cardiol.* 1995;49:159–166.

102. Torp-Pedersen C, Moller M, Bloch-Thomsen PE, et al. Dofetilide in patients with congestive heart failure and left ventricular dysfunction. Danish Investigations of Arrhythmia and Mortality on Dofetilide Study Group. *N Engl J Med.* 1999;341:857–865.

103. Singh S, Zoble RG, Yellen L, et al. Efficacy and safety of oral dofetilide in converting to and maintaining sinus rhythm in patients with chronic atrial fibrillation or atrial flutter: the symptomatic atrial fibrillation investigative research on dofetilide (SAFIRE-D) study. *Circulation.* 2000;102:2385–2390.

104. Kochiadakis GE, Igoumenidis NE, Solomou MC, et al. Efficacy of amiodarone for the termination of persistent atrial fibrillation. *Am J Cardiol.* 1999;83:58–61.

105. Galve E, Rius T, Ballester R, et al. Intravenous amiodarone in treatment of recent-onset atrial fibrillation: results of a randomized, controlled study. *J Am Coll Cardiol.* 1996;27:1079–1082.

106. Peuhkurinen K, Niemela M, Ylitalo A, et al. Effectiveness of amiodarone as a single oral dose for recent-onset atrial fibrillation. *Am J Cardiol.* 2000;85:462–465.

107. Singh BN, Singh SN, Reda DJ, et al. Amiodarone versus sotalol for atrial fibrillation. *N Engl J Med.* 2005;352: 1861–1872.

108. Benditt DG, Williams JH, Jin J, et al. Maintenance of sinus rhythm with oral d, l-sotalol therapy in patients with symptomatic atrial fibrillation and/or atrial flutter. d, l-Sotalol Atrial Fibrillation/Flutter Study Group. *Am J Cardiol.* 1999;84:270–277.

109. Wanless RS, Anderson K, Joy M, et al. Multicenter comparative study of the efficacy and safety of sotalol in the prophylactic treatment of patients with paroxysmal supraventricular tachyarrhythmias. *Am Heart J.* 1997;133: 441–446.

110. Juul-Moller S, Edvardsson N, Rehnqvist-Ahlberg N. Sotalol versus quinidine for the maintenance of sinus rhythm after direct current conversion of atrial fibrillation. *Circulation.* 1990;82:1932–1939.

111. Crijns HJ, Gosselink AT, Lie KI. Propafenone versus disopyramide for maintenance of sinus rhythm after electrical cardioversion of chronic atrial fibrillation: a randomized, double-blind study. PRODIS Study Group. *Cardiovasc Drugs Ther.* 1996;10:145–152.

112. Roy D, Talajic M, Dorian P, et al. Amiodarone to prevent recurrence of atrial fibrillation. Canadian trial of atrial fibrillation investigators. *N Engl J Med.* 2000;342:913–920.

113. Kochiadakis GE, Igoumenidis NE, Marketou ME, et al. Low dose amiodarone and sotalol in the treatment of recurrent, symptomatic atrial fibrillation: a comparative, placebo controlled study. *Heart.* 2000;84:251–257.

114. Chun SH, Sager PT, Stevenson WG, et al. Long-term efficacy of amiodarone for the maintenance of normal sinus rhythm in patients with refractory atrial fibrillation or flutter. *Am J Cardiol.* 1995;76:47–50.

115. The AFFIRM. First Antiarrythmic Drug Substudy Investigators. Maintenance of sinus rhythm in patients with atrial fibrillation: an AFFIRM substudy of the first antiarrhythmic drug. *J Am Coll Cardiol.* 2003;42:20–29.

116. Naccarelli GV, Wolbrette DL, Khan M, et al. Old and new antiarrhythmic drugs for converting and maintaining sinus rhythm in atrial fibrillation: comparative efficacy and results of trials. *Am J Cardiol.* 2003;91:15D–26D.

117. Niebauer MJ, Brewer JE, Chung MK, et al. Comparison of the rectilinear biphasic waveform with the monophasic damped sine waveform for external cardioversion of atrial fibrillation and flutter. *Am J Cardiol.* 2004;93:1495–1499.

118. Prasad SM, Maniar HS, Camillo CJ, et al. The Cox Maze III procedure for atrial fibrillation: long-term efficacy in patients undergoing lone versus concomitant procedures. *J Thorac Cardiovasc Surg.* 2003;126:1822–1827.

119. McCarthy PM, Gillinov AM, Castle L, et al. The Cox-Maze procedure: The Cleveland Clinic experience. *Semin Thorac Cardiovasc Surg.* 2000;12:25–29.

120. Raanani E, Albage A, David TE, et al. The efficacy of the Cox/Maze procedure combined with mitral valve surgery: a matched control study. *Eur J Cardiothorac Surg.* 2001;19:438–442.

121. Schaff HV, Dearani JA, Daly RC, et al. Cox-Maze procedure for atrial fibrillation: Mayo Clinic experience. *Semin Thorac Cardiovasc Surg.* 2000;12:30–37.

122. Khargi K, Hutten BA, Lemke B, Deneke T. Surgical treatment of atrial fibrillation; a systematic review. *Eur J Cardiothoracic Surg.* 2005;27:258–265.

123. Kottkamp H, Hindricks G, Autschbach R, et al. Specific linear left atrial lesions in atrial fibrillation: intraoperative radiofrequency ablation using minimally invasive surgical techniques. *J Am Coll Cardiol.* 2002;40:475–480.

124. Salenger R, Lahey SJ, Saltman AE. The completely endoscopic treatment of atrial fibrillation: report on the first 14 patients with early results. *Heart Surg Forum.* 2004;7:E555–E558.

125. Swartz JF, Pellersels G, Silvers J, et al. A catheter-based curative approach to atrial fibrillation in humans (abstract). *Circulation.* 1994;90(4):I-335.

126. Calkins H, Brugada J, Packer DL, et al. HRS/EHRA/ECAS expert consensus statement on catheter and surgical ablation of atrial fibrillation: recommendations for personnel, policy, procedures and follow-up a report of the Heart Rhythm Society (HRS) Task Force on Catheter and Surgical Ablation of Atrial Fibrillation Developed in partnership with the European Heart Rhythm Association (EHRA) and the European Cardiac Arrhythmia Society (ECAS); in collaboration with the American College of Cardiology (ACC), American Heart Association (AHA), and the Society of Thoracic Surgeons (STS). *Europace.* 2007;9:335–379.

127. Wazni OM, Marrouche NF, Martin DO, et al. Radiofrequency ablation vs antiarrhythmic drugs as first-line treatment of symptomatic atrial fibrillation: a randomized trial. *JAMA.* 2005;293:2634–2640.

128. Oral H, Pappone C, Chugh A, et al. Circumferential pulmonary-vein ablation for chronic atrial fibrillation. *N Engl J Med.* 2006;354:934–941.

129. Stabile G, Bertaglia E, Senatore G, et al. Catheter ablation treatment in patients with drug-refractory atrial fibrillation: a prospective, multi-centre, randomized, controlled study (Catheter Ablation for the Cure of Atrial Fibrillation Study). *Eur Heart J.* 2006;27:216–221.

130. Pappone C, Augello G, Sala S, et al. A randomized trial of circumferential pulmonary vein ablation versus antiarrhythmic drug therapy in paroxysmal atrial fibrillation: the APAF Study. *J Am Coll Cardiol.* 2006;48:2340–2347.

131. Jais P, Cauchemez B, MacLe L, et al. Atrial fibrillation ablation vs antiarrhythmic drugs: a multicenter randomized trial (abstract). *Heart Rhythm.* 2006;3(Suppl):1126.

132. Cappato R, Calkins H, Chen SA, et al. Worldwide survey on the methods, efficacy, and safety of catheter ablation for human atrial fibrillation. *Circulation.* 2005;111:1100–1105.

133. Jayam VK, Dong J, Vasamreddy CR, Lickfett L, et al. Atrial volume reduction following catheter ablation of atrial fibrillation and relation to reduction in pulmonary vein size: an evaluation using magnetic resonance angiography. *J Interv Card Electrophysiol.* 2005;13:107–114.

134. Tsao HM, Wu MH, Huang BH, et al. Morphologic remodeling of pulmonary veins and left atrium after catheter ablation of atrial fibrillation: insight from long-term follow-up of three-dimensional magnetic resonance imaging. *J Cardiovasc Electrophysiol.* 2005;16:7–12.

135. Lemola K, Desjardins B, Sneider M, et al. Effect of left atrial circumferential ablation for atrial fibrillation on left atrial transport function. *Heart Rhythm.* 2005;2:923–928.

136. Verma A, Kilicaslan F, Adams JR, et al. Extensive ablation during pulmonary vein antrum isolation has no adverse impact on left atrial function: an echocardiography and cine computed tomography analysis. *J Cardiovasc Electrophysiol.* 2006;17:741–746.

137. Chen MS, Marrouche NF, Khaykin Y, et al. Pulmonary vein isolation for the treatment of atrial fibrillation in patients with impaired systolic function. *J Am Coll Cardiol.* 2004;43:1004–1009.

138. Hsu LF, Jais P, Sanders P, et al. Catheter ablation for atrial fibrillation in congestive heart failure. *N Engl J Med.* 2004;351:2373–2383.

139. Tondo C, Mantica M, Russo G, et al. Pulmonary vein vestibule ablation for the control of atrial fibrillation in patients with impaired left ventricular function. *Pacing Clin Electrophysiol.* 2006;29:962–970.

140. Oral H, Pappone C, Chugh A, et al. Circumferential pulmonary-vein ablation for chronic atrial fibrillation. *N Engl J Med.* 2006;354:934–941.

141. Khan MN, Jais P, Cummings J, et al. Pulmonary-vein isolation for atrial fibrillation in patients with heart failure. *N Engl J Med.* 2008;359:1778–1785.

142. Haissaguerre M, Jais P, Shah DC, et al. Electrophysiological end point for catheter ablation of atrial fibrillation initiated from multiple pulmonary vein foci. *Circulation.* 2000;101(12):1409–1417.

143. Feinberg MS, Waggoner AD, Kater KM, Cox JL, Lindsay BD, Perez JE. Restoration of atrial function after the maze procedure for patients with atrial fibrillation. Assessment by Doppler echocardiography. *Circulation.* 1994;90 (5 Pt 2):II285–II292.

144. Prasad SM, Maniar HS, Camillo CJ, et al. The Cox maze III procedure for atrial fibrillation: long-term efficacy in patients undergoing lone versus concomitant procedures. *J Thorac Cardiovasc Surg.* 2003;126: 1822–1828.

145. Ninet J, Roques X, Seitelberger R, et al. Surgical ablation of atrial fibrillation with off-pump, epicardial, high-intensity focused ultrasound: results of a multicenter trial. *J Thorac Cardiovasc Surg.* 2005;130:803–809.

146. Pruitt JC, Lazzara RR, Dworkin GH, Badhwar V, Kuma C, Ebra G. Totally endoscopic ablation of lone atrial fibrillation: initial clinical experience. *Ann Thorac Surg.* 2006;81:1325–1330.

147. Wolf RK, Schneeberger EW, Osterday R, et al. Video-assisted bilateral pulmonary vein isolation and left atrial appendage exclusion for atrial fibrillation. *J Thorac Cardiovasc Surg.* 2005;130:797–802.

148. Melby SJ, Zierer A, Bailey MS, et al. A new era in the surgical treatment of atrial fibrillation: the impact of ablation technology and lesion set on procedural efficacy. *Ann Surg.* 2006;244:583–592.

149. Chen SA, Chiang CE, Wu TJ, et al. Radiofrequency catheter ablation of common atrial flutter: comparison of electrophysiologically guided focal ablation technique and linear ablation technique. *J Am Coll Cardiol.* 1996;27: 860–868.

150. Natale N, Newby KH, Pisanó E, et al. Prospective randomized comparison of antiarrhythmic therapy versus first-line radiofrequency ablation in patients with atrial flutter. *J Am Coll Cardiol.* 2000;35:1898–1904.

151. McAnulty JH, Rahimtoola SH, Murphy E, et al. Natural history of "high-risk" bundle-branch block: final report of a prospective study. *N Engl J Med.* 1982;307:137–143.

152. Dhingra RC, Wyndham C, Bauernfeind R, et al. Significance of block distal to the His bundle induced by atrial pacing in patients with chronic bifascicular block. *Circulation.* 1979;60:1455–1464.

153. Scheinman MM, Peters RW, Modin G, et al. Prognostic value of infranodal conduction time in patients with chronic bundle branch block. *Circulation.* 1977;56:240–244.

154. Denes P, Levy L, Pick A, Rosen KM. The incidence of typical and atypical A-V Wenckebach periodicity. *Am Heart J.* 1975;89:26–31.

155. Meytes I, Kaplinsky E, Yahini JH, et al. Wenckebach A-V block: a frequent feature following heavy physical training. *Am Heart J.* 1975;90:426–430.

156. Shaw DB, Kekwick CA, Veale D, et al. Survival in second degree atrioventricular block. *Br Heart J.* 1985;53:587–593.

157. Narula OS, Smet P. Wenckebach and Mobitz type II A-V block due to block within the His bundle and bundle branches. *Circulation.* 1970;41:947–965.

158. Miles Wm, Klein LS. Sinus nodal dysfunction and atrioventricular conduction disturbances. In: Naccarelli GV ed. *Cardiac Arrhythmias: A Practical Approach.* Mt. Kisco, NY: Futura; 1991:243–282.

159. Damato AN, Lau SH, Helfant RH, et al. A study of heart block in man using His bundle recordings. *Circulation.* 1969;39:297–305.

160. Rosen KM, Gunnar RM, Rahimtoola SH. Site and type of second degree AV block. *Chest.* 1972;61:99–100.

161. MacMurray FG. Stokes-Adams disease. *New Eng J Med.* 1957;256:643–652.

162. Lepeschkin E. The electrocardiographic diagnosis of bilateral bundle branch block in relation to heart block. *Progr Cardiovasc Dis.* 1964;6:445–451.

163. Pinsky W, Gillette PC, Garson AT. Diagnosis, management and long term results of patients with complete atrioventricular block. *Pediatrics.* 1982;69:728–733.

164. Zipes DP, Ackerman MJ, Estes MIII, et al. Task force 7: arrhythmias. *J Am Coll Cardiol.* 2005;45:1354–1363.

165. Hussain Z, Swindle J, Hauptman PJ. Digoxin use and digoxin toxicity in the post-DIG era. *J Card Fail.* 2006;12(5):343–346.

166. Josephson ME, Kastor JA. Supraventricular tachycardia: mechanisms and management. *Ann Intern Med.* 1977;87: 346–358.

167. Akhtar M. Supraventicular tachycardias. Electrophysiologic mechanisms, diagnosis, and pharmacologic therapy. In: Josephson ME, Wellens HJJ, eds. *Tachycardias: Mechanisms, Diagnosis, Treatment.* Philadelphia, PA: Lea & Febiger; 1984:137.

168. Josephson ME, Seides SE, Batsford WB, et al. The effects of carotid sinus pressure in reentrant paroxysmal supraventricular tachycardia. *Am Heart J.* 1974;88:694–695.

169. DiMarco JP, Sellers TD, Bere RM, West GA. Adenosine: electrophysiologic effects and therapeutic use for terminating paroxysmal supraventricular tachycardias. *Circulation.* 1983;68:1254–1263.

170. Belhassen B, Glick A, Laniado S. Comparative clinical and electrophysiologic effects of adenosine triphosphate and verapamil on paroxysmal reciprocating junctional tachycardia. *Circulation.* 1988;77:795–805.

171. Belhassen B, Pelleg A. Acute management of paroxysmal supraventricular tachycardia: verapamil, adenosine triphoshate or adenosine? *Am J Cardiol.* 1984;54:225–227.

172. Stevenson WG, Delacretaz E. Electrophysiology: radiofrequency catheter ablation of ventricular tachycardia. *Heart.* 2000;84:553–559.

173. Kuchar DL, Ruskin JN, Garan H. Electrocardiographic localization of the site of origin of ventricular tachycardia in patients with prior myocardial infarction. *J Am Coll Cardiol.* 1989;13:893–903.

174. Lown B, Wolf M. Approaches to sudden death from coronary heart disease. *Circulation.* 1971;44:130–142.

175. Flemming M, Oral H, Kim M, et al. Electrocardiographic predictors of successful ablation of tachycardia or bigeminy arising in the right ventricular outflow tract. *Am J Cardiol.* 1999;84:1266–1268.

176. Friedman PA, Asirvatham SJ, Grice S, et al. Noncontact mapping to guide ablation of right ventricular outflow tract tachycardia. *J Am Coll Cardiol.* 2002;39:1808–1812.

177. Takemoto M, Yoshimura H, Ohba Y, et al. Radiofrequency catheter ablation of premature ventricular complexes from right ventricular outflow tract improves left ventricular dilation and clinical status in patients without structural heart disease. *J Am Coll Cardiol.* 2005;45:125–165.

178. Kennedy HL, Underhill SJ. Frequent or complex ventricular ectopy in apparently healthy subjects. *Am J Cardiol.* 1976;38:141–148.

179. Bigger JT Jr, Fleiss JL, Kleiger R, Miller JP, Rolnitzky LM. The relationships among ventricular arrhythmias, left ventricular dysfunction, and mortality in the 2 years after myocardial infarction. *Circulation.* 1984;69:250–258.

180. The Multicenter Postinfarction Research Group. Risk stratification and survival after myocardial infarction. *N Engl J Med.* 1983;309:331–336.

181. Kotler MN, Tabatznik B, Mower MM, Tominaga S. Prognostic significance of ventricular ectopic beats with respect to sudden death in the late postinfarction period. *Circulation.* 1973;47:959–966.

182. Holmes J, Kubo SH, Cody RJ, Kligfield P. Arrhythmias in ischemic and nonischemic dilated cardiomyopathy: prediction of mortality by ambulatory electrocardiography. *Am J Cardiol.* 1985;55:146–151.

183. Prystowsky EN, Heger JJ, Zipes DP. The recognition and treatment of patients at risk for sudden death. In: Eliot RS, Saenz A, Forker AD, eds. *Cardiac Emergencies.* Mt. Kisco, NY: Futura Publishing Co; 1982:353–384.

184. Ruberman W, Weinblatt E, Goldberg JD, et al. Ventricular premature beats and mortality after myocardial infarction. *N Engl J Med.* 1977;297:750–757.

185. Moss AJ, David HT, DeCamilla J, Bayer LW. Ventricular ectopic beats and their relation to sudden and nonsudden cardiac death after myocardial infarction. *Circulation.* 1979;60:988–997.

186. Maggioni AP, Zuanetti G, Franzosi MG, et al. Prevalence and prognostic significance of ventricular arrhythmias after acute myocardial infarction in the fibrinolytic era. *Circulation.* 1993;87:312–322.

187. Buxton AE, Fisher JD, Josephson ME, et al. and the MUSTT Investigators. Prevention of sudden death in patients with coronary artery disease. *Prog Cardiovasc Dis.* 1993;36:215–226.

188. Epstein AW, Bigger JT Jr, Wyse DG, et al. Events in the Cardiac Arrhythmia Suppression Trial (CAST): mortality in the entire population enrolled. *J Am Coll Cardiol.* 1991;18:14–19.

189. Greene HL, Roden DM, Katz RJ, et al. The Cardiac Arrhythmia Suppression Trial: first CAST then CAST-II. *J Am Coll Cardiol.* 1992;19:894–898.

190. Julian DG, Camm AJ, Frangin G, et al. Randomized trial of effect of amiodarone on mortality in patients with left-ventricular dysfunction after recent myocardial infarction: EMIAT. *Lancet.* 1997;349:667–673.

191. Cairns JA, Connolly SJ, Roberts R, Gent M (for the Canadian Amiodarone Myocardial Infarction Arrhythmia Trial Investigators). Randomized trial of outcome after myocardial infarction in patients with frequent or repetitive ventricular premature depolarizations: CAMIAT. *Lancet.* 1997;349:675–682.

192. Nakagawa H, Beckman KJ, McClelland JH, et al. Radiofrequency catheter ablation of idiopathic left ventricular tachycardia guided by a Purkinje potential. *Circulation.* 1993;23:1333–1341.

193. Rodriguez LM, Smeets JL, Timmermans C, et al. Predictors of successful ablation of right- and left-sided idiopathic ventricular tachycardia. *Am J Cardiol.* 1997;79(3):309–314.

194. Belhassen B, Rotmensch HH, Laniado S. Response of recurrent sustained ventricular tachycardia to verapamil. *Br Heart J.* 1981;46:679–682.

195. Lin FC, Finley CD, Rahimtoola SH, Wu D. Idiopathic paroxysmal ventricular tachycardia with a QRS pattern of right bundle branch block and left axis deviation: a unique clinical entity with specific properties. *Am Cardiol.* 1983;52: 95–100.

196. Ohe T, Aihara N, Kamakura S, Kurita T, Shiniizu W, Shimomura K. Long-term outcome of verapamil-sensitive sustained left ventricular tachycardia in patients without structural heart disease. *J Am Coil Cardiol.* 1995;25: 54–58.

197. Corrado D, Basso C, Thiene G, et al. Spectrum of clinicopathologic manifestations of arrhythmogenic right ventricular cardiomyopathy/dysplasia: a multicenter study. *J Am Coll Cardiol.* 1997;30:1512–1520.

198. Daliento L, Rizzoli G, Thiene G, et al. . Diagnostic accuracy of right ventriculography in arrhythmogenic right ventricular cardiomyopathy. *Am J Cardiol.* 1997;66:741–745.

199. Ricci C, Longo R, Pagnan L, et al. Magnetic resonance imaging in right ventricular dysplasia. *Am J Cardiol.* 1992;70:1589–1595.

200. Blake LM, Scheinman MM, Higgins CB. MR features of arrhythmogenic right ventricular dysplasia. *Am J Radiol.* 1994;162:809–812.

201. Asimaki A, Tandri H, Huang H, et al. A new diagnostic test for arrhythmogenic right ventricular cardiomyopathy. *New Engl J Med.* 2009;360:1075–1084.

202. Zipes DP, Camm AJ, Borggrefe M, et al. ACC/AHA/ESC 2006 guidelines for management of patients with ventricular arrhythmias and the prevention of sudden cardiac death—executive summary: a report of the American College of Cardiology/American Heart Association Task Force and the European Society of Cardiology Committee for Practice Guidelines (Writing Committee to Develop Guidelines for Management of Patients With Ventricular Arrhythmias and the Prevention of Sudden Cardiac Death). *J Am Coll Cardiol.* 2006;48:1064–1108.

203. Maggioni AP, Zuanetti G, Franzosi MG, et al. Prevalence and prognostic significance of ventricular arrhythmias after acute myocardial infarction in the fibrinolytic era. GISSI-2 results. *Circulation.* 1993;87:312–322.

204. Blnck Z, Dhala A, Deshpande S, et al. Bundle branch reentrant ventricular tachycardia: cumulative experience in 48 patients. *J Cardiovasc Electrophysiol.* 1993;4:23–62.

205. Delacretaz E, Stevenson WG, Ellison KE, et al. Mapping and radiofrequency catheter ablation of the tree types of sustained monomorphic ventricular tachycardias in nonischemic heart disease. *J Cardiovasc Electrophysiol.* 2000;1: 11–17.

206. Sosa E, Scanavacca M, D'Avila A, et al. Endocardial and epicardial ablation guided by nonsurgical transthoracic epicardial mapping to treat recurrent ventricular tachycardia. *J Cardiovasc Electrophysiol.* 1998;9:229–239.

207. The Antiarrhythmics versus Implantable Defibrillators (AVID) Investigators. A comparison of antiarrhythmic-drug therapy with implantable defibrillators in patients resuscitated from near-fatal ventricular arrhythmias. *N Engl J Med.* 1997;337:1576–1583.

208. Connolly SJ, Gent M, Roberts RS, et al. Canadian implantable defibrillator study (CIDS): a randomized trial of the implantable cardioverter defibrillator against amiodarone. *Circulation.* 2000;101:1297–1302.

209. Kuck KH, Cappato R, Siebels J, et al. Randomized comparison of antiarrhythmic drug therapy with implantable defibrillators in patients resuscitated from cardiac arrest: the Cardiac Arrest Study Hamburg (CASH). *Circulation.* 2000;102:748–754.

210. Buxton AE, Lee KL, Fisher JD, et al. A randomized study of the prevention of sudden death in patients with coronary artery disease. Multicenter Unsustained Tachycardia Trial Investigators. *N Engl J Med.* 1993;341:1882–1890.

211. Moss AJ, Jackson Hall W, Canom DS, et al. Improved survival with an implanted defibrillator in patients with coronary disease at high risk for ventricular arrhythmia. *N Engl J Med.* 1996;335:1933–1940.

212. Bardy GH, Lee KL, Mark DB, et al. Amiodarone or an implantable cardioverter-defibrillator for congestive heart failure. *N Engl J Med.* 2005;352:225–237.

213. Moss AJ, Zareba W, Jackson Hall W, et al. Prophylactic implantation of a defibrillator in patients with myocardial infarction and reduced ejection fraction. *N Engl J Med.* 2002;346:877–883.

214. Akhtar M, Shenasa M, Jazayeri M, Caceres J. Wide QRS complex tachycardia. Reappraisal of a common clinical problem. *Ann Intern Med.* 1988;109:905–912.

215. Wellens HJ, Bar FW. The value of the electrocardiogram in the differential diagnosis of a tachycardia with a widened QRS complex. *Am J Med.* 1978;64:27–33.

216. Kindwall KE, Brown J, Josephson ME. Electrocardiographic criteria for ventricular tachycardia in wide complex left bundle branch block morphology tachycardias. *Am J Cardiol.* 1988;61:1279–1283.

217. Griffith MJ, de Belder MA, Linker NJ, Ward DE. Multivariate analysis to simplify the differential diagnosis of broad complex tachycardia. *Br Heart J.* 1991;66:166–174.

218. Brugada P, Brugada J, Mont L, Smeets J. A new approach to the differential diagnosis of a regular tachycardia with a wide QRS complex. *Circulation.* 1991;83:1649–1659.

219. Alberca T, Almendral J, Sanz P, Almazan A, Cantalapiedra JL. Evaluation of the specificity of morphological electro-cardiographic criteria for the differential diagnosis of wide QRS complex tachycardia in patients with intraventricular conduction defects. *Circulation.* 1997;96:3527–3533.

220. Vereckei A, Duray G, Szénási G, Altmose GT, Miller JM. Application of a new algorithm in the differential diagnosis of wide QRS complex tachycardia. *Eur Heart J.* 2007;28:589–600.

221. Dendi R, Josephson ME. A new algorithm in the differential diagnosis of wide complex tachycardia. *Eur Heart J.* 2007;28:525–526.

222. Roberts R. Genomics and cardiac arrhythmias. *J Am Coll Cardiol.* 2006;47:9–21.

223. Kaab S, Schulze-Bahr E. Susceptibility genes and modifiers for cardiac arrhythmias. *Cardiovasc Res.* 2005;6:397–413.

224. Wiesfeld ACP, Hemels MEW, VanTintelen P, Van den Berg MP, Van Veldhuisen DJ, Van Gelder IC. Genetic aspects of atrial fibrillation. *Cardiovasc Res.* 2005;67:414–418.

225. Maron BJ, McKenna WJ, Danielson GK, et al. ACC/ESC clinical expert consensus document on hypertrophic cardiomyopathy: a report of the American College of Cardiology Task Force on Clinical Expert Consensus Documents and the European Society of Cardiology Committee for Practice Guidelines (Committee to Develop an Expert Consensus Document on Hypertrophic Cardiomyopathy). *J Am Coll Cardiol.* 2003;42:1687–1713.

226. Panza JA, Maron BJ. Relation of electrocardiographic abnormalities to evolving left ventricular hypertrophy in hypertrophic cardiomyopathy during childhood. *Am J Cardiol.* 1989;63:1258–1265.

227. Brugada R, Brugada J, Antzelevitch C, et al. Sodium channel blockers identify risk for sudden death in patients with ST-segment elevation and right bundle branch block but structurally normal hearts. *Circulation.* 2000;101:510–515.

228. Yan GX, Antzelevitch C. Cellular basis for the Brugada syndrome and other mechanisms of arrhythmogenesis associated with ST-segment elevation. *Circulation.* 1999;100:1660–1666.

229. Wang K, Asinger RW, Marriott HJL. ST-Segment elevation in conditions other than acute myocardial infarction. *N Engl J Med.* 2003;349:2128–2135.

230. Goldenberg I, Moss AJ, Zareba W. QT Interval: how to measure it and what is "normal". *J Cardiovasc Electrophysiol.* 2006;17:333–336.

25 Evidence-Based Management of the Patient with Congestive Heart Failure

Nicolas W. Shammas

CONTENTS

Key Words: Congestive heart failure; Echocardiography; Systolic dysfunction; Diastolic dysfunction; Pulmonary edema.

KEY POINTS

- The sympathetic nervous system and the renin–angiotensin–aldosterone system are therapeutic targets in patients with congestive heart failure.
- Modifiable risk factors for the development of congestive heart failure include diabetes, coronary artery disease, valvular heart disease, hypertension, and excessive alcohol intake.
- Treatment of chronic symptomatic congestive heart failure consists of beta blockers, ACEI, and/or ARB, diuretics to induce a euvolemic state, and in advanced symptomatic patients (Class III or IV) aldosterone antagonists.
- Heart failure with normal systolic ejection fraction (HFNEF) is present in approximately 50% of heart failure patients. No evidence-based treatment for HFNEF exists to date. Aggressive blood pressure control is a Class I indication. The use of ACEI or ARB particularly in patients with diabetes and LV hypertrophy is recommended.
- Intravenous positive inotropes lead to increased mortality and are best avoided when possible except to achieve hemodynamic stability. In patients with atrial fibrillation, maintaining normal sinus rhythm in patients with congestive heart failure can help improve cardiac output.
- In patients with advanced congestive heart failure, mechanical devices such as biventricular pacing, implantable cardioverter defibrillator (ICD), or left ventricular assist devices are important therapies in eligible patients.

From: *Contemporary Cardiology: Comprehensive Cardiovascular Medicine in the Primary Care Setting*
Edited by: Peter P. Toth, Christopher P. Cannon, DOI 10.1007/978-1-60327-963-5_25
© Springer Science+Business Media, LLC 2010

25.1. EPIDEMIOLOGY OF CONGESTIVE HEART FAILURE

Congestive heart failure (CHF) is the result of either a weak heart muscle (systolic failure) or a stiff ventricle (diastolic failure). Systolic and diastolic failure may coexist in the same patient *(1)*. Irrespective of the etiology, it leads to an inadequate amount of oxygenated blood to meet cellular demand.

CHF is a growing problem in the United States and particularly in the elderly *(2)*. Over half a million cases are diagnosed on an annual basis with subsequent high mortality *(3)* and a large cost to our economic system *(4)*.

Although less studied, diastolic failure occurs in approximately 30–35% of all patients and 55% of the elderly with CHF *(5, 6)*. Recently heart failure with normal left ventricular function (HFNEF) is a term that has been more widely used than "diastolic heart failure" and describes a heterogeneous group of patients with a number of pathological mechanisms *(7)*. It is estimated that 50% of HF patients have HFNEF and display similar physiologic and neurohormonal phenotypes to patients with HF and reduced systolic function. Unless more effective acute and preventative therapies are implemented in treating CHF patients, the social burden in treating these patients will continue to rise *(8)*.

CHF appears to be on the rise in the United States *(4, 9)* and is partly due to the high prevalence of the metabolic syndrome, diabetes mellitus, hypertension, and obesity *(10)*. Although improvement in survival has been noted in the younger heart failure patient over the past two decades, this benefit has not been seen in the elderly and females *(11)*. Survival has improved however in both genders over the past 50 years *(12)*.

25.2. PATHOPHYSIOLOGY OF CONGESTIVE HEART FAILURE

There are multiple risk factors that lead to injury to the myocardium including coronary artery disease (CAD), hypertension, valvular heart disease, diabetes mellitus, congenital heart defects, anemia, metabolic syndrome, cardiotoxins, and alcoholism *(13, 14)*. Left ventricular remodeling with reduction of left ventricular function (as measured by the ejection fraction) and dilatation of the left ventricle subsequently occur. The remodeling process is initially an adaptation mechanism to reduce wall stress and increase cardiac output by hypertrophy of viable myocytes. Hypertrophy, however, eventually leads to an increase in mass-to-volume ratio and premature myocyte cell death *(15)*. As the syndrome of heart failure occurs, a patient presents with fatigue, increased weight, dyspnea, orthopnea, paroxysmal nocturnal dyspnea, and chest pain. A reduced left ventricular function increases the risk of arrhythmias and sudden cardiac death as well as pump failure *(16, 17)*.

Cardiac remodeling is mediated partly by the renin–angiotensin–aldosterone (RAAS) system and the sympathetic nervous system (SNS) (Fig. 1). Activation of the RAAS system leads to a rise in angiotensin II (AII); sodium retention and myocardial fibrosis mediated by angiotensin II and aldosterone; peripheral vasoconstriction; and endothelial injury *(18)*, which lead to programmed cell death (apoptosis), hypertrophy, and fibrosis. AII also promotes aldosterone secretion. In addition, vasoconstrictors such as endothelin-1 and reactive oxygen species (ROS) are increased and nitric oxide (NO) synthesis and release are reduced, all contributing to vasoconstriction *(18, 19, 20)*. Furthermore, endothelial dysfunction is further impaired by the increase in inflammatory markers and cytokines *(19, 21, 22)*.

Elevated sympathetic tone is part of the syndrome of heart failure with elevation of circulating catecholamines and suppression of adrenergic receptors *(23)*. Adrenaline has direct toxic effect on the myocardium *(24)*. Also, it induces cellular calcium overload *(25)*, decreases myocardial mechanical efficiency, precipitates arrhythmias, increases myocardial oxygen consumption and coronary blood flow requirements, and induces left ventricular hypertrophy *(26)*.

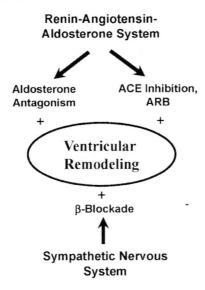

Fig. 1. The renin–angiotensin–aldosterone system and the sympathetic nervous system promote ventricular remodeling, a process that can be reversed with aldosterone antagonism, ACEI, or ARB and beta blockade.

The SNS and the RAAS systems are therapeutic targets, and blocking their activation has been shown to reduce mortality and morbidity in patients with CHF. Aldosterone is only partially produced as a result of angiotensin activation, and therefore, AII suppression *(27)* is not adequate to block its secretion. The addition of aldosterone blockers is, therefore, needed for optimal suppression of aldosterone, and it has been shown to provide additional reductions in mortality and morbidity in patients with CHF *(28, 29)* (Fig. 2). Finally, beta adrenergic blockade also contributes in reducing the activity of the RAAS *(30)*.

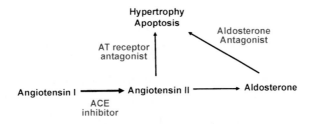

Fig. 2. Interventions to block the renin–angiotensin–aldosterone system.

Several other therapies have been tested in CHF patients and have shown conflicting results. These include vasopeptidase inhibitors, endothelin antagonists, immunomodulating agents, and growth hormone *(31)*. At the present time, interventions that modulate the SNS and RAAS remain the only proven treatment to reduce mortality and morbidity in patients with congestive heart failure.

HFNEF describes a heterogeneous pool of patients that make about 50% of HF patients with a unique set of pathophysiologic mechanisms. These patients are typically older with hypertension, obesity, renal failure, anemia, and atrial fibrillation and are more likely to be females. There is also a high incidence of diabetes and coronary artery disease in these patients *(7)*. In contrast to patients with impaired left ventricular EF, HFNEF patients have non-dilated left ventricular cavity size, concentric instead of eccentric left ventricular hypertrophy, and a normal EF *(32)*.

It is controversial whether LV systolic function is truly normal in patients with HFNEF because EF is an imprecise measure of left ventricular systolic function. However, invasive conductance studies suggested from pressure–volume loops that end-systolic pressure–volume relationship is steeper or normal in HFNEF suggesting a normal systolic function. On the other hand, end-diastolic pressure–volume relationship is shifted leftward and upward indicating diastolic dysfunction *(33, 34)*.

Diastolic dysfunction is not uncommon among elderly patients estimated at about 5.6%, but only 1% has HFNEF *(35)*. In one study, the product of left ventricular mass index and left atrial volume has the highest predictive accuracy for HFNEF *(36)*. In addition to ventricular stiffness, arterial stiffness has also been suggested to contribute to HFNEF, and the combined ventricular–arterial stiffness leads to an exaggerated hypertensive response after small increases in LV end-diastolic volume *(7)*.

25.3. ACC/AHA CLASSIFICATION OF CONGESTIVE HEART FAILURE

The current ACC/AHA classification for CHF *(3)* is complementary to the New York Heart classification (NYHC) *(37)* and helps define the evolution of symptoms of patients with CHF. In addition, the ACC/AHA classification focuses on the risk factors for CHF by identifying patients who have risk factors for CHF.

This classification includes four stages of CHF:

Stage A: Asymptomatic patients with no left ventricular dysfunction but are at risk of developing CHF including patients with coronary artery disease, hypertension, diabetes mellitus, family history of cardiomyopathy, and the metabolic syndrome.

Stage A is not represented in the NYHC.

Stage B: Asymptomatic patients with left ventricular dysfunction. This is equivalent to Class I of the NYHC.

Stage C: Symptomatic patients with exertion and with left ventricular dysfunction. This is equivalent to the NYHC Class II and Class III and includes about five million people in the United States.

Stage D: Symptomatic patients at rest. This is equivalent to Class IV of the NYHC and includes about 200,000 people in the United States.

25.4. PHARMACOLOGIC THERAPY OF CONGESTIVE HEART FAILURE

25.4.1. Heart Failure with Normal Ejection Fraction (HFNEF) and Diastolic Dysfunction

As noted above, one of the main pathophysiologic mechanisms of HFNEF is diastolic dysfunction, but not all patients with diastolic dysfunction have heart failure and not all patients with HF and diastolic dysfunction represent "true" HFNEF. "True" HFNEF does not include those with coronary artery disease, valvular heart disease, restrictive or constrictive cardiomyopathy, obesity, pulmonary hypertension and right-sided failure, high-output failure caused by anemia, thyrotoxicosis or arteriovenous fistula, constrictive pericarditis, or intracardiac shunt.

Diastolic dysfunction has been associated with many conditions including coronary artery disease, hypertension, valvular disease, age *(38)*, elevated triglyceride levels possibly secondary to intracellular lipid accumulation *(39)*, sleep apnea *(40)*, and hypertrophic cardiomyopathy. Treatment with an ARB (losartan) has yielded improvement in diastolic function but did not change left ventricular cavity size or mass *(41)*.

Isolated diastolic dysfunction is uncommon and has been identified in 11.5% of patients with no CAD or valvular disease with the use of echocardiography *(42)*. Increase in left atrial size and

N-terminal pro B-type natriuretic peptide (NT-proBNP) appears to be predictors of LV diastolic dysfunction (43). Also, varying degrees of diastolic dysfunction are seen with different left ventricular geometric patterns (44).

Recently an algorithm to diagnose HFNEF has been proposed by the Working Group of the European Society of Cardiology (45). In general, patients with signs and symptoms of HF, normal EF > 50%, LVEDVI < 97 mL/m^2, and with evidence of abnormal LV relaxation, filling, diastolic distensibility, and diastolic stiffness will meet the diagnosis of HFNEF if one of the following three criteria is met: mean PCWP > 12 mmHg or LVEDP > 16 mmHg by invasive testing; E/E' > 15 by tissue Doppler, or 8 < E/E' < 15 by tissue Doppler with a BNP > 200 pg/mL and/or NT-proBNP > 220 pg/mL or BNP > 200 pg/mL and/or NT-proBNP > 220 pg/mL and LVH or atrial fibrillation or left atrial dilation, or abnormal pulmonary venous return.

Patients with left ventricular diastolic dysfunction need to be treated with aggressive blood pressure control with the use of diuretics, beta blockers, or non-dihydropyridine calcium channel blockers (diltiazem or verapamil) (46). The ACC/AHA 2005 Guidelines recommend blood pressure control as a Class I, level A in patients with HFNEF (47).

ACE inhibitors or angiotensin receptor blockers (ARBs) can have long-term value in reducing left ventricular hypertrophy and theoretically may improve left ventricular compliance (48) and improve diastolic function in contrast to hydralazine and hydrochlorothiazide (49). In the Hong Kong Diastolic Heart Failure Study (50), diuretics in combination with an ACEI (ramipril) or ARB (irbesartan) marginally improved LV systolic and diastolic function and lowered BNP at 1 year.

Aldosterone antagonist appears to have a beneficial effect on diastolic function particularly in the elderly, possibly by reducing myocardial fibrosis (51). Losartan and amlodipine are currently being tested in The Effect of Losartan and Amlodipine on Left Ventricular Diastolic Function in Patients With Mild-to-Moderate Hypertension (J-ELAN) to determine their role in improving diastolic function (52).

Diastolic dysfunction also has been described in diabetic patients with impaired glucose tolerance and insulin resistance (53) and is associated with endothelial dysfunction and abnormalities on stress myocardial single-photon emission computed tomography (54). Glycemic control shows an improvement in diastolic parameters that was inversely correlated with percent changes in glycated hemoglobin (55).

In the Euro Heart Failure Survey I, preserved systolic function is also seen in elderly patients with HF (56). These patients typically have a high mortality. Measurements of EF and lifesaving therapies are quite often underutilized in this group of patients with multiple comorbidities. The use of beta blockers and ACEI was associated with a better outcome in these patients.

In conclusion, ACEI and ARB are important therapies in reducing left ventricular hypertrophy and improving left ventricular diastolic function. The role of beta blockers and calcium channel blockers remains unclear but may be considered. Diuretics reduce left ventricular filling pressures and improve symptoms. Risk factor modification is also important including treatment of hypertension, diabetes, sleep apnea, elevated triglycerides, coronary artery disease, and valvular disease.

25.4.2. Asymptomatic Left Ventricular Systolic Dysfunction

Asymptomatic left ventricular dysfunction (Stage B, ACC/AHA classification) is prevalent and typically identified by echocardiography (57). Asymptomatic left ventricular systolic dysfunction (ejection fraction ≤50%) was reported in 6.0% of men and 0.8% of women with a hazard ratio for CHF of 4.7 on 12 years follow-up (58). Neurohormonal activation is present in patients with asymptomatic left ventricular dysfunction and leads to worsening left ventricular function and progression to symptomatic failure *(59)*.

Risk factors modification is also important in these patients including treatment of hypertension, diabetes, sleep apnea, elevated triglycerides, coronary artery disease *(60)*, valvular disease, smoking cessation, reducing alcohol intake or illicit drug use, and routine exercise. Tachycardia-induced cardiomyopathy needs to be recognized and treated. Anemia has been associated with asymptomatic left ventricular dysfunction and progression to heart failure particularly when the hematocrit is $\leq 40\%$ *(61)*.

Beta blockers and ACEI are important therapy in Stage B CHF including the post-myocardial infarction patients *(61, 62)* and has been shown to improve left ventricular EF *(63)* and reduce progression to heart failure *(64)*. In the SOLVD trial *(65)*, asymptomatic patients with reduced left ventricular function (EF<35%) were randomized to enalapril ($n = 2,117$) versus placebo ($n = 2,111$) and followed for an average of 37.4 months. The reduction in cardiovascular mortality was larger in the enalapril group than placebo (risk reduction of 12%, $p = 0.12$). Also, the combined endpoint of death and heart failure was 36% lower in the enalapril group ($p < 0.001$).

ARBs are a reasonable alternative to ACEI *(66)*. The role of calcium channel blockers or digoxin in Stage B CHF is unclear. Endothelin A/B receptor antagonists (enrasentan) increases resting cardiac index, but was associated with more serious adverse events (16.7 and 2.8%, respectively, $p = 0.02$) than enalapril *(67)*.

As per *ACC/AHA Guideline Update 2005*, patients with asymptomatic left ventricular dysfunction post-myocardial infarction and an EF of $\leq 30\%$ despite optimal medical therapy for at least 40 days post-MI need to be considered for an implantable defibrillator (ICD) without requiring screening for ventricular arrhythmias, whether occurring spontaneously or induced by electrophysiologic testing *(68–70)*. ICD therapy in this population yielded a 31% reduction in mortality during an average follow-up of 20 months *(70)*.

Echocardiography or isotope ventriculography has been used for periodic follow-up of patients with asymptomatic left ventricular dysfunction. Patients with familial cardiomyopathy need to have their immediate family members screened for asymptomatic left ventricular dysfunction *(71)*.

25.4.3. Symptomatic Left Ventricular Systolic Dysfunction

Symptomatic left ventricular systolic dysfunction (Stage C, ACC/AHA classification) requires close follow-up and intense pharmacologic treatment (Table 1). In addition to risk factor modifications, patients will need to be treated with pharmacologic and mechanical means to improve their morbidity and mortality. Serial monitoring of ejection fraction is also important. A summary of therapies for Stage C CHF is presented below.

25.4.4. Angiotensin Converting Enzyme Inhibitors (ACEI)

ACEIs reduce mortality by 15–20% and rehospitalizations by 30–35% in patients with left ventricular systolic dysfunction (ejection fraction of <40%). The Cooperative North Scandinavian Enalapril Survival Study (CONSENSUS) compared the effects of enalapril versus placebo on mortality in patients with severe CHF. Enalapril reduced mortality by 31% at 1 year ($p = 0.001$) as well as congestive heart failure hospitalization *(72)*. The SOLVD trial also confirmed the same findings. Patients receiving conventional treatment for Class II and III heart failure were randomly assigned to receive either placebo ($n = 1,284$) or enalapril ($n = 1,285$). Enalapril reduced mortality by 16% ($p = 0.0036$) and mortality and congestive heart failure by 26% ($p < 0.0001$) at an average follow-up of 41.4 months *(73)*. Furthermore, SOLVD showed that enalapril attenuates progressive increases in left ventricular dilatation and hypertrophy in patients with reduced left ventricular function *(74)*. Finally, Pitt and colleagues also has shown that enalapril reduced development of heart failure by 37% and hospitalization from heart failure by 36% ($p < 0.001$) *(75)*.

Table 1

Commonly Used Drugs in the Treatment of Congestive Heart Failure

Angiotensin converting enzyme inhibitors
Accupril 5–40 mg PO QD, max 40 mg/day, start 5–10 mg PO QD
Captopril 12.5–50 mg PO TID, max 150 mg/day, start 6.25–12.5 mg PO TID
Enalapril 2.5–20 mg PO BID, max 40 mg/day, start at 2.5 mg QD
Lisinopril 5–20 mg PO QD, max 40 mg/day, start 2.5–5 mg PO QD
Monopril 10–40 mg PO QD/BID, max 80 mg/day, start 10 mg PO QD
Perindopril 4–16 mg PO QD, max 16 mg/day, start 2 mg PO QD
Ramipril 5 mg PO BID, max 10 mg/day, start at 2.5 mg PO BID

Angiotensin receptor blockers
Losartan 25–100 mg PO QD, max 100 mg/day, start 25–50 mg PO QD[a]
Candesartan 8–32 mg PO QD, max 32 mg/day, start 16 mg PO QD[a]
Valsartan 40–160 mg PO BID, max 320 mg/day, start 40 mg PO BID
Irbesartan 75–300 mg PO QD, max 300 mg/day, start 75 mg PO QD[a]

Beta blockers
Carvedilol 3.125–25 mg PO BID, max 50 mg PO QD, start 3.125 mg PO BID
Metoprolol succinate 12.5–200 mg PO QD, max 200 mg/day, start 12.5 mg PO QD
Bisoprolol 5–10 mg PO QD, max 10 mg PO QD, start 2.5 mg PO QD[a]

Aldosterone antagonists
Spironolactone 12.5–25 mg PO BID, max 50 mg/day, start 12.5 mg PO BID
Eplerenone 50 mg PO QD, Max 50 mg/day, start 25 mg PO QD[b]

[a]Off label use.
[b]For CHF patients post-myocardial infarction.

ACEI post-MI has also shown a significant mortality benefit. The Acute Infarction Ramipril Efficacy (AIRE) study *(76)* showed a 27% ($p = 0.002$) reduction in the 30-month cumulative mortality with ramipril over placebo in post-MI CHF patients. Also, in the Survival and Ventricular Enlargement (SAVE) trial *(77)*, captopril was administered 3–16 days after myocardial infarction in patients with asymptomatic left ventricular dysfunction (EF<40%) and followed for an average of 42 months. Captopril improved survival (risk reduction was 19%, $p = 0.019$) and morbidity. In addition, in the Trandolapril Cardiac Evaluation (TRACE) study, trandolapril reduced mortality by 22% ($p = 0.01$) in patients with reduced left ventricular function after an MI. Trandolapril reduced overall mortality, mortality from cardiovascular causes, sudden death, and the development of severe heart failure *(78)*. Finally, in the Survival of Myocardial Infarction Long-Term Evaluation (SMILE) study *(79)*, zofenopril reduced the risk of death or severe congestive heart failure by 34% ($p = 0.018$) at 6 weeks when initiated early after MI. At 1 year, the reduction in mortality risk was 29% ($p = 0.011$).

Early initiation of ACEI in hospital leads to a higher use of ACEI on an outpatient basis and, therefore, initiating ACEI early is important in all patients with CHF.

25.4.5. Angiotensin Receptor Blockers (ARB)

ARB is an effective treatment in patients with CHF. In the Randomized Evaluation of Strategies for Left Ventricular Dysfunction (RESOLVD) pilot study *(27)*, 768 patients in NYHC II to IV and EF <40% received candesartan, candesartan plus enalapril, or enalapril alone for 43 weeks. Left ventricular cavity size increased less and BNP levels decreased more with combination therapy compared to ARB or ACEI alone *(66)*.

In the Evaluation of Losartan in the Elderly (ELITE) trial *(80)*, 722 patients with EF $\leq$40%, $\geq$65 years of age, and in NYHC Class II–IV were included. The primary endpoint was death and/or hospital admission for heart failure and occurred at a rate of 9.4% in the losartan group compared to 13.2% in the captopril group (risk reduction 32%, $p = 0.075$). This risk reduction was primarily due to a decrease in all-cause mortality (4.8 versus 8.7%; risk reduction 46%, $p = 0.035$) with similar rates of hospital admissions in both groups (5.7%). ELITE II *(81)* randomized 3,152 patients aged 60 years or older with NYHC II–IV and ejection fraction of <40% to losartan ($n = 1,578$) titrated to 50 mg once daily or captopril ($n = 1,574$) titrated to 50 mg three times daily. ELITE II showed no differences in mortality between losartan and captopril and confirmed that ARB therapy can be a potential substitute to ACEI.

The Valsartan in Heart Failure Trial (Val-HeFT) *(82)* randomized 5,010 patients with heart failure of New York Heart Association (NYHA) Class II, III, or IV to receive 160 mg of valsartan or placebo twice daily. The primary outcomes were mortality and the combined endpoint of mortality and morbidity, defined as the incidence of cardiac arrest with resuscitation, hospitalization for heart failure, or receipt of intravenous inotropic or vasodilator therapy for at least 4 h. Mortality was similar in both groups, but the combined endpoint of morbidity and mortality was reduced by 13.2% with valsartan ($p = 0.009$), predominantly driven by a reduction in heart failure hospitalizations (13.8 versus 18.2%, $p < 0.001$). In patients intolerant to ACEI, valsartan (titrated to 160 mg twice daily) reduced both all-cause mortality and combined mortality and morbidity compared with placebo (17.3 versus 27.1%, $p = 0.017$ and 24.9 versus 42.5%, $p < 0.001$, respectively) *(83)*. In a substudy of this trial, Valsartan taken with either ACEI or beta blockers reversed left ventricular remodeling *(84)*. Of interest, in the Val-HeFT, valsartan with either a beta blocker or ACEIs showed a positive effect on outcome *(85)*, but an adverse effect in patients receiving both types of drugs *(82)*. This concern of adding an ARB to patients on both ACEI and beta blockers was not confirmed in the CHARM trial.

The Candesartan in Heart Failure Assessment of Reduction in Mortality and morbidity (CHARM) *(83)* was a randomized, double-blind, placebo-controlled, multicenter study in patients with NYHC Class II–IV. This trial had three complementary arms: CHARM-added—candesartan (titrated to 32 mg once daily) is added to an ACEI; CHARM-alternative—candesartan administered to patients who cannot tolerate ACEIs; CHARM-preserved—candesartan is administered to patients with preserved left ventricular function irrespective of whether they are on ACEI or not. In the CHARM-added and CHARM-alternative arms, patients with EF $\leq$ 40% were included. In the "overall programme" of this study *(84)*, which included both preserved and reduced left ventricular function, total mortality was not reduced compared to placebo. However, in a subgroup analysis of patients with symptomatic heart failure and reduced left ventricular function, candesartan significantly reduced all-cause mortality (28 versus 31%, $p = 0.0018$), cardiovascular death (22.8 versus 26.2%, $p = 0.005$), and CHF hospitalizations (22.5 versus 28.1%, $p < 0.001$) when added to standard therapies including ACEI, beta blockers, and aldosterone antagonists *(85)*. Candesartan also reduced progression to diabetes *(86)*, sudden cardiac death, and death from worsening heart failure in patients with symptomatic failure *(83)*.

The Valsartan in Acute Myocardial Infarction Trial (VALIANT) *(87)* randomized patients 0.5–10 days after an acute MI with reduced left ventricular function to valsartan (4,909 patients) titrated to 160 mg twice a day, valsartan (80 mg twice a day) plus captopril (50 mg three times a day) (4,885 patients), or captopril (4,909 patients) alone titrated to 50 mg three times a day in addition to standard therapy. The primary endpoint of the study was all-cause mortality at a median follow-up of 24.7 months. Valsartan was equally effective compared to captopril in reducing all-cause mortality. Also combining valsartan with captopril increased the rate of adverse events without improving survival.

In the Optimal Trial in Myocardial Infarction with Angiotensin II Antagonist Losartan (OPTI-MAAL), patients after an acute myocardial infarction were randomized to losartan versus captopril. The primary endpoint was reduction in all-cause mortality at a mean follow-up of 2.7 years.

A non-significant difference was seen in total mortality in favor of captopril (18 versus 16% in the losartan versus captopril, respectively, $p = 0.07$). However, there were significantly more cardiovascular deaths with losartan (15%) than with captopril (13%) ($p = 0.03$) *(88)*. Losartan was better tolerated than captopril with fewer patients discontinuing their medications (17 versus 23%, $p < 0.0001$) *(89)*. An echocardiographic substudy of the OPTIMAAL trial has shown that both losartan and captopril improve systolic function after an acute MI but the benefit is greater for captopril *(90)*.

A growing body of evidence suggests that an ARB can be an alternative to an ACEI in patients with CHF *(71)*.

25.4.6. Aldosterone Blockers

Angiotensin II is a dominant stimulus of aldosterone secretion *(91)*. Aldosterone secretion, however, continues to escape ACEI or ARB *(27, 92, 93)*. A reduction, however, in aldosterone plasma level is seen with angiotensin blockers *(94)*. Recent data confirms that aldosterone blockers are important to improve morbidity and mortality in patients with CHF and reduced left ventricular systolic function. Aldosterone blockade reduces myocardial fibrosis and ventricular remodeling and has important effects on autonomic balance, fibrinolysis, oxidative stress, and activation of the NF-kappaB and AP-1 signaling pathways *(95)*.

The Randomized Aldactone Evaluation Study (RALES) *(28)* randomized patients ($n = 1,663$) with advanced CHF and EF $\leq$ 35% to spironolactone 25 mg daily ($n = 822$) or placebo ($n = 841$) including ACEI, digoxin, and diuretics. After a mean follow-up of 24 months, the trial was stopped early. Spironolactone reduced the primary endpoint of mortality by 30% (46 versus 35%, $p < 0.001$) primarily due to reduction of progression of CHF and sudden cardiac death (Fig. 3). In addition, spironolactone significantly improved New York Heart Association functional class ($p < 0.001$) and reduced rehospitalization due to worsening CHF by 35% ($p < 0.001$). Spironolactone also increases the risk of hyperkalemia *(96)*, which accounted for an increase in hospitalization from 2.4 per 1,000 patients in 1994 to 11.0 per 1,000 patients in 2001 ($p < 0.001$) and a mortality increase from 0.3 per 1,000 to 2.0 per 1,000 patients ($p < 0.001$). Therefore, close follow-up of patients for serum potassium levels is needed when spironolactone is initiated. Avoiding spironolactone in patients with elevated potassium levels (>5 mEq/L) and high baseline creatinine (>2.0) is advised to avoid serious hyperkalemia problem.

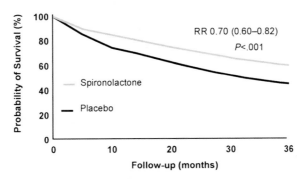

Fig. 3. The Randomized Aldactone Evaluation Study (RALES) showed that at 36 months of follow-up, spironolactone reduced mortality by 30% when added to conventional therapy in patients with symptomatic congestive heart failure (relative risk 0.70, 95% CI 0.60–0.82; $p < 0.0001$). Treating 1,000 heart failure patients with spironolactone for 1 year would prevent 52 deaths and 125 cardiovascular hospitalizations *(28)*.

Another recent trial, Eplerenone Post-AMI Heart Failure Efficacy and Survival Study (EPHESUS) *(29)*, randomized patients with CHF and an EF<40%, 3–14 days post-MI, to eplerenone (25–50 mg daily) or placebo. At a mean follow-up of 27 months, eplerenone, reduced total mortality by 15%

($p = 0.008$), cardiovascular mortality or cardiovascular hospitalizations by 13% ($p = 0.002$), and sudden cardiac death by 21% ($p = 0.03$). The EPHESUS established the importance of aldosterone antagonism in post-MI patients with reduced left ventricular function irrespective of the degree of heart failure.

25.4.7. β(Beta)-Blockade in Heart Failure

Multiple β(beta)-blockers have been shown to reduce mortality and morbidity in patients with heart failure and reduced left ventricular systolic function. Current guidelines support the use of carvedilol, metoprolol, and bisoprolol to treat patients with CHF. Beta blockers reduce mortality by approximately 35% when added to standard therapy in mild to moderate *(97–99)* or advanced CHF *(100)* and reduced hospitalizations by 33–38% *(97, 98, 101)*. Beta blockers have a positive impact on positive remodeling by reducing cavity size and improving ejection fraction *(102)*.

In the US Carvedilol Heart Failure Study *(97)* (Fig. 4), 1,094 patients were enrolled in a double-blind, placebo-controlled, stratified program in which they received one of four treatment protocols based on their exercise capacity. Patients with heart failure were randomized to placebo ($n = 398$) or carvedilol ($n = 696$) in addition to conventional therapy. The overall mortality at 6-month follow-up was reduced by 65% ($p < 0.001$) and rehospitalization by 27% with carvedilol ($p = 0.036$). This effect was seen in both black and non-black patients *(103)*. Carvedilol also reduced length of hospital stay and length of stay in the intensive care unit leading to a 57% reduction in inpatient care costs for cardiovascular admissions ($p = 0.016$) and 81% lower for heart failure admissions ($p = 0.022$) *(101)*. Finally, severe heart failure (EF < 22%, markedly reduced 6-min corridor walk test, and severe impairment of quality of life) had an improvement in EF with carvedilol ($p = 0.004$) *(104)*. In the Carvedilol Prospective Randomized Cumulative Survival (COPERNICUS) study group *(105)*, 2,289 patients with severe heart failure symptoms were randomly assigned to receive carvedilol ($n = 1,156$) or placebo ($n = 1,133$). The carvedilol group experienced no increase in cardiovascular risk and had fewer patients who died (19 versus 25; hazard ratio [HR] 0.75; 95% confidence interval [CI] 0.41–1.35) and were hospitalized (134 versus 153; HR 0.85; 95% CI 0.67–1.07). Carvedilol was well tolerated in euvolemic patients with fewer patients withdrawn from treatment than placebo.

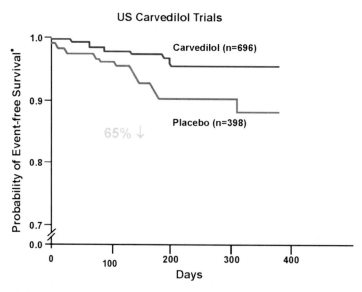

Fig. 4. US Carvedilol trials showing a significant reduction in mortality with carvedilol compared to placebo in patients with left ventricular systolic dysfunction.

In the Metoprolol CR/XL Randomized Intervention Trial in Congestive Heart Failure (MERIT-HF) study 991 patients with chronic heart failure in NYHC II–IV and EF$\leq$40% were enrolled in a double-blind, randomized, placebo-controlled study of metoprolol CR/XL versus placebo *(98)*. All-cause mortality and sudden death were reduced by 34% ($p = 0.00009$) and 41% ($p = 0.0002$) in the metoprolol group. Also, metoprolol CR/XL reduced the number of hospitalizations due to worsening heart failure ($p < 0.001$) and number of days in hospital due to worsening heart failure ($p < 0.001$). In post-MI patients with symptomatic CHF and an EF$\leq$40% and receiving contemporary management, metoprolol CR/XL reduced total mortality by 40% ($p = 0.0004$) and sudden death by 50% ($p = 0.0004$) *(106)*.

The Cardiac Insufficiency Bisoprolol II (CIBS-II) study was a double-blind, placebo-controlled trial in Europe that enrolled 2,647 symptomatic patient with Class III or IV heart failure and an EF$\leq$35% randomized to bisoprolol or placebo. At 1.3 years, all-cause mortality and sudden death were reduced by 34% ($p < 0.0001$) and 44% ($p = 0.0011$), respectively, with bisoprolol. Also, bisoprolol resulted in fewer hospital admissions per patient hospitalized, fewer hospital admissions overall, and fewer days spent in hospital or intensive care unit leading to a reduction in the cost of care by 5–10% compared to placebo *(107)*.

The Carvedilol Or Metoprolol European Trial (COMET) *(108, 109)* is the only randomized trial that compared two beta blockers in a randomized, double-blind study in the management of CHF patients. 3,029 patients with Class II–IV heart failure were recruited at 317 centers in 15 European countries. At 58 months, there was a 17% reduction in mortality with carvedilol compared to metoprolol tartrate ($p = 0.0017$). Recently, carvedilol (6.25–25 mg twice daily) was also shown in The Glycemic Effects in Diabetes Mellitus: Carvedilol-Metoprolol Comparison in Hypertensives (GEMINI) study not to alter glycemic control in diabetics when compared to metoprolol tartrate (50–200 mg twice a day). Furthermore, it did improve some components of the metabolic syndrome such as improving insulin sensitivity *(110)*.

Currently recommended beta blockers in the management of CHF are carvedilol, metoprolol succinate, and bisoprolol *(71)*. Adherence to the use of beta blockade is of paramount importance to reduce the economic burden of CHF. Beta blockers are currently underutilized in patients with CHF *(111)* and continued educational efforts are needed to promote guidelines in heart failure management.

Aggressive titration of beta blockers is needed in patients with CHF. Higher levels of beta blockade and ACEI are associated with better improvement of ejection fraction and greater reductions in cardiovascular hospitalizations *(112–114)*. In a substudy of the Assessment of Treatment with Lisinopril and Survival (ATLAS) trial, the composite endpoint of mortality or hospitalization decreased incrementally with the use of high-dose ACE inhibitors ($n = 475$) (adjusted odds ratio [aOR] 0.93; $p = $ NS), high-dose ACE inhibitors plus beta blockers ($n = 72$) (aOR 0.89; $p = $ NS), and high-dose ACE inhibitors plus beta blockers plus digoxin ($n = 77$) (aOR 0.47; $p = 0.006$) compared with low-dose ACE inhibitors ($n = 471$) *(114)*. A stepwise approach in titration of beta blockade is generally followed with an increase in the dose every 2 weeks as tolerated until achieving the maximum tolerable dose.

25.4.8. Digoxin Therapy in Congestive Heart Failure

Digoxin was introduced by William Withering and has been used therapeutically for more than 250 years *(115)*. It has been widely used in the treatment of atrial fibrillation as a rate control agent but its utility in CHF has been debated.

The Digitalis Investigation Group (DIG) *(116)* is a randomized, double-blind clinical trial that studied the effects of digoxin on mortality and hospitalization in patients with congestive heart failure. DIG showed no advantage of digoxin on mortality at 37 months follow-up. Digoxin, however, reduced the rate of hospitalization for worsening heart failure. A comprehensive post hoc analysis, however, of the DIG showed that digoxin at a serum concentration of 0.5–0.9 ng/mL did reduce mortality (29 versus 33%, adjusted hazard ratio (AHR) of 0.77) and heart failure hospitalizations (23 versus 33%, AHR of 0.68) in all heart failure patients with no interaction with EF > 45% ($p = 0.834$) or gender ($p = 0.917$) (*117*). In another substudy of the DIG trial, perceived health, quality of life measures, and the 6-min walk test were not statistically different between Digoxin and placebo in patients in normal sinus rhythm at 12 month follow-up (*118*). Furthermore, digoxin efficacy was not altered by renal glomerular filtration but renal dysfunction was a predictor of mortality in patients with GFR<50 ml/min (*119*).

Patients on digoxin and receiving standard treatment for congestive heart failure might experience a slight reduction in EF (*120–123*), worsening maximal exercise capacity, and increased incidence of treatment failure upon withdrawal of this drug (*121, 123*).

Currently, digoxin is indicated for the treatment of chronic heart failure in patients with left ventricular dysfunction and NYHC Class II–III despite optimal medical treatment with ACEI, beta blockers, and diuretics (ACC/AHA Class IIa indication). Digoxin is not indicated for the acute treatment of CHF, and serial measurements of digoxin levels are currently considered unnecessary. Digoxin dose needs to be reduced when administered with amiodarone.

25.4.9. Mechanical Treatment of Stage C Heart Failure

25.4.9.1. Cardiac Resynchronization Therapy

Cardiac resynchronization therapy (CRT) is indicated in patients with advanced heart failure symptoms (Class III or IV) despite optimal medical management, an EF $\leq$ 35%, sinus rhythm, and cardiac dyssynchrony defined as a wide QRS complex > 120 ms. The outcomes of CRT system implantation in 2,078 patients from a multicenter study program showed that the procedure is safe, well-tolerated, and has a high success rate (*124*).

In the Multicenter InSync Randomized Clinical Evaluation (MIRACLE) trial (*124*), 369 patients with EF $\leq$ 35%, QRS duration $\geq$ 130 ms, and Class III–IV NYHC, despite optimal medical treatment, were randomized to controls ($n = 182$, ICD activated, CRT off) and the CRT group ($n = 187$, ICD activated, CRT on). CRT improved quality of life, functional status, and exercise capacity without adversely influencing ICD function. In addition, in the InSyncIII study (*125*), a multicenter, prospective, non-randomized, 6-month trial of 422 patients with wide QRS complex and a Class III or IV heart failure, sequential CRT therapy provided a modest increase in stroke volume and improved exercise capacity but had no change in functional status or quality of life compared to a historic control from the MIRACLE trial. Furthermore, improvement in left ventricular function occurs with CRT is more prominent in patients with non-ischemic heart failure and less severe mitral insufficiency (*126*). Finally, in the Comparison of Medical Therapy, Pacing, and Defibrillation in Heart Failure (COMPANION) trial, the risk of the combined endpoint of death from, or hospitalization for, heart failure was reduced by 34% ($p < 0.002$). In the same trial, death from any cause was reduced by 24% ($p = 0.059$) in the pacemaker group compared to the medical therapy alone (*127*). In this trial, the addition of a defibrillator reduced mortality beyond that achieved with CRT therapy alone.

Current guidelines recommend CRT therapy in patients with advanced heart failure symptoms and wide QRS complex who are already optimized on medical treatment with the goal to improve exercise capacity, functional status, quality of life, and to help reverse left ventricular remodeling (*71*).

25.4.9.2. Implantable Cardioverter Defibrillators

Sudden death is a major cause of mortality in patients with left ventricular dysfunction. Implantable cardioverter defibrillators (ICD) are currently indicated in patients with moderate CHF and reduced EF <30% on optimal medical therapy and have a reasonable expectation of survival for more than 1 year who are at least 40 days post-myocardial infarction; or have non-ischemic cardiomyopathy; or have had a serious arrhythmia such as ventricular fibrillation, ventricular tachycardia, or cardiac arrest *(70, 128)*.

In the Sudden Cardiac Death in Heart Failure Trial (SCD-HeFT), 2,521 patients with moderate heart failure and an EF $\leq$35% were randomized to conventional therapy for CHF plus placebo, conventional therapy plus amiodarone, or conventional therapy plus ICD. Amiodarone had no favorable effect on survival whereas ICD reduced overall mortality by 23% at 45.5 months mean follow-up *(128)*. In addition, the COMPANION *(127)* trial showed that ICD therapy can reduce death by 36% ($p = 0.003$) in patients with advanced heart failure due to ischemic or non-ischemic cardiomyopathy and a QRS $\geq$120 ms when compared to optimal medical therapy. The Multicenter Automatic Defibrillator Implantation Trial II (MADIT-II) randomized 1,232 patients with EF $\leq$30% to ICD or conventional medical therapy. Death was the primary endpoint and the average follow-up was 20 months. The mortality rates were 19.8% in the conventional therapy group and 14.2% in the defibrillator group (hazard ratio for the risk of death in the ICD group was 0.69, $p = 0.016$) *(129)*. A long-term follow-up study from MADIT-II showed that the probability of survival after successful therapy with an ICD for ventricular fibrillation or tachycardia was 80% at 1 year *(130)*. The MADIT-II also indicated that benefit from ICD therapy is similar among all the different heart failure subgroups *(68)*. Currently the MADIT-CRT is ongoing and is testing whether CRT-D will reduce the risk of mortality in patients with reduced EF ($\leq$30%), prolonged QRS $\geq$ 130 ms and NYHC Class I–II *(68)*.

25.4.9.3. MISCELLANEOUS THERAPY

CHF patients need to be instructed on dietary salt restriction (2 g sodium/day), fluid restriction, daily weight monitoring, smoking cessation, regular exercise, avoidance of alcohol intake, and aggressive treatment of high blood pressure and dyslipidemia. Aggressive treatment of sleep apnea is also indicated *(132)*. In general CHF patients need to avoid non-steroidal anti-inflammatory drugs (NSAIDS), most calcium channel blockers, and antiarrhythmic agents. Finally, exercise testing and enrolment in an exercise structured program is advised in these patients.

25.4.9.4. MANAGEMENT OF THE ACC/AHA STAGE D CONGESTIVE HEART FAILURE PATIENT

Acutely decompensated CHF patients with severe left ventricular dysfunction require intense pharmacologic and mechanical management. Patients with advanced decompensated failure have a poor short-term prognosis. In the Initiation Management Pre-discharge Assessment of Carvedilol Heart Failure (IMPACT-HF) Registry *(133)*, mortality and rehospitalization rate was 31% at 60-day follow-up.

Positive inotropic agents such as dopamine and milrinone might be utilized for palliative reasons because they improve symptoms and increase functional capacity but they could worsen arrhythmias and possibly increase the risk of mortality *(134, 135)*. In a randomized trial of milrinone versus placebo in 951 patients with decompensated CHF, milrinone caused more sustained hypotension and atrial arrhythmias compared to placebo with no positive impact on mortality *(136)*. An analysis from the Acute Decompensated Heart Failure National Registry (ADHERE), a large retrospective registry of patients with acute decompensated CHF, patients who received milrinone and dobutamine had a higher in-hospital mortality than those who received nitroglycerin and nesiritide. Both nesiritide and nitroglycerin had similar in-hospital mortality *(137)*.

Current *ACC/AHA Guidelines* consider the use of intermittent positive inotropic agents for the management of decompensated heart failure as a Class III indication, indicating that their use should be discouraged.

Data on IV nesiritide suggest that this drug is effective in lowering wedge pressure and improving patient's symptoms *(138)*. In the Vasodilatation in the Management of Acute CHF (VMAC) trial, 489 inpatients with decompensated CHF were enrolled in a randomized trial of nesiritide versus nitroglycerin or placebo for 3 h followed by nesiritide or nitroglycerin for 24 h. The primary and secondary outcomes of the study are pulmonary capillary wedge pressure (PCWP) at 3 and 24 h, respectively. IV nesiritide was administered as a bolus of 2 μg/kg followed by continuous infusion of 0.01 μg/kg/min. At 3 h, dyspnea improved with nesiritide compared with placebo ($p = 0.03$), but there was no difference compared to nitroglycerin. At 24 h, the reduction in PCWP was greater in the nesiritide group (–8.2 mmHg) than the nitroglycerin group (–6.3 mmHg) with a modest improvement in clinical status (VMAC investigators). In VMAC, there was no significant difference between nesiritide and nitroglycerin subjects in 6-month mortality. The hemodynamic benefits and safety of nesiritide in patients with acutely decompensated CHF are maintained in patients receiving chronic beta blockers *(139)*.

In the Prospective Randomized Evaluation of Cardiac Ectopy with Dobutamine or Natrecor Therapy (PRECEDENT), 255 patients were randomized to dobutamine or nesiritide in the management of decompensated congestive heart failure. Dobutamine was associated with arrhythmia and tachycardia whereas nesiritide reduced ventricular ectopy and did not increase heart rate suggesting a safer profile of nesiritide over dobutamine *(140)*.

The 30-day mortality from pooled data from seven clinical trials (Table 2) *(138, 140–144)* was 5.3% for Natrecor and 4.3% for control (hazard ratio 1.27 [0.81–2.01]). In a recent pooled analysis of three randomized studies *(145)* 485 patients were randomized to nesiritide and 377 to control therapy. Death at 30 days occurred more frequently in patients treated with nesiritide than placebo at 30 days of follow-up (7.2 versus 4%, $p = 0.059$).

Table 2
Percent 30-Day Mortality in Seven Nesiritide Trials

Trial	Natrecor (%)	Control (%)	Hazard ratio	Confidence interval
Mills et al.	2.70	7.50	0.38	(0.05–2.67)
PRECEDENT	3.70	6.10	0.6	(0.18–1.97)
Efficacy	5.90	5.80	1.25	(0.24–6.45)
Comparative	6.90	4.90	1.43	(0.53–3.97)
VMAC	8.10	5.10	1.56	(0.75–3.24)
PROACTION	4.2	0.90	4.99	(0.58–42.73)
FUSION I	1.40	2.90	0.49	(0.07–3.47)
Pooled (all)	5.30	4.30	1.27	(0.81–2.01)

25.4.10. Mechanical Support of the Failing Heart

The Randomized Evaluation of Mechanical Assistance in Treatment of Chronic Heart Failure (REMATCH) trial *(146, 147)* randomized 129 patients with end-stage heart failure who were ineligible for cardiac transplantation to receive a left ventricular assist device ($n = 68$) or optimal medical management ($n = 61$). Survival (52 versus 25%, $p = 0.002$) and quality of life were significantly improved with the device compared to medical therapy at 1 year. Serious adverse events did occur in the group when compared to medical therapy and included infection, bleeding, and device malfunction. In this trial, patients undergoing inotropic support derived major mortality and quality of life benefits from the assist device compared to patients receiving medical therapy. Also, patients not undergoing inotropic support had an overall better survival rates both with and without the assist device, but differences did not reach significance.

Recent improvements in the HeartMate VE left ventricular assist device (LVAD) to the HeartMate XVE LVAD have recently led to significant improvements in outcomes *(148)* indicating that as technology and experience with LVAD evolve this therapy might become more accessible to the Class IV heart failure patient who is ineligible for cardiac transplantation.

25.5. CASE STUDIES

25.5.1. Case Study 1

P.S. is a 57-year-old male with history of old myocardial infarction, ischemic cardiomyopathy, and an ejection fraction of 32%. He has been short of breath with minimal home activity, placing him in a Class III New York Heart Classification for failure. Patient has been on carvedilol 25 mg PO BID, lisinopril 20 mg PO daily, furosemide 60 mg po daily, and spironolactone 25 mg PO BID. Patient is euvolemic on his current medical regimen. His electrocardiogram showed a normal sinus rhythm with a left bundle branch block and a QRS complex duration of 140 ms. Patient was referred for biventricular pacing-defibrillator placement. Two weeks post-procedure, the patient's symptoms markedly improved, and he was in Class II NYHC. Cardiac rehabilitation was initiated, and at 3 months follow-up he was in functional Class I NYHC. A MUGA scan was performed and his ejection fraction improved to 44%.

25.5.2. Case Study 2

M.S. is a 35-year-old female with a recent viral infection and subsequent congestive heart failure. Echocardiography showed an ejection fraction of 25% and no evidence of significant valvular disease. Blood testing showed normal thyroid function tests, negative antinuclear antibody, normal iron and iron saturation, normal liver function tests, and electrolytes. Computed tomography of the coronaries showed a calcium score of 0 and normal coronaries in a right dominant system. Patient was started on carvedilol 3.125 mg PO BID and titrated to 25 mg PO BID over a period of 2 months. She was also started on lisinopril 5 mg PO daily and increased to 20 mg PO QD. After 6 months patient's ejection fraction normalized to 56% and she was completely asymptomatic. She was maintained on her carvedilol and lisinopril, and at 2 years follow-up she continued to have stable left ventricular function. Patient was presumed to have a viral cardiomyopathy and experienced excellent recovery of cardiac function (Fig. 5).

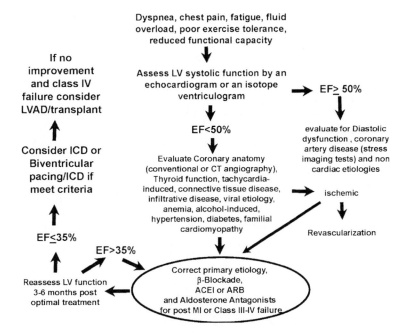

Fig. 5. Algorithm.

25.6. CONCLUSION

Treatment of heart failure starts with controlling risk factors; management of asymptomatic systolic dysfunction; and aggressive treatment of symptomatic failure with diuretics, beta blockers, ACEI (or ARB), and aldosterone antagonists. The use of IV inotropes should be discouraged except for hemodynamic stability. Eligible patients need to receive biventricular pacing, ICD, or LVAD. Diastolic dysfunction is often a neglected cause of CHF, and diagnosis needs to be considered when CHF is present in the setting of normal left ventricular systolic function. HFNEF diagnosis is a relatively new entity that needs to be considered in the symptomatic heart failure patient.

REFERENCES

1. Brush C. Doppler tissue analysis of mitral annular velocities: evidence for systolic abnormalities in patients with diastolic heart failure. *J Am Soc Echocardiogr.* 2003;16:1031–1036.
2. Haney S, Sur D, Xu Z. A review and primary care perspective. *J Am Bd Fam Prac.* 2005;18:189–198.
3. Hunt SA, Baker DW, Chin MH, et al. American College of Cardiology/American Heart Association Task Force on Practice Guidelines (Committee to Revise the *1995 Guidelines for the Evaluation and Management of Heart Failure*); International Society for Heart and Lung Transplantation; Heart Failure Society of America. *ACC/AHA Guidelines for the Evaluation and Management of Chronic Heart Failure in the Adult: Executive Summary A Report of the American College of Cardiology/American Heart Association Task Force on Practice Guidelines* (Committee to Revise the 1995 Guidelines for the Evaluation and Management of Heart Failure): Developed in Collaboration With the International Society for Heart and Lung Transplantation; Endorsed by the Heart Failure Society of America. *Circulation.* 2001;104:2996–3007.
4. O'Connell JB, Bristow M. Economic impact of heart failure in the United States: time for a different approach. *J Heart Lung Transplant.* 1993;13:S107–S112.
5. Senni M, Tribouilloy CM, Rodeheffer RJ, et al. Congestive heart failure in the community. A study of al incident cases in Olmsted County, Minnesota, in 1991. *Circulation.* 1998;98:2282–2289.
6. Kitzman DW, Gardin JM, Gottdiener JS, et al. Importance of heart failure with preserved systolic function in patients ≥65 years of age. *Am J Cardiol.* 2001;87:413–419.
7. Maeder MT, Kaye DM. Heart failure with normal left ventricular ejection fraction. *J Am Coll Cardiol.* 2009;53:905–918.
8. Stewart S, MacIntyre K, Capewell S, McMurray JJ. Heart failure and the aging population: an increasing burden in the 21st century? *Heart.* 2003;89:49–53.
9. Senni M, Tribouilloy CM, Rodeheffer RJ, et al. Congestive heart failure in the community: trends in incidence and survival in a 10-year period. *Arch Intern Med.* 1999;159:29–34.
10. Young JB, Dunlap ME, Pfeffer MA, et al. Mortality and morbidity reduction with Candesartan in patients with chronic heart failure and left ventricular systolic dysfunction: results of the CHARM low-left ventricular ejection fraction trials. *Circulation.* 2004;110:2618–2626.
11. Roger VL, Weston SA, Redfield MM, et al. Trends in heart failure incidence and survival in a community-based population. *JAMA.* 2004;292:344–350.
12. Levy D, Kenchaiah S, Larson MG, et al. Long-term trends in the incidence of and survival with heart failure. *N Engl J Med.* 2002;347:1397–1402.
13. Levy D, Larson MG, Vasan RS, et al. The progression from hypertension to congestive heart failure. *JAMA.* 1996;275:1557–1562.
14. Kannel WB, Ho K, Thom T. Changing epidemiological features of cardiac failure. *Br Heart J.* 1994;72(2 Suppl):S3–S9.
15. Blaufarb IS, Sonnenblick EH. The renin–angiotensin system in left ventricular remodeling. *Am J Cardiol.* 1996;77:8C–16C.
16. Solomon SD, Anavekar N, Skali H, et al. for the Candesartan in Heart Failure Reduction in Mortality (CHARM) Investigators. Influence of ejection fraction on cardiovascular outcomes in a broad spectrum of heart failure patients. *Circulation.* 2005;112:3738–3744.
17. Curtis JP, Sokol SI, Wang Y, et al. The association of left ventricular ejection fraction, mortality, and cause of death in stable outpatients with heart failure. *J Am Coll Cardiol.* 2003;42:736–742.
18. Opie LH. The neuroendocrinology of congestive heart failure. *Cardiovasc J S Afr.* 2002;13:171–178.
19. Tousoulis D, Charakida M, Stefanadis C. Inflammation and endothelial dysfunction as therapeutic targets in patients with heart failure. *Int J Cardiol.* 2005;100:347–353.

20. Bauersachs J, Schafer A. Endothelial dysfunction in heart failure: mechanisms and therapeutic approaches. *Curr Vasc Pharmacol.* 2004;2:115–124.

21. Francis GS. Neurohumoral activation and progression of heart failure: hypothetical and clinical considerations. *J Cardiovasc Pharmacol.* 1998;32(Suppl 1):S16–S21.

22. Blum A, Miller H. Pathophysiological role of cytokines in congestive heart failure. *Annu Rev Med.* 2001;52:15–27.

23. Bristow MR. Changes in myocardial and vascular receptors in heart failure. *J Am Coll Cardiol.* 1993;22 (4 Suppl A):61A–71A.

24. Mann DL, Kent RL, Parsons B, Cooper G. 4th Adrenergic effects on the biology of the adult mammalian cardiocyte. *Circulation.* 1992;85:790–804.

25. Mann DL. Basic mechanisms of disease progression in the failing heart: the role of excessive adrenergic drive. *Prog Cardiovasc Dis.* 1998;41(1 Suppl 1):1–8.

26. Nikolaidis LA, Trumble D. Hentosz, et al. Catecholamines restore myocardial contractility in dilated cardiomyopathy at the expense of increased coronary blood flow and myocardial oxygen consumption (MvO2 cost of catecholamines in heart failure). *Eur J Heart Fail.* 2004;6:409–419.

27. McKelvie RS, Yusuf S, Pericak D, et al. Comparison of candesartan, enalapril, and their combination in congestive heart failure: randomized evaluation of strategies for left ventricular dysfunction (RESOLVD) pilot study. The RESOLVD Pilot Study Investigators. *Circulation.* 1999;100:1056–1064.

28. Pitt B, Zannad F, Remme WJ, et al. The effect of spironolactone on morbidity and mortality in patients with severe heart failure. Randomized Aldactone Evaluation Study Investigators. *N Engl J Med.* 1999;341:709–717.

29. Pitt B, Williams G, Remme W, et al. The EPHESUS trial: eplerenone in patients with heart failure due to systolic dysfunction complicating acute myocardial infarction. Eplerenone Post-AMI Heart Failure Efficacy and Survival Study. *Cardiovasc Drugs Ther.* 2001;15:79–87.

30. Goldsmith SR. Interactions between the sympathetic nervous system and the RAAS in heart failure. *Curr Heart Fail Rep.* 2004;1:45–50.

31. van de Wal RM, Voors AA, Plokker HW, van Gilst WH, van Veldhuisen DJ. New pharmacological strategies in chronic heart failure. *Cardiovasc Drugs Ther.* 2004;18:491–501.

32. Aurigemma GP, Zile MR, Gaasch WH. Contractile behavior of the left ventricle in diastolic heart failure with emphasis on regional systolic function. *Circulation.* 2006;113:296–304.

33. Baicu CF, Zile MR, Aurigemma GP, Gaasch WH. Left ventricular systolic performance, function and contractility in patients with diastolic heart failure. *Circulation.* 2005;111:2306–2312.

34. Kawaguchi M, Hay I, Fetics B, Kass DA. Combined ventricular systolic and arterial stiffening in patients with heart failure and preserved ejection fraction: implications for systolic and diastolic reserve limitations. *Circulation.* 2003;107:714–720.

35. Redfiled MM, Jacobsen SJ, Burnett JC Jr, Mahoney DW, Bailey KR, Rodeheffer RJ. Burden of systolic and diastolic ventrciular dysfunction in the community: appreciating the scope of heart failure epidemic. *JAMA.* 2003;289: 194–202.

36. Tsang TS, Barnes ME, Gersh BJ, Bailey KR, Seward JB. Left atrial volume as a morphophysiologic expression of left ventricular diastolic dysfunction and relation to cardiovascular risk burden. *Am J Cardiol.* 2002;90:1284–1289.

37. Ahmed A. American College of Cardiology/American Heart Association Chronic Heart Failure Evaluation and Management guidelines: relevance to the geriatric practice. *J Am Geriatr Soc.* 2003;51:123–126.

38. Ewy GA. Diastolic dysfunction. *J Insur Med.* 2004;36:292–297.

39. de Las Fuentes L, Waggoner AD, Brown AL, Davila-Roman VG. Plasma triglyceride level is an independent predictor of altered left ventricular relaxation. *J Am Soc Echocardiogr.* 2005;18:1285–1291.

40. Kasikcioglu HA, Karasulu L, Durgun E, Oflaz H, Kasikcioglu E, Cuhadaroglu C. Aortic elastic properties and left ventricular diastolic dysfunction in patients with obstructive sleep apnea. *Heart Vessels.* 2005;20:239–244.

41. Araujo AQ, Arteaga E, Ianni BM, Buck PC, Rabello R, Mady C. Effect of Losartan on left ventricular diastolic function in patients with nonobstructive hypertrophic cardiomyopathy. *Am J Cardiol.* 2005;96:1563–1567.

42. Mottram PM, Short L, Baglin T, Marwick TH. Is "diastolic heart failure" a diagnosis of exclusion? Echocardiographic parameters of diastolic dysfunction in patients with heart failure and normal systolic function. *Heart Lung Circ.* 2003;12:127–134.

43. Lim TK, Ashrafian H, Dwivedi G, Collinson PO, Senior R. Increased left atrial volume index is an independent predictor of raised serum natriuretic peptide in patients with suspected heart failure but normal left ventricular ejection fraction: implication for diagnosis of diastolic heart failure. *Eur J Heart Fail.* 2006;8:38–45; Epub 2005 Aug 22.

44. Qu P, Ding Y, Xia D, Wang H, Tian X. Variations in cardiac diastolic function in hypertensive patients with different left ventricular geometric patterns. *Hypertens Res.* 2001;24(5):601–604.

45. Paulus WJ, Tschope C, Sanderson JE, et al. How to diagnose diastolic heart failure: a consensus statement on the diagnosis of heart failure with normal left ventricular ejection fraction by the Heart Failure and Echocardiography Associations of the European Society of Cardiology. *Eur Heart J.* 2007;28:2539–2550.

46. Morris SA, Van Swol M, Udani B. The less familiar side of heart failure: symptomatic diastolic dysfunction. *J Fam Pract.* 2005;54:501–511.

47. Hunt SA. ACC/AHA 2005 guideline update for the diagnosis and management of chronic heart failure in the adult: a report of the American College of Cardiology/American Heart Association Task Force on Practice Guidelines (Writing Committee to update the *2001 Guidelines for the Evaluation and Management of Heart Failure*). *J Am Coll Cardiol.* 2005;46:e1–e82.

48. Mandinov L, Eberli FR, Seiler C, Hess OM. Diastolic heart failure. *Cardiovasc Res.* 2000;45:813–825.

49. Chang NC, Shih CM, Bi WF, Lai ZY, Lin MS, Wang TC. Fosinopril improves left ventricular diastolic function in young mildly hypertensive patients without hypertrophy. *Cardiovasc Drugs Ther.* 2002;16:141–147.

50. Yip GWK, Wang M, Wang T, Chan S, Fung JWH, Yeung L, Yip T, Lau ST, Lau CP, Tang MO, Yu CM, Sanderson JE. The Hong Kong diastolic heart failure study: a randomised controlled trial of diuretics, irbesartan and ramipril on quality of life, exercise capacity, left ventricular global and regional function in heart failure with a normal ejection fraction. *Heart.* 2008;94(5):573–580; Epub 2008 Jan 20.

51. Roongsritong C, Sutthiwan P, Bradley J, Simoni J, Power S, Meyerrose GE. Spironolactone improves diastolic function in the elderly. *Clin Cardiol.* 2005;28:484–487.

52. The J-ELA N. investigators. Effect of Losartan and Amlodipine on Left Ventricular Diastolic Function in Patients With Mild-to-Moderate Hypertension (J-ELAN). *Circ J.* 2006;70:124–128.

53. Bajraktari G, Koltai MS, Ademaj F, et al. Relationship between insulin resistance and left ventricular diastolic dysfunction in patients with impaired glucose tolerance and type 2 diabetes. *Int J Cardiol.* 2006;110:206–211; Epub 2005 Nov 17.

54. Charvat J, Michalova K, Chlumsky J, Valenta Z, Kvapil M. The association between left ventricle diastolic dysfunction and endothelial dysfunction and the results of stress myocardial SPECT in asymptomatic patients with type 2 diabetes. *J Int Med Res.* 2005;33:473–482.

55. Grandi AM, Piantanida E, Franzetti I, et al. Effect of glycemic control on left ventricular diastolic function in type 1 diabetes mellitus. *Am J Cardiol.* 2006;97:71–76.

56. Komajda M, Hanon O, Hochadel M, Follath F, Swedberg K, Gitt A, Cleland JG. Management of octogenarians hospitalized for heart failure in Euro Heart Failure Survey I. *Eur Heart J.* 2007;28:1310–1318.

57. Rodeheffer RJ. The new epidemiology of heart failure. *Curr Cardiol Rep.* 2003;5:181–186.

58. Wang TJ, Evans JC, Benjamin EJ, et al. Natural history of left ventricular systolic dysfunction in the community. *Circulation.* 2003;108:977–982.

59. Francis GS, Benedict C, Johnstone DE, et al. Comparison of neuroendocrine activation in patients with left ventricular dysfunction with and without congestive heart failure. A substudy of the Studies of Left Ventricular Dysfunction (SOLVD). *Circulation.* 1990;82:1724–1729.

60. Das SR, Drazner MH, Yancy CW, Stevenson LW, Gersh BJ, Dries DL. Effects of diabetes mellitus and ischemic heart disease on the progression from asymptomatic left ventricular dysfunction to symptomatic heart failure: a retrospective analysis from the Studies of Left Ventricular Dysfunction (SOLVD) Prevention trial. *Am Heart J.* 2004;148:883–888.

61. Das SR, Dries DL, Drazner MH, Yancy CW, Chae CU. Relation of lower hematocrit to progression from asymptomatic left ventricular dysfunction to symptomatic heart failure (from the Studies of Left Ventricular Dysfunction Prevention trial). *Am J Cardiol.* 2005;96:827–831.

62. Dries DL, Strong MH, Cooper RS, Drazner MH. Efficacy of angiotensin-converting enzyme inhibition in reducing progression from asymptomatic left ventricular dysfunction to symptomatic heart failure in black and white patients. *J Am Coll Cardiol.* 2002;40:311–317.

63. Konstam MA, Kronenberg MW, Rousseau MF, et al. Effects of the angiotensin converting enzyme inhibitor enalapril on the long-term progression of left ventricular dilatation in patients with asymptomatic systolic dysfunction. SOLVD (Studies of Left Ventricular Dysfunction) Investigators. *Circulation.* 1993;88(5 Pt 1):2277–2283.

64. Jessup M, Brozena S. Heart failure. *N Engl J Med.* 2003;348:2007–2018.

65. SOLVD investigators. Effect of enalapril on mortality and the development of heart failure in asymptomatic patients with reduced left ventricular ejection fractions. The SOLVD Investigattors. *N Engl J Med.* 1992;327:685–691.

66. Eisenberg MJ, Gioia LC. Angiotensin II Receptor Blockers in Congestive Heart Failure. *Cardiol Rev.* 2006;14:26–34.

67. Prasad SK, Dargie HJ, Smith GC, et al. Comparison of the dual receptor endothelin antagonist enrasentan with enalapril in asymptomatic left ventricular systolic dysfunction: a cardiovascular magnetic resonance study. *Heart.* 2006;92:798–803; Epub 2005 Dec 9.

68. Zareba W, Piotrowicz K, McNitt S. Moss AJ; MADIT II Investigators. Implantable cardioverter–defibrillator efficacy in patients with heart failure and left ventricular dysfunction (from the MADIT II population). *Am J Cardiol.* 2005;95:1487–1491.

69. Moss AJ. MADIT-I and MADIT-II. *J Cardiovasc Electrophysiol.* 2003;14(9 Suppl):S96–S98.

70. Moss AJ, Zareba W, Hall WJ, et al. Multicenter Automatic Defibrillator Implantation Trial II Investigators. Prophylactic implantation of a defibrillator in patients with myocardial infarction and reduced ejection fraction. *N Engl J Med.* 2002;346:877–883.

71. ACC/AHA 2005 Guideline Update. Diagnosis and management of chronic heart failure in the adult. *Circulation.* 2005 Sep 20;112:e154–e235; Epub 2005 Sep 13.

72. Trial Study CONSENSUS. Group. Effects of enalapril on mortality in severe congestive heart failure. Results of the Cooperative North Scandinavian Enalapril Survival Study (CONSENSUS). *N Engl J Med.* 1987;316:1429–1435.

73. SOLVD investigators. Effect of enalapril on survival in patients with reduced left ventricular ejection fractions and congestive heart failure. *N Engl J Med.* 1991;325:293–302.

74. Greenberg B, Quinones MA, Koilpillai C, et al. Effects of long-term enalapril therapy on cardiac structure and function in patients with left ventricular dysfunction. Results of the SOLVD echocardiography substudy. *Circulation.* 1995;91:2573–2581.

75. Pitt B. Use of converting enzyme inhibitors in patients with asymptomatic left ventricular dysfunction. *J Am Coll Cardiol.* 1993;22(4 Suppl A):158A–161A.

76. AIRE investigators. Effect of ramipril on mortality and morbidity of survivors of acute myocardial infarction with clinical evidence of heart failure. The Acute Infarction Ramipril Efficacy (AIRE) Study Investigators. *Lancet.* 1993;342:821–828.

77. Pfeffer MA, Braunwald E, Moye LA, et al. Effect of captopril on mortality and morbidity in patients with left ventricular dysfunction after myocardial infarction. Results of the survival and ventricular enlargement trial. The SAVE Investigators. *N Engl J Med.* 1992;327:669–677.

78. Kober L, Torp-Pedersen C, Carlsen JE, et al. A clinical trial of the angiotensin-converting-enzyme inhibitor trandolapril in patients with left ventricular dysfunction after myocardial infarction. Trandolapril Cardiac Evaluation (TRACE) Study Group. *N Engl J Med.* 1995;333:1670–1676.

79. Ambrosioni E, Borghi C, Magnani B. The effect of the angiotensin–converting–enzyme inhibitor zofenopril on mortality and morbidity after anterior myocardial infarction. The Survival of Myocardial Infarction Long-Term Evaluation (SMILE) Study Investigators. *N Engl J Med.* 1995;332:80–85.

80. Pitt B, Segal R, Martinez FA, et al. Randomised trial of losartan versus captopril in patients over 65 with heart failure (Evaluation of Losartan in the Elderly Study, ELITE). *Lancet.* 1997;349:747–752.

81. Pitt B, Poole-Wilson PA, Segal R, et al. Effect of losartan compared with captopril on mortality in patients with symptomatic heart failure: randomised trial—the Losartan Heart Failure Survival Study ELITE II. *Lancet.* 2000;355:1582–1587.

82. Cohn JN. Tognoni G; Valsartan Heart Failure Trial Investigators. A randomized trial of the angiotensin-receptor blocker valsartan in chronic heart failure. *N Engl J Med.* 2001;345:1667–1675.

83. Maggioni AP, Anand I, Gottlieb SO, et al. Effects of valsartan on morbidity and mortality in patients with heart failure not receiving angiotensin-converting enzyme inhibitors. *J Am Coll Cardiol.* 2002;40:1414–1421.

84. Wong M, Staszewsky L, Latini R, et al. Val-HeFT Heart Failure Trial Investigators. Valsartan benefits left ventricular structure and function in heart failure: Val-HeFT echocardiographic study. *J Am Coll Cardiol.* 2002;40:970–975.

85. Young JB. The global epidemiology of heart failure. *Med Clin North Am.* 2004;88:1135–1143.

86. Yusuf S, Ostergren JB, Gerstein HC, et al. Candesartan in Heart Failure-Assessment of Reduction in Mortality and Morbidity Program Investigators. Effects of candesartan on the development of a new diagnosis of diabetes mellitus in patients with heart failure. *Circulation.* 2005;112:48–53.

87. Solomon SD, Wang D, Finn P, et al. Effect of candesartan on cause-specific mortality in heart failure patients: the Candesartan in Heart failure Assessment of Reduction in Mortality and morbidity (CHARM) program. *Circulation.* 2004;110:2180–2183.

88. Doggrell SA. ACE inhibitors or AT-1 antagonists—which is OPTIMAAL after acute myocardial infarction? *Expert Opin Pharmacother.* 2003;4:407–409.

89. Dickstein K, Kjekshus J. OPTIMAAL Steering Committee of the OPTIMAAL Study Group. Effects of losartan and captopril on mortality and morbidity in high-risk patients after acute myocardial infarction: the OPTIMAAL randomised trial. Optimal Trial in Myocardial Infarction with Angiotensin II Antagonist Losartan. *Lancet.* 2002;360:752–760.

90. Moller JE, Dahlstrom U, Gotzsche O, et al. OPTIMAAL Study Group. Effects of losartan and captopril on left ventricular systolic and diastolic function after acute myocardial infarction: results of the Optimal Trial in Myocardial Infarction with Angiotensin II Antagonist Losartan (OPTIMAAL) echocardiographic substudy. *Am Heart J.* 2004;147:494–501.

91. Weber KT. Aldosterone in congestive heart failure. *N Engl J Med.* 2001;345:1689–1697.

92. Schjoedt KJ, Andersen S, Rossing P, et al. Aldosterone escape during blockade of the renin-angiotensin-aldosterone system in diabetic nephropathy is associated with enhanced decline in glomerular filtration rate. *Diabetologia.* 2004;47:1936–1939.

93. Deswal A, Yao D. Aldosterone Receptor Blockers in the Treatment of Heart Failure. *Curr Treat Options Cardiovasc Med.* 2004;6:327–334.

94. Cohn JN, Anand IS, Latini R, Masson S, Chiang YT, Glazer R; Valsartan Heart Failure Trial Investigators. Sustained reduction of aldosterone in response to the angiotensin receptor blocker valsartan in patients with chronic heart failure: results from the Valsartan Heart Failure Trial. *Circulation.* 2003;108:1306–1309.

95. Pitt B. Effect of aldosterone blockade in patients with systolic left ventricular dysfunction: implications of the RALES and EPHESUS studies. *Mol Cell Endocrinol.* 2004;217:53–58.

96. Masoudi FA, Gross CP, Wang Y, et al. Adoption of spironolactone therapy for older patients with heart failure and left ventricular systolic dysfunction in the United States, 1998–2001. *Circulation.* 2005;112:39–47.

97. Packer M, Bristow MR, Cohn JN, et al. The effect of carvedilol on morbidity and mortality in patients with chronic heart failure. US Carvedilol Heart Failure Study Group. *N Engl J Med.* 1996;334:1349–1355.

98. Study Group MERIT-HF. Effect of metoprolol CR/XL in chronic heart failure: Metoprolol CR/XL Randomised Intervention Trial in Congestive Heart Failure (MERIT-HF). *Lancet.* 1999;253:2001–2007.

99. Investigators CIBIS-II. The Cardiac Insufficiency Bisoprolol Study II (CIBIS-II): a randomised trial. *Lancet.* 1999;353:9–13.

100. Packer M, Coats AJ, Fowler MB, et al. Carvedilol Prospective Randomized Cumulative Survival Study Group. Effect of carvedilol on survival in severe chronic heart failure. *N Engl J Med.* 2001;344:1651–1658.

101. Fowler MB, Vera-Llonch M, Oster G, et al. Influence of carvedilol on hospitalizations in heart failure: incidence, resource utilization and costs. US Carvedilol Heart Failure Study Group. *J Am Coll Cardiol.* 2001;37:1692–1699.

102. Remme WJ, Riegger G, Hildebrandt P, et al. The benefits of early combination treatment of carvedilol and an ACE-inhibitor in mild heart failure and left ventricular systolic dysfunction. The carvedilol and ACE-inhibitor remodelling mild heart failure evaluation trial (CARMEN). *Cardiovasc Drugs Ther.* 2004;18:57–66.

103. Yancy CW, Fowler MB, Colucci WS, et al. US Carvedilol Heart Failure Study Group. Race and the response to adrenergic blockade with carvedilol in patients with chronic heart failure. *N Engl J Med.* 2001;344:1358–1365.

104. Cohn JN, Fowler MB, Bristow MR, et al. Safety and efficacy of carvedilol in severe heart failure. The US Carvedilol Heart Failure Study Group. *J Card Fail.* 1997;3:173–179.

105. Krum H, Roecker EB, Mohacsi P, et al. Carvedilol Prospective Randomized Cumulative Survival (COPERNICUS) Study Group. Effects of initiating carvedilol in patients with severe chronic heart failure: results from the COPERNICUS Study. *JAMA.* 2003;289:712–718.

106. Janosi A, Ghali JK, Herlitz J, et al. MERIT-HF Study Group. Metoprolol CR/XL in postmyocardial infarction patients with chronic heart failure: experiences from MERIT-HF. *Am Heart J.* 2003;146:721–728.

107. CIBIS-II Investigators. Reduced costs with bisoprolol treatment for heart failure: an economic analysis of the second Cardiac Insufficiency Bisoprolol Study (CIBIS-II). *Eur Heart J.* 2001;22:1021–1031.

108. Torp-Pedersen C, Poole-Wilson PA, Swedberg K, et al. Effects of metoprolol and carvedilol on cause-specific mortality and morbidity in patients with chronic heart failure—COMET. *Am Heart J.* 2005;149:370–376.

109. Poole-Wilson PA, Swedberg K, Cleland JG, et al. Comparison of carvedilol and metoprolol on clinical outcomes in patients with chronic heart failure in the Carvedilol Or Metoprolol European Trial (COMET): randomised controlled trial. *Lancet.* 2003;362:7–13.

110. Bakris GL, Fonseca V, Katholi RE, et al. Metabolic effects of carvedilol vs metoprolol in patients with type 2 diabetes mellitus and hypertension: a randomized controlled trial. *JAMA.* 2004;292:2227–3226.

111. Lenzen MJ, Boersma E. Scholte Op Reimer WJ, et al. Under-utilization of evidence-based drug treatment in patients with heart failure is only partially explained by dissimilarity to patients enrolled in landmark trials: a report from the Euro Heart Survey on Heart Failure. *Eur Heart J.* 2005;26:2706–2713.

112. Hori M, Sasayama S, Kitabatake A, et al. Low-dose carvedilol improves left ventricular function and reduces cardiovascular hospitalization in Japanese patients with chronic heart failure: the Multicenter Carvedilol Heart Failure Dose Assessment (MUCHA) trial. *Am Heart J.* 2004;147:324–330.

113. Bristow MR, Gilbert EM, Abraham WT, et al. Carvedilol produces dose-related improvements in left ventricular function and survival in subjects with chronic heart failure. MOCHA Investigators. *Circulation.* 1996;94:2807–2816.

114. Majumdar SR, McAlister FA, Cree M. Do evidence-based treatments provide incremental benefits to patients with congestive heart failure already receiving angiotensin-converting enzyme inhibitors? A secondary analysis of one-year outcomes from the Assessment of Treatment with Lisinopril and Survival (ATLAS) study. *Clin Ther.* 2004;26:694–703.

115. Wade OL. Digoxin 1785–1985. I. Two hundred years of digitalis. *J Clin Hosp Pharm.* 1986;11:3–9.

116. Digitalis Investigation Group. The effect of digoxin on mortality and morbidity in patients with heart failure. The Digitalis Investigation Group. *N Engl J Med.* 1997;336:525–533.

117. Ahmed A, Rich MW, Love TE, et al. Digoxin and reduction in mortality and hospitalization in heart failure: a comprehensive post hoc analysis of the DIG trial. *Eur Heart J.* 2006;27:178–186.

118. Lader E, Egan D, Hunsberger S, Garg R, Czajkowski S, McSherry F. The effect of digoxin on the quality of life in patients with heart failure. *J Card Fail.* 2003;9:4–12.

119. Shlipak MG, Smith GL, Rathore SS, Massie BM, Krumholz HM. Renal function, digoxin therapy, and heart failure outcomes: evidence from the digoxin intervention group trial. *J Am Soc Nephrol.* 2004;15:2195–2203.

120. Shammas NW, Harris ML, McKinney D, Hauber WJ. Digoxin withdrawal in patients with dilated cardiomyopathy following normalization of ejection fraction with beta blockers. *Clin Cardiol.* 2001;24:786–787.

121. Uretsky BF, Young JB, Shahidi FE, Yellen LG, Harrison MC, Jolly MK. Randomized study assessing the effect of digoxin withdrawal in patients with mild to moderate chronic congestive heart failure: results of the PROVED trial. PROVED Investigative Group. *J Am Coll Cardiol.* 1993;22:955–962.

122. DiBianco R, Shabetai R, Kostuk W, Moran J, Schlant RC, Wright R. A comparison of oral milrinone, digoxin, and their combination in the treatment of patients with chronic heart failure. *N Engl J Med.* 1989;320:677–683.

123. Packer M, Gheorghiade M, Young JB, et al. Withdrawal of digoxin from patients with chronic heart failure treated with angiotensin-converting-enzyme inhibitors. RADIANCE Study. *N Engl J Med.* 1993;329:1–7.

124. Leon AR, Abraham WT, Curtis AB, et al. MIRACLE Study Program. Safety of transvenous cardiac resynchronization system implantation in patients with chronic heart failure: combined results of over 2,000 patients from a multicenter study program. *J Am Coll Cardiol.* 2005;46:2348–2356.

125. Leon AR, Abraham WT, Brozena S, et al. InSync III Clinical Study Investigators. Cardiac resynchronization with sequential biventricular pacing for the treatment of moderate-to-severe heart failure. *J Am Coll Cardiol.* 2005;46: 2298–2304.

126. Woo GW, Petersen-Stejskal S, Johnson JW, Conti JB, Aranda JA Jr, Curtis AB. Ventricular reverse remodeling and 6-month outcomes in patients receiving cardiac resynchronization therapy: analysis of the MIRACLE study. *J Interv Card Electrophysiol.* 2005;12:107–113.

127. Bristow MR, Saxon LA, Boehmer J, et al. Comparison of Medical Therapy, Pacing, and Defibrillation in Heart Failure (COMPANION) Investigators. Cardiac-resynchronization therapy with or without an implantable defibrillator in advanced chronic heart failure. *N Engl J Med.* 2004;350:2140–2150.

128. Bardy GH, Lee KL, Mark DB, et al. Sudden Cardiac Death in Heart Failure Trial (SCD-HeFT) Investigators. Amiodarone or an implantable cardioverter-defibrillator for congestive heart failure. *N Engl J Med.* 2005;352:225–237.

129. Moss AJ, Daubert J, Zareba W. MADIT-II: clinical implications. *Card Electrophysiol Rev.* 2002;6:463–465.

130. Moss AJ, Greenberg H, Case RB, et al. Multicenter Automatic Defibrillator Implantation Trial-II (MADIT-II) Research Group. Long-term clinical course of patients after termination of ventricular tachyarrhythmia by an implanted defibrillator. *Circulation.* 2004;110(25):3760–3765.

131. Moss AJ, Brown MW, Cannom DS, et al. Multicenter automatic defibrillator implantation trial-cardiac resynchronization therapy (MADIT-CRT): design and clinical protocol. *Ann Noninvasive Electrocardiol.* 2005;10(4 Suppl):34–43.

132. Naughton MT. The link between obstructive sleep apnea and heart failure: underappreciated opportunity for treatment. *Curr Cardiol Rep.* 2005;7:211–215.

133. O'Connor CM, Stough WG, Gallup DS, Hasselblad V, Gheorghiade M. Demographics, clinical characteristics, and outcomes of patients hospitalized for decompensated heart failure: observations from the IMPACT-HF registry. *J Card Fail.* 2005;11:200–205.

134. Levine BS. Intermittent positive inotrope infusion in the management of end-stage, low-output heart failure. *J Cardiovasc Nurs.* 2000;14:76–93.

135. Felker GM, O'Connor CM. Inotropic therapy for heart failure: an evidence-based approach. *Am Heart J.* 2001;142:393–401.

136. Cuffe MS, Califf RM, Adams KF Jr, et al. Outcomes of a Prospective Trial of Intravenous Milrinone for Exacerbations of Chronic Heart Failure (OPTIME-CHF) Investigators. Short-term intravenous milrinone for acute exacerbation of chronic heart failure: a randomized controlled trial. *JAMA.* 2002;287:1541–1547.

137. Abraham WT, Adams KF, Fonarow GC, et al. ADHERE Scientific Advisory Committee and Investigators; ADHERE Study Group. In-hospital mortality in patients with acute decompensated heart failure requiring intravenous vasoactive medications: an analysis from the Acute Decompensated Heart Failure National Registry (ADHERE). *J Am Coll Cardiol.* 2005;46:57–64.

138. Colucci WS, Elkayam U, Horton DP, et al. Intravenous nesiritide, a natriuretic peptide, in the treatment of decompensated congestive heart failure. Nesiritide Study Group. *N Engl J Med.* 2000;343:246–253.

139. Abraham WT, Cheng ML. Smoluk G; Vasodilation in the Management of Acute Congestive Heart Failure (VMAC) Study Group. Clinical and hemodynamic effects of nesiritide (B-type natriuretic peptide) in patients with decompensated heart failure receiving beta blockers. *Congest Heart Fail.* 2005;11:59–64.

140. Burger AJ, Horton DP, LeJemtel T, et al. Prospective randomized evaluation of cardiac ectopy with dobutamine or natrecor therapy. Effect of nesiritide (B-type natriuretic peptide) and dobutamine on ventricular arrhythmias in the treatment of patients with acutely decompensated congestive heart failure: the PRECEDENT study. *Am Heart J.* 2002;144:1102–1108.

141. Mills RM, LeJemtel TH, Horton DP, et al. Sustained hemodynamic effects of an infusion of nesiritide (human b-type natriuretic peptide) in heart failure: a randomized, double-blind, placebo-controlled clinical trial. Natrecor Study Group. *J Am Coll Cardiol.* 1999;34:155–162.

142. VMAC Investigators (Vasodilatation in the Management of Acute CHF). Intravenous nesiritide vs nitroglycerin for treatment of decompensated congestive heart failure: a randomized controlled trial. *JAMA.* 2002;287: 1531–1540.

143. Peacock WF, Emerman CL, Silver MA. Nesiritide added to standard care favorably reduces systolic blood pressure compared with standard care alone in patients with acute decompensated heart failure. *Am J Emerg Med.* 2005;23: 327–331.

144. Yancy CW, Saltzberg MT, Berkowitz RL, et al. Safety and feasibility of using serial infusions of nesiritide for heart failure in an outpatient setting (from the FUSION I trial). *Am J Cardiol.* 2004;94:595–601.

145. Sackner-Bernstein JD, Kowalski M, Fox M, Aaronson K. Short-term risk of death after treatment with nesiritide for decompensated heart failure: a pooled analysis of randomized controlled trials. *JAMA.* 2005;293:1900–1905.

146. Rose EA, Gelijns AC, Moskowitz AJ, et al. Randomized Evaluation of Mechanical Assistance for the Treatment of Congestive Heart Failure (REMATCH) Study Group. Long-term mechanical left ventricular assistance for end-stage heart failure. *N Engl J Med.* 2001;345:1435–1443.

147. Stevenson LW, Miller LW, Desvigne-Nickens P, et al. REMATCH Investigators. Left ventricular assist device as destination for patients undergoing intravenous inotropic therapy: a subset analysis from REMATCH (Randomized Evaluation of Mechanical Assistance in Treatment of Chronic Heart Failure). *Circulation.* 2004;110:975–981.

148. Long JW, Kfoury AG, Slaughter MS, et al. Long-term destination therapy with the HeartMate XVE left ventricular assist device: improved outcomes since the REMATCH study. *Congest Heart Fail.* 2005;11:133–138.

150. Francis GS. Pathophysiology of chronic heart failure. *Am J Med.* 2001;110(Suppl 7A):37S–46S.

V CARDIAC IMAGING

26 Screening for Coronary Artery Calcium

Nikolaos Alexopoulos, Dalton S. McLean, Stamatios Lerakis, and Paolo Raggi

CONTENTS

Key Words: Calcific atherosclerotic plaque; Coronary calcium; Computed tomography; Risk stratification; Vascular age.

KEY POINTS

- Most risk stratification tools are not completely accurate, and many patients considered to be at low risk suffer coronary events, while some intermediate- to high-risk patients may be at lower than predicted risk. The focus has, therefore, turned to imaging tools to identify atherosclerosis in its pre-clinical stages.
- Calcium deposition accompanies the formation of atherosclerotic plaque from its inception, and it proceeds via active processes of mineralization similar to bone formation. The extent of coronary artery calcium is a good marker of the presence of atherosclerosis, although it represents only 15–20% of the total atheroma volume.
- There is a large amount of data to show that coronary artery calcium is an independent predictor of cardiovascular events among patients at intermediate risk in the general population. It also adds incremental prognostic information beyond traditional risk factors in this segment of the population.
- There are no data to support calcium imaging in low-risk patients, while there are good initial data to support its use even in high-risk individuals such as diabetic patients and the elderly.
- Women benefit from calcium screening even more than men because the accuracy of risk prediction models based on traditional risk factors is lower in women.

From: *Contemporary Cardiology: Comprehensive Cardiovascular Medicine in the Primary Care Setting*
Edited by: Peter P. Toth, Christopher P. Cannon, DOI 10.1007/978-1-60327-963-5_26
© Springer Science+Business Media, LLC 2010

- The ability of coronary artery calcium to predict risk has been shown to be equal for patients of different ethnicities (Caucasian, African-American, Asian, and Hispanic).
- Extent of coronary calcium can be used to adjust the age of the individual patient according to the extent of subclinical atherosclerosis detected. The concept of vascular age can be applied to predict the number of life years lost by the individual.
- Calcium screening in low-risk symptomatic patients helps discriminate patients in need of further testing from those that can be managed medically and discharged from the emergency department.
- Regression of coronary artery calcium has not yet been conclusively shown to be attainable. However, continued accumulation of large amounts of calcium has been clearly shown to be linked with unfavorable cardiovascular events.

26.1. INTRODUCTION

The striking improvement in cardiovascular therapies during the last several decades has caused a marked decrease in mortality linked to atherosclerotic diseases in Western societies. Nonetheless, coronary artery disease (CAD) remains the main cause of non-fatal events, and it is associated with substantial functional impairment in survivors of acute events, imposing a very large economic burden on societies. The use of risk scoring tools helps to identify patients both at higher risk of disease and those who are most likely to benefit from therapeutic intervention. Unfortunately, it has become apparent that most of these tools are not completely accurate, and many patients considered to be at low risk suffer coronary events, and, on the contrary, intermediate- to high-risk patients may actually be at a much lower risk than predicted. The attention of several investigators, therefore, turned to the development of imaging tools to identify atherosclerosis or its *signature* in its pre-clinical stages. Coronary artery calcium (CAC) imaging (Fig. 1) is one of the imaging modalities that has received the most attention in the past 15 years and the one that has raised significant controversy among experts. That calcium deposition accompanies the formation of atherosclerotic plaque from its inception has been well known for two centuries. More recently, it has become apparent that CAC deposition occurs via active processes of calcification of the interstitium resembling bone formation. Furthermore, the

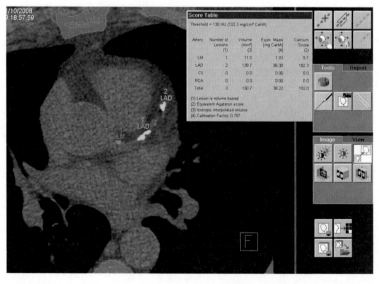

Fig. 1. Axial chest CT image showing calcification of the left main trunk (LM) and left anterior descending coronary artery (LAD). The total (Agatston) coronary artery calcium score is 192.

extent of CAC has been shown to be a good marker of the burden of atherosclerosis, although it may only represent 15–20% of the total atheroma volume. In this chapter we will review the most relevant literature on the use of CAC as a risk stratification tool of asymptomatic and symptomatic patients as well as the utility of sequential CAC scanning to follow the evolution of coronary atherosclerosis.

26.2. PROGNOSTIC ROLE OF CORONARY ARTERY CALCIUM IN ASYMPTOMATIC PATIENTS

26.2.1. General Population

Several major reports have highlighted the independent and incremental prognostic value of CAC over traditional risk factor assessment (Table 1). Kondos et al. *(1)* followed 5,635 asymptomatic, middle-aged patients, with predominantly low to moderate Framingham risk score (FRS), for 37 months for the occurrence of "soft" events (angina pectoris and revascularization) and "hard" events (death and myocardial infarction). Among men, they described a significant increase in risk of both hard events and combined events for each quartile increase in CAC score. For hard events the relative risk increased from 1.76 in the first quartile, compared to no CAC, to 7.2 in the fourth CAC score quartile. Women suffered very few hard events, and, to run statistically meaningful calculations, the investigators had to consider the impact of CAC on combined soft and hard events. The relative risk increased from 1.3 to 10.3 in the first to the fourth quartile of CAC score *(1)*.

After ranking, according to baseline CAC score of 10,377 asymptomatic patients followed for a mean of 5 years, Shaw et al. *(2)* reported that the adjusted relative risk for all-cause death was 1.64, 1.74, 2.54, and 4.03 for CAC scores of 11–100, 101–400, 401–1,000 and greater than 1,000, compared to a CAC score of 1–10. The area under the receiver operating characteristic curve (AUC) to predict death was greater for CAC than for traditional risk factors (0.78 vs 0.72, $p < 0.001$). The incremental predictive value of CAC score to predict all-cause death, using the same cut-off values, was recently confirmed by Budoff et al. *(3)* in 25,253 asymptomatic subjects followed for 6.8 years.

In the St. Francis Heart Study *(4)*, 4,613 asymptomatic middle-aged subjects were followed for 4.3 years after CAC screening. The baseline CAC score was higher in the patients who suffered cardiovascular events than in those without events during follow-up. The best predictor of cardiac death during follow-up was a CAC score >100. CAC score predicted cardiovascular events independently of standard risk factors and CRP and was superior to the Framingham risk score. Similarly, Greenland et al. *(5)*, LaMonte et al. *(6)*, Taylor et al. *(7)*, Detrano et al. *(8)*, and Becker et al. *(9)* added further evidence that CAC works well in intermediate-risk patients to improve risk prediction (Table 1). Additionally, Detrano et al. *(8)* demonstrated that CAC maintains its predictive ability in patients of different ethnicities (Caucasian, African-American, Asian, and Hispanic) living in North America. In view of the evidence that CAC screening improves risk prediction in patients at intermediate risk of hard events at 10 years (10–20% risk according to the Framingham risk score categories), both European and American guidelines support CAC screening in this population subset *(10, 11)*. In asymptomatic subjects at intermediate risk, a low CAC score may help reclassify these patients as low-risk, whereas a high CAC score would reclassify them as high-risk. In the latter case, more aggressive preventive measures and pharmacological interventions should be instituted to manage risk for disease progression and acute cardiovascular events. This would include, for example, an LDL goal much lower than the one used in intermediate-risk patients (usually set at 130 mg/dL), and similar to those of patients with established CAD (<100 mg/dL). The CAC score cut-off value used to discriminate high- from intermediate-risk patients is >100, as implicated by the Francis Heart Study results *(4)*, or a score >75th percentile for age as suggested by the ATP III NCEP guidelines *(12)*. However, a CAC score >400 or >90th percentile denotes even higher annual risk of cardiovascular events (4.8% and 6.5%, respectively) *(13, 14)* and should prompt far more aggressive therapy goals (for example, LDL<70 mg/dL).

Table 1
Synopsis of the Main Studies Demonstrating the Value of Coronary Artery Calcium as an Independent and Incremental Marker of Risk

Primary author	Study type	No of patients	Mean follow-up (years)	Type of events	No of events	Incremental prognostic value of coronary calcium
Shaw L 2	Observational	10,377	5	All-cause death	249	Yes
Kondos G 1	Observational	5,635	3	Myocardial infarction, death, and revascularizations	224	Not assessed
Greenland P 5	Prospective	1,029	7.0 (median)	Myocardial infarction and death	84	Yes
LaMonte M 6	Prospective	10,746	3.5	Myocardial infarction and cardiovascular death	81	Yes
Arad Y 4	Prospective	4,613	4.3	Atherosclerotic cardiovascular events	119	Yes
Taylor A 7	Prospective	1,983	3	Acute coronary syndrome and sudden cardiac death	9	Yes
Detrano R 8	Prospective	6,722	3.8	Myocardial infarction and cardiovascular death	89	Yes
Becker A 9	Prospective	1,726	3.4	Myocardial infarction and cardiovascular death	179	Yes

Importantly, when using CAC screening, Kalia et al. *(15)* demonstrated an increased patient adherence to recommended medical management and statin therapy.

As opposed to intermediate-risk patients, the clinical utility of CAC screening is not well documented in low- and high-risk patients. Most physicians would consider high-risk patients (>20% 10-year risk of hard events) candidates for aggressive risk modification independent of CAC score findings. On the other hand, in most low-risk patients CAC is either absent or the score is low and the majority of these patients would not be reclassified to a higher risk category, rendering CAC screening not cost-effective in this subset. Thus, CAC measurement is not currently indicated in low-risk asymptomatic patients *(10, 11)*. However, some patients with a low FRS may benefit from CAC screening, such as younger (35–45-year-old) patients with a positive family history of premature CAD *(16)*, although specific data on these patients are not yet available.

A degree of uncertainty surrounds the need for stress testing in asymptomatic patients found to harbor large amounts of CAC. Given the low positive predictive value of stress testing in patients with low pretest probability of CAD, most authorities do not recommend the use of stress testing in these patients *(11)*. However, a CAC score >400 has been associated with a positive result on stress testing with myocardial perfusion imaging (Fig. 2) in a proportion varying between 8.9% and 46% of patients

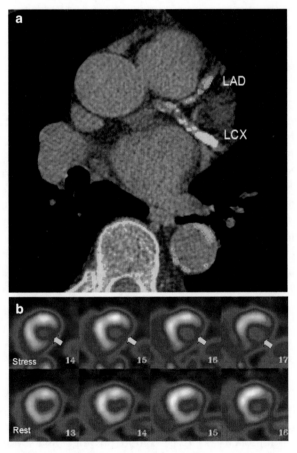

Fig. 2. (a) Axial chest CT image showing dense calcification of the left anterior descending coronary artery (LAD) and left circumflex coronary artery (LCX). **(b)** Corresponding stress and rest short-axis myocardial perfusion images showing an inferolateral perfusion defect during stress (*yellow arrow*) that resolves with rest. This suggests the presence of obstructive coronary artery disease in the left circumflex coronary artery.

(17, 18). This suggests that in such patients there may be adequate pretest probability to justify stress testing. In no case, however, should a high CAC score (>400) justify the performance of an invasive coronary angiogram to exclude the presence of obstructive CAD without having first performed a functional stress test.

26.3. VASCULAR AGE

The seventeenth century physician Thomas Sydenham once wrote "a man is as old as his arteries" *(19)*. In accordance with this notion, the extent of CAC could potentially be used to calculate the vascular age of a given subject. The measurement of a CAC score in large populations without apparent cardiovascular disease has led to the development of nomograms of CAC scores according to age and gender *(20, 21)*. By comparing a subject's CAC score to that of others of the same age and gender, a CAC percentile rank for the individual under study can be determined. A percentile higher than the median for the individual under exam is an index not only of severity, but also of prematurity of atherosclerosis and hence a measure of increased biological age in the face of a younger chronological age *(22)*. Using this approach, Shaw et al. *(12)* were able to assess the number of life years lost or gained in a large population sample based on the amount of CAC measured on a screening EBCT about 5 years prior. The concept of coronary age is very self intuitive and may therefore constitute a more effective way to communicate to an individual his actual risk ("you are 49 but your arteries are 60 years old") rather than simply providing an absolute CAC score.

26.4. SPECIAL POPULATIONS

26.4.1. The Elderly

Several reports supported the independent and incremental prognostic value of CAC in the elderly. In a subgroup of patients older than 70 years of age in the Rotterdam study, subjects with CAC scores of 401–1,000 and >1,000 had a relative risk of myocardial infarction or cardiovascular death of 5.5 and 8.2, respectively, compared to those with low CAC score (0–100) *(21)*. The predictive power of CAC was independent of the FRS category (low, intermediate, or high). Raggi et al. *(23)* followed 35,388 patients, among whom 3,570 subjects were ≥70 year old at screening, for an average period of 5.8 ± 3 years. Increasing CAC scores were associated with decreasing survival rates across all age deciles ($p < 0.0001$), suggesting that CAC is predictive of outcome even in older age. Additionally, using CAC score categories, more than 40% of elderly patients were reclassified to either lower or higher risk FRS categories compared to their original ranking. This was likely due to a reduction in weight attributed to age, the variable carrying most weight in the Framingham algorithm, in the absence of subclinical atherosclerosis *(23)*.

26.4.2. Patients with Diabetes Mellitus

Diabetic patients are less likely to experience classic ischemic symptoms despite a high prevalence of CAD as evidenced by the finding of a similar prevalence of myocardial perfusion defects in diabetic patients without known CAD and non-diabetic patients with known CAD *(24–26)*. Therefore, the identification of pre-clinical CAD may be a very desirable goal, and assessment of CAC with functional imaging performed when the CAC score is very high (Agatston score ≥ 400) appears to be a reasonable risk stratification approach *(27)*. CAC is more prevalent and severe in diabetic patients than the general population *(28, 29)*, and it reflects the larger atherosclerotic burden of these patients. In a study of 9,474 non-diabetic and 903 diabetic asymptomatic individuals, the diabetic patients had a significantly higher CAC score and a higher death rate *(29)*. In addition, for any given CAC score, the diabetic patients had a greater rate of mortality than non-diabetic patients. Importantly, there was no significant difference in survival between diabetic (98.8% at 5 years) and non-diabetic patients (99% at 5 years) with no CAC, underlying the powerful negative predictive value of the absence of this marker of atherosclerosis. In a more recent study, doubling of the CAC score increased cardiovascular event risk by 32% (30). Finally, among diabetic patients, CAC has been shown to predict cardiovascular events more accurately than the Framingham or UKPDS risk scores (31). Investigators have shown that among type 2 diabetic patients, increasing CAC scores are associated with a higher probability of abnormalities on myocardial perfusion imaging (MPI) (32), and, for the same level of CAC, the risk of an abnormal MPI is greater than for patients without diabetes mellitus. Wong et al. (33) showed that the presence of diabetes mellitus or the metabolic syndrome significantly increased the risk of MPI defects among patients with CAC scores ≥100. For a score of 100–399, 13% of diabetic patients had inducible ischemia versus 3.6% among non-diabetic subjects, and for a score ≥400, 23.4% of diabetic patients had inducible ischemia versus 13.6% of non-diabetic subjects. For a score <100, the risk of inducible ischemia by MPI was similarly low for diabetic and non-diabetic patients. This suggests that if CAC screening were to be implemented for asymptomatic type 2 diabetic patients, it would be reasonable to restrict MPI to patients with CAC scores ≥100 in the hope of detecting silent ischemia. This notion is supported by the findings of a study conducted by Anand et al. (32) in which the investigators performed CAC screening in 510 asymptomatic diabetic patients and MPI in those with CAC score >100. During a mean follow-up of 2.2 years, CAC scores and abnormal MPI were equally predictive of cardiovascular morbidity and mortality and demonstrated a statistically significant interaction for the prediction of an adverse cardiovascular outcome.

26.4.3. Screening of Asymptomatic Women

CAD is the leading cause of mortality among both men and women in the United States. Compared to men, women are more likely to have atypical symptoms, and diagnostic testing is often delayed (34). Almost 40% of initial cardiac events are fatal among women (35), and they also have a worse prognosis after a non-fatal myocardial infarction or revascularization procedures compared to men (36, 37). Furthermore, current risk prediction algorithms, such as the Framingham risk score, perform poorly in women compared to men (38). Therefore, alternative risk stratification methods have been investigated, including CAC screening. CAC accumulation in women lags 10 years behind men until around the age of 70, when the gender difference in prevalence of CAC effectively disappears (11). In a cohort of 10,377 asymptomatic patients (40% women) followed for 5±3.5 years, CAC was an independent predictor of death and added incremental prognostic value to the Framingham risk score in both genders (39). Of note, for a given absolute CAC score, women demonstrated a higher mortality than men (39). Among 2,684 asymptomatic women from the Multi-Ethnic Study of Atherosclerosis (MESA), a CAC score > 0 (found in approximately 30% of this population) was predictive of cardiovascular events, while a CAC score ≥ 300 was associated with an 8.6% absolute risk of events over 3.75 years (23% event rate at 10 years) (40). A meta-analysis of two observational registries and three prospective studies showed that CAC screening is equally accurate for risk stratification in men and women (41). Importantly, for a CAC score of 0, men and women had an equivalent minimal risk of cardiovascular events (41).

26.4.4. Patients with Chronic Kidney Disease

Cardiac CT has been utilized to investigate the natural history and pathogenesis of CAC as well as the impact of different therapeutic strategies in chronic kidney disease (CKD). Evidence indicates that the prevalence of CAC increases as the estimated glomerular filtration rate (eGFR) declines (42). In a prospective study of 313 high-risk hypertensive patients, a reduced eGFR was shown to be a major determinant of the rate of progression of CAC *(43)*. Additionally, Sigrist et al. *(44)* reported a prevalence of CAC of 46% in 46 pre-dialysis patients compared to 70% and 73%, respectively, in 60 hemodialysis and 28 peritoneal dialysis patients ($p = 0.02$). Finally, in two randomized studies, CAC was reported in 57% of adult patients who just initiated hemodialysis *(45)* and in 80–85% of established hemodialysis patients *(46)*.

A number of factors have been associated with CAC in dialysis patients. Associations with age and duration of dialysis *(46, 47)*, diabetes mellitus *(46)*, abnormalities of mineral metabolism *(48–50)*, and use and dose of calcium-based phosphate binders *(51, 52)* have all been reported. Hyperphosphatemia and its therapeutic approach appear to be particularly important in patients with end-stage renal disease. To investigate the impact of therapy for hyperphosphatemia on the progression of CAC, two randomized clinical trials compared the effect of sevelamer (a non-absorbable polymer with phosphate-binding ability in the gut) and calcium-based phosphate binders in hemodialysis patients *(51)*. In both studies, the drugs provided a comparable phosphate control, although a significantly higher serum calcium concentration was noted in the calcium salt-treated arm. At the end of follow-up, sevelamer-treated subjects experienced a significantly smaller CAC progression in both studies *(51)*. Importantly, in the more recent of these two trials, all-cause mortality was significantly lower in the sevelamer arm after 4.5 years of follow-up ($p = 0.02$) *(45)*. CAC scores were shown to be predictive of an unfavorable outcome in dialysis patients by Matsuoka et al. *(53)* The authors followed 104 chronic hemodialysis patients for an average of 43 months after a screening EBT. Patients were divided into two groups according to a baseline CAC score falling below or above the median for the group (score = 200). The 5-year cumulative survival was significantly lower for patients with a CAC score >200 than for those with a score<200 (67.9% versus 84.2%, $p = 0.0003$).

In summary, CAC appears to be predictive of unfavorable outcomes even in high-risk subjects such as CKD patients. However, the studies published so far are small and larger trials will need to be conducted to more fully delineate the relationship between CAC and CKD.

26.5. THE PROGNOSTIC VALUE OF NO CORONARY ARTERY CALCIUM (CALCIUM SCORE 0)

Except for patients with advanced renal failure in whom calcification of the muscular media can occur, calcium in the coronary arteries is found only in association with atherosclerosis in the subintimal space *(11, 54)*. Furthermore, as already discussed, the extent of CAC correlates closely with total atherosclerotic plaque burden *(55–57)*. It may be logical to conclude that a CAC score of 0 would suggest minimal risk of coronary atherosclerosis and thus minimal risk of cardiovascular events. Indeed, a CAC score of 0 has consistently been shown to have a high negative predictive value among asymptomatic patients. In a cohort of 25,253 asymptomatic subjects the 10-year survival for patients with a CAC score of 0 (44% of the sample) was 99.4% *(3)*. Similarly, in a cohort of 10,377 asymptomatic patients, the 5-year survival was 99% for those with a calcium score ≤10 *(2)*. In a meta-analysis including 35,765 asymptomatic patients with a mean follow-up of 4.7 years, 45% had a CAC score of 0 *(58)*. The investigators recorded 48 hard cardiovascular events among those with no CAC for an estimated 10-year risk of events of 0.3% and a negative predictive value of 99.9%. In addition to suggesting an excellent clinical prognosis, a CAC score of 0 in a low- to intermediate-risk asymptomatic population suggests a very low risk of obstructive non-calcified plaque (0.5%) on invasive angiography *(59)*. However, the risk of obstructive disease rises significantly with even low CAC scores in symptomatic subjects *(18)*. As mentioned in the previous sections, the benefit of low risk with a CAC of 0 extends even to high-risk patients such as those with diabetes mellitus and advanced renal failure *(29, 45, 58)*.

26.6. CALCIUM SCREENING IN SYMPTOMATIC PATIENTS

As a measure of subclinical atherosclerosis, CAC has been utilized to predict the presence of obstructive CAD in the general population but has demonstrated only a modest positive predictive value despite its high sensitivity. Nonetheless, its high negative predictive value has been employed to address the diagnosis of chest pain in acute and sub-acute settings. In an early study, 105 patients with angina-like chest pain but negative ECG and cardiac enzymes underwent CAC screening by EBCT in the emergency department before admission or discharge from the hospital. All patients were managed according to the standard approach at that institution and 100 of the 105 underwent other cardiac testing. The presence of a CAC > 0 showed 100% sensitivity but only 63% specificity for detection of obstructive CAD. No patient discharged home with CAC of 0 had an event after 4 months of follow-up *(60)*. In a second study, Georgiou et al. *(61)* followed 192 patients who reported to a single institution emergency department with chest pain; all patients were submitted to CAC screening but the results were not used to make any clinical decision on patient disposition. After an average follow-up of 50 months, the cardiovascular event rate for patients with a CAC score of 0 was 0.6% per year, with a progressive increase in risk as the CAC score increased ($\sim$14% per year with CAC $\geq$ 400). All myocardial infarctions and cardiac deaths occurred among patients with CAC score > 0. Taken together, these results suggest that patients with chest pain, negative cardiac enzymes, a normal EKG, and a CAC score of 0 have very low event rates and can be safely discharged from the emergency department. As confirmation of this assertion, in a population of 1,347 patients with symptoms suggestive of CAD who underwent both CAC scoring and invasive coronary angiography, only 0.6% of 720 patients with critical stenoses on angiography had CAC scores of 0, for a negative predictive value of 98% *(62)*. Interestingly, the false negative CAC results were found in patients below age 50, suggesting that a CAC score of 0 is a stronger predictor of the absence of obstructive CAD in patients > 50 years. Other angiographic *(63)* and nuclear stress testing *(18, 64)* studies in symptomatic patients have shown similarly high negative predictive accuracy for a CAC of 0 in ruling out obstructive CAD. However, a recent study of 291 symptomatic patients referred for coronary angiography and CAC scoring questioned the validity of this concept. In fact, the negative predictive value of CAC score = 0 to exclude a >50% luminal stenosis was 68%, suggesting a lower degree of confidence in this approach *(65)*. Overall, however, there is fairly good evidence to suggest that among low risk symptomatic patients with negative markers of ongoing myocardial ischemia, CAC can be used to screen patients in whom invasive angiography can be safely avoided.

26.7. CORONARY ARTERY CALCIUM PROGRESSION

Since CAC is a sensitive marker of subclinical atherosclerosis, a decade ago researchers started to investigate whether serial changes in CAC score were helpful in monitoring the response to medical therapy. The underlying assumption was that changes in CAC reflect changes in atherosclerotic disease burden. In this view, an increase in CAC above a certain threshold signifies progressive disease, while minimal or no change in CAC identifies stable disease. However, a reliable interpretation of change in CAC score between scans requires that the variability of serial CAC scores be very low. Although initially very poor, the interscan variability has now improved significantly on sequential scans performed within minutes of each other ($\sim$10% with 64-slice MDCT scanners) *(66–68)*. An important consideration as one sets up a sequential CT scanning program is the radiation dose provided with each cardiac CT that mandates that the benefit/risk ratio of repeat scanning be carefully weighed. Progression of CAC is generally calculated as a percent or absolute change from the baseline score. The absolute score change is usually greater in patients with a higher baseline CAC score, although the absolute differences may be small compared to the baseline score (hence a small relative score change). On the contrary, larger percent score changes are expected in patients with a low initial CAC score (e.g., a CAC score change from 10 to 20 is equal to 10 points absolute increase but relative progression of 100%) and do not necessarily reflect a clinically relevant change. In subjects at average Framingham risk the annual CAC progression typically ranges from 20% to 25% using either the Agatston or the volume score *(69–78)*. Factors that may significantly modify rate of change include the patient's baseline CAC score, gender, age, family history of premature CAD, ethnicity, diabetes and glycemic control, body mass index, hypertension, and renal insufficiency *(79–84)*. Most patients will exhibit some increase in CAC scores over time *(69, 70, 72, 74, 75, 77)* although a baseline score of 0 is usually associated with a very slow and delayed growth *(72)*. Therefore, in patients with CAC score of 0 a CT scan should not be repeated prior to 5 years from the initial scan *(72)*.

A number of observational studies and randomized clinical trials have evaluated change in CAC following treatment with statin therapy. Although there was no prior evidence that CAC progression may be influenced by serum lipids, statins were the therapeutic agents of choice due to their strong impact on atherosclerosis events. In four observational reports untreated patients had an average CAC score progression of 36% *(83, 85–87)*, while statin therapy attenuated CAC progression to about 13% *(83, 85–87)*. Unfortunately, these promising initial data were not confirmed by large randomized clinical trials that showed a similar change in CAC scores following placebo and moderate or intensive statin therapy *(88, 89)*. Indeed, except for a small, cross over, prospective trial *(90)*, all other randomized trials failed to confirm the observational data. The lack of an effect in these clinical trials suggests that a longer observational time period may be warranted and/or that statins may reduce cardiac events independent of an effect on calcified plaque. One concern is that these trials often did not aggressively treat other CV risk factors that may confound the lack of therapeutic benefit of statins. Other treatments have also been tested to slow CAC progression. In the Women's Health Initiative (WHI), menopausal women between the ages of 50–59 years were randomized to treatment with conjugated estrogens or placebo *(91)*. In a sub-study of the WHI, 1,064 women underwent CAC screening 8.7 years from trial initiation. Women receiving estrogens showed a lower CAC score compared to those receiving placebo (83.1 versus 123.1, $p = 0.02$). Finally, several reports have noted that a rapid change in CAC score is associated with worse clinical outcomes, including incident MI *(74, 92)*. It would appear that patients exhibiting significant CAC progression from their index scan ($\geq$15% per year) and those with baseline CAC scores $\geq$400 have a shorter lag time to the development of acute MI compared to those with a progression < 15% per year and CAC scores $\leq$100. Thus, the baseline CAC score provides an insight into not only the expected rate of progression but also the timeline of conversion to symptomatic CAD.

26.8. CONCLUSIONS

The field of preventive cardiology has advanced greatly over the past few decades. New and more potent medications aimed at slowing the development and progression of atherosclerosis have become available. The success of preventive efforts is reflected by the reduction in fatal events as recently reported by the American Heart Association, although non-fatal events with substantial consequences for families and society continue to occur at a high rate. The field of atherosclerosis imaging developed with the hope that early detection of subclinical disease and aggressive modification of risk (i.e., accurate risk stratification) could significantly reduce the incidence of acute cardiovascular events. The field has witnessed enormous advancements in just a few years and CAC imaging has played a substantial role. It remains to be clearly demonstrated that patients benefit not only from knowing their actual risk but from the subsequent "graded therapeutic approach" to this newly discovered risk factor. Indeed, a large asymptomatic atherosclerosis burden could be seen as an additional risk factor, probably even more important that other factors used to predict risk. While the field deserves support, it is important to educate the public and physicians as to its advantages and disadvantages for the most proper use of these powerful imaging tools. In the meantime, the screening of asymptomatic intermediate-risk patients for refinement of risk stratification and imaging in stable patients with chest discomfort to exclude obstructive CAD may constitute the best current indications.

REFERENCES

1. Kondos GT, Hoff JA, Sevrukov A, et al. Electron-beam tomography coronary artery calcium and cardiac events: a 37-month follow-up of 5,635 initially asymptomatic low- to intermediate-risk adults. *Circulation.* 2003;107: 2571–2576.
2. Shaw LJ, Raggi P, Schisterman E, Berman DS, Callister TQ. Prognostic value of cardiac risk factors and coronary artery calcium screening for all-cause mortality. *Radiology.* 2003;228:826–833.
3. Budoff MJ, Shaw LJ, Liu ST, et al. Long-term prognosis associated with coronary calcification: observations from a registry of 25,253 patients. *J Am Coll Cardiol.* 2007;49:1860–1870.
4. Arad Y, Goodman KJ, Roth M, Newstein D, Guerci AD. Coronary calcification, coronary disease risk factors, C-reactive protein, and atherosclerotic cardiovascular disease events: the St. Francis Heart Study. *J Am Coll Cardiol.* 2005;46(1):158–165.
5. Greenland P, LaBree L, Azen SP, Doherty TM, Detrano RC. Coronary artery calcium score combined with Framingham score for risk prediction in asymptomatic individuals. *JAMA.* 2004;29:210–215.
6. LaMonte MJ, FitzGerald SJ, Church TS, et al. Coronary artery calcium score and coronary heart disease events in a large cohort of asymptomatic men and women. *Am J Epidemiol.* 2005;162(5):421–429.
7. Taylor AJ, Bindeman J, Feuerstein I, Cao F, Brazaitis M, O'Malley PG. Coronary calcium independently predicts incident premature coronary heart disease over measured cardiovascular risk factors: mean three-year outcomes in the Prospective Army Coronary Calcium (PACC) project. *J Am Coll Cardiol.* 2005;46:807–814.
8. Detrano R, Guerci AD, Carr JJ, et al. Coronary calcium as a predictor of coronary events in four racial or ethnic groups. *N Engl J Med.* 2008;358:1336–1345.
9. Becker A, Leber A, Becker C, Knez A. Predictive value of coronary calcifications for future cardiac events in asymptomatic individuals. *Am Heart J.* 2008;155:154–160.
10. De Backer G, Ambrosioni E, Borch-Johnsen K, et al. European guidelines on cardiovascular disease prevention in clinical practice. Third Joint Task Force of European and Other Societies on Cardiovascular Disease Prevention in Clinical Practice. *Eur Heart J.* 2003;24:1601–1610.
11. Budoff MJ, Achenbach S, Blumenthal RS, et al. Assessment of coronary artery disease by cardiac computed tomography: a scientific statement from the American Heart Association Committee on Cardiovascular Imaging and Intervention, Council on Cardiovascular Radiology and Intervention, and Committee on Cardiac Imaging, Council on Clinical Cardiology. *Circulation.* 2006;114:1761–1791.
12. Shaw LJ, Raggi P, Berman DS, Callister TQ. Coronary artery calcium as a measure of biologic age. *Atherosclerosis.* 2006;188:112–119.
13. Raggi P, Callister TQ, Cooil B, et al. Identification of patients at increased risk of first unheralded acute myocardial infarction by electron-beam computed tomography. *Circulation.* 2000;101:850–855.
14. Raggi P, Cooil B, Callister TQ. Use of electron beam tomography data to develop models for prediction of hard coronary events. *Am Heart J.* 2001;141:375–382.
15. Kalia NK, Miller LG, Nasir K, Blumenthal RS, Agrawal N, Budoff MJ. Visualizing coronary calcium is associated with improvements in adherence to statin therapy. *Atherosclerosis.* 2006;185:394–399.
16. Nasir K, Budoff MJ, Wong ND, et al. Family history of premature coronary heart disease and coronary artery calcification: Multi-Ethnic Study of Atherosclerosis (MESA). *Circulation.* 2007;116:619–626.
17. He ZX, Hedrick TD, Pratt CM, et al. Severity of coronary artery calcification by electron beam computed tomography predicts silent myocardial ischemia. *Circulation.* 2000;101:244–251.
18. Berman DS, Wong ND, Gransar H, et al. Relationship between stress-induced myocardial ischemia and atherosclerosis measured by coronary calcium tomography. *J Am Coll Cardiol.* 2004;44:923–930.
19. Garrison FH. On Thomas Sydenham (1624–1689). *NY Acad Med.* 1928;4:993.
20. Hoff JA, Chomka EV, Krainik AJ, Daviglus M, Rich S, Kondos GT. Age and gender distributions of coronary artery calcium detected by electron beam tomography in 35,246 adults. *Am J Cardiol.* 2001;87:1335–1339.
21. Vliegenthart R, Oudkerk M, Hofman A, et al. Coronary calcification improves cardiovascular risk prediction in the elderly. *Circulation.* 2005;112:572–577.
22. Sirineni GK, Raggi P, Shaw LJ, Stillman AE. Calculation of coronary age using calcium scores in multiple ethnicities. *Int J Cardiovasc Imag.* 2008;24:107–111.
23. Raggi P, Gongora MC, Gopal A, Callister TQ, Budoff M, Shaw LJ. Coronary artery calcium to predict all-cause mortality in elderly men and women. *J Am Coll Cardiol.* 2008;52:17–23.

24. Margolis JR, Kannel WS, Feinleib M, Dawber TR, McNamara PM. Clinical features of unrecognized myocardial infarction—silent and symptomatic. Eighteen year follow-up: the Framingham study. *Am J Cardiol.* 1973;32:1–7.

25. Miller TD, Rajagopalan N, Hodge DO, Frye RL, Gibbons RJ. Yield of stress single-photon emission computed tomography in asymptomatic patients with diabetes. *Am Heart J.* 2004;147:890–896.

26. Nesto RW, Phillips RT, Kett KG, et al. Angina and exertional myocardial ischemia in diabetic and nondiabetic patients: assessment by exercise thallium scintigraphy. *Ann Intern Med.* 1988;108:170–175.

27. Bax JJ, Young LH, Frye RL, Bonow RO, Steinberg HO, Barrett EJ. Screening for coronary artery disease in patients with diabetes. *Diabetes Care.* 2007;30:2729–2736.

28. Iwasaki K, Matsumoto T, Aono H, Furukawa H, Samukawa M. Prevalence of subclinical atherosclerosis in asymptomatic diabetic patients by 64-slice computed tomography. *Coron Artery Dis.* 2008;19:195–201.

29. Raggi P, Shaw LJ, Berman DS, Callister TQ. Prognostic value of coronary artery calcium screening in subjects with and without diabetes. *J Am Coll Cardiol.* 2004;43:1663–1669.

30. Elkeles RS, Godsland IF, Feher MD, et al. Coronary calcium measurement improves prediction of cardiovascular events in asymptomatic patients with type 2 diabetes: the PREDICT study. *Eur Heart J.* 2008;29:2244–2251.

31. Anand DV, Lim E, Lahiri A, Bax JJ. The role of non-invasive imaging in the risk stratification of asymptomatic diabetic subjects. *Eur Heart J.* 2006;27:905–912.

32. Anand DV, Lim E, Hopkins D, et al. Risk stratification in uncomplicated type 2 diabetes: prospective evaluation of the combined use of coronary artery calcium imaging and selective myocardial perfusion scintigraphy. *Eur Heart J.* 2006;27:713–721.

33. Wong ND, Rozanski A, Gransar H, et al. Metabolic syndrome and diabetes are associated with an increased likelihood of inducible myocardial ischemia among patients with subclinical atherosclerosis. *Diabetes Care.* 2005;28: 1445–1450.

34. Shaw LJ, Miller DD, Romeis JC, Kargl D, Younis LT, Chaitman BR. Gender differences in the noninvasive evaluation and management of patients with suspected coronary artery disease. *Ann Intern Med.* 1994;120:559–566.

35. Mosca L, Grundy SM, Judelson D, et al. AHA/ACC scientific statement: consensus panel statement. Guide to preventive cardiology for women. American Heart Association/American College of Cardiology. *J Am Coll Cardiol.* 1999;33:1751–1755.

36. Vaccarino V, Abramson JL, Veledar E, Weintraub WS. Sex differences in hospital mortality after coronary artery bypass surgery: evidence for a higher mortality in younger women. *Circulation.* 2002;105:1176–1181.

37. Vaccarino V, Parsons L, Every NR, Barron HV, Krumholz HM. Sex-based differences in early mortality after myocardial infarction. National Registry of Myocardial Infarction 2 Participants. *N Engl J Med.* 1999;341:217–225.

38. Michos ED, Nasir K, Braunstein JB, et al. Framingham risk equation underestimates subclinical atherosclerosis risk in asymptomatic women. *Atherosclerosis.* 2006;184:201–206.

39. Raggi P, Shaw LJ, Berman DS, Callister TQ. Gender-based differences in the prognostic value of coronary calcification. *J Womens Health.* 2004;13:273–283.

40. Lakoski SG, Greenland P, Wong ND, et al. Coronary artery calcium scores and risk for cardiovascular events in women classified as "low risk" based on Framingham risk score: the Multi-Ethnic Study of Atherosclerosis (MESA). *Arch Intern Med.* 2007;167:2437–2442.

41. Bellasi A, Lacey C, Taylor AJ, et al. Comparison of prognostic usefulness of coronary artery calcium in men versus women (results from a meta- and pooled analysis estimating all-cause mortality and coronary heart disease death or myocardial infarction). *Am J Cardiol.* 2007;100:409–414.

42. Baber U, de Lemos JA, Khera A, et al. Non-traditional risk factors predict coronary calcification in chronic kidney disease in a population-based cohort. *Kidney Int.* 2008;73:615–621.

43. Bursztyn M, Motro M, Grossman E, Shemesh J. Accelerated coronary artery calcification in mildly reduced renal function of high-risk hypertensives: a 3-year prospective observation. *J Hypertens.* 2003;21:1953–1959.

44. Sigrist M, Bungay P, Taal MW, McIntyre CW. Vascular calcification and cardiovascular function in chronic kidney disease. *Nephr Dial Transplant.* 2006;21:707–714.

45. Block GA, Raggi P, Bellasi A, Kooienga L, Spiegel DM. Mortality effect of coronary calcification and phosphate binder choice in incident hemodialysis patients. *Kidney Intl.* 2007;71:438–441.

46. Raggi P, Boulay A, Chasan-Taber S, et al. Cardiac calcification in adult hemodialysis patients. A link between end-stage renal disease and cardiovascular disease? *J Am Coll Cardiol.* 2002;39:695–701.

47. Goodman WG, Goldin J, Kuizon BD, et al. Coronary-artery calcification in young adults with end-stage renal disease who are undergoing dialysis. *N Engl J Med.* 2000;342:1478–1483.

48. Oh J, Wunsch R, Turzer M, et al. Advanced coronary and carotid arteriopathy in young adults with childhood-onset chronic renal failure. *Circulation.* 2002;106:100–105.

49. Wang AY, Wang M, Woo J, et al. Cardiac valve calcification as an important predictor for all-cause mortality and cardiovascular mortality in long-term peritoneal dialysis patients: a prospective study. *J Am Soc Nephr.* 2003;14: 159–168.

50. Chertow GM, Raggi P, Chasan-Taber S, Bommer J, Holzer H, Burke SK. Determinants of progressive vascular calcification in haemodialysis patients. *Nephr Dial Transplant.* 2004;19:1489–1496.

51. Chertow GM, Burke SK, Raggi P. Sevelamer attenuates the progression of coronary and aortic calcification in hemodialysis patients. *Kidney Int.* 2002;62:245–252.

52. Guerin AP, London GM, Marchais SJ, Metivier F. Arterial stiffening and vascular calcifications in end-stage renal disease. *Nephr Dial Transplant.* 2000;15:1014–1021.

53. Matsuoka M, Iseki K, Tamashiro M, et al. Impact of high coronary artery calcification score (CACS) on survival in patients on chronic hemodialysis. *Clin Experimental Nephr.* 2004;8:54–58.

54. Budoff MJ, Gul KM. Expert review on coronary calcium. *Vasc Health Risk Manag.* 2008;4:315–324.

55. Baumgart D, Schmermund A, Goerge G, et al. Comparison of electron beam computed tomography with intracoronary ultrasound and coronary angiography for detection of coronary atherosclerosis. *J Am Coll Cardiol.* 1997;30:57–64.

56. Mintz GS, Pichard AD, Popma JJ, et al. Determinants and correlates of target lesion calcium in coronary artery disease: a clinical, angiographic and intravascular ultrasound study. *J Am Coll Cardiol.* 1997;29:268–274.

57. Rumberger JA, Simons DB, Fitzpatrick LA, Sheedy PF, Schwartz RS. Coronary artery calcium area by electron-beam computed tomography and coronary atherosclerotic plaque area. A histopathologic correlative study. *Circulation.* 1995;92:2157–2162.

58. Shareghi S, Ahmadi N, Young E, Gopal A, Liu ST, Budoff MJ. Prognostic significance of zero coronary calcium scores on cardiac computed tomography. *J Cardiovasc Comput Tomogr.* 2007;1:155–159.

59. Cheng VY, Lepor NE, Madyoon H, Eshaghian S, Naraghi AL, Shah PK. Presence and severity of noncalcified coronary plaque on 64-slice computed tomographic coronary angiography in patients with zero and low coronary artery calcium. *Am J Cardiol.* 2007;99:1183–1186.

60. Laudon DA, Vukov LF, Breen JF, Rumberger JA, Wollan PC, Sheedy PF 2nd. Use of electron-beam computed tomography in the evaluation of chest pain patients in the emergency department. *Ann Emerg Med.* 1999;33:15–21.

61. Georgiou D, Budoff MJ, Kaufer E, Kennedy JM, Lu B, Brundage BH. Screening patients with chest pain in the emergency department using electron beam tomography: a follow-up study. *J Am Coll Cardiol.* 2001;38:105–110.

62. Becker A, Leber A, White CW, Becker C, Reiser MF, Knez A. Multislice computed tomography for determination of coronary artery disease in a symptomatic patient population. *Int J Cardiovasc Imaging.* 2007;23:361–367.

63. Budoff MJ, Diamond GA, Raggi P, et al. Continuous probabilistic prediction of angiographically significant coronary artery disease using electron beam tomography. *Circulation.* 2002;105:1791–1796.

64. Esteves FP, Sanyal R, Nye JA, Santana CA, Verdes L, Raggi P. Adenosine stress rubidium-82 PET/computed tomography in patients with known and suspected coronary artery disease. *Nucl Med Commun.* 2008;29:674–678.

65. Gottlieb I, Miller JM, Arbab-Zadeh A, Dewey M, Clouse ME, Sara L, Niinuma H, Bush DE, Paul N, Vavere AL, Texter J, Brinker J, Lima JA, Rochitte CE. The absence of coronary calcification does not exclude obstructive coronary artery disease or the need for revascularization in patients referred for conventional coronary angiography. *J Am Coll Cardiol.* 2010;55(7):627–634.

66. Groen JM, Greuter MJ, Schmidt B, Suess C, Vliegenthart R, Oudkerk M. The influence of heart rate, slice thickness, and calcification density on calcium scores using 64-slice multidetector computed tomography: a systematic phantom study. *Invest Radiol.* 2007;42:848–855.

67. Horiguchi J, Matsuura N, Yamamoto H, et al. Variability of repeated coronary artery calcium measurements by 1.25-mm- and 2.5-mm-thickness images on prospective electrocardiograph-triggered 64-slice CT. *Eur Radiol.* 2008;18: 209–216.

68. Horiguchi J, Yamamoto H, Hirai N, et al. Variability of repeated coronary artery calcium measurements on low-dose ECG-gated 16-MDCT. *AJR.* 2006;187:W1–W6.

69. Becker A, Leber A, von Ziegler F, Becker C, Knez A. Comparison of progression of coronary calcium in postmenopausal women on versus not on estrogen/progestin therapy. *Am J Cardiol.* 2007;99:374–378.

70. Budoff MJ, Chen GP, Hunter CJ, Takasu J, Agrawal N, Sorochinsky B, Mao S. Effects of hormone replacement on progression of coronary calcium as measured by electron beam tomography. *J Women's Health.* 2005;14: 410–417.

71. Budoff MJ, Raggi P. Coronary artery disease progression assessed by electron-beam computed tomography. *Am J Cardiol.* 2001;88:46E–50E.

72. Gopal A, Nasir K, Liu ST, Flores FR, Chen L, Budoff MJ. Coronary calcium progression rates with a zero initial score by electron beam tomography. *International J Cardiol.* 2007;117:227–231.

73. Hsia J, Klouj A, Prasad A, Burt J, Adams-Campbell LL, Howard BV. Progression of coronary calcification in healthy postmenopausal women. *BMC Cardiovasc Disord.* 2004;4:21.

74. Raggi P, Cooil B, Shaw LJ, et al. Progression of coronary calcium on serial electron beam tomographic scanning is greater in patients with future myocardial infarction. *Am J Cardiol.* 2003;92:827–829.

75. Rasouli ML, Nasir K, Blumenthal RS, Park R, Aziz DC, Budoff MJ. Plasma homocysteine predicts progression of atherosclerosis. *Atherosclerosis.* 2005;181:159–165.

76. Shemesh J, Apter S, Stolero D, Itzchak Y, Motro M. Annual progression of coronary artery calcium by spiral computed tomography in hypertensive patients without myocardial ischemia but with prominent atherosclerotic risk factors, in patients with previous angina pectoris or healed acute myocardial infarction, and in patients with coronary events during follow-up. *Am J Cardiol.* 2001;87:1395–1397.

77. Sutton-Tyrrell K, Kuller LH, Edmundowicz D, et al. Usefulness of electron beam tomography to detect progression of coronary and aortic calcium in middle-aged women. *Am J Cardiol.* 2001;87:560–564.

78. Yoon HC, Emerick AM, Hill JA, Gjertson DW, Goldin JG. Calcium begets calcium: progression of coronary artery calcification in asymptomatic subjects. *Radiology.* 2002;224:236–241.

79. Cassidy AE, Bielak LF, Zhou Y, Sheedy PF 2nd, et al. Progression of subclinical coronary atherosclerosis: does obesity make a difference? *Circulation.* 2005;111:1877–1882.

80. Kawakubo M, LaBree L, Xiang M, et al. Race-ethnic differences in the extent, prevalence, and progression of coronary calcium. *Ethn Dis.* 2005;15:198–204.

81. Kronmal RA, McClelland RL, Detrano R, et al. Risk factors for the progression of coronary artery calcification in asymptomatic subjects: results from the Multi-Ethnic Study of Atherosclerosis (MESA). *Circulation.* 2007;115: 2722–2730.

82. Mehrotra R, Budoff M, Christenson P, et al. Determinants of coronary artery calcification in diabetics with and without nephropathy. *Kidney Intl.* 2004;66:2022–2031.

83. Raggi P, Cooil B, Ratti C, Callister TQ, Budoff M. Progression of coronary artery calcium and occurrence of myocardial infarction in patients with and without diabetes mellitus. *Hypertension.* 2005;46:238–243.

84. Snell-Bergeon JK, Hokanson JE, Jensen L, et al. Progression of coronary artery calcification in type 1 diabetes: the importance of glycemic control. *Diabetes Care.* 2003;26:2923–2928.

85. Budoff MJ, Lane KL, Bakhsheshi H, et al. Rates of progression of coronary calcium by electron beam tomography. *Am J Cardiol.* 2000;86:8–11.

86. Budoff MJ, Yu D, Nasir K, et al. Diabetes and progression of coronary calcium under the influence of statin therapy. *Am Heart J.* 2005;149:695–700.

87. Callister TQ, Raggi P, Cooil B, Lippolis NJ, Russo DJ. Effect of HMG-CoA reductase inhibitors on coronary artery disease as assessed by electron-beam computed tomography. *N Engl J Med.* 1998;339:1972–1978.

88. Raggi P, Davidson M, Callister TQ, et al. Aggressive versus moderate lipid-lowering therapy in hypercholesterolemic postmenopausal women: Beyond Endorsed Lipid Lowering with EBT Scanning (BELLES). *Circulation.* 2005;112: 563–571.

89. Schmermund A, Achenbach S, Budde T, et al. Effect of intensive versus standard lipid-lowering treatment with atorvastatin on the progression of calcified coronary atherosclerosis over 12 months: a multicenter, randomized, double-blind trial. *Circulation.* 2006;113:427–437.

90. Achenbach S, Ropers D, Pohle K, et al. Influence of lipid-lowering therapy on the progression of coronary artery calcification: a prospective evaluation. *Circulation.* 2002;106:1077–1082.

91. Manson JE, Allison MA, Rossouw JE, et al. Estrogen therapy and coronary-artery calcification. *N Engl J Med.* 2007;356:2591–2602.

92. Raggi P, Callister TQ, Shaw LJ. Progression of coronary artery calcium and risk of first myocardial infarction in patients receiving cholesterol-lowering therapy. *Arterioscler Thromb Vasc Biol.* 2004;24:1272–1277.

27 Cardiac Computed Tomography

Patrick Donnelly and Udo Hoffmann

CONTENTS

Key Words: Cardiac computed tomography; Cardiac and coronary anatomy; Electrocardiographic synchronization; Contrast nephropathy.

KEY POINTS

- Multislice CT, with its high spatial and temporal resolution, has the unique capability to non-invasively visualize coronary artery plaque and stenosis.
- Cardiac CT uses ECG triggering and is a robust, fast (10 s), and relatively simple imaging test.
- Adequate patient selection and preparation are key for diagnostic image quality.
- Radiation exposure (7–20 mSv) and iodinated contrast administration (60–100 mL) are the risks associated with cardiac CT; the newest CT scanners allow a low radiation dose protocol (<5 mSv).
- Adequate use of post-processing and knowledge about artifacts are essential to achieve high diagnostic accuracy and to avoid unnecessary subsequent tests.
- The strength of cardiac CT is the exclusion of significant CAD in patients with an intermediate likelihood of CAD.
- Cardiac CT is limited in patients with known CAD.
- Cardiac CT may improve the management of patients with acute chest pain.
- Plaque assessment will potentially provide useful information for risk stratification and preventive therapy.

From: *Contemporary Cardiology: Comprehensive Cardiovascular Medicine in the Primary Care Setting*
Edited by: Peter P. Toth, Christopher P. Cannon, DOI 10.1007/978-1-60327-963-5_27
© Springer Science+Business Media, LLC 2010

27.1. INTRODUCTION

Computed tomography (CT) is one of the greatest innovations of the twentieth century, and it has revolutionized clinical practice. Sir Godfrey Hounsfield, an English engineer working for EMI, and Allan Cormack of Tufts University, Massachusetts, a South African-born physicist, developed the concept and the first computed axial tomographic (CAT) scanner in 1972. For the first time, a large volume of data could be collected in an orthogonal plane by using a thin X-ray beam to rotate around a region of interest. The earliest scanners took hours to acquire data and several days to reconstruct the final image for analysis. Subsequent advances such as "slip-ring" technology removed the need for a rigid mechanical linkage between the power cables and the X-ray tube. This enabled the X-ray tube to rotate indefinitely and resulted in spiral CT. CT imaging has become a cornerstone of clinical practice, and it is thought that over 62 million CT scans are performed each year in the USA *(1)*.

Cardiac imaging with CT represents a relatively new application for this well-established technique. One percent of all CT examinations performed per annum in the USA are thought to have a cardiac indication. While this represents a small proportion of the total number of CT examinations performed each year, interest in cardiac CT has been unprecedented, and this has directly contributed to rapid CT platform development. Before cardiac CT could be applied to the clinical arena, challenges such as respiratory motion, cardiac motion, heart rate variability, and the relative motion of submillimeter coronary arteries had to be overcome. Eight years passed from the introduction of "slip-ring" technology to the introduction of mechanical cardiac CT imaging.

In 1998, "multidetector" CT technology became commercially available by enlarging the imaging platform from the traditional single detector to a design with four detector channels. X-ray data acquisition was synchronized with the electrocardiograph (EKG), and respiratory motion was negated by a 40–60-s breath-hold. Although not yet ready for prime time, these innovative concepts produced the earliest mechanical cardiac CT images *(2)*. Biannual advances in CT technology have revolutionized how the heart is assessed.

27.2. TECHNICAL BACKGROUND

Cardiac CT has been made possible by improvements in CT platform design, EKG-gated image acquisition, faster post-processing, and improved image archiving capabilities. All mechanical CT scanners have three core components: a gantry, an X-ray source, and a detector array. The gantry houses both the X-ray tube and the detector array (Fig. 1).

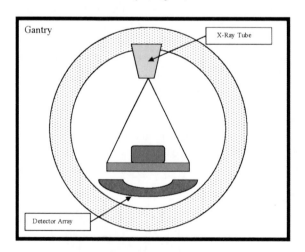

Fig. 1. Anatomy of a CT scanner.

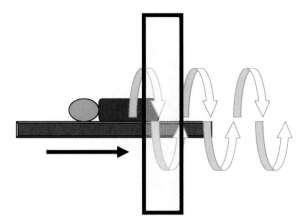

Fig. 2. Helical CT. The patient table (*purple*) moves through the center of the CT scanner (*black rectangle*). In the scanner, the X-ray source rotates around the patient in a circular path. The relative motion of the patient table to the X-ray source creates a helical path (*green arrow*).

The X-ray tube rotates around the patient as the table on which the patient is placed moves through the gantry. This relative movement of the patient through the gantry and the continuous rotation of the X-ray tube effectively produce a spiral path (Fig. 2).

X-rays are generated within the X-ray tube by high-energy electrons, which bombard a metal target made from a heavy atomic material. On striking the metal target, the electrons lose 99% of their energy in low-energy collisions with the atoms of the target. Most of this energy is lost as heat; a small proportion will generate X-ray radiation.

The X-ray beam generated by the source passes through the patient, and some of the constituent photons are absorbed or scattered. This reduction in X-ray photons is called attenuation, and it is dependent on the initial photon energy and the tissue density and atomic characteristics that the X-ray beam encounters.

The emergent X-ray beam strikes the detector array where the photon energy is converted into electronic impulses. The detector array may be fixed or adaptive. In a fixed array, detectors are of equal size and are evenly spaced. The adaptive array is more common in commercial systems and incorporates detectors of different sizes. The detectors can be utilized in a variety of configurations (Fig. 3).

The electronic impulses are converted into digital information from which the attenuation value can be calculated. The attenuation value is described in Hounsfield units (HU) and is relative to the attenuation value of water, which is calibrated to 0 (range –1024 to 3071 HU). The final image is composed of a matrix of tiny squares or pixels, with each pixel designated an attenuation value that corresponds to the tissue from which it originated. The greater the tissue density through which the X-ray beam passes, the higher the attenuation value. Cardiac CT images are displayed on an image matrix of 512 × 512 pixels. A single 3D pixel is called a voxel.

The time it takes for the X-ray source to complete one full 360° rotation of the patient is called the gantry rotation time. The temporal resolution can be thought of as the frequency by which the data that generates an image is acquired. Therefore, if it takes one full gantry rotation time of 500 ms to acquire all of the information, the temporal resolution would be 500 ms. In practice, data can be acquired using an 180° rotation. Current systems have gantry rotation times of less than 330 ms, and, therefore, a minimum temporal resolution of 165 ms can be achieved.

Several innovative methods have been developed to improve the temporal resolution. Multi-segment reconstruction involves the acquisition of smaller packages of data during a single gantry rotation. The

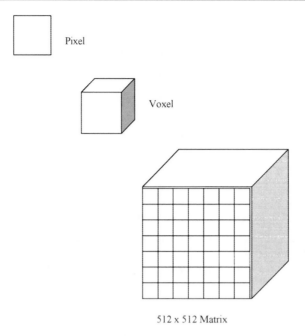

Pixel

Voxel

512 x 512 Matrix

Fig. 3. Image reconstruction, pixel–voxel–matrix.

trade-off for this method is the requirement to sample data over more heartbeats. More heartbeats equate to longer breath-hold requirements and increased susceptibility of the test to heart-rhythm and breath-hold artifacts. A second but significant limitation with this technique is that it is based on the assumption that the coronary artery will return to the same anatomical position at the same time point in the cardiac cycle. In practice, this is not the case and small variations in the anatomical position of the coronary arteries can create significant reconstruction artifact when multi-segment reconstruction algorithms are utilized.

A second technique uses a novel CT platform design. Two X-ray tubes and two detectors placed at 90° to each other rotate at 330 ms. The effective temporal resolution is 83 ms. If a multi-segment (dual) reconstruction algorithm is applied, the effective temporal resolution can be 42 ms *(3)*.

The recent introduction of full-volume coverage scanners represents an exciting innovation. Two-hundred and fifty-six detectors image approximately 12 cm in a single rotation. Cardiac CT of the native coronary arteries with 64-detector technology typically takes 8–10 s. A 256-detector-based scanner can acquire images in 1–2 s or a single heartbeat. If the potential of this technology is realized, cardiac CT could be suitable for most clinical scenarios. EKG synchronization may be rendered obsolete, and breath-hold, heart rate, and arrhythmia artifacts may no longer limit cardiac CT analysis.

The spatial resolution of CT is a measure of how close together two lines can be and still be resolved independently in the image generated. These line pairs, and not the total number of pixels within an image, define the spatial resolution. The smaller the detector size, the greater the potential for a higher spatial resolution due to the creation of an image matrix composed of smaller voxels (the smallest 3D element in the CT data set). In the current context, cardiac CT has a maximal spatial resolution of 0.3–0.4 mm. This resolution is sufficient to visualize the major epicardial coronary arteries but inadequate to overcome the artifact associated with high-density structures such as calcified atherosclerotic plaque.

27.3. ELECTROCARDIOGRAPHIC SYNCHRONIZATION

The current generation of cardiac CT scanners requires the robust acquisition of X-ray generated data to be synchronized with the cardiac cycle. This EKG synchronization allows the reconstruction of data sets that have been acquired over a series of heartbeats but at a specific time point within the cardiac cycle.

The cardiac cycle is composed of two phases—systole and diastole. Systole consumes two-thirds of the duration of a cardiac cycle and varies little with heart rate. This period represents significant cardiac and coronary artery motion and pushes current CT platforms to their limits of temporal resolution. There are three recognized systolic phases—isovolumetric contraction, rapid ejection, and reduced ejection. Isovolumetric contraction corresponds with the EKG QRS complex. In this phase, there is virtually no cardiac motion, but the duration of isovolumetric contraction is too narrow for cardiac CT data acquisition. Late systole, a period of slower ventricular ejection, is a potential target for data acquisition in cardiac CT, particularly in patients with higher heart rates (>65 bpm).

Diastole represents only one-third of the cardiac cycle, but it is favored imaging. Ideally, cardiac CT should reconstruct images in mid-diastole *(4)*; unfortunately, with increased heart rates, the diastolic time window contracts, and the optimal temporal window for acquisition advances from 75% of the R–R interval for subjects with heart rates <70 bpm to 85% of the R–R interval in subjects with heart rates >80 bpm (Table 1) *(4, 5)*.

Table 1
Heart Rate and Temporal Resolution Requirements

Heart rate (bpm)	Temporal resolution (ms)	Imaging phase
40	500	Diastole
50	400	Diastole
60	300	Diastole
70	200	Diastole
80	150	Diastole
90	120	Late systole
100	100	Late systole
120	50–100	Late systole

There are two basic EKG synchronization techniques—prospective and retrospective. Both methods involve the analysis of a single heartbeat as defined by the R–R interval of the EKG signal. The intention of each algorithm is to acquire isocardiophasic reconstruction of the coronary arteries. Each artery is sampled at the same time point in the same anatomical position within each heartbeat. A scan can be triggered prospectively or retrospectively by three basic methods; the absolute delay method involves data collection at a fixed time interval after the preceding R wave. An absolute reverse delay involves data collection at a fixed time interval from the succeeding R wave. A relative delay involves data collection as a percentage of the R–R interval; therefore, it is relative to the heart rate of the patient. The ability of current algorithms to utilize both fixed and relative delay protocols facilitates robust clinical imaging over a greater range of heart rates (Fig. 4).

Prospective triggering ensures a rapid scan time and reduced radiation exposure to the patient. The R wave of the EKG is recognized by the algorithm, and after a pre-specified time interval and for a specific duration, data is acquired. The process is repeated until the heart is imaged. A series of axial scans are generated. The major limitation of this technique is the lack of flexibility during postprocessing. If an inappropriate time interval has been selected, image quality may be suboptimal. A significant change in the R–R interval will also contribute to image degradation.

Retrospective synchronization allows the clinician to review data acquired over the entire cardiac cycle and to choose only the highest quality data sets for analysis. The time interval selected can be defined as a percentage of the R–R interval or as a specific time interval after or before the R wave (Fig. 5). This technique acquires data in a continuous spiral. Comprehensive data sets are available

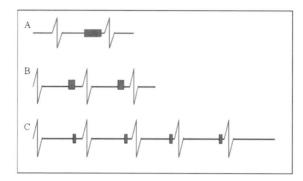

Fig. 4. Single versus multi-sector reconstruction. (**a**) Single-sector reconstruction. The image is reconstructed for data that is generated from a single cardiac cycle and utilizes a full 180° rotation. (**b**) Dual-sector reconstruction. Images are acquired at a pre-specified time points in the cardiac cycle and acquired over two heartbeats. This requires two 90° rotations. (**c**) Multi-sector reconstruction. Images are acquired rapidly over many heartbeats.

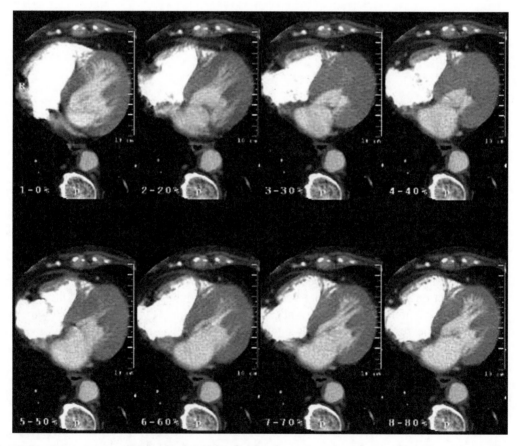

Fig. 5. EKG synchronization. Simultaneous EKG synchronization with image acquisition allows reconstruction of images from any time point in the cardiac cycle.

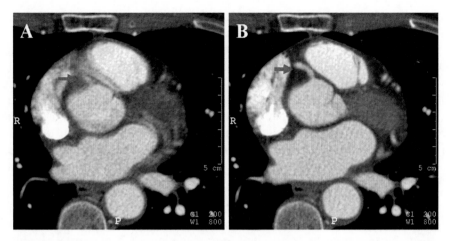

Fig. 6. Optimal temporal phase for reconstruction. (**a**) Axial image that demonstrates RCA motion artifact (*red arrow*) when imaged at 10% of the R–R interval. (**b**) Axial image of the same RCA but imaged at 40% of the R–R interval. The proximal coronary artery is easily identified.

for review but at the cost of a significantly higher radiation exposure to the patient, prolonged post-processing, and image archiving (Fig. 6).

27.4. HOW TO PERFORM A CARDIAC CT EXAMINATION

In recent years, cardiac CT has made the transition from an operator-dependant procedure to a semi-automated technique with variables in patient size, heart rate, and rhythm automatically adjusted for by advanced software algorithms. Despite these developments, there are some important steps that should be strictly adhered to if images of diagnostic quality are to be consistently achieved.

27.4.1. Step 1

Patient selection is key and probably the most important step for successful imaging. The referring clinician must have a clear understanding of the strengths and limitations of the technique and the indications that have recently been issued by professional bodies. If a subject is considered suitable for cardiac CT, screening for contraindications should be undertaken. In general contrast allergy, severe renal impairment, pregnancy, orthopnoea, claustrophobia, and arrhythmias with poorly controlled ventricular response should be considered absolute contraindications to the procedure.

27.4.2. Step 2

The heart rate, breath-hold capacity, renal function, and medications should all be documented. Heart rates <65 bpm and sinus rhythm are desirable for optimal CT image quality. Recently, the latest generation of high temporal resolution scanners (data acquisition 83 ms) can acquire diagnostic images for heart rates up to 100 bpm. In general heart rates <80 bpm for dual-source CT and <70 bpm for conventional 64 multidetector platforms are desirable. Optimal heart rates can be achieved by the administration of heart rate-lowering medication, such as beta-blockers, calcium, and/or If channel antagonists.

Conventional 64-detector platforms require an 8–10 s breath-hold for native coronary artery imaging and 15 s for coronary artery bypass graft evaluation. This requirement is easily achieved by most subjects; however, we recommend instruction on breath-hold technique, with specific instructions to avoid the "valsalva maneuver." As the breath-hold duration increases, some subjects find it difficult to maintain. They begin to forcibly exhale against a closed glottis. This contributes to diaphragmatic drift, and stimulation of the parasympathetic nervous system. These alterations in the cardiac anatomical position and shifts in the R–R interval cause image artifact. This can be avoided by observation of a number of breath-hold practices to ensure patient eligibility and clarify patient expectation.

The relative risk of contrast nephropathy needs to be considered before a contrast-enhanced cardiac CT angiogram. It is perhaps best avoided in patients with a serum creatinine levels >1.8 mL/dL. Patients with mild to moderate renal impairment should be encouraged to hydrate before the procedure to reduce the small risk of contrast-induced nephropathy. Subjects with a history of mild contrast material allergy may be administered steroids and antihistamines pre-examination. Medication should be documented and all nephrotoxic medication omitted on the day of the CT examination.

27.4.3. Step 3: Scanner Technology

Cardiac CT should be performed on a CT platform that is capable of the simultaneous acquisition of at least 16 slices. Scans are more consistently reproducible on CT platforms capable of 64 slices or more.

27.4.4. Step 4: Scan Protocols

The rapid evolution of cardiac CT had contributed to the development of numerous protocols—non-contrast-enhanced calcium score, contrast-enhanced coronary artery angiogram, comprehensive cardiothoracic (triple rule out), and cardiac morphology and function evaluation. Protocol selection and scan parameters are determined by the clinical question and patient characteristics. Careful consideration of the effective radiation dose to the patient should lead to protocol refinements that spare radiation exposure such as prospective triggering and tube current modulation.

27.4.5. Step 5: Immediate Pre-scan Requirements

Venous access is achieved with a minimum 16-gauge catheter in the right median antecubital vein. Three plastic electrocardiograph electrodes should be placed on the torso. Metal electrodes may cause significant streak artifact. Two electrodes are placed beneath the right and left clavicle, and the third is placed on the abdomen. All electrodes are positioned to ensure a high-quality electrocardiogram trace with a sizable R wave for EKG synchronization.

Sublingual nitrate immediately pre-test may be administered to vasodilate the coronary vascular bed and improve image quality. Subjects that are nitrate naïve may experience a reflex tachycardia and presyncope.

27.4.6. Step 6: Protocol Initiation

A scout scan is performed to determine the field of view and scan range. This may be followed by a non-contrast-enhanced, prospective triggered coronary artery calcium scan 120 kV, 80 mAs, 3 mm slice thickness, and a calcium threshold of 130 HU.

A CT coronary angiogram (CTA) is usually performed with 50–100 mL of non-ionic contrast media. The volume of contrast should be minimized. The contrast is injected at a rate of 4–6 mL/s. A bolus of saline is administered to wash contrast out of the right ventricle, which can cause artifact. CTA may be initiated by a test bolus or automated bolus scan technique.

A test bolus involves the administration of 20 mL of contrast. The transit time is assessed by a series of dynamic low-dose (120 kV, 20 mAs) monitoring scans at the level of the aortic root. The delay between each monitoring scan acquisition is approximately 1 s. Acquisition of the dynamic monitoring scans started 10 s after the beginning of the injection of intravenous contrast material. The region of interest in the aortic root is monitored to generate an enhancement curve. The time needed to reach the peak of maximum enhancement equates to the delay applied prior to the manual triggering of the CT angiogram.

An automated bolus tracking technique monitors in real time a region of interest in the ascending aorta. A pre-defined threshold of 120–150 HU defines the threshold for automated scan initiation. A scan delay of 5–6 s facilitates breath-hold instruction and inspiration, and ensures that the peak contrast attenuation is achieved prior to EKG data acquisition. Vascular enhancement should be uniform and contrast attenuation within the lumen should be in excess of 200 HU.

27.4.7. Step 7: Data Reconstruction and Post-processing

A single cardiac CT study can generate over 1,500 images and requires 500 MB of storage. The final data set can be post-processed using a number of different algorithms. Typically, a slice thickness of 0.6–0.75 mm is utilized with a 50% overlap between images. The smaller image slice improves the spatial resolution, but this is at the expense of noisier images. In large subjects, thicker slices may improve image quality but at the expense of the spatial resolution.

Reconstruction kernels are used to convert the raw data from the spiral scan into interpretable images. Kernels are filters that balance the sharpness of the image with the image noise. High-resolution (sharp) kernels increase the resolution of the image but at the expense of image noise. Low-resolution (smooth) kernels reduce the noise but at the cost of resolution. The choice of smooth or sharp kernel will depend on the clinical requirement. For example, calcium and stents would require a sharp reconstruction kernel to improve image quality.

27.4.8. Step 8: Scan Reporting

A cardiac CT report should contain appropriate identifying information on both patient and referrer. The date and time of the examination should be recorded. The date, time, indication, and author of the report should be clearly visible. The technical limitations and image quality should be defined. The CT reader should comment on coronary artery anatomy and the presence, location, and type of coronary atheroma. Where possible, the functional significance of the atheroma should be defined. Cardiac structure and function, including regional wall motion abnormalities and perfusion defects, should be assessed. Additional information on non-coronary structures such as pulmonary venous anatomy, cardiac veins, and valves can be commented on where appropriate. Incidental findings should be reported.

27.5. RADIATION DOSE

The annual background radiation in the USA is 1–4 mSv. A single cardiac CT can expose the patient to five times this radiation dose (Table 2). The effective radiation exposure of cardiac CT is considered a major limitation of this technique. The American Heart Association scientific statement on cardiac CT suggests that a 10 mSv cardiac CT examination may be associated with an increased lifetime risk of a fatal malignancy. The possibility of fatal malignancy has been quoted as 1 in 2,000 cases (7).

The complex theories of cancer risk estimation are beyond the scope of this chapter. However, there is considerable discussion within the scientific community on how this lifetime risk can be best modeled. There are some basic points of consensus; the risk of low-level radiation, such as that used in CT, is largely unknown. There is data present that suggests that for exposures greater than 100 mSv there is a significant lifetime risk of a fatal malignancy as a direct consequence of this level of radiation exposure. For CT with doses consistently less than 20 mSv, the evidence is less robust. Repeated and unnecessary CT examinations should be avoided. The effective radiation dose of a cardiac CT examination is greater in women than in men due to the exposure of radiation-sensitive breast tissue that lies within the scan range. The lifetime cancer risk should be considered in the patient context.

Table 2
Effective Radiation Exposure for Cardiac Examinations

Radiation source	Effective radiation dose (mSv)
Annual background radiation	2–5
Chest X-ray	0.1
Coronary angiography (no ventriculogram)	2–6
SPECT	6–15
Coronary CT calcium	1–3
Coronary CT angiogram (retrospective)	7–25
Coronary CT angiogram (ETCM)	6–10
Coronary CT angiogram (prospective)	1–3

ETCM, EKG tube current modulation.

Older patients have a lower associated risk, and for those patients with a cardiomyopathy, discussion of cancer risk may be a moot point given that the 5-year survival rate is less than 50%. In younger subjects, the associated lifetime attributable cancer risk may be estimated based on age, gender, and the scan protocol utilized *(8)*.

An acceptable radiation exposure for a cardiac CT examination would be <12 mSv. This is slightly higher than a conventional angiogram without left ventriculography, which is thought to be approximately 7 mSv. This is not representative of current interventional practice where an increasing number of cardiac catheterizations are performed through a radial artery vascular access site. This change in practice has been driven by the relatively high femoral access site complication rate but at the cost of increased radiation exposure to both patient and staff *(9)*.

At present, myocardial perfusion imaging is considered the non-invasive imaging test of choice for patients with suspected coronary artery disease. However, approximately 50% of the studies performed in the USA use thallium or a dual-isotope imaging protocol. This practice can expose patients to between 17 and 24 mSv of radiation. When technetium radioisotope is used, the radiation exposure may be much lower, between 7 and 12 mSv *(10)*. Sixty-four-detector cardiac calcium score examinations expose patients to approximately 2 mSv. A 64-detector cardiac CTA using a retrospective gating algorithm can expose patients to an effective radiation dose of between 8 and 24 mSv. Comprehensive cardiothoracic and coronary artery bypass graft evaluations may expose patients to radiation doses in excess of 30 mSv. The application of effective dose sparing algorithms can reduce the dose of CTA by 50–60%.

The challenge for cardiac CTA is to lower the radiation dose further. If cardiac CT can generate consistently diagnostic images with radiation exposures <5 mSv, it is likely to be considered the imaging investigation of choice for the majority of patients with suspected coronary artery disease. This would represent a seismic shift in conventional practice and secure a central niche for cardiac CT in the assessment of patients.

The radiation exposure is dependant on the scan parameters utilized. The tube current, slice scan time, and peak tube kilovoltage (kVp) are major contributors to the effective radiation dose. Tube current and slice scan time influence the mAs. There is a linear relationship between the radiation dose and the mAs. Increasing the mAs from 100 to 200 delivers twice the dose. Increasing kVp can increase the radiation dose, because the X-ray beam has more energy. This increases penetration and more radiation reaches the detectors. Often an increase in kVp will require a reduction in mAs to maintain image integrity. This mAs reduction limits or may reduce the radiation exposure to the patient. The slice thickness, slice spacing, and helical pitch may affect dose as well. In single-slice CT with well-designed collimators, dose (as indicated by CT dose index, CTDI) is relatively independent of slice thickness for contiguous slices. Of course, the total length of the area scanned, as well as slice spacing, will determine how much total energy is deposited in the patient. For the same techniques, doses for helical scans with a pitch of 1.0 are equivalent to axial scans with contiguous slices. Pitches greater or less than 1 influence the CT dose index values proportionally.

Radiation reduction can be achieved by several methods. The exact determination of the scan length and narrow field of view can directly reduce the radiation dose. Alteration of scan parameters such as the kVp and mAs will also reduce dose. A reduction of the tube current from 120 to 100 kV can result in a radiation dose reduction from 8.8 to 16.9 mSv for 120 kV to 4.9–11.9 mSv for 100 kV *(11)*. A reduction in mAs from 300 to 150 could reduce the dose by 50%.

Two automated techniques facilitate radiation dose reduction. EKG controlled tube current modulation reduces the tube current between 4 and 25% of the nominal value but restores the maximal current at a time point pre-specified as optimal for coronary artery imaging. High-quality images can be acquired at a single time point at the cost of noisier images at other phases. Similarly, sequential prospectively triggered protocols can reduce the radiation exposure by reducing the overlap associated with retrospective gated spiral scanning. These studies provide ultra-low radiation doses but at the potential expense suboptimal image quality for interpretation *(12)*.

A multicenter observational study *(13)* (Protection 1) demonstrated a wide variation in the effective radiation exposure of patients that underwent cardiac CT by institution and CT platform utilized. Significant factors that influence dose included patient weight, scan length, lower tube voltage 100 kV versus 120 kV, tube current modulation, and sequential versus spiral protocols. Tube current modulation or sequential prospective triggered scan protocols should be considered for all cardiac CT examinations. The radiation dose for CT angiograms that utilize automated dose reduction protocols may be as low as 2–10 mSv. In the Protection 1 study, 70% of examinations were performed using these dose sparing algorithms. The median radiation dose for a cardiac CT was found to be 12 mSv. Despite the recent introduction of these algorithms, clinical practice has already changed. Future dose reductions may be achieved by the addition of appropriate organ, improved detector efficiency, advanced organ shields, advanced filters, and post-processing algorithms.

All cardiac CT examinations should be performed with a dose that is as low as reasonably achievable (ALARA). This goal must be weighted against the requirement to achieve a diagnostic scan. Radiation dose reduction at the expense of diagnostic image quality should be avoided. A cardiac CTA should be viewed as a definitive diagnostic technique for the majority of patients assessed. It should provide accurate diagnostic information and inform treatment strategies. Further diagnostic imaging investigations should rarely be required. The radiation dose should be adjusted for each patient

27.6. CARDIAC ANATOMY

Knowledge of normal coronary artery anatomy and cardiac morphology is essential for CT analysis. Normal cardiac morphology is described as situs solitus (Fig. 7). This means that the right atrium is connected to the right ventricle, which in turn is connected to the right ventricular outflow tract and common pulmonary artery. The left atrium is connected to the left ventricle, which in turn is connected to the aorta. Variations in this basic anatomical design exist but are beyond the scope of this chapter.

Normal coronary artery anatomy (Fig. 8) is defined as a left main, which originates superior to the right coronary artery from the left coronary sinus. The left main usually bifurcates but may trifurcate beneath the left atrial appendage to form the left anterior descending (LAD), the left circumflex (LCX), and/or the ramus intermedius. The LAD follows the anterior interventricular groove until it reaches the left ventricular apex. The LAD supplies two important side branch groups. The septal perforators originate from the right ventricular side of the LAD. They supply the anterior two-thirds of the septum. The diagonal branches arise from the left ventricular side of the LAD and supply the lateral wall of the left ventricle. Typically, there are two or three important diagonal branches. The LCX is often a short and recessive vessel. It follows a course laterally in the left atrioventricular groove and supplies

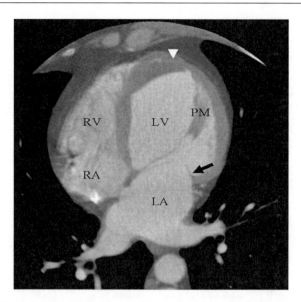

Fig. 7. Situs solitus. RA, right atrium; RV, right ventricle; LA, left atrium; LV, left ventricle; PM, papillary muscle; black arrow, posterior mitral valve leaflet; white arrowhead, apical thrombus.

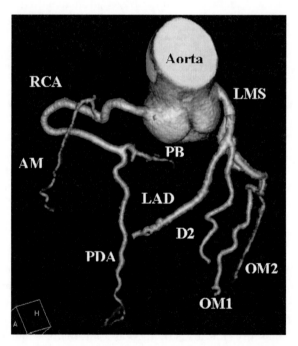

Fig. 8. Normal coronary artery anatomy. RCA, right coronary artery; AM, acute marginal; PDA, posterior descending branch; PB, posterobasal branch; LMS, left main stem; LAD, left anterior descending; D2, second diagonal; OM1, first marginal; OM2, second marginal.

the lateral and posterior walls of the left ventricle with a variable number of obtuse marginal branches. The ramus intermedius may be present in 30% of people and originates between the LAD and the LCX coronary arteries to supply the anterolateral wall of the left ventricle. When present the diagonal and marginal systems are less well developed. The RCA arises from the right coronary cusp, descends in the right atrioventricular groove, continues to the inferior surface of the heart, and bifurcates at the posterior interventricular groove. There are two major branches, the posterior descending (PDA) and the posterolateral (PL). The PDA arises from the RCA in 80% of cases. This is described as a right dominant system. In 15% of subjects, the PDA originates from the LCX system. In the remainder (5%), the posterior interventricular septum is supplied by both the RCA and the LCX. This variation of anatomy is described as co-dominant. The second branch that arises at the crux is the posterolateral branch and this supplies the posterior and inferior wall of the left ventricle.

27.7. POST-PROCESSING TECHNIQUES

Axial images are considered the source data, and axial scrolling is considered the cornerstone for the evaluation of a cardiac CT study. Multiplanar reconstructions (MPR) are created by reconstruction from a stack of axial images. The images can be displayed in axial, sagittal, and coronal sections and

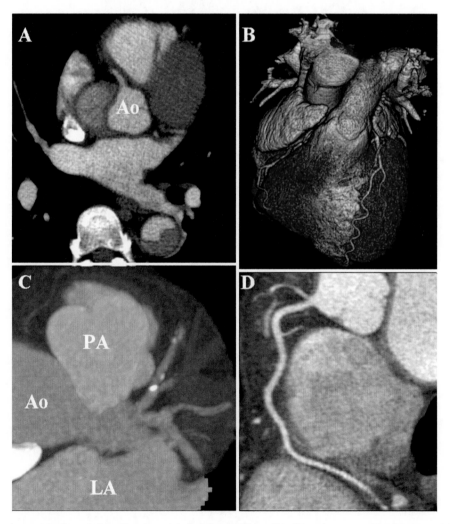

Fig. 9. Image interpretation and projection. (**a**) Axial scrolling. (**b**) 3D volume rendered image. (**c**) Maximum intensity projection. (**d**) Curved multi-planar reconstruction.

can be easily generated. Curved multiplanar reconstructions (cMPR) allow the tortuous longitudinal course of a coronary artery to be displayed in a single image. cMPR utilizes an algorithm that distorts the natural anatomical geometry. Coronary artery stenosis quantification using this technique may lead to misinterpretation of the anatomy. Assessment should always be performed in at least two orthogonal planes. Maximum intensity projections (MIP) use a similar principle to invasive angiography (Fig. 9). Voxels with the highest attenuation values are utilized to create the final 2D images, which can often display long coronary artery segments. This technique is particularly useful when non-coronary structures obscure coronary artery visualization. The high-density contrast within the lumen can be extracted and the rest of the non-contrast-enhanced data discarded. MIPs should not be used when coronary artery calcification is present. The calcium frequently is of a comparable or higher density than the coronary artery lumen. The calcium will be most prominent, and the lower density lumen or

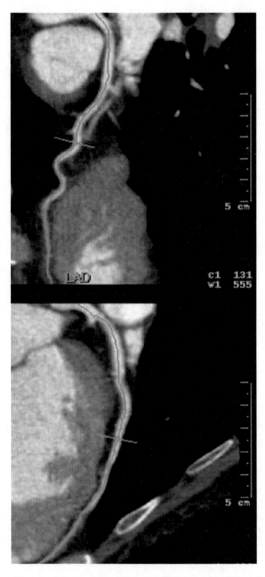

Fig. 10. Orthogonal projections. Two orthogonal projections of the LAD. Note the lack of mid-vessel tortuosity in the *lower image*.

non-calcified atherosclerotic plaque will be obscured. Three dimensional volume-rendered images of the heart are visually impressive. They provide a rapid impression of the cardiac CT. Image voxels are prescribed specific attenuation values based on major tissue densities. The operator has full control over the voxel number specified; therefore the final image can be adjusted to make certain types of tissue more transparent or opaque as required.

For stenosis quantification, two 3–6 mm-long orthogonal maximum intensity projections should be reconstructed (Fig. 10). A comparison of the lumen size proximal and distal to the stenosis should be made and defined as a percentage diameter stenosis. Lesions with lumen reduction of >70% are thought to be of hemodynamic significance. For left main stem lesions, the threshold for significance is much lower. A 50% diameter stenosis is considered functionally significant. Semi-quantitative software packages may allow semi-automated stenosis analysis; however, many are not sufficiently robust to be utilized in clinical practice.

27.8. CARDIAC CT ARTIFACTS

Image artifacts are often multifactorial (Fig. 11). Technical limitations of the current generation of cardiac CT platforms, limitations in scan protocol preparation, and patient-related factors can all conspire to reduce image quality and influence the accuracy of analysis.

Coronary arteries are submillimeter structures that require the highest possible spatial resolution for accurate analysis. The current technology has a spatial resolution of 0.4–0.6 mm. Accurate quantitative stenosis assessment would require a spatial resolution of 0.2 mm.

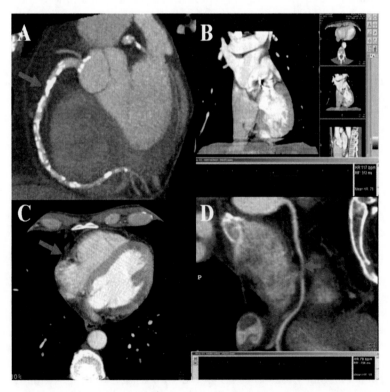

Fig. 11. Cardiac CT artifacts. (**a**) Calcification. Sheet calcification limits visualization of the vessel lumen (*red arrow*). (**b**) Premature atrial ectopic (*green line*) creates a step artifact in the reconstruction of the inferior cardiac border (*red arrow*). (**c**) Intrinsic motion of the right coronary artery (*red arrow*). (**d**) Inappropriate EKG synchronization (*green line*) contributes to reconstruction artifact (*red arrow*).

In order to freeze cardiac motion, the temporal resolution must be faster than the intrinsic cardiac motion. Cardiac CT exploits the physiology of the cardiac cycle. Images are optimal if acquired at low heart rates (<65 bpm) and are captured at end-systole or mid-diastole. These time points represent the period of least cardiac motion. For robust cardiac CT imaging, the next generation of scanners will require a temporal resolution of <50 ms.

Cardiac, respiratory, and involuntary patient movements contribute to motion artifacts. Cardiac motion includes excessive heart rate variability and arrhythmias. Adequate heart rate control pre-procedure can be achieved with the administration of negatively chronotropic medication. Heart rates <65 bpm reduce motion and provide an optimal diastolic window for data acquisition. ECG editing can facilitate the removal of short-lived extrasystoles or arrhythmias from the final data set that is utilized for image reconstruction. The introduction of high temporal resolution and full-volume coverage CT scanners may make the issue of heart rate motion obsolete. Respiratory motion can be avoided by care-ful patient instruction and breath-hold practice. There must be an adequate delay between breath-hold instruction and scan initiation. Barriers to comprehension such as language difficulties and auditory impairment can be overcome with appropriate planning. A shallow breath is all that is required and it is important that the Valsalva maneuver is prevented. Patients that are dyspneic when supine can be oxygenated.

Involuntary patient motion can be avoided by education, optimization of patient position, and increased awareness of the normal sensation of contrast administration, and stressed patients can be given water to avoid throat dryness and cough reflex. Poor contrast enhancement of the coronary arteries can occur as a consequence of inappropriate and small-caliber cannula placement, contrast extravasation, low-contrast injection rate, insufficient contrast concentration and volume, and inac-curate scan triggering. All of these factors can be avoided with appropriate attention to protocol planning.

Dose reduction is important. Low dose that contributes to a poor contrast-to-noise ratio is unaccept-able and exposes patients to further testing that may not otherwise be required.

Finally, high-density structures such as calcium, pacemaker wires, intracardiac occluder devices, and surgical clips cause beam-hardening artifacts. Increased tube current and the utilization of an appropriate reconstruction filter can limit the impact of this artifact on the final data set.

27.9. INDICATIONS FOR CARDIAC CT

Comprehensive guidelines for the clinical utilization of cardiac CT were issued in 2006 and 2007. They are summarized in the following top five cardiac CT indications.

27.9.1. Assessment of Suspected Coronary Artery Anomaly

Coronary artery anomalies are a rare form of congenital heart disease and are reported to affect <0.1% of the general population. Although the majority of coronary artery anomalies are benign and of no hemodynamic significance, a small proportion is responsible for 20% of all sudden cardiac deaths reported in the less-than-35 age-group (14–19).

An anomalous origin of a coronary artery from an opposite coronary sinus associated with an inter-arterial path, a single coronary artery, and a coronary artery fistula have all been associated with adverse cardiovascular outcomes. Basso et al. (15) demonstrated that, in as many as 30% of young athletes, symptoms can occur. They concluded that investigation should be mandatory, particularly in symptomatic athletes who are at greatest risk of sudden cardiac death.

In the current context, there is no real consensus for the classification, investigation, manage-ment, and follow-up of these patients (20). Most are detected at autopsy or coincidently at cardiac catheterization. Cardiac catheterization is invasive, and it is challenging even with appropriate catheter selection. The determination of the course of an anomalous artery will require multiple projections and experienced interpretation. In contrast, cardiac CT is non-invasive and can facilitate rapid determination of the course of an anomalous coronary artery and thereby determine the significance if any (Fig. 12).

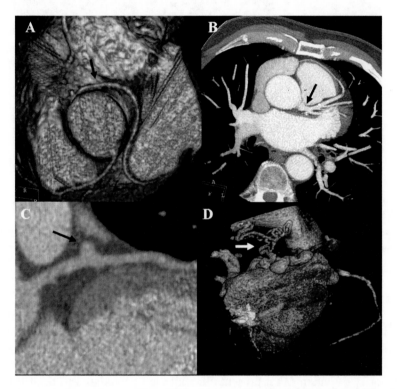

Fig. 12. Coronary artery variation and anomalies. (**a**) Left circumflex coronary artery which arises from the right coronary sinus. (**b**) Single coronary artery arises from the left coronary sinus. (**c**) Aneurysm of the left anterior descending coronary artery caused by Kawasaki disease. (**d**) Aorta–left circumflex fistula.

27.9.2. Assessment of Coronary Artery Calcium

Coronary artery calcification is a surrogate marker of atherosclerotic plaque burden. High coronary calcium scores correlate with greater plaque burdens and higher cardiovascular event rates (Fig. 13). The assessment of coronary calcium burden is useful in asymptomatic patients thought to be at intermediate risk of a cardiovascular event. This is defined as a 10–20% 10-year risk of a cardiovascular event based on traditional risk factor assessment. There is no role for coronary calcium assessment in low- (<10%) and high-risk patients (>20%). A calcium score of 0 indicates an extremely low probability of a 3–5-year cardiovascular event, but this score in an intermediate risk patient should not reduce the therapeutic measures taken to reduce traditional risk factors (e.g. hypertension, hypercholesterolemia). In patients with atypical symptoms, coronary calcium assessment may be helpful in the rule out of a cardiac etiology. Patients with a dilated cardiomyopathy may have a calcium score to rule out an ischemic etiology. Finally, coronary calcium may be useful in the assessment of patients with acute chest pain and non-specific EKGs. Three major single-center observational studies have been reported and one study found in a 7-year follow-up that the annualized event rate for a 0 calcium score was 0.6%.

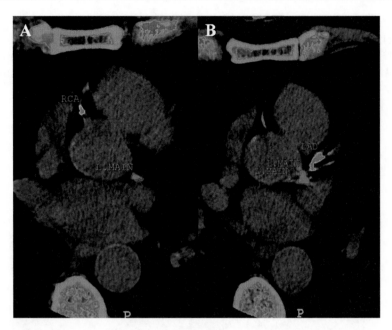

Fig. 13. Coronary artery calcium score. (**a**) Non-contrast CT scan demonstrates calcium in the proximal LMS and RCA (*blue area*). (**b**) Calcified coronary atheroma is present in both the LMS and the LAD (*blue area*).

27.9.3. Elective Assessment of Native Coronary Artery Disease

Coronary artery disease presents as chest pain or exertional angina in 50% of patients. The prevalence of non-specific chest pain is much greater than the incidence of angina. The need for the further assessment of chest pain to rule out coronary heart disease is determined by the physician, based on the characteristics of symptoms and the patient's pre-test probability of underlying coronary artery disease (Table 3). The majority of patients that present clinically are considered to be at least at intermediate risk of coronary artery disease and merit further investigation.

Table 3
Pre-test Probability of Coronary Artery Disease (72)

Age	Gender	Typical angina	Atypical probable angina	Non-anginal chest pain	Asymptomatic
30–39	Man	Intermediate	Intermediate	Low	Very low
	Woman	Intermediate	Very low	Very low	Very low
40–49	Man	High	Intermediate	Intermediate	Low
	Woman	Intermediate	Low	Very low	Very low
50–59	Man	High	Intermediate	Intermediate	Low
	Woman	Intermediate	Intermediate	Low	Very low
60–69	Man	High	Intermediate	Intermediate	Low
	Woman	High	Intermediate	Intermediate	Low

The niche for cardiac CT in this patient population is continuing to evolve. Established non-invasive tests such as dobutamine stress echocardiography and myocardial stress perfusion imaging using single-photon emission CT are well validated, clinically reliable, and inform clinical decisions. However, they are not without limitation; they provide functional rather than anatomical information, and high interobserver variability rates have been reported.

The invasive coronary angiogram remains the gold standard for the assessment of patients with suspected coronary artery disease. Twenty to forty percent of all diagnostic angiograms demonstrate no evidence of obstructive coronary disease. Cardiac CT has evolved rapidly in the last 10 years, and rapid advances in technology have required repetitive validation studies with each technical breakthrough. The advent of 64-detector CT technology has ushered in an era of technical stability, and numerous studies have reported on the clinical efficacy of this technique. The development of 64-detector CT has significantly increased the specificity of the test. A comparison of 16- and 64-detector CT on a per-patient basis observed an increase in specificity from 69 to 90%, and in the increase in the PPV from 79 to 93%. In a meta-analysis of cardiac CT examinations performed between 2002 and 2006, the number of unnecessary invasive angiograms was reduced by approximately 30% due to the introduction of 64-detector technology (21).

Cardiac CT can accurately identify coronary artery anatomy and determine the extent of coronary artery stenosis severity. The consistently high negative predictive value allows significant coronary artery pathology to be reliably excluded. Symptomatic patients that are considered to have an intermediate probability of coronary artery disease and have an inconclusive exercise stress test should be considered suitable for cardiac CT angiography.

Accurate coronary artery stenosis quantification by cardiac CT is a greater challenge (Fig. 14). Several studies have demonstrated the feasibility of this technique in both calcified and non-calcified atheroma. Correlation with intravascular ultrasound and invasive coronary angiography is moderate to good (22, 23). These studies have evaluated culprit coronary lesions that cause >50% stenosis. Few studies have evaluated the accuracy of quantitative cardiac CT in the quantification of non-culprit lesions. CT can accurately quantify the stenosis grade in coronary arteries with a caliber in excess of 3 mm. For vessels <3 mm correlation with conventional angiography is poor. The plaque composition also appears to influence stenosis assessment. There is a poor correlation when the plaque is predominantly calcified, a moderate correlation for non-calcified plaque, and a good correlation for mixed plaque (24).

Clinicians remain unclear about the functional relevance of coronary artery stenosis quantification by cardiac CT. Myocardial perfusion imaging (MPI) is considered the non-invasive investigation for the determination of hemodynamically significant coronary artery stenosis. Patients with stable angina

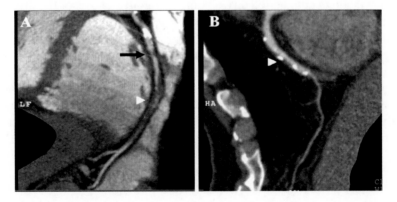

Fig. 14. CT angiography. (**a**) 53-year-old, acute coronary syndrome presentation with inferolateral ST segment elevation. Curved MPR demonstrates mild ostial RCA disease. Significant sheet calcification in the proximal RCA limits lumen assessment. Immediately distal to this calcified plaque there is a non-occlusive mixed plaque. Beyond this in the mid-RCA there is a significant stenosis (*black arrow*). There is a short section of normal caliber vessel that terminates in a total occlusion (*white arrowhead*). (**b**) 46-year-old, acute coronary syndrome presentation with non-ST elevation infarction. Curved MPR RCA demonstrates moderate proximal mixed plaque disease (*white arrowhead*).

and normal MPI findings have a low risk for future cardiac events *(25)*. This is a valuable information that guides clinical management. A recent study compared CT lesion severity with MPI. If cardiac CT demonstrated a lesion <60%, then functional ischemia was rare. If CT defined a lesion >80%, then functional ischemia at MPI was frequently observed. For intermediate lesions by CT 60–80% hemodynamic significance by MPI was observed in <50%. The accuracy of CT to define a hemodynamically significant stenosis, applying a stenosis threshold of >70%, resulted in a 79% sensitivity, 92% specificity, 66% positive predictive value, and 96% negative predictive value *(26)*.

Conventional wisdom suggests that qualitative assessment of stenosis severity by invasive coronary angiography may overestimate lesion severity by 20%. A recent study compared qualitative CT angiography (CTA), quantitative CT angiography (QCTA), qualitative invasive angiography (CA), and quantitative coronary angiography (QCA) to measurement of the fractional flow reserve (FFR). The diagnostic accuracy of CTA, QCTA, CA, and QCA to detect a hemodynamically significant coronary stenosis was 49, 71, 61, and 67%, respectively. Correlation between QCT and QCA with FFR measurement was poor *(27)*.

Cardiac CT provides anatomical information on lesion severity, but it cannot assess the hemodynamic severity of a lesion. Improvements in detector design, spatial resolution, and the development of stress CT for the detection of regional wall motion abnormalities will be required before cardiac CT can provide both anatomical and functional information.

27.9.4. Elective Assessment of Coronary Artery Bypass Grafts

Coronary artery bypass grafts are considered the best revascularization strategy for patients with multi-vessel or left main stem obstructive coronary disease. However, vein graft occlusion rates can exceed 20% in the first year after surgery and are thought to occlude at a rate of 4% per year after 4 years. Vein graft occlusion is a major cause for readmission after surgery. Invasive catheter angiography in these patients can be difficult. Vascular access limitations, poor catheter engagement of the grafts, prolonged screening times, and significant morbidity and mortality risk have made cardiac CT an attractive alternative.

Conventional CT platforms have demonstrated the feasibility of CT for imaging coronary artery bypass grafts *(28–34)*. Initial results demonstrated that the proximal anastomosis site could be assessed, but no information could be reliably obtained on graft stenosis or the distal anastomosis site (one of the commonest areas for disease recurrence). Improvements in CT technology have created increasing interest in CT evaluation of grafts (Fig. 15). Saphenous vein grafts are less challenging for CT than the native coronary arteries due to their large caliber, thin wall, absence of calcified atheroma, and relative immobility. Arterial grafts, however, continue to be challenging due to their size, tortuosity, mobility, and metallic clips. In patients where graft disease is considered, cardiac CT can rapidly identify the bypass graft anatomy and determine the suitability for a graft percutaneous revascularization. A meta-analysis of 723 patients with 2,023 bypass grafts demonstrated a high accuracy of CT for the detection of graft obstruction (occlusion and >50% stenosis). The sensitivity was 97.6% [95% confidence interval (CI): 96–98.6%]; specificity 96.7% (95% CI: 95.6–97.5%); positive predictive value 92.7% (95% CI: 90.5–94.6%); and negative predictive value 98.9% *(35)*.

27.9.5. Emergency Assessment of Non-specific Chest Pain and Acute Coronary Syndromes

Chest pain is one of the most frequent causes of presentation to the emergency department. Five million emergency department visits result in 2 million hospitalizations at a cost of $8 billion. Over 60% of admissions are not cardiac and 2% of emergency department discharges are. A rapid and effective method to identify or rule out an acute coronary syndrome is highly desirable *(36)*.

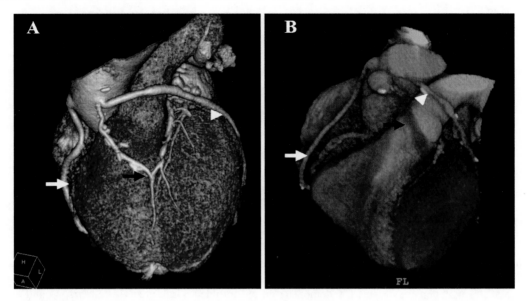

Fig. 15. Coronary artery bypass grafts. (**a**) 3D volume rendered reconstruction. There are three patent coronary artery bypass grafts. There is a saphenous vein graft to the RCA (*white arrow*), a saphenous vein graft to the LCX territory (*white arrowhead*), and a left internal mammary artery graft to the distal LAD (*black arrow*). Note the distal anastomosis site of the LIMA graft to the LAD is patent with good distal run-off. (**b**) There are three Saphenous vein grafts. The SVG to RCA is patent (*white arrow*). The SVG to D2 has a proximal occlusion (*black arrow*). The SVG to the LCX territory has a significant proximal stenosis (*white arrowhead*).

The high negative predictive value of contrast-enhanced CCT for the detection of coronary artery disease makes it an attractive tool to rule out myocardial infarction. The utility of contrast-enhanced CCT has been reported in three single-center studies. Hoffmann et al. *(37)* in a prospective double-blind observational cohort study demonstrated the feasibility of CCT in 103 consecutive patients awaiting hospital admission to rule out myocardial infarction. All patients were at low risk. Forty percent of patients had no CT evidence of atherosclerotic plaque. None of these patients were determined to have ACS. Sixty percent of patients had demonstrable atheroma including all 14 patients with ACS. The presence of a significant stenosis (>50%) was excluded in 71% of these patients, none of whom has ACS. In 13 patients, a significant stenosis was detected, 8 of whom had ACS (Fig. 16). In 17 patients, a significant stenosis could not be excluded. Six of these patients were determined to have ACS. The overall positive and negative predictive value of CCT for the detection of ACS was 47 and 100%, respectively. In a registry-based observational study Rubinshtein et al. *(38, 39)* assessed the impact of CCT on clinical decision making in 58 intermediate risk patients. This represented one half of the potential intermediate risk population presenting to their ED with chest pain. Forty-one patients were considered by two physicians to have ACS. Nineteen of these patients had established coronary heart disease. Only 10 of the 22 patients with no prior diagnosis of coronary heart disease were considered to have ACS after CCT. CCT detected ACS with a sensitivity of 100% and a specificity of 92%. The initial diagnosis of ACS was revised in 44%, and after diagnostic revision, hospitalization was considered unnecessary in 45% of the ACS cohort. Goldstein et al. *(40)* performed a randomized trial in 197 low-risk patients to compare the efficiency of CCT with single-photon emission tomography (SPECT). Ninety-nine patients underwent CCT, of which 67 were considered normal and discharged. Twenty-four patients were considered to have moderate plaque (>25 and <70%) or non-diagnostic. This cohort underwent SPECT evaluation. Three studies were considered functionally

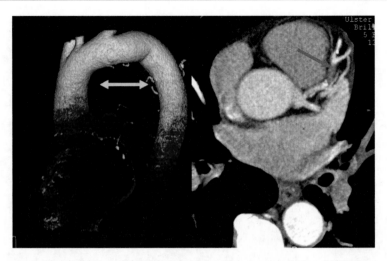

Fig. 16. CT for the triage of acute chest pain. 46-year-old male, no conventional risk factors for CAD. Acute presentation to ED 40 min after the onset of chest-back pain. No EKG changes, CXR suggested a widened mediastinum. Comprehensive cardiac CT demonstrated an unfolded aortic arch (*yellow arrow*) and an acute occlusion of the proximal LAD (*red arrow*).

abnormal. The remaining eight patients were considered to have severe stenoses (>70%) at CCT and all were found to be severe stenoses at invasive catheter angiography. In the population assessed with CCT an immediate diagnosis and discharge was achieved in 68% of patients. Eighty-seven percent of the patients with moderate plaque or non-diagnostic scans were discharged after SPECT imaging. There were no events in the entire population. Interestingly the rate of discharge was greater in the standard of care group. In both diagnostic studies, CCT increased the demand for invasive coronary angiography.

An alternative strategy for patients with non-specific acute chest pain is the comprehensive thoracic CT evaluation. This protocol facilitates the rapid rule out of the major cardiothoracic causes of chest pain. CT can identify an acute coronary syndrome, pulmonary embolism, and acute aortic syndromes. A single study performed rapidly to exclude the major causes of life-threatening chest pain could make a significant impact on ED chest pain triage.

White et al. *(41)*, in an observational case series of 69 stable patients with chest pain, demonstrated the feasibility of a comprehensive cardio-thoracic CT protocol. An initial CT assessment was made of non-cardiac disease and for the contrast-enhanced presence of coronary artery calcification using the extended field of view images (ECG-gated 75% R–R interval). Further post-processing and analysis of the cardiac CT data set for coronary artery anatomy, cardiac function, and myocardial perfusion abnormalities were performed. The consensus group reviewed the discharge diagnoses, clinical records, and all relevant standard care test results. The CT was normal in 75% of the cases; coronary heart disease was found in 14% and non-cardiac findings in 4%. The sensitivity and specificity for a diagnosis of a cardiac cause of chest pain were 83 and 96%, respectively. Unique to this study is the fact that no pre-scan beta-blockade was administered. Vessel attenuation of different thoracic vascular territories was measured, and two independent readers semi-quantitatively analyzed image quality. With a mean scan time of 12 s and diagnostic image quality for the aorta, coronary, and pulmonary arteries in 58 of the 60 patients enrolled, it is possible that at last there is a realistic possibility of ED triple rule out without rate-lowering medication.

Further prospective trials are required; however, a synergistic cardiac CT and biomarker strategy for the rapid assessment of emergency department chest pain appears to hold significant promise.

27.10. EMERGING INDICATIONS

27.10.1. Radiofrequency Pulmonary Venous Ablation

Atrial fibrillation (AF) is the most common sustained cardiac arrhythmia and a major risk factor for cerebrovascular ischemia. It is present in 10% of the population more than 80 years old and has a mortality rate twice that of control subjects. AF presents with short episodes of arrhythmia, which self-terminate. Forty percent of patients develop persistent atrial fibrillation, which requires chemical or electrical cardioversion to restore a normal heart rhythm. Half of these patients will have a recurrent episode within 1 year, and many will develop permanent AF. AF is most commonly seen in structurally abnormal hearts; however, it may occur in normal hearts in times of stress, infection, or after stimulants such as caffeine, alcohol, cocaine, or amphetamines. Medical treatments with antiarrhythmics, which can reduce the heart rate, suppress the arrhythmia recurrence. Refractory symptomatic atrial fibrillation can be treated by percutaneous or surgical ablation.

Radiofrequency ablation of the pulmonary veins is increasingly considered for patients with AF. Over 90% of AF arises from sleeves of ectopic atrial tissue found around the pulmonary veins. Fifty percent of these ectopic foci originate from the left superior pulmonary vein. Traditional imaging techniques such as echocardiography and pulmonary venography can be difficult to perform and often only limited views of the pulmonary veins can be obtained. Cardiac CT can map the anatomical distribution of the pulmonary veins and left atrium both before and after the procedure; it can also assess the pulmonary vein size, which can influence the size of the ablation catheter *(42, 43)* (Fig. 17). Knowledge of the distance from the ostium of the pulmonary vein to the first side branch is also helpful to the electrophysiologist as ablation within 5 mm of the ostium or the first bifurcation increases the risk for pulmonary vein stenosis. Specialist electrophysiology laboratories have the capability to fuse the anatomical cardiac CT information with the electrophysiological map. This image fusion may improve the procedural success rate.

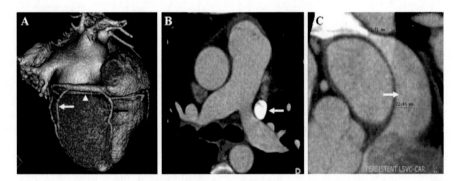

Fig. 17. Coronary venous anatomy. (**a**) 3D volume rendered reconstruction of cardiac venous anatomy. The identification of an appropriate lateral wall cardiac vein target can determine the success of cardiac resynchronization therapy. CT demonstrates the middle cardiac vein (*white arrow*), great cardiac vein (*white arrowhead*) in the left atrioventricular groove, and a lateral cardiac vein, which is a suitable target for the left ventricular lead. (**b**) Axial image that demonstrates a persistent left superior vena cava. (**c**) Aneurysmal coronary artery sinus with a significant great cardiac vein stenosis.

27.10.2. Preoperative Valvular Replacement Assessment

Cardiac CT is increasingly utilized in the preoperative evaluation of patients who are to undergo cardiac surgery *(44)*. By convention, all male patients aged 35 or more and post-menopausal and premenopausal females with risk factors that require cardiac surgery for severe valvular heart disease undergo an invasive angiogram to determine if bypass graft revascularization is also required. Many patients have a low probability for a significant coronary artery stenosis. It has been estimated that in patients with a low-intermediate probability of coronary artery disease as many as 70% could avoid an invasive angiogram preoperatively. In addition, the accuracy of information on the aortic valve, aorta, and left ventricular size may make it more attractive "one-stop shop" in younger subjects with severe aortic valve disease *(45, 46)* (Fig. 18). Cardiac CT facilitates 3D and multiplanar reconstructions. This allows for accurate orientation of the parasternal short-axis views of the aortic valve in mid-late systole.

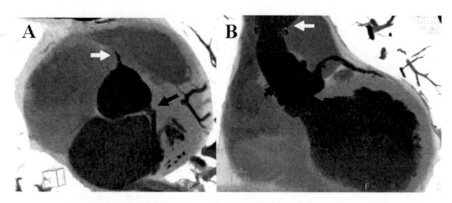

Fig. 18. Preoperative valve assessment. (**a**) Axial short-axis view of a tricuspid aortic valve. The right coronary artery (*white arrow*) and left main stem (*black arrow*) can also be identified. Moderate–severe calcification of all three aortic valve leaflets is present (*central black area*). (**b**) Sagittal view of the ascending aorta and aortic valve. This reconstruction allows accurate quantification of the size of the aorta at leaflet (*green arrow*), sinus of valsalva (*red arrow*), sinotubular junction (*blue arrow*), and ascending aorta (*white arrow*). Note prior ascending aorta aneurysmal repair and severely dilated left ventricle (LV). This information is very valuable to the surgeon preoperatively.

For older patients, the application of a preoperative cardiac CT is more complex. Older patients are more likely to have degenerative valvular disease, which is associated with extensive calcification. This limits image quality and impairs accurate quantification. In addition, the prevalence of co-existent coronary artery disease will be in excess of 50%. The accuracy of cardiac CT to determine the functional significance of a moderate coronary artery anatomical lesion is at best 50%. If coronary atheroma is predominantly calcified, quantification of lumen encroachment may be impossible.

Cardiac CT may be helpful in the assessment and planning of transcutaneous aortic valve insertions. CT can accurately quantify the size of the aorta, which would facilitate accurate prosthesis sizing. The unique ability to orientate the aortic root and valve plane may provide information on the optimal invasive angiographic projection pre-procedure. This would reduce scan time, contrast requirements, and radiation exposure to the patient during the procedure.

27.10.3. Left Ventricular Function

Cardiac CT is unlikely to replace echocardiography to assess left ventricular systolic function. CT may be a suitable option to determine cardiac morphology and function in subjects with poor acoustic images or limited echocardiographic windows. Multiple temporal phases within the cardiac cycle are reconstructed. Ideally, these should be at 5% time points through the R–R interval. The end-systolic and end-diastolic time points are identified from the EKG and visually from images that identify the largest and smallest left ventricular cavity area (Fig. 19).

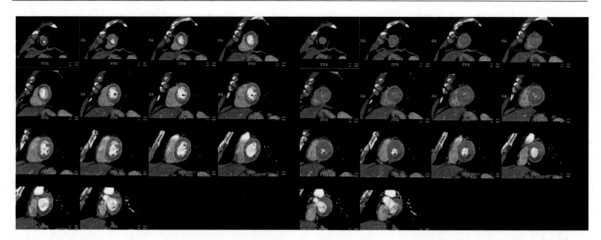

Fig. 19. Cardiac function. Cardiac function can be assessed by the determination of the time points in the cardiac cycle that correspond to end systole and diastole. Correct alignment along the cardiac axis and knowledge of the slice thickness allows for the determination of the stroke volume, ejection fraction, and cardiac output. Tracing of the endocardial and epicardial contours facilitates the assessment of wall thickness and left ventricular wall mass. Cine imaging can determine regional wall motion abnormalities.

CT utilizes two established methods to assess ventricular function. The area length method applied to long-axis images and the Simpson's method applied to short-axis views. The area length method utilizes the area (A) defined within the endocardial contour trace in long-axis two-chamber view and the length (L) from the left ventricular apex to the level of the mitral valve ring. The left ventricular volume is calculated by the following formula:

$$\text{Long-axis volume} = (8/3) \times A^2/(3.125 \times L)$$

Simpson's method utilizes the endocardial contours if the entire short-axis images of the left ventricular cavity. The cross-sectional area of each left ventricular image is calculated. Left ventricular volume is calculated by adding all the cross-sectional areas and multiplied by the distance between each slice thickness.

Left ventricular ejection fraction is calculated from the end-diastolic and end-systolic volumes and is given by

$$\text{Ejection fraction} = [(\text{LVedv} - \text{LVesv})/\text{LVedv}] \times 100\%$$

The correlation between cardiac CT and cardiac MRI or gated myocardial perfusion imaging is good *(47, 48)*.

27.10.4. Perfusion Imaging

The introduction of hybrid CT–PET and CT–SPECT scanners allows the integration of anatomical information acquired with CT imaging and the functional information obtained form SPECT or PET imaging. However, the scan capital investment cost, protocol incompatibility, and the radiation dose of the scan protocols have generated interest in the utilization of cardiac CT as a stand-alone test for myocardial perfusion imaging.

Preliminary studies, both ex vivo and in vivo, have demonstrated that CT perfusion is feasible *(49–54)* (Fig. 20). A recent study utilized the first pass of iodinated contrast material to assess myocardial perfusion and detect microvascular obstruction (no reflow) in patients within 5 days of their

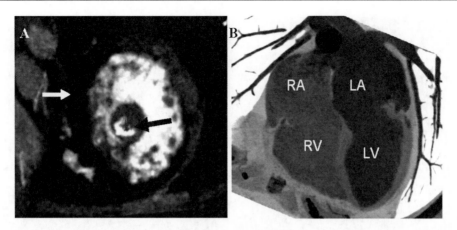

Fig. 20. CT and myocardial perfusion. (**a**) Short-axis view of the left ventricle. Note full thickness LAD infarction (*white arrow*). A spherical lesion is visualized in the LV cavity (*black arrow*). This is an organized thrombus with calcification. (**b**) Apical four-chamber view. RA, right atrium; RV, right ventricle; LA, left atrium; LV, left ventricle.

myocardial infarction *(55)*. In a sub-group of 15 patients, a second scan was performed 7 min later to assess total infarct size by using delayed hyperenhancement. Early hypoenhancement and delayed hyperenhancement were compared between multidetector CT and cardiac MR. Early hypoenhancement was recognized on all multidetector CT and cardiac MR images. Delayed hyperenhancement was observed with cardiac MR imaging at all examinations and with multidetector CT at 11 of 15 examinations. While signal intensity differences between hypoperfused and normal myocardium were comparable for first-pass cardiac CT and MR imaging, cardiac MR imaging had a significantly better contrast-to-noise ratio (CNR) for delayed acquisitions. Hypoenhanced areas (as a percentage of left ventricular mass) at first-pass CT demonstrated a good correlation with those at first-pass cardiac MR imaging. Delayed enhancement CT demonstrated a moderate correlation with delayed enhancement MR imaging. Quantification of delayed hypoenhancement had very good correlation between CT and MR. A further study defined the accuracy of cardiac CT for the assessment of cardiac function, regional wall motion abnormalities (RWMA), and perfusion defects in 32 subjects with an acute myocardial infarction *(56)*. Global LV function and RWMA were compared with transthoracic echocardiography. Perfusion defects were correlated with cardiac biomarkers and single-photon emission CT (SPECT). Cardiac CT demonstrated a good correlation with TTE for the assessment of LV function. A moderate correlation was demonstrated when the perfusion defect size was compared with SPECT.

This early work demonstrates promise but technical limitations, namely insufficient temporal resolution, beam-hardening artifacts, and excessive radiation dose, need to be overcome before robust clinical CT perfusion becomes a reality. A prospective gating protocol can substantially reduce the dose but at the cost to the contrast-noise ratio of the images *(57)*. A single imaging modality that can determine atherosclerotic plaque burden, anatomical location, and severity of stenosis and its functional significance within 12 min could revolutionize non-invasive cardiac imaging.

27.10.5. Atherosclerotic Plaque Assessment

Coronary artery disease is a major cause of mortality in the Western world. Atherosclerotic plaque rupture or erosion can result in a sudden cardiac death or presentation with a major adverse coronary event. These vulnerable plaques have a thin fibrous cap (<65 μm), are predominantly composed of lipid (>40%), and are not visible with invasive angiography.

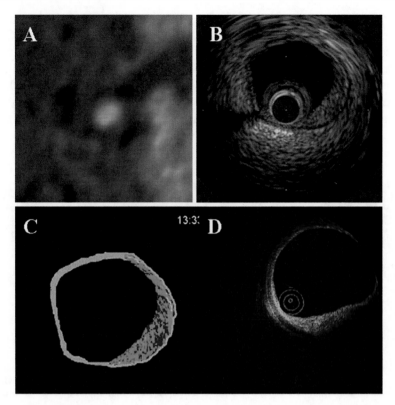

Fig. 21. Atherosclerotic plaque imaging. (**a**) Cardiac CT demonstrates a non-calcified plaque (3–7 o'clock position). (**b**) The non-calcified plaque correlates with intravascular ultrasound (IVUS) *gray scale*. (**c**) IVUS radiofrequency backscatter determines that the plaque is predominantly fibrous (*green color*). (**d**) Optical coherence tomography (OCT), which is the in vivo gold standard for plaque characterization confirms both the presence and the character of the plaque.

The spatial resolution of current CT platforms is approximately 400 μm. The pre-requisite sixfold increase in resolution to determine plaque cap thickness is not foreseeable in the near future. However, cardiac CT can detect atherosclerotic plaque and markers of plaque vulnerability (Fig. 21). In a series of small in vivo studies, cardiac CT was compared to intravascular ultrasound (IVUS) for plaque detection. Cardiac CT can reliably detect atherosclerotic plaque with sensitivities of 83–96% *(59, 60)*. Calcified plaque can consistently be detected with sensitivities >95%. Further plaque characterization is more difficult. Early papers suggested that CT attenuation values could reliably determine the predominant constituent of atherosclerotic plaque. Calcified plaque >130 HU, fibrous plaque 70–110 HU, and lipid-rich plaque <60 HU *(61, 62)*. Despite this promise, subsequent papers have demonstrated that differentiation of non-calcified plaque into lipid and fibrous by attenuation value is an oversimplification of the complexity of atherosclerotic plaque components *(63)*. There is significant overlap between fibrous and lipid plaque when compared to plaque identified on IVUS. This in part is attributable to the arbitrary definition of atherosclerotic plaque to facilitate comparison between CT and IVUS, and it is influenced by the contrast enhancement of the coronary artery lumen *(64)*. Non-calcified plaque detection is limited by reader experience, motion, noise, calcification, and lack of ex vivo validation.

Numerous studies have demonstrated that CT angiograms with high diagnostic image quality can detect and quantify surrogate markers of plaque vulnerability *(65–67)*. The plaque area, volume, and remodeling index defined by CT have demonstrated a moderate correlation with IVUS. Plaque area measurements appear to be consistently overestimated. This is attributable to the inadequate spatial resolution of current CT platforms to differentiate between the contrast-enhanced lumen and the coronary artery vessel wall. Post-processing techniques such as voxel analysis of CT plaque images may allow more accurate plaque quantification *(68)*.

CT may be able to demonstrate atherosclerotic plaque progression. Our group followed patients for 2 years and demonstrated de novo plaque development despite medical treatment (Fig. 22). Recently a report suggested that CT may be able to monitor changes in plaque characterization after treatment *(69)*. If this capability is realized at a low-radiation exposure CT plaque imaging may be suitable to act as a surrogate cardiovascular endpoint in clinical trails or to facilitate optimization of medical management.

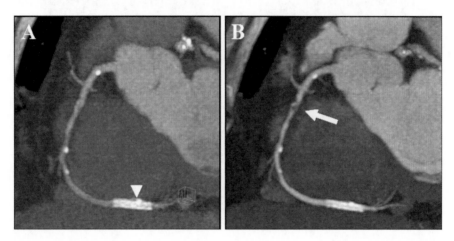

Fig. 22. Atherosclerotic plaque progression. (**a**) Index cardiac CT examination. This demonstrated mild proximal and mid-vessel RCA atheroma. A stent was present pre-crux (*arrowhead*). (**b**) CT performed 2 years after the index scan. Despite optimal medical treatment, there is evidence of plaque progression. A significant obstructive lipid-rich atherosclerotic plaque is present in the second part.

27.10.6. Pericardial Assessment

The pericardium is a thin, two-layered structure that envelops the heart. The parietal and visceral pericardia are separated by <50 mL of serous fluid. The pericardium reduces friction and limits infection between the heart and the adjacent mediastinal structures. In subjects with limited echocardiography windows, cardiac CT may be an attractive diagnostic alternative (Fig. 23). Pericardial effusions commonly develop with infection, myocardial infarction, cardiac dysfunction, and malignancy. Loculated pericardial effusions, particularly if located anteriorly, are difficult to identify by echocardiography. CT attenuation values may help differentiate the cause of the effusion. Cardiac CT may be useful in assessing patients with suspected constrictive pericarditis. The presence of pericardial calcification, a pericardial thickness >4 mm, reduced right ventricular volume, a paradoxical septal bounce, and systemic venous dilatation may all correlate with pericardial constriction in symptomatic patients. CT may be useful in the identification and characterization of pericardial cysts and neoplasm.

27.11. CARDIAC CT PRESENT AND FUTURE

Cardiac CT has evolved beyond the expectations of most clinicians. Feasibility studies have consistently demonstrated that this imaging technique is robust and operator independent. The consistently high negative predictive value of cardiac CT to exclude coronary artery disease (95–99%) supersedes existing non-invasive imaging. The need for clinical studies with an emphasis of long-term follow-up

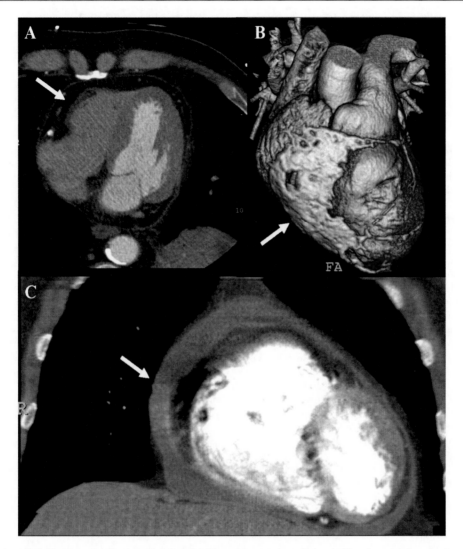

Fig. 23. Pericardial disease. (**a**) Pericardial fat. (**b**) Extensive pericardial calcification. (**c**) Large circumferential pericardial effusion.

has been recognized by the CT research world. Prognostic information comparable to that, which exists for alternative imaging modalities, is highly desirable. Within the last year, promising reports suggest that a normal cardiac CT scan is associated with a low cardiovascular event rate. There appears to be a <1% chance of a cardiovascular event in the subjects followed for 6 years. Additional prognostic information may be acquired by defining the location, extent, and character of coronary atherosclerotic plaque *(70)*. This, in addition to left ventricular systolic function and regional wall motion abnormalities, may facilitate the development of a cardiac CT risk score, which could influence but more importantly individualize patient management.

Scientific guidelines provide unequivocal recommendations for standards on clinical competency and reporting, technical specifications and protocol selection for cardiac CT examinations, and appropriateness criteria/indications for cardiac CT examinations *(7, 71)*. These are likely to be revised in the face of ongoing technological advances and the publication of prospective, multicenter clinical trials.

Manufacturers have addressed the concerns of radiation dose with the introduction of advanced algorithms that allow coronary angiography to be performed with exposures less than 2 mSv. Further technical innovations in CT platform and detector design, in addition to advanced post-processing algorithms, may improve the spatial resolution to 0.2 mm. If this is achieved, cardiac CT will have "crossed the Rubicon" and a new era in non-invasive cardiac imaging and patient-centric treatment will be defined.

REFERENCES

1. Brenner DJ, Hall EJ. Computed tomography—an increasing source of radiation exposure. *N Engl J Med.* 2007;357:2277–2284.
2. Achenbach S, Giesler T, Ropers D, et al. Detection of coronary artery stenoses by contrast-enhanced, retrospectively electrocardiographically-gated, multislice spiral computed tomography. *Circulation.* 2001;103:2535–2538.
3. Flohr TG, McCollough CH, Bruder H, et al. First performance evaluation of a dual-source CT (DSCT) system. *Eur Radiol.* 2006;16:256–268.
4. Herzog C, Arning-Erb M, Zangos S, et al. Multi-detector row ct coronary angiography: influence of reconstruction technique and heart rate on image quality. *Radiology.* 2006;238:75–86.
5. Hoffmann MHK, Shi H, Manzke R, et al. Noninvasive coronary angiography with 16-detector row CT: effect of heart rate. *Radiology.* 2005;234:86–97.
6. Seifarth H, Wienbeck S, Pusken M, et al. Optimal systolic and diastolic reconstruction windows for coronary ct angiography using dual-source CT. *Am J Roentgenol.* 2007;189:1317–1323.
7. Budoff MJ, Achenbach S, Blumenthal RS, et al. Assessment of coronary artery disease by cardiac computed tomography: a scientific statement from the American Heart Association Committee on Cardiovascular Imaging and Intervention, Council on Cardiovascular Radiology and Intervention, and Committee on Cardiac Imaging, Council on Clinical Cardiology. *Circulation.* 2006;114:1761–1791.
8. Einstein AJ, Henzlova MJ, Rajagopalan S. Estimating risk of cancer associated with radiation exposure from 64-slice computed tomography coronary angiography. *JAMA.* 2007;298:317–323.
9. Brasselet C, Blanpain T, Tassan-Mangina S, et al. Comparison of operator radiation exposure with optimized radiation protection devices during coronary angiograms and ad hoc percutaneous coronary interventions by radial and femoral routes. *Eur Heart J.* 2008;29:63–70.
10. Einstein AJ. Radiation risk from coronary artery disease imaging: how do different diagnostic tests compare? *Heart.* 2008;94:1519–1521.
11. Pflederer T, Rudofsky L, Ropers D, et al. Image quality in a low radiation exposure protocol for retrospectively ECG-gated coronary CT angiography. *Am J Roentgenol.* 2009;192:1045–1050.
12. Husmann L, Valenta I, Gaemperli O, et al. Feasibility of low-dose coronary CT angiography: first experience with prospective ECG-gating. *Eur Heart J.* 2008;29:191–197.
13. Hausleiter J, Meyer T, Hermann F, et al. Estimated radiation dose associated with cardiac CT angiography. *JAMA.* 2009;301:500–507.
14. Angelini P, Velasco JA, Flamm S. Coronary anomalies: incidence, pathophysiology, and clinical relevance. *Circulation.* 2002;105:2449–2454.
15. Basso C, Maron BJ, Corrado D, Thiene G. Clinical profile of congenital coronary artery anomalies with origin from the wrong aortic sinus leading to sudden death in young competitive athletes. *J Am Coll Cardiol.* 2000;35:1493–1501.
16. Cheitlin MD, De Castro CM, McAllister HA. Sudden death as a complication of anomalous left coronary origin from the anterior sinus of valsalva: a not-so-minor congenital anomaly. *Circulation.* 1974;50:780–787.
17. Liberthson RR. Sudden death from cardiac causes in children and young adults. *N Engl J Med.* 1996;334:1039–1044.
18. Maron BJ, Shirani J, Poliac LC, Mathenge R, Roberts WC, Mueller FO. Sudden death in young competitive athletes. Clinical, demographic, and pathological profiles. *JAMA.* 1996;276:199–204.
19. Taylor A, Rogan K, Virmani R. Sudden cardiac death associated with isolated congenital coronary artery anomalies. *J Am Coll Cardiol.* 1992;20:640–647.
20. Angelini P. Coronary artery anomalies: an entity in search of an identity. *Circulation.* 2007;115:1296–1305.
21. Hamon M, Morello R, Riddell JW, Hamon M. Coronary arteries: diagnostic performance of 16- versus 64-section spiral CT compared with invasive coronary angiography meta-analysis. *Radiology.* 2007;245:720–731.
22. Cury RC, Ferencik M, Achenbach S, et al. Accuracy of 16-slice multi-detector CT to quantify the degree of coronary artery stenosis: assessment of cross-sectional and longitudinal vessel reconstructions. *Eur J Radiol.* 2006;57:345–350.
23. Ricardo CC, Eugene VP, Maros F, et al. Comparison of the degree of coronary stenoses by multidetector computed tomography versus by quantitative coronary angiography. *Am J Cardiol.* 2005;96:784–787.
24. Dodd JD, Rieber J, Pomerantsev E, et al. Quantification of nonculprit coronary lesions: comparison of cardiac 64-MDCT and Invasive coronary angiography. *Am J Roentgenol.* 2008;191:432–438.

25. Iskander S, Iskandrian AE. Risk assessment using single-photon emission computed tomographic technetium-99m sestamibi imaging. *J Am Coll Cardiol.* 1998;32:57–62.

26. Sato A, Hiroe M, Tamura M, et al. Quantitative measures of coronary stenosis severity by 64-slice CT angiography and relation to physiologic significance of perfusion in nonobese patients: comparison with stress myocardial perfusion imaging. *J Nucl Med.* 2008;49:564–572.

27. Meijboom WB, Van Mieghem CAG, van Pelt N, et al. Comprehensive assessment of coronary artery stenoses: computed tomography coronary angiography versus conventional coronary angiography and correlation with fractional flow reserve in patients with stable angina. *J Am Coll Cardiol.* 2008;52:636–643.

28. Malagutti P, Nieman K, Meijboom WB, et al. Use of 64-slice CT in symptomatic patients after coronary bypass surgery: evaluation of grafts and coronary arteries. *Eur Heart J.* 2007;28:1879–1885.

29. Martuscelli E, Romagnoli A, D'Eliseo A, et al. Evaluation of venous and arterial conduit patency by 16-slice spiral computed tomography. *Circulation.* 2004;110:3234–3238.

30. Meyer TS, Martinoff S, Hadamitzky M, et al. Improved noninvasive assessment of coronary artery bypass grafts with 64-slice computed tomographic angiography in an unselected patient population. *J Am Coll Cardiol.* 2007;49: 946–950.

31. Nieman K, Pattynama PMT, Rensing BJ, van Geuns R-JM, de Feyter PJ. Evaluation of patients after coronary artery bypass surgery: CT angiographic assessment of grafts and coronary arteries. *Radiology.* 2003;229:749–756.

32. Pache G, Saueressig U, Frydrychowicz A, et al. Initial experience with 64-slice cardiac CT: non-invasive visualization of coronary artery bypass grafts. *Eur Heart J.* 2006;27:976–980.

33. Ropers D, Pohle F-K, Kuettner A, et al. Diagnostic accuracy of noninvasive coronary angiography in patients after bypass surgery using 64-slice spiral computed tomography with 330-ms gantry rotation. *Circulation.* 2006;114: 2334–2341.

34. Schlosser T, Konorza T, Hunold P, Kuhl H, Schmermund A, Barkhausen Jo. Noninvasive visualization of coronary artery bypass grafts using 16-detector row computed tomography. *J Am Coll Cardiol.* 2004;44:1224–1229.

35. Hamon M, Lepage O, Malagutti P, et al. Diagnostic performance of 16- and 64-section spiral CT for coronary artery bypass graft assessment: meta-analysis. *Radiology.* 2008;247:679–686.

36. Hoffmann U, Pena AJ, Moselewski F, et al. MDCT in early triage of patients with acute chest pain. *Am J Roentgenol.* 2006;187:1240–1247.

37. Hoffmann U, Nagurney JT, Moselewski F, et al. Coronary multidetector computed tomography in the assessment of patients with acute chest pain. *Circulation.* 2006;114:2251–2260.

38. Rubinshtein R, Halon DA, Gaspar T, et al. Impact of 64-slice cardiac computed tomographic angiography on clinical decision-making in emergency department patients with chest pain of possible myocardial ischemic origin. *Am J Cardiol.* 2007;100:1522–1526.

39. Rubinshtein R, Halon DA, Gaspar T, et al. Usefulness of 64-slice cardiac computed tomographic angiography for diagnosing acute coronary syndromes and predicting clinical outcome in emergency department patients with chest pain of uncertain origin. *Circulation.* 2007;115:1762–1768.

40. Goldstein JA, Gallagher MJ, O'Neill WW, Ross MA, O'Neil BJ, Raff GL. A randomized controlled trial of multi-slice coronary computed tomography for evaluation of acute chest pain. *J Am Coll Cardiol.* 2007;49:863–871.

41. White CS, Kuo D, Kelemen M, et al. Chest pain evaluation in the emergency department: can MDCT provide a comprehensive evaluation? *Am J Roentgenol.* 2005;185:533–540.

42. Jongbloed MRM, Dirksen MS, Bax JJ, et al. Atrial Fibrillation: multi-detector row CT of pulmonary vein anatomy prior to radiofrequency catheter ablation—initial experience. *Radiology.* 2005;234:702–709.

43. Paul C, Aine Marie K, Benoit D, et al. Normative analysis of pulmonary vein drainage patterns on multidetector CT with measurements of pulmonary vein ostial diameter and distance to first bifurcation. *Acad Radiol.* 2007;14:178–188.

44. Gilard M, Cornily J-C, Pennec P-Y, et al. Accuracy of multislice computed tomography in the preoperative assessment of coronary disease in patients with aortic valve stenosis. *J Am Coll Cardiol.* 2006;47:2020–2024.

45. Feuchtner GM, Dichtl W, Friedrich GJ, et al. Multislice computed tomography for detection of patients with aortic valve stenosis and quantification of severity. *J Am Coll Cardiol.* 2006;47:1410–1417.

46. LaBounty TM, Sundaram B, Agarwal P, Armstrong WA, Kazerooni EA, Yamada E. Aortic valve area on 64-MDCT correlates with transesophageal echocardiography in aortic stenosis. *Am J Roentgenol.* 2008;191:1652–1658.

47. Mahnken AH, Koos R, Katoh M, et al. Sixteen-slice spiral CT versus MR imaging for the assessment of left ventricular function in acute myocardial infarction. *Eur Radiol.* 2005;15:714–720.

48. Henneman M, Bax J, Schuijf J, et al. Global and regional left ventricular function: a comparison between gated SPECT, 2D echocardiography and multi-slice computed tomography. *Eur J Nuc Med Mol Imag.* 2006;33:1452–1460.

49. Baks T, Cademartiri F, Moelker AD, et al. Multislice computed tomography and magnetic resonance imaging for the assessment of reperfused acute myocardial infarction. *J Am Coll Cardiol.* 2006;48:144–152.

50. George RT, Silva C, Cordeiro MAS, et al. Multidetector computed tomography myocardial perfusion imaging during adenosine stress. *J Am Coll Cardiol.* 2006;48:153–160.

51. Gerber BL, Belge B, Legros GJ, et al. Characterization of acute and chronic myocardial infarcts by multidetector computed tomography: comparison with contrast–enhanced magnetic resonance. *Circulation.* 2006;113:823–833.

52. Habis M, Capderou A, Ghostine S, et al. Acute myocardial infarction early viability assessment by 64-slice computed tomography immediately after coronary angiography: comparison with low-dose dobutamine echocardiography. *J Am Coll Cardiol.* 2007;49:1178–1185.

53. Hoffmann U, Millea R, Enzweiler C, et al. Acute myocardial infarction: contrast-enhanced multi-detector row CT in a porcine model. *Radiology.* 2004;231:697–701.

54. Mahnken AH, Koos R, Katoh M, et al. Assessment of myocardial viability in reperfused acute myocardial infarction using 16-slice computed tomography in comparison to magnetic resonance imaging. *J Am Coll Cardiol.* 2005;45: 2042–2047.

55. Nieman K, Shapiro MD, Ferencik M, et al. Reperfused myocardial infarction: contrast-enhanced 64-section CT in comparison to MR imaging. *Radiology.* 2008;247:49–56.

56. Cury RC, Nieman K, Shapiro MD, et al. Comprehensive assessment of myocardial perfusion defects, regional wall motion, and left ventricular function by using 64-section multidetector CT. *Radiology.* 2008;248:466–475.

57. Chang H-J, George RT, Schuleri KH, et al. Prospective electrocardiogram-gated delayed enhanced multidetector computed tomography accurately quantifies infarct size and reduces radiation exposure. *J Am Coll Cardiol Img.* 2009;2: 412–420.

58. Leber AW, Becker A, Knez A, et al. Accuracy of 64-Slice computed tomography to classify and quantify plaque volumes in the proximal coronary system: a comparative study using intravascular ultrasound. *J Am Coll Cardiol.* 2006;47: 672–677.

59. Leber AW, Knez A, Becker A, et al. Accuracy of multidetector spiral computed tomography in identifying and differentiating the composition of coronary atherosclerotic plaques: a comparative study with intracoronary ultrasound. *J Am Coll Cardiol.* 2004;43:1241–1247.

60. Achenbach S, Moselewski F, Ropers D, et al. Detection of calcified and noncalcified coronary atherosclerotic plaque by contrast-enhanced, submillimeter multidetector spiral computed tomography: a segment-based comparison with intravascular ultrasound. *Circulation.* 2004;109:14–17.

61. Becker CR, Knez A, Ohnesorge B, Schoepf UJ, Reiser MF. Imaging of noncalcified coronary plaques using helical CT with retrospective ECG gating. *Am J Roentgenol.* 2000;175:423–424.

62. Schroeder S, Kopp AF, Baumbach A, et al. Noninvasive detection and evaluation of atherosclerotic coronary plaques with multislice computed tomography. *J Am Coll Cardiol.* 2001;37:1430–1435.

63. Karsten P, Stephan A, Briain M, et al. Characterization of non-calcified coronary atherosclerotic plaque by multi-detector row CT: comparison to IVUS. *Atherosclerosis.* 2007;190:174–180.

64. Cademartiri F, La Grutta L, Palumbo A, et al. Coronary plaque imaging with multislice computed tomography: technique and clinical applications. *Eur Radiol Suppl.* 2006;16:M44–M53.

65. Moselewski F, Ropers D, Pohle K, et al. Comparison of measurement of cross-sectional coronary atherosclerotic plaque and vessel areas by 16-slice multidetector computed tomography versus intravascular ultrasound. *Am J Cardiol.* 2004;94:1294–1297.

66. Hoffmann U, Moselewski F, Nieman K, et al. Noninvasive assessment of plaque morphology and composition in culprit and stable lesions in acute coronary syndrome and stable lesions in stable angina by multidetector computed tomography. *J Am Coll Cardiol.* 2006;47:1655–1662.

67. Achenbach S, Ropers D, Hoffmann U, et al. Assessment of coronary remodeling in stenotic and nonstenotic coronary atherosclerotic lesions by multidetector spiral computed tomography. *J Am Coll Cardiol.* 2004;43:842–847.

68. Brodoefel H, Burgstahler C, Sabir A, et al. Coronary plaque quantification by voxel analysis: dual-source MDCT angiography versus intravascular sonography. *Am J Roentgenol.* 2009;192:W84–W89.

69. Moroi M, Kunimasa T, Furuhashi T, Fukuda H, Sugi K. Possible assessment of coronary plaque morphology before and after treatment with statin by multislice spiral computed tomographic coronary angiography—a case report. *Int J Angiol.* 2005;14:225–227.

70. Min JK, Lin FY, Saba S. Coronary CT angiography: clinical utility and prognosis. *Curr Cardiol Rep.* 2009;11:47–53.

71. Hendel RC, Patel MR, Kramer CM, et al. ACCF/ACR/SCCT/SCMR/ASNC/NASCI/SCAI/SIR 2006 appropriateness criteria for cardiac computed tomography and cardiac magnetic resonance imaging: a report of the American College of Cardiology Foundation Quality Strategic Directions Committee Appropriateness Criteria Working Group, American College of Radiology, Society of Cardiovascular Computed Tomography, Society for Cardiovascular Magnetic Resonance, American Society of Nuclear Cardiology, North American Society for Cardiac Imaging, Society for Cardiovascular Angiography and Interventions, and Society of Interventional Radiology. *J Am Coll Cardiol.* 2006;48:1475–1497.

72. Diamond GA, Forrester JS. Analysis of probability as an aid in the clinical diagnosis of coronary-artery disease. *N Engl J Med.* 1979;300:1350–1358.

28 Cardiac Magnetic Resonance Imaging

David A. Carballo, Judith L. Meadows,
Otavio R. Coelho-Filho, and Raymond Y. Kwong

CONTENTS

Key Words: Congenital heart disease; Late gadolinium enhancement; Magnetic resonance imaging; Shunt size; T2 measurements.

KEY POINTS

- A cardiac magnetic resonance (CMR) examination consists of a selection set of pulse sequence techniques. Each pulse sequence technique can evaluate different cardiac structures or physiologies in any arbitrary scan planes of interests. CMR, therefore, may provide a "one-stop shop" evaluation of cardiac conditions of interest within acceptable scan times for most patients, typically of 1 h or less.
- The pulse sequence techniques most commonly employed in clinical studies include cine steady-state free precession (SSFP) for imaging cardiac function, T1-weighted black-blood fast spin-echo imaging to determine cardiac structure, first-pass myocardial perfusion for detection of ischemia, late gadolinium enhancement (LGE) imaging for myocardial scar, phase-contrast imaging for cardiac blood flow, T2*-weighted gradient-echo imaging to assess iron content, and T2-weighted black-blood fast spin-echo for imaging of myocardial edema.
- Most common clinical indications to CMR examination include (a) assessment of ventricular function, size, and myocardial mass; (b) stress CMR function and perfusion for detection of myocardial ischemia; (c) myocardial viability for assessment of risk versus benefit for coronary revascularization; (d) assessment of etiology of cardiomyopathy (including differentiation of ischemic versus non-ischemic cardiomyopathy, pericardial disease, and infiltrative cardiomyopathy); (e) congenital heart disease; and (f) structural mapping to assist ablation treatment of arrhythmias (e.g., pulmonary vein and ventricular ablation).

From: *Contemporary Cardiology: Comprehensive Cardiovascular Medicine in the Primary Care Setting*
Edited by: Peter P. Toth, Christopher P. Cannon, DOI 10.1007/978-1-60327-963-5_28
© Springer Science+Business Media, LLC 2010

- With proper pre-test screening procedure, CMR has an impeccable record of performance safety. Currently, contraindications to performing CMR include presence of hazardous ferromagnetic metallic device and severe claustrophobia not controlled by sedatives. CMR does not involve the use of any ionizing radiation.
- While a development of a serious condition known as nephrogenic systemic fibrosis (NSF) has been associated with the use of high-dose gadolinium contrast agent among patients with reduced renal function, current evidence indicates that those at high risk are primarily the patients with severe renal dysfunction (eGFR < 30 mL/kg/min).
- There is a growing but robust body of evidence that supports the strong prognostic implication provided by CMR in assessment of coronary artery disease.

28.1. INTRODUCTION

Cardiovascular morbidity and related mortality are a major public health concern, and indeed coronary artery disease (CAD) remains the leading cause of death in adults both in Europe and in the United States with over 13,000,000 Americans estimated to have chronic CAD *(1)*. With its non-invasiveness and no need for use of ionizing radiation, cardiac magnetic resonance (CMR) imaging can be used to assess myocardial morphology, function, ischemia, and viability, and its clinical role has been expanding in clinical cardiology.

Several CMR techniques are currently in clinical use. In this chapter, we illustrate some of these techniques as well as the expanding roles of CMR in the non-invasive diagnosis of various cardiac disorders by case scenarios followed by a brief discussion.

28.2. GENERAL INDICATIONS

The current recognized indications of cardiac magnetic resonance imaging have recently been summarized by Pennell et al. *(2)* (Table 1), and appropriateness criteria have also been put forward by the joint collaboration of the American College of Cardiology Foundation *(3)*, as have standardized acquisition protocols (refer to website of the Society of Cardiovascular Magnetic Resonance, www.scmr.org). Of particular importance is that CMR is now acknowledged as providing clinically relevant information when used as a first-line imaging technique (a Class I level of evidence) for the assessment of global ventricular (left and right) function and mass, for the assessment of nascent coronary anomalies, and for the detection and assessment of myocardial viability. CMR is also well suited to the diagnosis of cardiac and pericardiac tumors, hypertrophic cardiomyopathy, arrhythmogenic right ventricular cardiomyopathy, and in the overall evaluation of congenital heart disease.

With technological advances in hardware and software, increasing magnet strengths, and novel acquisition sequences, current scan times have been reduced and are typically under 1 h in most clinical cases. Multiple techniques can be performed within a single imaging session to assess myocardial structure and physiology, valvular function, and at-rest or stress hemodynamics. In fact, CMR is able to complement or replace a number of existing common imaging modalities. Many quantitative CMR techniques use three-dimensional acquisition without the need for geometric assumptions (such as the modified Simpson's equation for calculation of ventricular volumes) and also reduce error attributable to observer bias. In addition, the lack of ionizing radiation use also allows truly non-invasive serial follow-up studies applicable in many clinical settings as well as creating an opportunity to study patient response to medical therapies.

Current relative contraindications to CMR include patients with permanent pacemakers and automated implantable cardiac defibrillators, although in specific situations the risk–benefit might warrant

Table 1
Indications for CMR

Indication	Class
Congenital heart disease	
General indications	
Initial evaluation and follow-up of adult congenital heart disease	I
Specific indications (e.g., assessment of shunt size [Qp/Qs])	I
Acquired diseases of the vessels (e.g., diagnosis and follow-up of thoracic aortic aneurysm including Marfan syndrome)	I
Coronary artery disease	
1. Assessment of global ventricular (left and right) function and mass	I
2. Detection of coronary disease (e.g., regional left ventricular function at rest and during dobutamine stress)	II
Assessment of myocardial perfusion	II
Arterial wall imaging	Inv
3. Acute and chronic myocardial infarction (e.g., detection and assessment)	
Myocardial viability	I
Ventricular thrombus	I
Acute coronary syndromes	II Inv
In patients with pericardial disease, cardiac tumors, cardiomyopathies, and cardiac transplants	
1. Pericardial effusion	III
2. Constrictive pericarditis	II
3. Detection and characterization of cardiac and pericardiac tumors	I
4. Ventricular thrombus	II
5. Hypertrophic cardiomyopathy: apical/non-apical	I/II
6. Dilated cardiomyopathy: differentiation from dysfunction related to CAD	I
7. Arrhythmogenic right ventricular cardiomyopathy (dysplasia)	I
8. Restrictive cardiomyopathy	II
9. Siderotic cardiomyopathy (in particular, thalassemia)	I
10. Non-compaction	II
11. Post-cardiac transplantation rejection	Inv
In patients with valvular heart disease (e.g., quantification of stenosis)	I

Class I: Provides clinically relevant information and is usually appropriate; may be used as first-line imaging technique; and usually supported by substantial literature.

Class II: Provides clinically relevant information and is frequently useful; other techniques may provide similar information; and supported by limited literature.

Class III: Provides clinically relevant information and is infrequently used because information from other imaging techniques is usually adequate.

Class IV: Potentially useful, but still investigational.

Adapted from *(2)*, *(27)*.

its use. In the latter part of this chapter we briefly discuss safety and claustrophobia, and the current methods to manage these issues.

28.3. SPECIFIC INDICATIONS

28.3.1. Discussion of Technique

In a strong magnetic field inside the magnetic resonance scanner (the scanner is always on), atomic spins align and precess around the axis of this field. CMR utilizes the phenomenon of magnetic resonance of atomic nuclei within such a magnetic field when they are subjected to radiofrequency waves. Because of the predominance of hydrogen atoms and its single-nucleus proton, current CMR relies on disrupting and then receiving the signals from protons as they realign themselves after this disruption. The three key parameters that describe this realignment are the T1, T2, and T2* (pronounced T2 star) relaxation times, corresponding to longitudinal, transverse, and translational magnetization, respectively. Living tissues are characterized by their chemical and biochemical compositions and, as such, have distinct signatures when viewed by CMR. By imaging such tissues through the prism of their distinct relaxation times, CMR enables us to distinguish tissues with extreme precision and resolution. Imaging pulse sequences have been designed to give preferential weight to the different characteristic relaxation times and by doing so allow for unprecedented tissue discrimination.

There are two fundamental CMR sequences from which all others are based, namely the spin-echo (SE) and gradient-echo (GE) sequences. In general, the former is often referred to as black-blood imaging with blood appearing black contrary to the latter, which is referred to as white-blood imaging in which both blood and fat appear bright. SE sequences are generally used for static anatomical imaging, while GE and its variants are useful for functional imaging. Two further noteworthy techniques referred to as "cine" (such as steady-state free precession or SSFP) and inversion recovery imaging are variants of GE sequences and form the basis of the functional sequences used in perfusion and late gadolinium enhancement imaging. Advances in cardiac imaging have also been in great part due to ECG gating, although more rapid real-time acquisition sequences are currently being developed.

The evaluation of global and regional LV function, size, and LV mass, therefore, relies on a combination of SE and GE sequences, with stress perfusion mainly using "cine" or moving sequences. Another widespread feature of stress perfusion imaging is the preparation or saturation pulse that is applied to null the myocardium, allowing the inversion recovery period to then discriminate between scarred and normal tissue. Late gadolinium enhancement (LGE) imaging is the current gold-standard technique in detecting and sizing myocardial infarction *(4, 5)*. For patients with coronary artery disease being considered for mechanical revascularization, the transmural extent of LGE can stratify the potential benefit from medical therapy or revascularization procedure by providing accurate prediction of segmental recovery of contractile function *(5–7)*. A recent multi-center trial illustrated the excellent accuracy and the robustness of the LGE technique in detection of myocardial infarction when this technique is applied in a multi-center setting with MRI scanners manufactured by different vendors *(8)*. In addition, the clinical application of this technique has recently been shown to contribute important prognostic information in patients with ischemic heart disease. For instance, evaluations of unrecognized myocardial scarring and assessments of the peri-infarct zone in patients with recognized or unrecognized MI have suggested a high cardiac risk with the potential of providing novel methods of patient risk stratification *(9–11)*. This growing body of evidence indicates that the prognostic information provided by CMR is capable of independent and robust prediction of patient adverse events.

CMR is proving to be a robust imaging modality for evaluation of myocardial iron overload with T2* sequences having been validated in the evaluation disorders such as thalassemia. These sequences are now currently used to gauge myocardial involvement, both qualitatively and quantitatively, and have, in effect, become the reference non-invasive standard. The T2* relaxation parameter has the characteristic of being most shortened in tissues containing particulate iron. In a study of 32 patients, measurements of myocardial T2* using a single breath-hold multiecho constant repetition (TR) technique compared with the standard multiple breath-hold variable TR technique showed good agreement of values between both methods paving the way for more rapid acquisition times *(12)*. This has recently allowed the non-invasive monitoring of patients suffering from thalassemia or asymptomatic myocardial siderosis undergoing iron-chelating therapy *(13, 14)*.

Other techniques visualizing atrial and pulmonary vein anatomy using three-dimensional acquisition sequences have found crucial roles in aiding pre-procedural planning of electrophysiological RF ablations of atrial or ventricular arrhythmias.

28.3.2. Imaging Cases

These CMR techniques allow for the assessment of many variables. Areas of particular interest are as follows:

- Anatomical characterization and functional evaluation of myocardium,
- Myocardial perfusion and stress CMR to detect ischemia,
- Assessment of myocardial viability,
- Characterization of heart valve disease, and
- Evaluation of cardiac masses and tumors.

Other cardiovascular diseases not specifically discussed here, but to which CMR greatly contributes, include adult congenital heart disease, arrhythmogenic right ventricular dysplasia, and pericardial disease.

Through chosen cases, Figs. 1, 2, 3, 4, 5, and 6 illustrate part of the range of practical CMR applications in clinical practice.

These cases underscore the importance of the specific CMR protocols, tailoring them to the clinical question at hand. Concerning anatomical characterization and functional evaluation, they illustrate how the anatomical characterization and the evaluation of function are not based on geometrical assumptions as in echocardiography. With respect to myocardial perfusion and stress CMR to detect ischemia, a recent multi-center trial suggested that CMR stress perfusion imaging was a valuable alternative to single-photon emission computed tomography (SPECT) for CAD detection showing equal performance in head-to-head comparisons in all patient groups, but, in fact, CMR stress perfusion imaging performed better than SPECT in patients with two or more vessel CAD *(15)*. This is not surprising given that the current CMR perfusion technique can operate at a substantially higher in-plane spatial resolution (1.5–2.0 mm as compared to 10–12 mm for SPECT) at high contrast–noise ratio. A recent meta-analysis reviewing 37 studies comprising 2,191 patients demonstrated that stress cardiac MRI, using either perfusion imaging or stress-induced wall motion abnormalities imaging, had overall good sensitivity and specificity for the diagnosis of CAD *(16)*. In this meta-analysis, CMR stress cine function had a sensitivity of 83% and a specificity of 86%, whereas CMR stress perfusion imaging has a sensitivity of 91% and a specificity of 81% in detecting significant coronary artery disease. Klem et al. *(17)* recently reported that combined perfusion and infarction CMR examination with a visual interpretation algorithm can accurately diagnose CAD in the clinical setting, the combination being superior to perfusion CMR alone. These studies together have validated the clinical role of CMR stress perfusion imaging to be a powerful diagnostic and prognosticating tool for patients with suspected or confirmed CAD *(18)*.

The assessment of myocardial viability and the detection of previous myocardial necrosis have come to represent a cornerstone of the value of CMR. LGE is a marker of tissue necrosis and fibrosis in the assessment of both ischemic and non-ischemic cardiomyopathies. In patients with coronary artery disease, our group has recently shown that unrecognized myocardial scarring and peri-infarct tissue heterogeneity identified by LGE imaging are markers of high cardiac risk beyond patient demographical, ECG, and left ventricular function variables *(9, 11, 19)*. Numerous reports from experienced centers have demonstrated the strong prognostic implication of stress CMR in the prediction of major adverse cardiac events from CAD such as death or acute myocardial infarction. Assessing traditional atherogenic risk factors allows a certain degree of risk prediction and prognosis but does not discern those at specific risk of sudden cardiac death.

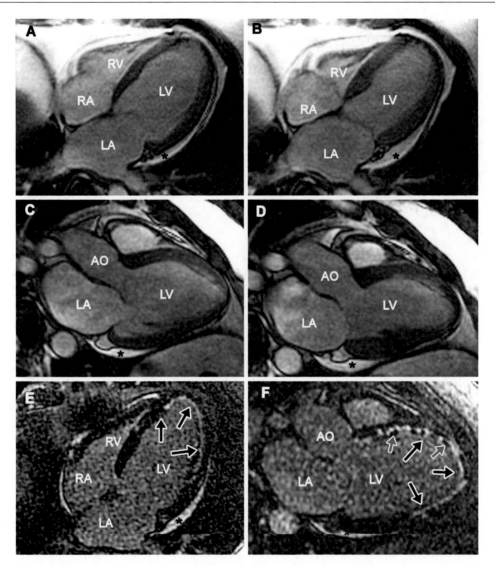

Fig. 1. Case of a 59-year-old man with a recent history of an anterior ST elevation myocardial infarction referred to CMR for left ventricular function assessment as well as further evaluation of a new pericardial effusion seen on an echocardiogram. The four-chamber and three-chamber cine SSFP images (**a–d**) show moderate left ventricular systolic dysfunction (LVEF = 37%) with akinesis of the mid-anterior wall, the mid-antero-septum, and the entire distal LV and LV apex. The late gadolinium enhancement (LGE) images (**e, f**) show an extensive area of transmural infarction (*black arrows*) involving the entire mid- to distal anterior wall, the anteroseptal wall, and the left ventricle apex associated with patchy areas of microvascular obstruction (*red arrow*). This extensive transmural extent of myocardial infarction in the left anterior descending arterial territory indicates a low likelihood of segmental wall motion contractile recovery despite revascularization of the left anterior descending coronary stenosis. The imaging of the small circumferential pericardial effusion (*asterisk*) does not show evidence of acute or subacute blood by signal intensity criteria. LA, left atrium; RA, right atrium; LV, left ventricle; RV, right ventricle.

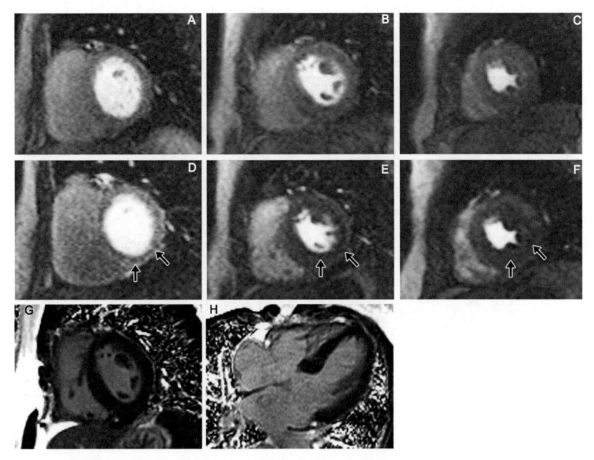

Fig. 2. Adenosine stress CMR of a 57-year-old woman with a history of hypertension who complained of atypical chest pain and had a non-diagnostic exercise ECG test. Myocardial perfusion during adenosine stress (**d–f**) revealed hypoperfusion evidenced by a stress perfusion defect involving the mid- to distal inferolateral wall; this perfusion defect is not seen at rest (**a–c**). The LGE images (**g, h**) showed no evidence of myocardial infarction. These findings therefore are consistent with a region of inducible myocardial ischemia. These findings were confirmed by severe stenoses of the left circumflex and right coronary artery on invasive angiography.

28.4. SAFETY CONSIDERATIONS

CMR (including 1.5 and 3 T) has been shown to be safe in the vast majority of clinical settings including common situations involving cardiac patients having had previous coronary stents. Although experience with 3 T magnets is only growing, there does not appear to be any documented major increased risk compared to 1.5 T studies. A recent consensus document published by the American Heart Association and endorsed by the American College of Cardiology suggests that patients with coronary stents are safe to undergo CMR at 3 T or lower magnetic field *(20)*. Gadolinium-based contrast agents (GBCAs) are the most common contrast agents used in magnetic resonance imaging and had demonstrated a very low incidence of serious adverse side effects. More common side effects are in general mild and include headaches of short duration, fatigue, and nausea and vomiting. In June of 2006, the US Food and Drug Administration (FDA) issued a public health advisory concerning a rare but serious condition known as nephrogenic systemic fibrosis (NSF) (or nephrogenic fibrosing dermopathy), which was linked to the use of gadolinium-based contrast agents (GBCAs). Nephrogenic

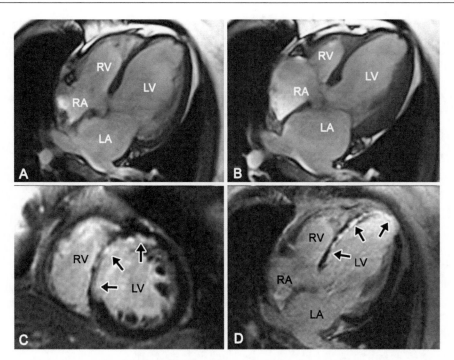

Fig. 3. CMR of a patient with a history of a large anterior myocardial infarction. The *upper panels* (**a**, **b**) show the diastolic (**a**) and systolic (**b**) cine SSFP images demonstrating moderate left ventricular dysfunction (LVEF = 38%) with akinesis of the mid- to distal anterior wall as well as dyskinesis of the apex. The LGE images (Figure **c** and **d**) show a full-thickness myocardial infarction matching the wall motion abnormality. The transmural extent of late gadolinium enhancement signifies a very low likelihood of recovery after eventual revascularization. LA, left atrium; RA, right atrium; LV, left ventricle; RV, right ventricle.

systemic fibrosis is a serious scleroderma-like reaction that may occur after exposure to GBCAs, particularly in patients with renal insufficiency and in patients receiving gadodiamide (Omniscan; GE Health Diagnostic). NSF was first identified in 1997, and its incidence linked to gadolinium use in the literature in 2006 *(21)*. It was originally described as nephrogenic fibrosing dermatopathy based upon its presentation as sub-acute swelling of the distal extremities followed by weeks of severe skin induration and extension of skin distribution. The skin induration may be associated with persistent pain, muscle restlessness, and loss of skin/joint flexibility. While initially observed to affect primarily skin, it is now known that there may be involvement of lungs, skeletal muscle, heart, and renal tubules, and it is associated with an increased frequency of thrombotic events. The name of the entity has, therefore, been expanded to describe its systemic manifestations. The median time between GBCA exposure and onset of symptoms is 25 days, with a range of 2–75 days *(22)*.

Worldwide, there have been more than 200 cases of NSF reported *(23)*. All reports occurred in patients who had chronic kidney disease stage 4 or 5 (glomerular filtration rate <30 mL/min/1.73 m^2) or end-stage renal disease and who were on dialysis. Marckmann et al. *(22)* documented 13 patients with ESRD who developed NSF after gadodiamide-enhanced MRI. No other common exposure was identified in this patient series. The approximate incidence of NSF is 3–5% in patients with severe renal dysfunction. At the time of preparation of this chapter, there has been no report of NSF in patients with normal renal function. Ninety-five percent of NSF patients with linkage to GBCAs reported exposure to a GBCA in the 2–3 months prior to symptom onset, with 80% of NSF patients reporting exposure to gadodiamide *(24)*. While it remains unclear if this is a GBCA class-type reaction, there have been

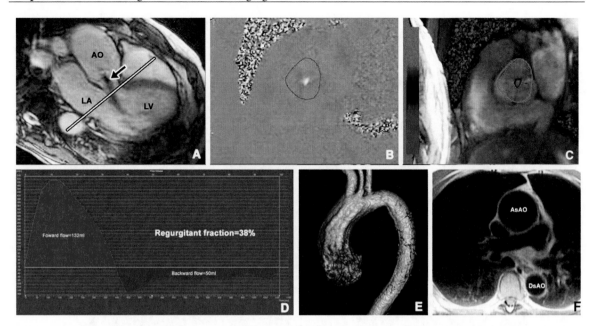

Fig. 4. CMR of a 70-year-old male with a history of ascending aortic dilation and moderate aortic insufficiency. (**a**) Three-chamber cine SSFP showing a mildly dilated left ventricle with an aortic regurgitant jet (*black arrow*). The *white line* perpendicular to the regurgitant jet represents the plane through which the phase-contrast images were acquired to assess the aortic regurgitation. (**b, c**) Phase-contrast images of the aortic valve revealing a central regurgitant jet. The *red circle* represents the area used for the flow measurement. (**d**) Graph showing the forward and backward flows measured by the phase-contrast images. (**e**) Three-dimensional volume reconstruction of gadolinium-enhanced MRA. Note that the ascending aorta is dilated compared to the descending aorta. (**f**) Axial T1-weighted double inversion recovery fast spin-echo imaging demonstrating dilatation of the ascending aorta.

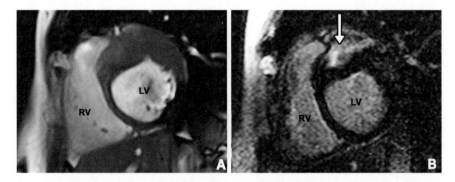

Fig. 5. CMR of a 28-year-old asymptomatic male with a family history of hypertrophic cardiomyopathy, which revealed hyperdynamic left ventricular systolic function with an LVEF of 65%. The basal anteroseptum was markedly thickened and measured 23 mm; the basal inferolateral wall measured 12 mm (ratio = 1.9) (**a**). There was extensive, heterogeneous epicardial and myocardial late gadolinium enhancement involving the anterior and anteroseptal walls (**b**).

rare cases linked to gadopentetate dimeglumine (Magnevist, Berlex Imaging) and gadoversetamide (OptiMARK; Mallinckrodt). The number of reported cases remains quite small in proportion to the more than 200 million patients who have been administered GBCAs and the more than 30 million patients who have received gadodiamide.

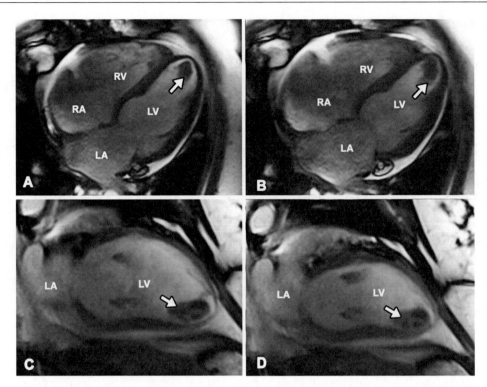

Fig. 6. A 58-year-old male with newly diagnosed idiopathic dilated cardiomyopathy referred to CMR for assessment of left ventricular function. (**a, b**) and (**c, d**) represent four- and two-chamber cine SSFP images in diastole and systole, respectively, showing a severely enlarged left ventricle with global hypokinesis (LVEF = 18%). The *white arrows* point to a large thrombus located in the LV apex. LA, left atrium; RA, right atrium; LV, left ventricle; RV, right ventricle.

The pathophysiology of this entity is as yet unknown, but current hypotheses suggest that circulating CD34-positive fibroblasts and procollagen are probably implicated, migrating out of the blood circulation and into neighboring tissues before undergoing "fibroblastic" differentiation. However, while the precise cause of NSF remains unclear, the causal relationship between gadodiamide exposure and NSF appears convincing. Gadolinium has been identified as a potential trigger in patients with severe renal insufficiency, currently defined as a glomerular filtration rate of under 30 mL/min. The pathology of NSF skin lesions demonstrates increased tissue deposition of collagen. In addition, there is a recent report of the detection of gadolinium in a biopsy taken from an NSF patient *(25)*. Gadodiamide is renally excreted and has a half-life that may be 20 times longer in patients with renal insufficiency as compared to patients with normal renal function, in whom the half-life for clearance is 1.5 h. As compared to the other GBCAs, gadodiamide is less stable and undergoes more transmetallation (release of free gadolinium from the chelated form) resulting in greater amounts of toxic free gadolinium. The release of free gadolinium is likely increased in the setting of slower excretion time and an altered acid–base balance due to renal insufficiency.

Unfortunately, there is no established treatment for NSF, but there may be some benefits of rapid correction of renal dysfunction by either hemodialysis or kidney transplantation. Based on the revised FDA advisory in 2007, stating that gadolinium-containing agents should be used only when absolutely necessary in patients with end-stage renal disease or with severely decreased glomerular filtration rates, this advisory recommends the following:

1. Exposure to GBCAs increases the risk of NSF in patients with acute or chronic severe renal insufficiency (glomerular filtration rate <30 mL/min/1.73 m^2) or acute renal insufficiency of any severity due to hepato-renal syndrome or in the peri-operative liver transplantation period.
2. If the use of these agents is deemed absolutely necessary, the lowest possible dose of GBCA should be used.
3. For patients receiving hemodialysis, health-care professionals may consider prompt hemodialysis following GBCA administration in order to enhance the contrast agent's elimination. However, it is unknown if hemodialysis prevents NSF.

28.5. TRAINING IN CMR AND OTHER PRACTICAL ISSUES

The Society of Cardiovascular Magnetic Resonance (SCMR) has been pivotal in establishing training guidelines for physicians with a strong interest in learning CMR. As published in a 2008 article, the *Journal of the American College of Cardiology* (JACC) detailed an outline of the current training *(26)*. The current recommendation for each of the three levels of training in CMR is detailed in Table 2. Information about current certified training centers can be found on the website www.scmr.org.

Table 2
Current (2008) Training Guideline Endorsed by the Society of Cardiovascular Magnetic Resonance (SCMR)

Level	Duration of training in months	Number of cases
1	1	25 mentored interpretations by a level 2- or level 3-trained physician
2	3–6	150 mentored interpretations by a certified level 2- or level 3-(preferred) qualified CMR physician, including at least 50 as primary interpreter (and operator, if possible)
3	At least 12	300 mentored interpretations by a level 3-qualified CMR physician including 100 as primary interpreter (and operator, if possible)

In the clinical setting, certain practical aspects of CMR need to be considered before proceeding and merit a direct discussion with the patient. These include, for instance, the total duration of the CMR scan and the duration of patient breath-holding during sequence acquisition. The latter can, in some cases, be reduced using parallel imaging techniques.

The management of patients suffering from claustrophobia is also of particular importance. Usually patient reassurance and sometimes the use of single-dose anxiolytics are sufficient to allow the scan to proceed. The need for conscious sedation is relatively uncommon—less than 1% of all clinical cases. As has been referred to previously, certain advances in CMR technology have allowed for shorter scan times. Furthermore, the introduction of larger bore whole magnets has also rendered the scan less challenging and problematic for those suffering from claustrophobia.

As with other imaging modalities, a careful appreciation of artifacts is necessary for correct image interpretation, and this becomes more important when image quality is suboptimal. Special consideration is needed to discern artifacts related to motion, metallic and magnetic field susceptibility, wraparound effects linked to relatively small fields of view, shimming artifacts related to magnetic field inhomogeneities, chemical shift artifacts appearing at specific tissue interfaces, and partial volume artifacts related to image resolution.

In planning a CMR scan, a systematic approach should be adopted in order to ensure the best patient care and most efficient use of the technical hardware. This may involve several steps which include the following:

1. Defining the clinical question to be answered,
2. Considering which CMR pulse sequence is best suited to characterizing a given cardiac abnormality,
3. Checking for CMR safety contraindications (e.g., presence of ferromagnetic foreign bodies, pace setting medical devices, and severe renal dysfunction), and
4. Planning the specific CMR protocol.

28.6. FUTURE PROSPECTS

The increasing public health and economic burden of cardiovascular disease means that primary and secondary prevention is becoming the cornerstone of clinical practice. CMR's ability to provide significant prognostic information in a single exam makes it an invaluable tool in this regard, and, with its high spatial resolution and aptitude at tissue characterization, it has been shown to provide complementary and, in some cases, incremental prognostic findings when compared to other conventional imaging techniques.

As the cases presented here illustrate, be it in the differentiation of ischemic and non-ischemic cardiomyopathies, in the identification of CAD, myocardial ischemia, and prior infarction, or in the evaluation of specific cardiomyopathies, the information provided by CMR not only enhances the understanding of the underlying condition but also contributes to patient management. For instance, with the wide availability and increasing use of implantable cardioverter defibrillators, it is becoming important to identify high-risk subgroups of patients in order to potentially limit implantation-related morbidity.

CMR hardware and novel pulse sequences are continuously being developed and refined. Areas of promise include real-time and three-dimensional acquisition sequences that may improve current interpretation and herald the next generation of images paving the way for improved coronary artery visualization. Beyond the quality of the images, however, the central goal is improved patient care through enhanced diagnostic accuracy and ultimately improved outcomes. It is in this context that beyond its already established indications, CMR is likely to gain a fundamental role in future cardiovascular disease management.

REFERENCES

1. Writing Group Members. Heart disease and stroke statistics 2009 update: a report from the American Heart Association Statistics Committee and Stroke Statistics Subcommittee. *Circulation.* 2009;119:e21–e181 (originally published online Dec. 15, 2008).
2. Pennell DJ, Sechtem UP, Higgins CB, et al. Clinical indications for cardiovascular magnetic resonance (CMR): consensus panel report. *J Cardiovasc Magn Reson.* 2004;6:727–765.
3. Hendel RC, Patel MR, Kramer CM, et al. ACCF/ACR/SCCT/SCMR/ASNC/NASCI/SCAI/SIR 2006 appropriateness criteria for cardiac computed tomography and cardiac magnetic resonance imaging: a report of the American College of Cardiology Foundation Quality Strategic Directions Committee Appropriateness Criteria Working Group, American College of Radiology, Society of Cardiovascular Computed Tomography, Society for Cardiovascular Magnetic Resonance, American Society of Nuclear Cardiology, North American Society for Cardiac Imaging, Society for Cardiovascular Angiography and Interventions, and Society of Interventional Radiology. *J Am Coll Cardiol.* 2006;48:1475–1497.
4. Kim RJ, Fieno DS, Parrish TB, et al. Relationship of MRI delayed contrast enhancement to irreversible injury, infarct age, and contractile function. *Circulation.* 1999;100:1992–2002.
5. Kim RJ, Wu E, Rafael A, et al. The use of contrast-enhanced magnetic resonance imaging to identify reversible myocardial dysfunction. *N Engl J Med.* 2000;343:1445–1453.

6. Choi KM, Kim RJ, Gubernikoff G, Vargas JD, Parker M, Judd RM. Transmural extent of acute myocardial infarction predicts long-term improvement in contractile function. *Circulation.* 2001;104:1101–1107.

7. Selvanayagam JB, Kardos A, Francis JM, et al. Value of delayed-enhancement cardiovascular magnetic resonance imaging in predicting myocardial viability after surgical revascularization. *Circulation.* 2004;110:1535–1541.

8. Kim RJ, Albert TS, Wible JH, et al. Performance of delayed-enhancement magnetic resonance imaging with gadoversetamide contrast for the detection and assessment of myocardial infarction: an international, multicenter, double-blinded, randomized trial. *Circulation.* 2008;117:629–637.

9. Kwong RY, Sattar H, Wu H, et al. Incidence and prognostic implication of unrecognized myocardial scar characterized by cardiac magnetic resonance in diabetic patients without clinical evidence of myocardial infarction. *Circulation.* 2008;118:1011–1020.

10. Yan AT, Shayne AJ, Brown KA, et al. Characterization of the peri-infarct zone by contrast-enhanced cardiac magnetic resonance imaging is a powerful predictor of post-myocardial infarction mortality. *Circulation.* 2006;114:32–39.

11. Kwong RY, Chan AK, Brown KA, et al. Impact of unrecognized myocardial scar detected by cardiac magnetic resonance imaging on event-free survival in patients presenting with signs or symptoms of coronary artery disease. *Circulation.* 2006;113:2733–2743.

12. Westwood M, Anderson LJ, Firmin DN, et al. A single breath-hold multiecho T2* cardiovascular magnetic resonance technique for diagnosis of myocardial iron overload. *J Magn Reson Imaging.* 2003;18:33–39.

13. Tanner MA, Galanello R, Dessi C, et al. Myocardial iron loading in patients with thalassemia major on deferoxamine chelation. *J Cardiovasc Magn Reson.* 2006;8:543–547.

14. Westwood MA, Sheppard MN, Awogbade M, Ellis G, Stephens AD, Pennell DJ. Myocardial biopsy and T2* magnetic resonance in heart failure due to thalassaemia. *Br J Haematol.* 2005;128:2.

15. Schwitter J, Wacker CM, van Rossum AC, et al. MR-IMPACT: comparison of perfusion-cardiac magnetic resonance with single-photon emission computed tomography for the detection of coronary artery disease in a multicentre, multivendor, randomized trial. *Eur Heart J.* 2008;29:480–489.

16. Nandalur KR, Dwamena BA, Choudhri AF, Nandalur MR, Carlos RC. Diagnostic performance of stress cardiac magnetic resonance imaging in the detection of coronary artery disease: a meta-analysis. *J Am Coll Cardiol.* 2007;50: 1343–1353.

17. Klem I, Heitner JF, Shah DJ, et al. Improved detection of coronary artery disease by stress perfusion cardiovascular magnetic resonance with the use of delayed enhancement infarction imaging. *J Am Coll Cardiol.* 2006;47:1630–1638.

18. Jahnke C, Nagel E, Gebker R, et al. Prognostic value of cardiac magnetic resonance stress tests: adenosine stress perfusion and dobutamine stress wall motion imaging. *Circulation.* 2007;115:1769–1776.

19. Yan AT, Gibson CM, Larose E, et al. Characterization of microvascular dysfunction after acute myocardial infarction by cardiovascular magnetic resonance first-pass perfusion and late gadolinium enhancement imaging. *J Cardiovasc Magn Reson.* 2006;8:831–837.

20. Levine GN, Gomes AS, Arai AE, et al. Safety of magnetic resonance imaging in patients with cardiovascular devices: an American Heart Association scientific statement from the Committee on Diagnostic and Interventional Cardiac Catheterization, Council on Clinical Cardiology, and the Council on Cardiovascular Radiology and Intervention: endorsed by the American College of Cardiology Foundation, the North American Society for Cardiac Imaging, and the Society for Cardiovascular Magnetic Resonance. *Circulation.* 2007;116:2878–2891.

21. Grobner T. Gadolinium—a specific trigger for the development of nephrogenic fibrosing dermopathy and nephrogenic systemic fibrosis? *Nephrol Dial Transplant.* 2006;21:1104–1108.

22. Marckmann P, Skov L, Rossen K, et al. Nephrogenic systemic fibrosis: suspected causative role of gadodiamide used for contrast-enhanced magnetic resonance imaging. *J Am Soc Nephrol.* 2006;17:2359–2362.

23. Vitti RA. Gadolinium-based contrast agents and nephrogenic systemic fibrosis. *Radiology.* 2009;250:959; author reply-60.

24. Kuo PH, Kanal E, Abu-Alfa AK, Cowper SE. Gadolinium-based MR contrast agents and nephrogenic systemic fibrosis. *Radiology.* 2007;242:647–649.

25. High WA, Ayers RA, Chandler J, Zito G, Cowper SE. Gadolinium is detectable within the tissue of patients with nephrogenic systemic fibrosis. *J Am Acad Dermatol.* 2007;56:21–26.

26. Pohost GM, Kim RJ, Kramer CM, Manning WJ. Task Force 12: training in advanced cardiovascular imaging (cardiovascular magnetic resonance [CMR]) endorsed by the Society for Cardiovascular Magnetic Resonance. *J Am Coll Cardiol.* 2008;51:404–408.

27. Pennell DJ, Sechtem UP, Higgins CB, et al. Clinical indications for cardiovascular magnetic resonance (CMR): consensus panel report. *Eur Heart J.* 2004;25:1940–1965.

Index

From: *Contemporary Cardiology: Comprehensive Cardiovascular Medicine in the Primary Care Setting*
Edited by: Peter P. Toth, Christopher P. Cannon, DOI 10.1007/978-1-60327-963-5
© Springer Science+Business Media, LLC 2010